Social Epidemiology

Social Epidemiology

Edited by

LISA F. BERKMAN, Ph.D.
Professor and Chair of Health and Social Behavior
Professor of Epidemiology
Harvard School of Public Health

ICHIRO KAWACHI, M.D., Ph.D.
Associate Professor of Health and Social Behavior
Harvard School of Public Health

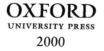

OXFORD
UNIVERSITY PRESS
2000

OXFORD

UNIVERSITY PRESS

Oxford   New York
Athens   Auckland   Bangkok   Bogotá   Buenos Aires   Calcutta
Cape Town   Chennai   Dar es Salaam   Delhi   Florence   Hong Kong   Istanbul
Karachi   Kuala Lumpur   Madrid   Melbourne   Mexico City   Mumbai
Nairobi   Paris   São Paulo   Singapore   Taipei   Tokyo   Toronto   Warsaw

and associated companies in
Berlin   Ibadan

Library of Congress Cataloging-in-Publication Data
Social epidemiology / edited by Lisa F. Berkman, Ichiro Kawachi.
p.   cm.
Includes bibliographical references and index.
ISBN 978-0-19-508331-6
1. Social medicine.   2. Epidemiology—Social aspects.
I. Berkman, Lisa F.   II. Kawachi, Ichiro.
RA418.S64228   2000   306.4′61—dc21   99-29249

The following page is regarded as an extension of the copyright page.

16 18 20 19 17 15

Printed in the United States of America
on acid-free paper

Copyright Acknowledgments

*This book is dedicated to
Sol Levine,
who was a source of inspiration
to many working in this field.*

Foreword

S. LEONARD SYME

In 1955, I was admitted to a new doctoral program at Yale University; it was called Medical Sociology. To my knowledge, this was the first formal training program ever offered in this new field. There were four students in our group at that time and the major decision we faced was whether we wanted to focus on the sociology *of* medicine or sociology *in* medicine. The logical choice was to study the sociology of medicine because there already existed a relatively large and interesting literature on this topic dealing with the institution of medicine and medical care, the sick role, and attitudes and beliefs of patients regarding illness, pain, and medical treatment. Three members of our group followed the logical path. However, I was more interested in the study of sociology *in* medicine: the study of how social factors affect health and well-being. This interest in studying sociology *in* medicine was recognized to be a risky decision because there was almost no literature in this field and no one was sure whether there ever would be. Nevertheless, I thought it was important to see if the study of social factors actually could shed light on the etiology of disease. During the last 40 years, it has been fascinating to watch this area of work grow and develop, and it is especially wonderful to now be able to write a foreword for this first textbook in social epidemiology. I suppose it is fair to say that this field now exists.

The maturation of social epidemiology is of great importance because it provides several perspectives upon epidemiologic research that are crucial to its mission. Two of these perspectives are of special significance. One of them involves a much-needed focus on the family, neighborhood, community, and social group. The second perspective involves a more appropriate way to study risk factors and diseases that can fundamentally change our approach to the concepts of etiology and intervention. These are nontrivial contributions and each deserves to be considered in more detail.

Let us consider the first issue, the focus on the group. A major purpose of epidemiology is to contribute information relevant to the prevention of disease and the promotion of health. To accomplish this goal, epidemiologists study the distribution of disease in populations and attempt to identify the factors that explain that distribution. As is evident throughout this book, the special perspective of social epidemiology brings to the field of epidemiology more than just an additional set of factors that can be studied. This perspective emphasizes the fact that health and disease are influenced by factors not only at the individual level but also at the group or community level. This approach is in startling contrast to most epidemiologic studies, which are still centered around individuals and individual risk factors. Thus, many so-called "community" studies in epidemiology really seem to consist of careful descriptions of individual behaviors and characteristics as these are related to the occurrence of disease. This research might more properly be seen as clinical research in large groups of people.

I have always considered the work of Émile Durkheim on suicide as providing a remarkable and valuable illustration of the importance of a social epidemiologic approach. As is well known, Durkheim demonstrated the importance of the social environment by studying one of the most individual and intimate behaviors imaginable—suicide. In his work, Durkheim noted that suicide rates in countries and groups exhibit a patterned regularity over time, even though individuals in these groups come and go. If suicide is a product of anguishing intimate and deeply personal problems, it is puzzling to see that rates of suicide in these groups remain higher or lower even though individuals move in and out of the groups. The answer, Durkheim suggested, was to be found in the social environment of these groups. These social factors in the environment would not, of course, determine which individuals in the group would commit suicide but they would help to explain group differences in the rate over time.

The perspective that Durkheim offered was to see that the health and well-being of a *community* were affected by the social milieu within which people lived. As noted above, most research in epidemiology today nevertheless continues to focus on the individual. We tend to study risk factors in individuals and we tend to focus *interventions* on individual behavior. The problem with this approach is that even if these interventions were completely successful, new people would continue to enter the at-risk population at an unaffected rate since we have done nothing to influence those forces in the community that caused the problem in the first place.

Scholars in epidemiology are increasingly coming to recognize this problem and they are calling for a "new epidemiology." It is therefore very pleasing to note the major emphasis in this book on such topics as inequalities, neighborhood, community, work, and family. For the first time in a major textbook, to my knowledge, we are offered here a chance to think about the social determinants of disease in a community context.

This approach to community also has important implications for efforts to prevent disease and promote health. As is well known, interventions directed toward reducing disease risk in individuals have not been successful; it is also becoming increasingly clear that community-based interventions that focus on individual risk factors are failing as well. With this book, we have a new opportunity to think more clearly and creatively about the real meaning of the social environment. This focus hopefully will encourage us to approach the issues of etiology *and* intervention in a fresh and more meaningful way.

The second perspective that social epidemiology helps us address is how we classify disease. Epidemiology is failing to solve the main problem it is intended to address. A major task of epidemiology is to identify risk factors for disease. The failure of the field to successfully accomplish this objective for many chronic diseases can be illustrated by the work that has been done on coronary heart disease—the number 1 cause of death in the industrialized countries of the world. Coronary heart disease has been studied by epidemiologists since the early 1950s in the most aggressive, well-financed manner the world has ever seen. During these years of massive worldwide effort, a large number of important risk factors have been identified. The three that everyone agrees on are cigarette smoking, high blood pressure, and high serum cholesterol. Dozens of other risk factors have been proposed, but not everyone agrees about them: obesity, physical inactivity, diabetes, blood lipid and clotting factors, stress, and various hormone factors. Nevertheless, when *all* of these risk factors are considered together, they explain only about 40% of the coronary heart disease that occurs.

How is it possible that after 50 years of effort, all of the risk factors we know about, combined, account for less that half of the disease that is identified? Is it possible that we have somehow missed one or two crucial risk factors? This is, of course, conceivable, but the relative risk of these missing risk factors would have to be enormous to account for the other 60% of the coronary heart disease that occurs. It seems not very likely that we would have missed one or two risk factors of such enormous power and importance. And, it must be said, our record in identifying risk factors for coronary heart disease is one of the very best; the results for other disease are far less impressive.

An early pioneer in the field of social epidemiology, John Cassel, suggested an explanation for this problem in a classic paper he wrote in 1976, just before his death. In this article, Cassel noted that a wide variety of disease outcomes were associated with similar circumstances. For example, he cited the remarkably similar set of risk factors that characterized people who developed tuberculosis or schizophrenia, people who became alcoholics, and those who were victims of multiple accidents or who committed suicide. Cassel also noted that this phenomenon generally had escaped comment, because, he suggested, investigators usually are "concerned with only one clinical entity, so that features common to multiple disease manifestations have tended to be overlooked."

We in epidemiology have adopted a disease classification scheme that is based on a clinical approach to disease. This approach, of course, is yet another legacy of our focus on the individual instead of the group. There is no question that this clinical approach is of value in diagnosing and treating disease in sick people, but it is not as useful if our goal is to *prevent* disease. Infectious disease epidemiologists of an earlier era solved this problem by classifying disease in a far more appropriate and useful way. They studied water-borne diseases, air-borne diseases, food-borne diseases, and vector-borne diseases. This classification scheme helped us think about interventions in a more effective way by targeting those elements of the environment that were responsible for the disease problem. We have not yet developed a comparable set of categories for the study of such noninfectious diseases and conditions as heart disease, cancer, injuries, and suicide.

Part of the difficulty here is that our major source of research funds, the National Institutes of Health (NIH), is so fundamentally organized around the clinical model of disease. To which NIH institute would one send a grant proposal on poverty diseases? Smoking diseases? Sexually transmitted diseases? Or nutritional deficiencies? The NIH would send such proposals to the Institute interested in the *clinical* outcome most relevant to the proposal. In doing so, it would transform the epidemiologic focus of the research to a more conventional clinical focus.

This book on social epidemiology offers a fresh approach to the problem. Not one chapter is organized around a clinical disease. Instead, the book focuses on those major social forces and concepts that influence the occurrence of disease and that perhaps can be used to think more creatively about new ways to classify disease and new ways to think about interventions. This is a major innovation and contribution to our thinking.

While thinking about what I might say in this foreword, I glanced at a volume that Leo Reeder and I edited in 1967 called *Social Factors and Cardiovascular Disease*. Contributors to that book were some of the most distinguished scholars in the field at the time, including Sol Levine, John Cassel, Adrian Ostfeld, Norman Scotch, Bruce Dohrenwend, and David Jenkins. When I compared the state of our science 30 years ago to what is contained in the present volume, I was in awe. While the material in the earlier book is primitive compared to our present knowledge, it is clear that the work we were doing at that time was on the right track. I hope that 30 years from now, in the year 2030, one of the editors of this book will write a foreword to a new volume on social epidemiology, and I hope that a similar leap will be seen in creativity, methodology, and sophistication. But I hope it will be clear also that this 2000 book laid an outstanding foundation for that future achievement. Our ability to progress in health promotion and disease prevention depends on it.

Preface

> Although we set out primarily to study reality, it does not follow that we do not wish to improve it; we should judge our researches to have no worth at all if they were to have only speculative interest. If we separate carefully the theoretical from the practical problems, it is not to the neglect of the latter, but on the contrary, to be in a better position to solve them.
>
> Emile Durkheim, *The Division of Labor*

Over the last 30 years there has been an explosion of interest in how society and different forms of social organization influence health and well-being. The field of social epidemiology has emerged during this time, drawing heavily on public health work done during the early part of this century by Frost, Goldberger, and Sydenstricker; on work on stress by Cannon and Selye; and on the blossoming fields of medical sociology and health psychology. Where epidemiology was once comfortable in assessing only the role of the physical environment in determining health outcomes, we now have the tools with which to assess the impact of the social environment. This volume represents one of the first attempts to bring together leading social epidemiologists to define collectively this new area of epidemiology. It moves beyond a focus on behavioral risk factors to examine the social context in which they occur and, even more importantly, to identify and describe a range of social conditions that appear to influence a broad range of health outcomes. Our aim is to provide the reader, from graduate student to active investigator, with a guide to the major social conditions of importance and to new approaches in statistics, physiology, public policy, and social psychology. Contributors have generally provided both theoretical and methodological overviews of their respective areas that should help investigators launch their own research, building on the most up-to-date information available.

The book is organized in five sets of chapters. After a foreword by S. L. Syme that embeds *Social Epidemiology* in a historical context, our introduction deals with overarching issues in the field. The first group of chapters deals with socioeconomic inequalities and the impact of discrimination on health. It begins with a chapter by Lynch and Kaplan that covers individual-based measures of the influence of social class and socioeconomic position on health. Krieger then explores the role of discrimination largely related to race and ethnicity but also to gender, sexual orientation, and age. Finally, Kawachi reviews the growing literature on area-based socioeconomic inequalities in mortality. Together, these three chapters provide the latest theories and evidence on the pervasive impact that socioeconomic position and discrimination have on health outcomes. They contribute to our understanding of the racial and ethnic disparities in health that are so prevalent in the United States by analyzing the social conditions which underlie them.

The next two chapters examine the work environment and the labor market in relation to health status. Theorell reviews the development of major concepts in work stress. Kasl and Jones discuss the influence of unemployment, labor market trends, and retirement policies on health status. These two chapters bring us up to date on current theory, measures, and methodologic problems in the study of work and health.

The role of community and social relations in health is the theme of the third set of chapters. Berkman and Glass tie together theoretical approaches and evidence concerning the effect on health of social integration, social networks, and social support. Then Kawachi and Berkman review the relatively new concept of social capital as it relates to health. As in the first section, area-based and individual-level assessments are discussed here.

The fourth section discusses psychological factors that are associated with health outcomes, especially cardiovascular disease. Carney and Freedland review the data related to depression and discuss detailed assessment strategies and biological mechanisms linked primarily to heart disease. Kubzansky and Kawachi cover other emotional states, both positive and negative. These psychological states are important in their own right and as pathways that mediate the influence of social circumstances on health.

The final set of chapters covers a number of issues that are central to social epidemiology and that require a truly multidisciplinary perspective. Emmons discusses the social context of health-promoting and health-damaging behaviors and how behavioral interventions might benefit from a deeper integration of the social organization into behavioral interventions. Glass presents new psychosocial models of intervention where the aim is to modify the social milieu as well as the psychological condition of individuals and groups. Brunner discusses the biological mechanisms that may mediate the influence of the social structure on health status. Macintyre and Ellaway review novel approaches to studying the social environment that directly characterize "place," neighborhood, and community. With these methods, both individual and ecologic conditions may be examined. Marmot discusses multilevel approaches to the investigation of social influences on health. Clearly, if we are to understand more about how social and psychological factors exert their influence, we must blend epidemiological investigations with experimental research. In the last chapter Heymann shows how social and economic policies are central to improving population health. This is critical to social epidemiology since we have little hope of improving health if we cannot influence public and private sector policy. The underlying theme of the volume is that in order to improve health, we must move beyond traditional medical or health care policy to understand the impact of social organization, social structure, and the policies that shape them on the health of the public.

Boston, Mass.   L.F.B.
June 1999

Acknowledgments

We owe an enormous debt of gratitude to the intellectual pioneers in the field of social epidemiology. Among the many we would like to acknowledge, Sol Levine stands out as a mentor among mentors. His enthusiasm and spirit of scientific inquiry live on in everyone who was taught by him (and almost anyone who worked with him would claim him as their mentor). If Sol were with us today (he passed away on November 17, 1996), he might well have been pleased with the progress that has been made in the field he helped to create.

We are also indebted to the many teachers and colleagues whose guidance, counsel, and insights we have benefited from over the years. I (L.F.B.) would like to especially acknowledge Len Syme. Some people serve as lifelong mentors. Len Syme has been such a person to me—always a step ahead, always there when needed. Len has truly been a guiding force demanding intellectual rigor and honesty for my entire career. It is impossible to fully acknowledge the debt of gratitude I owe him. This book literally would never have been written without him since he has trained the largest cluster of scholars in this field and a good many authors of chapters in this volume, including George Kaplan, Michael Marmot, Nancy Krieger, and myself.

The ideas essential to this book were developed while I was still a graduate student in epidemiology at U.C. Berkeley. Both supporters and skeptics moved along the critical thinking essential to this volume. I would like to acknowledge the important role that Warren Winkelstein and Bill Reeves from the Department of Epidemiology played in my intellectual development. Their creativity in pushing the boundaries of epidemiology while understanding its historical roots has been a source of inspiration. Claude Fischer (Sociology), Richard Lazarus (Psychology), and Lester Breslow (from UCLA) provided essential elements to the developmet of my sense of social epidemiology. Phil Lee has been a longtime friend to the field, even in its nascent stages, and at important moments in my career, he has consistently been there. I thank them all.

In 1979 I moved to Yale. I owe enormous thanks to Adrian Ostfeld, my department chair. His broad perspective, goodwill, and quiet support gave me freedom to explore the field. Ralph Horwitz, Al Evans, Burt Singer, Stan Kasl, close colleagues at Yale, have provided major challenges to this work that forced me to clarify and tighten many approaches. Even before I moved to Harvard in 1995, Leon Eisenberg had provided guidance for over twenty years. Some of my closest colleagues were part of the MacArthur Foundation Network on Successful Aging. Jack Rowe taught me the necessity of integrating a biological perspective into social epidemiology. His insightfulness and strategic thinking have helped advance my thinking in innumerable ways. I can't find words to thank Teresa Seeman, Marilyn Albert, Dan Blazer, Bob Kahn, and the many other colleagues in the network who struggled with me to translate the psychological and social experiences of older people into issues we could investigate using epidemiological methods. It has been my good fortune to work with such wonderful people.

Ichiro Kawachi would like to especially acknowledge Neil Pearce and Ian Prior from Wellington, New Zealand, who taught him everything he knows about epidemiology; as well as Graham Colditz and Diana Chapman Walsh in Boston, who encouraged him to explore the links between society and health.

The editors and authors have collectively benefited from the support and stimulation provided by three groups of colleagues: first, the international network of investigators devoted to the study of the social determinants of health, among them the Canadian Institute for Advanced Research (Fraser Mustard, Clyde Hertzman, Jonathan Lomas); the International Centre for Health and Society (Michael Marmot, Richard Wilkinson, Mel Bartley, David Blane); and the MacArthur Foundation Network on Socioeconomic Status and Health (Nancy Adler [chair], David Williams, Michael Marmot, Teresa Seeman, Katherine Newman, Mark Cullen, Karen Matthews, Bruce McEwen, Sheldon Cohen, Shelly Taylor).

A second group of colleagues from whom we have drawn inspiration and advice include members of the Program in Society and Health, established in 1992 as a joint venture of the Harvard School of Public Health and Tufts–New England Medical Center under the codirection of Sol Levine and Diana Chapman Walsh. We thank colleagues from this Program for their generous feedback, support, and criticism. We would especially like to thank Al Tarlov for the numerous ways in which he lent his generous support for this program. We would also like to thank Mike Miller, Pat Rieker, Phil Brown, Kathryn Lasch, Benjamin Amick III, Peter Conrad, Chloe Bird, and many others for the energy and thoughtfulness they brought to this important agenda.

Last but not least, we would like to thank our colleagues within the Department of Health and Social Behavior as well as within the wider Harvard community who have not actually contributed chapters to this volume. They include Glorian Sorensen, Camara Jones, Steve Gortmaker, Delores Acevedo-Garcia, Rima Rudd, Henry Wechsler, Bill De Jong, Lawren Daltroy, Bruce Kennedy, Dick Levins, and many others whose individual and collaborative efforts have contributed so much to advancing the field of social epidemiology.

This book would not have been possible without generous support from The Henry J. Kaiser Family Foundation, The John D. and Catherine T. MacArthur Foundation, The Rockefeller Foundation and The Robert Wood Johnson Foundation. In addition to our research support from the National Institutes of Health, these foundations have lent long-term support to efforts to develop the field of social epidemiology. Of course, no book on social epidemiology would be complete without acknolwedging the support of our families. I (LFB) would like to acknowledge all the support of my husband Miklos Pogany, my two children Andrei and Alex, and my father. Ichiro Kawachi would like to thank his wife, Cathy, three children Emily, Kenneth, Katie, and his parents.

Contents

Contributors

LISA F. BERKMAN, PhD
Professor and Chair
Department of Health and Social Behavior
Professor of Epidemiology
Harvard School of Public Health
Boston, MA

ERIC J. BRUNNER, MSc, PhD
Senior Lecturer
Department of Epidemiology and
  Public Health
International Centre for Health and Society
University College London
London, UK

ROBERT M. CARNEY, PhD
Professor of Medical Psychology
Department of Psychiatry
Washington University School of Medicine
St. Louis, MO

ANNE ELLAWAY, BA, MSc
Researcher
Medical Research Council
Social and Public Health Sciences Unit
Glasgow, UK

KAREN M. EMMONS, PhD
Division of Community-Based Research
Dana-Farber Cancer Institute
and Associate Professor
Department of Health and Social Behavior
Harvard School of Public Health
Boston, MA

KENNETH E. FREEDLAND, PhD
Associate Professor of Medical Psychology
Department of Psychiatry
Washington University School of Medicine
St. Louis, MO

THOMAS A. GLASS, PhD
Assistant Professor
Department of Health and Social Behavior
Harvard School of Public Health
Boston, MA

S. JODY HEYMANN, MD, PhD
Associate Professor
Department of Health and Social Behavior
Harvard School of Public Health
Boston, MA

BETH A. JONES, PhD, MPH
Assistant Professor of Epidemiology
Department of Epidemiology and
  Public Health
Yale University School of Medicine
New Haven, CT

GEORGE KAPLAN, PhD
Professor and Chair
Department of Epidemiology
School of Public Health
and Senior Research Scientist
Institute for Social Research
University of Michigan, Ann Arbor, MI

STANISLAV V. KASL, PhD
Professor of Epidemiology
Department of Epidemiology and
  Public Health
Yale University School of Medicine
New Haven, CT

ICHIRO KAWACHI, MD, PhD
Associate Professor
Department of Health and Social Behavior
Harvard School of Public Health
Boston, MA

NANCY KRIEGER, PhD
Associate Professor
Department of Health and Social Behavior
Harvard School of Public Health
Boston, MA

LAURA D. KUBZANSKY, PhD, MPH
Associate Director
Harvard Center for Society and Health
Harvard University
Harvard School of Public Health
Boston, MA

JOHN LYNCH, PhD, MPH, MEd
Assistant Research Scientist
Department of Epidemiology
School of Public Health and Institute for
  Social Research
University of Michigan
Ann Arbor, MI

SALLY MACINTYRE, MSc, PhD
Director
Medical Research Council
Social and Public Health Sciences Unit
Glasgow, UK

MICHAEL MARMOT, FRCP, PhD
Professor
International Centre for Health and Society
Department of Epidemiology and
  Public Health
University College London
London, UK

S. LEONARD SYME, PhD
Professor Emeritus
Epidemiology
University of California
Berkeley School of Public Health
Berkeley, CA

TÖRES THEORELL, MD, PhD
National Institute of Psychosocial Factors and
  Health and the Divisions for Occupational
  Health and Stress Research
Department of Public Health Sciences
Karolinska Institute
Stockholm, Sweden

Social Epidemiology

1

A Historical Framework for Social Epidemiology

LISA F. BERKMAN AND ICHIRO KAWACHI

Epidemiology is the study of the distribution and determinants of states of health in populations (Susser 1973). Ever since John Graunt (1662) counted deaths in county parishes in England in the seventeenth century, social variations in morbidity and mortality have been observed. Early studies often centered on the ill effects of poverty, poor housing conditions, and work environments. By the nineteenth century, physicians such as Villerme (1830) and Virchow (1848) refined observations identifying social class and work conditions as crucial determinants of health and disease (Rosen 1963). Durkheim wrote eloquently about another profound social experience, that of social integration and how it was related to patterns of mortality, especially suicide (1897). So, in many ways, the idea that social conditions influence health is not new. Social epidemiology, however, is.

As the public health movement developed in the United States and Great Britain in the nineteenth and early twentieth centuries, attention was drawn to the increased risk of disease among the poor (Rosen 1975; Duffy 1990). Efforts to improve their physical environments (e.g., housing, noxious work environments and water supply), sanitation, nutrition, and access to immunization were the primary focus of public health professionals. With broad improvements in the physical environment in the United States, Great Britain, and much of northern Europe, countrywide increases in life expectancy occurred. Based on this observation, many scientists forecast large-scale reductions of social disparities in health (Kadushin 1964). Perhaps no other phenomenon has augured the need for the perspective of social epidemiology as clearly, however, as the continued maintenance and recent growth of social inequalities in health in many countries. Thus, while diseases have come and gone, some infectious diseases have been eradicated, others have emerged, and a host of noninfectious diseases have dominated the profile of causes of death and disability, social inequalities in health remain. These persistent patterns call for an epidemiologic approach to understanding disease etiology that incorporates social experiences as more direct causes of disease and disability than is the customary view.

Fortunately, many forces have converged to permit the development of this field. Among the most critical has been the development of work on stress and physiologic responses to stressful experiences. Building on the fundamental work by Cannon (1935) and Selyé and Wolff (1973), health psychologists, neuroendocrinologists, and physiologists have made it clear that stressful conditions may exact a direct toll on the body, offering powerful biological models that link external stressors to physiologic responses capable of influencing disease development and prognosis. Work on psychophysiology, psychoneuroimmunology, and most recently on allostatic load has helped trace biologic pathways as well as specific behaviors and exposures to noxious agents that link social conditions to important health outcomes. (Cohen 1988; Kiecolt-Glaser et al. 1996, 1997; McEwen 1998).

The second factor has been a progressive increased blurring of the distinction between "psychosomatic" illness and other physical illnesses. Whereas it was formerly believed that some diseases were caused by psychological states with little biological basis and others were purely "physical," we now understand that in almost all cases this distinction is false. Most psychosomatic diseases involve varied genetic and environmental determinants, and all states of health and disease are influenced to some extent by psychosocial conditions. Rarely for any disorders is there a single necessary and sufficient cause of disease. The breakdown of this artificial dichotomy is critical to advancing knowledge in the coming decades: Diseases are no longer classified as psychosomatic or not.

A third theoretical development in understanding the distribution of risk in populations further enhances our ability to launch a solid investigation of social factors and health. In 1992, Geoffrey Rose (1992), an eminent epidemiologist, wrote a small book on the strategy of preventive medicine. In this landmark work, small only in size, Rose pointed out that rarely are either risk factors or disease binary in nature. In most cases, risks are distributed along a continuum and small shifts in the distribution of risk throughout a population can make large differences in the health status of that population. Furthermore, understanding the dynamics of why some populations have certain distributions leads to very different etiologic questions than asking why some individuals are in the tails of the distribution. Pursuing this population-based strategy, rather than a high-risk strategy, leads to framing very different questions and utilizing very different preventive approaches. The population strategy is of central importance to social epidemiology and it has been traditionally the mainstay of public health.

The fields of physiology and psychosomatic, social, and preventive medicine as well as medical sociology and health psychology have all made important contributions to the development of social epidemiology (See Rosen 1975 for an excellent history of preventive medicine in the United States). But the seeds of social epidemiology have also grown from within epidemiology itself. In the late 1960s and 1970s, epidemiologists such as John Cassel, Mervyn Susser, S. Leonard Syme, Saxon Graham, Lawrence Hinkle, Al Tyroler, Sherman James, and Leo Reeder started to develop a distinct area of investigation in epidemiology centered on the health impact of social conditions, particularly cultural change, social status and status inconsistency, and life transitions. Their work drew heavily on that of epidemiologists who worked earlier in the century such as Goldberger and Sydenstricker (Goldberger et al. 1929), who investigated the etiology of pellagra, and Wade Hampton Frost, whose work on tuberculosis was seminal (Maxcy 1941). They also drew deeply from medical sociology (Freeman et al. 1963) and the work of psychiatric epidemiologists (Faris and Dunham 1939; Hollingshead and Redlich 1958; Leighton 1959; Srole et al. 1962). Syme (1965) explained that investigations of the "social etiology of disease attempted to systematically examine variations in the incidence of particular diseases among people differentially located in the social structure and attempt[ed] to explore the ways in which their position in the social structure tended to make them more vulnerable, or less, to particular disease."

In a seminal article, Saxon Graham (1963) discussed the social epidemiology of selected chronic illnesses. While never giving an explicit definition of social epidemiology, he suggested that a union of sociology with the medical sciences would produce a new and more successful epidemiology. Graham went on to say that achieving a coherent and complete theory of disease causation would require obtaining social and biological data that are consistent with each other with regard to a specific disease (Graham 1963, p. 72). Thus, he argued, one must understand how membership in a social group relates to behavior patterns, to exposure to "vehicles" for transmitting agents, to direct tissue changes, and finally to disease. Graham aimed to identify specific social circumstances that led to a chain of events in which specific behaviors were linked to specific diseases. His classic example involved Percival Pott's analysis of scrotal cancer in chimney sweeps. Parallel to his analysis of Pott's studies, much of his early work dealt with smoking and dietary and sexual behaviors that were associated with different social groups and thus more proximally linked to specific diseases. In seeking to understand the large-scale social patterning of disease in terms of individual behaviors of group members, Graham's great contribution to epidemiology was his ability to incorporate this multilevel thinking into the field.

Almost a decade later, in the mid-1970s, two epidemiologists, John Cassel and Mervyn Susser, more explicitly tackled the methodologic controversies and paradigm shifts inherent in incorporating a deeper understanding of the social influences of disease into epidemiologic thinking. Armed with evidence from the previous decade,

John Cassel (1976) in the fourth Wade Hampton Frost Lecture to the American Public Health Association stated that "the question facing epidemiologic inquiry is, are there categories or classes of environmental factors that are capable of changing human resistance in important ways and making subsets of people more or less susceptible to ubiquitous agents in our environment." In this classic paper "The Contribution of the Social Environment to Host Resistance," he argued that environmental conditions capable of "producing profound effects on host susceptibility" involve the presence of other members of the same species, or more generally, certain aspects of the social environment (Cassel 1976, p. 108).

Building on the work of Hinkle (1973) and stress researchers such as Cannon (1935), Dubos (1965), and Selyé and Wolff (1973), Cassel posited that at least one of the properties of stressful situations might be that the actor is not receiving adequate evidence that his actions are leading to anticipated consequences. Today we might cite situations of powerlessness brought on by social disorganization, migration, discrimination, poverty, and low support at work as prime examples of this situation. Cassel also outlined a series of protective factors that might buffer the individual from the deleterious consequences of stressful situations. The property common to these processes is "the strength of the social supports provided by the primary groups of most importance to the individual" (Cassel 1976, p. 113). Thus, consolidating the findings gathered by epidemiologists doing empirical work on status and status incongruity (Syme et al. 1965; Hinkle 1973), rapid social change and disorganization (Cassel et al. 1961; James and Kleinbaum 1976), acculturation and migration (Marmot and Syme 1976), and social support and family ties (Nuckolls et al. 1972; Pless and Satterwaite 1972), Cassel laid out an intellectual agenda for social epidemiology that provided the groundwork for decades to come.

In a provocative series of articles, Mervyn

Susser has written that epidemiology must broaden its base and move beyond its focus on individual-level risk factors and "black box epidemiology" to a new "multilevel ecoepidemiology" (Susser 1994a,b, 1998; Susser et al. 1996a,b). The foundations for much of this framework can be seen in his 1973 book, *Causal Thinking in the Health Sciences: Concepts and Strategies in Epidemiology.* In the introduction to that volume, Susser stated that epidemiology shares the study of populations, in a general way, with other population sciences such as sociology, human biology, and population genetics. In affirming common methodologic and conceptual ground with other sciences involved in the study of society, he explained that "states of health do not exist in a vacuum apart from people. People form societies and any study of the attributes of people is also a study of the manifestations of the form, the structure and the processes of social forces" (Susser 1973, p. 6). In other chapters, Susser discussed how agent, host, and environment models, the most basic organizing principles of epidemiology, could be framed as an ecological system with different levels of organization.

Susser's recent work again emphasizes that epidemiology is, in essence, ecological since the biology of organisms is determined in a multilevel, interactive environment. Identifying risks at the individual level, even multiple risks, does not sufficiently explain interactions and pathways at that level, nor does it incorporate the social forces that influence risks to individuals.

GUIDING CONCEPTS IN SOCIAL EPIDEMIOLOGY

We define social epidemiology as the branch of epidemiology that studies the social distribution and social determinants of states of health. Defining the field in this way implies that we aim to identify socioenvironmental exposures that may be related to a broad range of physical and mental health outcomes. Our orientation is similar to other subdisciplines of epidemiology focused on exposures (e.g., environmental or nutritional epidemiology) rather than those areas devoted to the investigation of specific diseases (e.g., cardiovascular, cancer, or psychiatric epidemiology). We focus on specific social phenomena such as socioeconomic stratification, social networks and support, discrimination, work demands, and control rather than on specific disease outcomes. While future studies may reveal that some diseases are more heavily influenced by social experiences than others, we suspect that the vast majority of diseases and other health outcomes such as functional status, disability, and well-being are affected by the social world surrounding us all.

Like environmental and nutritional epidemiology, social epidemiology must integrate phenomena at the margins of what is defined as its domain. For instance, psychological states, behaviors, and aspects of the physical or built environment are influenced by social environments and vice versa. Borders at the periphery of any field, and social epidemiology is no exception, are bound to be fuzzy. We make no attempt to draw clean lines encircling the field. Because it is important for social epidemiologists to consider related areas, we have included sections in this volume on psychological states and behaviors that are closely related to the social experiences which are our primary concern. If we err on the side of blurring boundaries, we must balance that with precision in defining explicit testable hypotheses in our work. Without hypotheses that can be clearly supported or refuted, without having a clear understanding of temporal sequencing or biological plausibility, and without articulated theories and specific concepts to guide empirical investigation, we will not be able to make progress.

The rest of this chapter outlines several concepts that are important to the field of social epidemiology. These concepts are not offered as universals to be uncritically accepted but rather as useful and sometimes challenging guides that transcend the study of any single exposure.

A POPULATION PERSPECTIVE

Individuals are embedded in societies and populations. The crucial insight provided by Rose's (1992) population perspective is that an individual's risk of illness cannot be considered in isolation from the disease risk of the population to which she belongs. Thus, a person living in Finland is more likely to die prematurely of a heart attack compared to someone living in Japan, not just because any particular Finnish individual happens to have a high level of cholesterol, but because the population distribution of cholesterol levels in Finnish society *as a whole* is shifted to the right of the Japanese distribution. The level of cholesterol that might be considered "normal" in Finnish society would be grossly abnormal and a cause for alarm in Japan. Moreover, we know from detailed studies of migrants that the basis for these population differences are not genetic (Marmot and Syme 1976). For instance, Japanese immigrants to America take on the coronary risk profiles of their adopted country.

Although Rose's initial examples involved the examination of risk factors for heart disease, we now recognize that his insight has broad applicability to a swath of public health problems, ranging from aggression and violence, mental health, to the effects of poverty and material deprivation on health. Fundamentally, Rose's insight harks back to Durkheim's discovery about suicide: that the rate of suicide in a society is linked to collective social forces. There are a myriad reasons why any individual commits suicide, yet such individuals come and go while the *social* rate of suicide remains predictable.

The crucial implication of Rose's theory for social epidemiology is that we must incorporate the social context into explanations about why some people stay healthy while others get sick. Applying the population perspective into epidemiological research means asking "Why does *this* population have *this* particular distribution of risk?", in addition to asking "Why did this

particular individual get sick?" Furthermore, as Rose pointed out, the greatest improvements in population health are likely to derive from answering the first question, because the majority of cases of illness arise within the bulk of the population who are outside the tail of high risk.

THE SOCIAL CONTEXT OF BEHAVIOR

Over the last several decades, a huge number of clinical trials have been launched to modify individual behavioral risk factors such as alcohol and tobacco consumption, diet, and physical activity. By and large, the most successful have been those which incorporated elements of social organizational changes into interventions. We now understand that most behaviors are not randomly distributed in the population. Rather, they are socially patterned and often cluster with one another. Thus, many people who drink also smoke cigarettes, and those who follow health-promoting dietary practices also tend to be physically active. People who are poor, have low levels of education, or are socially isolated are more likely to engage in a wide range of risk-related behaviors and less likely to engage in health-promoting ones (Matthews et al. 1989; Adler et al. 1994). This patterned behavioral response has led Link and Phelan (1995) to speak of situations that place individuals "at risk of risks."

Understanding why "poor people behave poorly" (Lynch et al. 1997) requires a shift in understanding—specific behaviors once thought of as falling exclusively within the realm of individual choice occur in a social context. The social environment influences behavior by (1) shaping norms, (2) enforcing patterns of social control (which may be health-promoting or health-damaging), (3) providing or not providing environmental opportunities to engage in certain behaviors, and (4) reducing or producing stress for which certain behaviors may be an effective coping strategy, at least in the short term. Environments place constraints on individual choice. Incorporating the social context into behavioral interventions has led to a whole new range of clinical trials that take advantage of communities, schools, and work sites to achieve behavioral change (see Sorensen et al. 1998 and Chapter 11).

CONTEXTUAL MULTILEVEL ANALYSIS

The understanding that behavior is conditioned by society yields a more general appreciation of the need for contextual analysis in epidemiology. As Susser (1998) noted, "risk factor epidemiology in its pure form exploits neither the depth and precision of micro-levels nor the breadth and compass of macro-levels." Conceptions of how culture, policy, or the environment influences health remain fuzzy and speculative if one analyzes only the independent effects of individual-level risk factors. Ecological analysis, a central part of both epidemiology and sociology early in this century, offered an approach to the study of environments, but it lost a great deal of respectability because of problems related to the ecological fallacy (e.g., drawing individual inferences from grouped data; see Chapter 14). It was difficult, if not impossible, to rule out reverse causation (that the illness influenced residential relocation) in many studies. In fact, it was this latter problem that plagued many of the early studies on psychiatric disorder and community disorganization.

In the past few years, however, it has become apparent that just as there are ecologic-level exposures in environmental and infectious disease epidemiology, so are there valid ecologic-level exposures related to the social environment that are not adequately captured by investigation at an individual level (Macintyre et al. 1993; Kaplan 1996; Kawachi and Kennedy 1997; Kawachi et al. 1997). For example, the number of grocery stores, parks, the condition of housing stock, and voter participation may be critical determinants of behaviors, access to care, or illness. These ecologic-level expo-

sures call for innovative methods (Jones and Moon 1993; DiezRoux et al. 1997). The assessment of exposures at an environmental or community level may lead to an understanding of social determinants of health that is more than the sum of individual-level measures. Although important questions remain about the appropriate level of environmental assessment (e.g., neighborhood, city, state, country), the disentangling of compositional versus contextual effects, and the pathways linking such environmental exposures to individual health outcomes, ecological analyses offer a valuable research tool to epidemiologists. When coupled with individual-level data, they offer the critical advantages available in the form of multilevel analyses.

A DEVELOPMENTAL AND LIFE-COURSE PERSPECTIVE

In general, epidemiologists have only crude tools with which to explore developmental and lifecourse issues. Cumulative risk and latent periods are familiar terms but we often lack methods to deal with them adequately. Yet there is intriguing evidence that such perspectives may yield valuable insights. In fact, social epidemiologists working in the 1960s and 1970s implicitly adopted a lifecourse perspective in testing theories about status incongruity in which the stressful experiences being studied resulted from having grown up in one situation or as a member of one status group and then having shifted to either a higher or lower status. (See Syme et al. 1965 for an excellent discussion of this.)

Three hypotheses have been proposed (Power and Hertzman 1997) to explain early life influences the onset of disease in middle and late life. The first is that some exposure in early childhood could influence developmental processes—particularly brain development during periods of great plasticity. By molding patterns of response during these "critical stages," early life experiences would then make the individual vulnerable or resistant to various diseases in adulthood (Barker 1992). This model is similar to that of latency models. The second hypothesis is one of cumulative disadvantage and is outlined by several medical sociologists (Ross and Wu 1995). Disadvantage in early life sets in motion a series of subsequent experiences that accumulate over time to produce disease after 30, 40, 50, or 60 years of disadvantage. The third hypothesis is that while early experiences set the stage for adult experiences, it is really only the adult experiences that are directly related to health outcomes. For instance, low educational attainment in earlier life might matter only in so far as it constrains the range of job opportunities and job experiences. These three models lay out a framework within which to examine life-course issues. Our aim here is not to conclude that there is strong evidence to support one or another of them, nor in fact to advocate an overly deterministic, developmental model of disease causation at all, but rather to suggest that this perspective provides a lens through which to examine how social factors may influence adult health.

GENERAL SUSCEPTIBILITY TO DISEASE

Wade Hampton Frost (1937) noted that at the turn of the 20th century there was nothing that changed "nonspecific resistance to disease" as much as poverty and poor living conditions. In referring to this altered resistance, Frost suggested that it was not just increased risk of exposure among the poor that produced high prevalence rates of tuberculosis: It was something about their inability to fight off the disease—their increased susceptibility to disease *once* exposed—that contributed to high rates of disease in poor populations.

Cassel, Syme, and Berkman (Cassel 1976; Syme and Berkman 1976; Berkman and Syme 1979) built on this idea when they observed that many social conditions were linked to a very broad array of diseases and disabilities. They speculated that social factors influence disease processes by creating a vulnerability or susceptibility to disease in general rather than to any specific disorder. According to the general susceptibility hypothesis, whether individuals developed one disease or another depended on their behavioral or environmental exposures as well as their biological or genetic makeup. But whether they became ill or died at earlier ages or whether specific socially defined groups had greater rates of disease depended on socially stressful conditions.

As originally proposed, the concept of general susceptibility or psychosocial "host resistance" was a powerful and intuitively appealing metaphor but not well grounded biologically. It was not until research in social epidemiology became more integrated with research in neuroscience and psychoneuroimmunology that clear biological mechanisms were defined, at least as potential pathways leading from stressful social experiences to poor health. Neuroendocrinologists had identified classic stress mediators such as cortisol and catecholamines as well as less well understood mediators such as dehydroepiandrosterone (DHEA), prolactin, and growth hormone, and they knew that these affected multiple physiologic systems. By linking evidence from both fields, researchers showed that some stressful experiences activate multiple hormones and thus might not only affect multiple systems but could also produce wide-ranging end-organ damage. Furthermore, recent advances in understanding variable patterns of neuroendocrine response with age suggest that the cumulative effects of stress, or even stressful experiences that have taken place during development, may alter neuroendocrine-mediated biological pathways and lead to a variety of disorders from cardiovascular disease to cancer and infectious disease (Meany et al. 1988; Sapolsky 1996; McEwen 1998).

These developments in aging research suggest new ways in which stressful experiences may be conceptualized as accelerating the rate at which we age or changing the aging process itself (Berkman 1988). This conceptual shift relates well to earlier notions of general susceptibility.

CONCLUSION

In recent decades, the discipline of epidemiology has witnessed the birth of multiple subspecialties such as environmental, nutritional, clinical, reproductive, and most recently, genetic epidemiology (Rothman and Greenland 1998). The central question of social epidemiology—how social conditions give rise to patterns of health and disease in individuals and populations—has been around since the dawn of public health. But the rediscovery of this question through the lens of epidemiology is a relatively recent phenomenon. As demonstrated in the contributions to this volume, social epidemiologists are now applying concepts and methods imported from a variety of disciplines ranging from sociology, psychology, political science, economics, demography, and biology. The multidisciplinary nature of the venture makes the research both new and suited to tackle the problems at hand. Social epidemiology has already yielded many important findings during the relatively brief period of its existence, yet important discoveries remain to be made. By sharpening the tools we have to capture the powerful social forces experienced by individuals and communities, as well as by strengthening our methods of inquiry, we may look forward to further decades of insight into how society shapes the health of people. With rigorous attention to issues related to the social context, biological mechanisms, and the timing and accumulation of risk, we can hope to identify the ways in which the structure of society influences the public's health.

REFERENCES

Adler, N., Boyce, T., Chesney, M., Cohen, S., Folkman, S., Kahn, R., et al. (1994). Socioeconomic Status and Health: the challenge of the gradient. *Am Psychol* 49:15–24.

Barker, D.J.P. (1990). Fetal and infant origins of adult disease. *Br Med J*, 301(6761):1111.

Berkman, L. (1988). The changing and heterogeneous nature of aging and longevity: a social and biomedical perspective. *Annu Rev Ger Geriatr,* 8:37–68.

Berkman, L., and Syme, S. (1979). Social networks, host resistance, and mortality: a nine-year follow-up of Alameda County residents. *AJE,* 109:186–204.

Cannon, W.B. (1935). Stresses and strains of homeostasis. *Am J Med Sci,* 189:1–14.

Cassel, J. (1976). The contribution of the social environment to host resistance. *AJE,* 104:107–23.

Cassel, J., and Tyroler, H. (1961). Epidemiological studies of culture change: I. Health status and recency of industrialization. *Arch Environ Health,* 3:25–33.

Cohen, S. (1988). Psychosocial models of the role of social support in the etiology of physical disease. *Health Psychol.* 7:265–97.

DiezRoux, A.V., Nieto, F.J., Muntaner, C., Tyroler, H.A., Comstock, G.W., Shahar, E., et al. (1997). Neighborhood environments and coronary heart disease: a multilevel analysis. *Am J Epidemiol,* 146(1):48–63.

Dubos, R. (1965). *Man adapting.* New Haven: Yale University Press.

Duffy, J. (1990). *The sanitarians: a history of American public health.* Chicago: University of Illinois Press.

Durkheim, E. (1897). *Suicide.* New York: Free Press.

Faris, R.E.L., and Dunham, H.W. (1939). *Mental disorders in urban areas.* Chicago: University of Chicago Press.

Freeman, H.E., Levine, S., and Reeder, L.G. (1963). *Handbook of medical sociology.* Englewood Cliffs, NJ: Prentice Hall.

Frost, W.H. (1937). How much control of tuberculosis?" *Am J Public Health,* 27:759–66.

Goldberger, J., Wheeler, E., Sydenstricker, E., and King, W.I., et al. (1929). A study of endemic pellagra in some cotton-mill villages of South Carolina. Washington, DC, Hygenienic Laboratory Bulletin, No. 153, pp. 1–66.

Graham, S. (1963). Social factors in relation to chronic illness. In Freeman, H., Levine, S., Reeder, L.G. (eds.), *Handbook of medical sociology.* New Jersey: Prentice Hall.

Graunt, J. (1662). *Natural and political observations mentioned in a following index, and made upon the bills of mortality.* London. Reprinted Johns Hopkins University Press, Baltimore, 1939.

Hinkle, L.E. (1973). The concept of "stress" in the biological and social sciences. *Sci Med Man,* 1:31–48.

Hollingshead, A.B., and Redlich, F.C. (1958).

Social class and mental illness. New York: John Wiley.

James, S., and Kleinbaum, D. (1976). Socio-ecologic stress and hypertension related mortality rates in North Carolina. *AJPH,* 66:354–8.

Jones, K., and Moon, G. (1993). Medical geography; taking space seriously. *Prog Hum Geography,* 17(4):515–24.

Kadushin, C. (1964). Social class and the experience of ill health. *Sociol Inquiry,* 35:67–80.

Kaplan, G. (1996). People and places—contrasting perspectives on the association between social class and health. *Int J Health Serv,* 26(3):507–19.

Kawachi, I., and Kennedy, B.P. (1997). Health and social cohesion: why care about income inequality? *BMJ,* 314:1037–40.

Kawachi, I., Kennedy, B., Lochner, K., and Prothrow-Stith, D. (1997). Social capital, income inequality, and mortality. *Am J Public Health,* 87:1491–9.

Kiecolt-Glaser, J.K., Glaser, R., Gravenstein, S., Malarkey, W.B., and Sheridan, J.F., (1996). Chronic stress alters the immune response to influenza virus vaccine in older adults. *PNAS,* 93:3043–7.

Kiecolt-Glaser, J.K., Glaser, R., and Cacioppo, J.T. (1997). Marital conflict in older adults: endocrinological andimmunological correlates. *Psychosom Med,* 59:339–49.

Leighton, A.H. (1959). *My name is legion.* New York: Basic Books.

Link, B., and Phelan, J. (1995). Social conditions as fundamental causes of disease. *J Health Soc Behav,* (special issue) 80–94.

Lynch, J.W., Kaplan, G.A., and Salonen, J.T. (1997). Why do poor people behave poorly? Variation in adult health behaviors and psychological characteristics by stages of the socioeconomic life course. *Soc Sci Med,* 44:809–19.

Macintyre, S., Maciver, S., and Sooman, A. (1993). Area, class and health; should we be focusing on places or people? *J Soc Policy,* 22:213–34.

Marmot, M., and Syme, S. (1976). Acculturation and coronary heart disease in Japanese-Americans. *AJE,* 104:225–47.

Matthews, K., Kelsey, S., Meilahn, E., and et al. (1989). Educational attainment and behavioral and biologic risk factors for coronary heart disease in middle-aged women. *Am J Epidemiol,* 129:1132–44.

Maxcy, K.F. (ed.). (1941). *Papers of Wade Hampton Frost.* New York: Commonwealth Fund.

McEwen, B.S. (1998). Protective and damaging effects of stress mediators. *NEJM,* 338: 171–9.

Meany, M., Aitken, D., Berkel, C., Bhatnagar, S., and Sapolsky, R. (1988). Effect of neonatal handling on age-related impairments associated with the hippocampus. *Science,* 239: 766–8.

Nuckolls, K., Cassel, J., and Kaplan, B. (1972). Psychosocial assets, life crisis and the prognosis of pregnancy. *AJE,* 95:431–41.

Pless, I.B., and Satterwaite, B. (1972). Chronic illness in childhood: selection, activities and evaluation of non-professional family counselors. *Clin Pediatr,* 11:403–10.

Power, C., and Hertzman, C. (1997). Social and biological pathways linking early life and adult disease. In Marmot, M. and Wadsworth, M.E.J. (eds.), *Fetal and early childhood environment: long-term health implications.* London: Royal Society of Medicine Press Limited/British Medical Bulletin, 53: 1:210–22.

Rose, G. (1992). *The strategy of preventive medicine.* Oxford, England: Oxford University.

Rosen, G. (1963). The evolution of social medicine. In Freeman, H.E., Levine, S., and Reeder, L.G. (eds.), *Handbook of medical sociology.* Englewood Cliffs, NJ: Prentice Hall. pp. 1–61.

Rosen, G. (1975). *Preventive medicine in the United States 1900–1975: trends and interpretation.* New York: Science History.

Ross, C.E., and Wu, C.L. (1995). The links between education and health. *Am Sociol Rev,* 60:719–45.

Rothman K.J, Greenland S. (1998). *Modern Epidemiology,* second edition. Philadelphia, PA: Lipincott-Raven Publishers.

Sapolsky, R.M. (1996). Why stress is bad for your brain. *Science,* 273:749–50.

Selyé, H., and Wolff, H.G. (1973). The concept of "stress" in the biological and social sciences. *Sci Med Man,* 1:31–48.

Sorensen, G., Emmons, K., Hunt, M.K., and Johnston, D. (1998). Implications of the results of community intervention trials. *Annu Rev Public Health,* 19:379–416.

Srole, L. and et al. (1962). *Mental health in the metropolis.* New York: McGraw Hill.

Susser, M. (1973). *Causal thinking in the health sciences: concepts and strategies in epidemiology.* New York: Oxford Press.

Susser, M. (1994a). The logic in ecological: I. the logic of analysis. *Am J Public Health,* 84:825–9.

Susser, M. (1994b). The logic in ecological: II. The logic of design. *Am J Public Health,* 84:830–5.

Susser, M. (1998). Does risk factor epidemiology put epidemiology at risk? Peering into the near future. *J Epidemiol Community Health,* 52(10):608–11.

Susser, M., and Susser, E. (1996a). Choosing a

future for epidemiology: I. Eras and paradigms. *Am J Public Health*, 86:668–73.

Susser, M., and Susser, E. (1996b). Choosing a future for epidemiology: II. From black box to Chinese boxes and eco-epidemiology. *Am J Public Health*, 86:674–7.

Syme, S., and Berkman, L. (1976). Social class, susceptibility and sickness. *AJE*, 104:1–8.

Syme, S., Hyman, M., and Enterline, P. (1965). Cultural mobility and the occurrence of coronary heart disease. *J Health Hum Behav*, 6:178–89.

Villerme, L.R. (1830). De la mortalité dans divers quarters de la ville de Paris. *Annales d'hygiene publique*, 3:294–341.

Virchow, R. (1848). Report on the typhus epidemic in Upper Silesia. In Rather, L.J. (ed.), *Rudolph Virchow: collected essays on public health and epidemiology*. Canton, MA: Science History, 1:205–20.

2

Socioeconomic Position

JOHN LYNCH AND GEORGE KAPLAN

The relationship between the socioeconomic position of individuals and populations and their health is well established—the socioeconomically better-off doing better on most measures of health status. Indeed, this direct association between socioeconomic position, measured in various ways, and health status has been recognized for centuries (Antonovsky 1967). In medieval Europe, for example, Paracelsus noted unusually high rates of disease in miners (1567). By the 19th century, systematic investigations were being conducted by Villermè into the relationship between rent levels of areas and mortality in Paris (Susser et al. 1985). In 1848, Virchow reported on the relationship between poor living conditions and typhus in Upper Silesia (Rather 1988). In England, Farr examined differences in mortality by occupation (Rosen 1993), while Engels (1848) deplored the impact of the new working conditions of the Industrial Revolution on the health of the poor in England.

These differences in morbidity and mortality between socioeconomic groups have been observed in many studies and constitute one of the most consistent findings in epidemiologic research (Lynch et al. 1996, 1997c; Davey Smith et al. 1996; Sorlie et al. 1995; Link and Phelan 1995; Marmot et al. 1987). The general pattern of better health among those socioeconomically better off is found across time periods, demographic groups, most measures of health and disease, and various measures of socioeconomic position. This is not to say that relationships between socioeconomic factors and health are completely invariant or play out precisely the same way in all contexts. There are important political, cultural, and institutional factors that affect how socioeconomic conditions influence health (Kunitz 1994; Szreter 1997). Measures of socioeconomic position indicate particular structural locations within society. These structural positions are powerful determinants of the likelihood of health damaging exposures and of possessing particular health enhancing resources. This is perhaps the most basic principle in understanding how and why socioeconomic position is linked to health. For instance, the reason that women travelling in Third Class on the Titanic were 20 times more likely to drown compared to women in First Class (Lord 1955), was due to the socioeconomic distribution of the health protective resources—in this case, the lifeboats.

In recent years there has been an explosion of interest in socioeconomic inequalities in health (Kaplan and Lynch 1997), and the evidence has been comprehensively reviewed in a number of places (Townsend and Davidson 1982; Syme and Berkman 1976; Kaplan et al. 1987; Haan et al. 1989; Williams 1990; Kaplan and Keil 1993; Feinstein 1993; Macintyre 1997; Carroll et al. 1996). Rather than duplicating the substance of these reviews, our aim in this chapter is to shed light on some subterranean conceptual and methodological issues that are not often discussed in the social epidemiologic literature on socioeconomic position and health and to suggest some directions that might guide future research.

Before proceeding we should say a word or two about terminology. We use the phrase "socioeconomic position" to mean the social and economic factors that influence what position(s) individuals and groups hold within the structure of society, i.e., what social and economic factors are the best indicators of location in the social structure that may have influences on health. A variety of other terms have been used in epidemiologic literature including social class, social stratification, social inequality, social status, and socioeconomic status (Krieger et al. 1997). To a large extent these terms reflect different historical, conceptual, and disciplinary roots. Our use of the term "socioeconomic position" incorporates features from many of these traditions.

Humans probably have always developed social structures that differentiate particular groups according to characteristics valued in their society. Similar observations from animal studies suggest that this may have a biological and evolutionary dimension (Manuck 1988; Sapolsky 1993). While our understanding of the impact of socioeconomic position on health may benefit from such perspectives, it remains to be seen if this dimension will be any more than a minor adjunct to analyses of equity of resource allocation, social exclusion, and power relations, and how those factors play out in everyday life to influence the onset and progression of disease. From this perspective, we are less interested in the underlying phenomenon of hierarchy and its possible evolutionary roots than in the historical, cultural, and economic forces that shape the nature of the social hierarchies in which we live and their impact on life experiences and health.

We will briefly review some of the sociological traditions that shed light on social stratification. These provide a rich and diverse set of ideas which can inform our efforts to better understand the relations between socioeconomic position and health. One of the main aims of sociological research on stratification has been to identify and understand the principal lines of cleavage that structurally define society. While very little of this work was intended to directly inform understanding of the determinants of health, the structural fault lines that stratify societies according to socioeconomic position, race, ethnicity, and gender also turn out to be some of the most significant factors in determining patterns of population health. In general, sociologists are concerned with explaining the generation and reproduction of social stratification. Social epidemiologists, on the other hand, have been concerned with explaining its health consequences.

THE SOCIOLOGICAL BACKGROUND

In this section we will briefly discuss three major sociological traditions—Marxian, Weberian, and Functionalist—that have influenced the measurement and understanding of socioeconomic position in regard to health. At the risk of great oversimplification, we will argue that (1) the Marxian tradition presents a view of society stratified into "classes" that are determined by the nature of exploitative production relations, *(2)* the Weberian tradition views society as stratified in multiple ways—by class, status and political power—and this stratification leads to the unequal distribution of economic resources and skills, and finally *(3)* the Functionalist tradition in U.S. sociology views the stratification of society as a natural and necessary feature of complex modern societies.

Karl Marx believed that an understanding of social class "reveals the innermost secret, the hidden basis, of the entire social structure" (1894, p. 791). For Marx, "class" was defined by the relationship to the means of production, or in other words, the relationship to productive resources (Wright 1985).

For Marx, social development resulted from the productive interaction of humans and nature. This productive activity was at the root of all societies and each system of production established particular social relations between individuals and the productive process. Capitalism is a system of commodity production in which people engage in a process which not only meets their needs and the needs of their immediate others but also is supposed to produce surplus commodities which can be exchanged in a market. Classes emerge from this set of social relations of production when a differentiated division of labor allows any accumulated surplus of production to be appropriated by a small number of people. These people then stand in exploitative relations to those whose labor produces the surplus. Under capitalism this exploitation is an inherently structural element of the capitalist system (Wright 1985). According to this view, domination and exploitation are not an inherent part of the human condition but are processes which arise from concrete features of the mode of production. Classes are constituted in the relationship between groups who own property in the means of production (factories, financial institutions, etc.) and those who do not. This yields a dichotomous model of class relations, an exploiting "owning" class and a subordinate nonpropertied class who are of necessity in conflict. However, it is worth noting that this model was the pure type—a theoretical construct which would only be actualized in a fully bourgeois society.

The Marxian tradition has been carried forward by sociologists like Wright (1985, 1994) who have argued that the essence of class distinctions can be seen in the tensions of a middle class simultaneously exploiting and being exploited. It is a focus on the managerial functions of the middle class which leads to Wright's formulation—that the whole middle class is both exploited and exploiter. There is an inevitable tension in the middle class between those who act in the service of capital and those whose managerial activities are more closely aligned with the working class. This idea of "contradictory location" is not revealed by analyzing traditional occupational groups but by more sensitive differentiation of the particular mechanisms of exploitation evident in production relations. In its strictest interpretation, exploitation occurs through the social relations of production, but Wright argued that in practice, exploitation in contemporary capitalism is much more complex. He identified three forms of exploitation based on ownership of capital assets, control of organizational assets, and ownership of skill or credential assets. Control over these assets enables a particular group to appropriate surplus value and exclude those who might lay claim to this surplus. Wright's ideas have not been extensively tested in social epidemiology but do suggest a potentially fruitful avenue of social epidemiologic inquiry (Muntaner and Parsons 1996; Wohlfarth 1997; Muntaner et al. 1998).

In Weberian sociology, the focus was not on the structural relations imposed by capitalism; rather, the notion was that this system created groups, such as a working class, who were at a competitive disadvantage in the marketplace because they had fewer goods, abilities, and skills that they might exchange for income. Weber placed much

more emphasis on the role of individual social actors engaging in volitional activity in
a competitive marketplace. Classes could be
seen as groups of people who shared common sets of beliefs, values, and circumstances, or to use Weber's term, "life
chances" (1958). Class position is not primarily determined by relations in production but by the free-market opportunities
generated by these productive relations.
Weber recognized the relationship to productive resources was important—not because it was inherently exploitative but because it influenced the distribution of
economic opportunities, knowledge, assets,
and skills with which individuals arrived in
the market. Given a particular economic order, such as a capitalist system, class situation referred to the typical set of probabili-
ties that a particular array of economic
goods, living conditions, and personal life
experiences were available to any group.

Weber altered the focus from the dynamics of exploitation in capitalist modes of
production to the distributive aspects of
how production relations generated different life chances in the marketplace. Marxian scholars have suggested that studying
phenomena of distribution rather than of
production is to examine the wrong level of
reality (Poulantzas 1975). Furthermore, the
inevitable realities of exploitative production relations impose systemic priorities and
characteristics independent of the individuals who fill those roles. The idea that exploitative structural relations exist independent of individuals is consistent with
epidemiological evidence that class-related
health inequalities persist despite the fact
that particular individuals come and go out
of the various class groups over time.

Weber suggested that while there are
clearly economic determinants to social
stratification, any individual's fate—their
life chances, should be understood in terms
of the distributive forces of the market
which were subject to social and political as
well as economic power. In contrast to
classes, groups defined by their social status
were usually composed of communities of

people whose situation could be understood
by their "social honor." Social honor was
associated with a particular "style of life"
which these communities shared and was
not necessarily coincident with their economic circumstances. Weber suggested that
not all power differentials could be understood by reference to purely economic distinctions. Weber's point was that there are
other elements related to the distribution of
power that lie in some sense of social privilege unaccounted for by the naked possession of wealth. While the status order and
the purely functional order of class were not
contingent upon one another, Weber recognized that having social honor and economic advantage produced more power
than having social honor alone.

The Functionalist approach to social
stratification that developed in the United
States built on and altered aspects developed by Weber and to a lesser extent by
Marx. The contributions made by Davis
and Moore (1945), Warner (1960), and Parsons (1970) represented a "naturalist" conception of social stratification which has
often been implicit in justifications for differences in health status between sectors of
the society. In general, Functionalists argued that complex societies, of necessity, require stratification into sectors which are
more or less valuable to the progress of that
society. This rationale continues to be used
as a reason to intervene or to not intervene
in the health of some part of the social hierarchy. In fact, the implicit rationale for
many public health interventions has been
to ensure a healthy, functional workforce
which would play its role in the accumulation of wealth and the progress of society as
a whole.

While the Functionalists follow a more
Weberian approach to social stratification,
they share the Marxian view of the importance of structural features such as authority, position in the division of labor, and
property relations in determining social position. Social stratification was related to a
system of positions, not to the characteristics of individuals who occupied the posi-

tions. The primary driving forces of stratification were hardwired into the structure of a bureaucratically managed capitalist system so that the values, motives, and aspirations of the social actors involved were secondary in determining the nature of stratification.

However, in stark contrast to Marx, the Functionalist position implied a certain acquiescence over the existence of social inequality, so Davis and Moore (1945) argued meritocratically that social stratification was an unconsciously evolved device which ensured that those most qualified occupied the positions of power. While there are obvious weaknesses in this formulation it still forms one of the conceptual bases for contemporary arguments that social inequality is somehow the result of "natural" forces. Suffice it to say that this approach was, and continues to be used to legitimize the status quo. Warner demonstrated this orientation to social inequality by expressing hopes about how his book would be used:

The lives of many are destroyed because they do not understand the workings of social class. It is the hope of the authors that this book will provide a corrective instrument which will permit men and women better to evaluate their social situations and thereby better adapt themselves to social reality and fit their dreams and aspirations to what is possible. (1960, p. 5)

Even on the basis of these oversimplified positions, it should already be apparent that Marx was highly critical of capitalism as a system of social organization. In contrast, while Weber was not a champion of capitalism, his approach meant he was certainly not a critic of the system. Marx focused on how the social relations of capitalist production inevitably brought exploitation and conflict between the owners of the means of production and the workers who supplied the labor. Weber recognized the importance of production relations not because they exploited and alienated workers but because capitalist relations of production generated different sets of skills, knowledge, and assets that determined what Weber called an individual's "life chances" (1958). The issue

was not the hardwiring of exploitation in the capitalist system but the unequal distribution of "opportunity" produced by this system. This opportunity orientation implied that individuals could improve their market situation and life chances via strategies such as collective bargaining or obtaining more skills and knowledge.

It is this individualist Weberian focus that has led most epidemiological researchers to use indicators of "life chances" such as education, occupation, and income. The assumption here is that it is mechanisms linked to aspects of distribution that are most important for health—the skills, knowledge, and resources held by individuals that form the key linkage between social stratification and the health of those individuals. While Marx was deeply concerned with the human costs of exploitation, the locus of study was not individuals but the structural relations imposed by a capitalist economy. A Marxian approach focusing on exploitation as the link between socioeconomic position and health has not been well developed in social epidemiology but has been successfully applied in other disciplines (Boswell and Dixon 1993).

THE MEASUREMENT OF SOCIOECONOMIC POSITION

In Table 2–1 we have briefly described most of the major individual and area-level indicators of socioeconomic position that have been used in the epidemiologic literature. More extensive discussions of the details, potential advantages, and disadvantages of certain approaches to measurement have been presented in excellent reviews by Liberatos et al.(1988), Krieger et al. (1997), and Berkman and Macintyre (1997).

The measures of socioeconomic position presented in Table 2–1 reflect, to a greater or lesser degree, the Marxian, Weberian, or Functionalist schools of thought. Many of the measures in Table 2–1 are based on a Weberian framework concerned with measuring individual knowledge, credentials, skills, and assets. For instance, education,

Table 2–1. Compendium of individual and area-based measures of socioeconomic position

Individual-Level Measures

Occupation

Edwards—U.S. Census Classification (U.S. Census Bureau 1963; Haug 1977)	Categories of occupations that form the basis of the U.S. Census Classifications - basic scheme was devised on the conceptual distinction between manual and non-manual occupations. These types of scales exist for many countries
Registrar General's Classification—UK (Szreter 1984)	Categorization into 5 classes based on occupation
Occupational Grade (Rose and Marmot 1981)	Categorization of job types that reflects the occupational hierarchy within a specific working population, e.g., the Whitehall studies
Nam-Powers OSS (Nam and Powers 1983)	Continuous ranking of occupations based on average education and income of people in particular U.S. occupations—updated to 1980 Census
Nam-Powers SES (Nam and Terrie 1986)	Continuous score that includes the Nam-Powers OSS score plus education and family income—updated to 1980 Census
Duncan Socioeconomic Index—SEI (Duncan 1961)	Continuous score based on 45 occupational prestige rankings from U.S. National Opinion Polls. Income and education weights used to create scores for all occupations—updated to 1980 Census
Hollingshead (Hollingshead and Redlich 1958)	Continuous occupational prestige scale similar to Duncan SEI but could also be used as categorically as "social classes"—updated to 1970 Census
Siegel (Siegel 1971)	Continuous score based on occupational prestige rankings from U.S. National Opinion Polls—not updated past 1960 Census; males only
Warner—Index of Status Characteristics (Miller 1983)	Continuous score that combines information on occupation, source of income, housing type and area of residence—based on information from the 1940s
Erikson Goldthorpe—EGP (Erikson and Goldthorpe 1992; Kunst et al. 1998)	Clustering of occupational titles into 7 categories. Intended to be used in cross-national comparisons
Treiman (Treiman 1977)	Based on occupational prestige rankings from a number of countries. Designed to allow cross-country comparisons—males only
Wright's Social Class Scheme (Wright 1985, 1996; Wohlfarth 1997; Muntaner et al., 1998)	Categorization based on occupational hierarchy of managers, supervisors, and workers, plus information on supervision of other workers, and control over decision making
Unemployment (Bartley 1994)	Categorization based on exclusion from the workforce

Income

Self-reported Income (Backlund et al. 1996)	Continuous or categorical self-reports of income at the personal, family, or household level. Income definition is also important in regard to whether income is gross or net of taxes and transfers, or "disposable." It is also possible in some cases to gain access to administrative records such as the IRS or Social Security to get income information
Income in Relation to Poverty Level (Lynch et al. 1997c)	Categorization of income as a percentage of the official poverty-level income for a specific year, e.g., above and below 200% of the poverty level income

(continued)

18

Table 2–1.—Continued

Education

Self-reported Education (Feldman et al. 1989; Elo and Preston 1996)	Continuous information collected from self-reports of total number of years of education, or categorically as attainment of particular educational milestones such as completing high school

Wealth

Total Assets (Smith and Kington 1997; Muntaner et al., 1998)	Continuous measure of the value of housing, cars, investments, inheritance, pension rights, liquid vs. nonliquid assets
Population-specific scales (Dye and Lee 1994)	Developed for specific contexts where other measures may not be applicable. e.g., in remote Kashmiri villages the number of cows and sheep indicates control of valued resources

Area-Based Measures*

Occupational Structure (Wing et al. 1992; Armstrong and Castorina 1998)	Information on % white collar employment; % unemployed; average wage in manufacturing or other economic sectors; % unionized workforce
Educational Structure (Morris et al. 1996)	Information on % college graduates; % high school graduates; % with less than primary education; average reading and math scores
Economic Structure (Kaplan et al. 1996; Lynch et al. 1998; Jargowsky 1996)	Information on income distribution; average income, "economic segregation"; % in poverty; housing values; home ownership; car ownership; % welfare and other government assistance; % children in single-headed households; source of income; mortgage as % income
Economic Exploitation (Boswell and Dixon 1993)	Ratio of value added to wages in certain sectors of the economy
Housing Characteristics (Koopman et al. 1991; Polednak 1997)	Information on age of construction; vector infestation; population density per room; access to plumbing; kitchen; telephone; water; sewerage; residential segregation
Resource Base (Troutt 1993)	Information on the number of supermarkets, liquor outlets, parks, playgrounds, medical facilities, banks and other public and private services
Poverty Area—U.S. (Haan et al. 1987)	More than 20% households below poverty-level income
Material Hardship—U.S. (Mayer and Jencks 1989)	Combines information on unmet needs for food, housing and medical care
Deprivation Area—UK (Townsend et al. 1988; Eames et al. 1993; Carstairs 1995)	Combines information on unemployment, car and home ownership, overcrowding, etc.

* Many of these are Census-derived measures and can be gathered from other administrative and private sources.

income, wealth, and to a lesser extent the occupational classifications are all indicators of what resources individuals hold and what sort of "life chances" they have. The occupational prestige scales are more related to the Functionalist tradition. Only Wright's (1985) formulation and the area measure of exploitation rate attempt to directly tap the Marxian understanding of socioeconomic position. In theory, the choice of measure of socioeconomic position should depend on how you believe socioeconomic position is linked to health damaging exposures and health protective resources and ultimately to health. Is it exploitation, few tangible resources, or lack of prestige that causes poor health, or some combination of these? In any event, claims that one measure is universally better than another are conceptually and methodologically unhelpful (Winkleby et al. 1992), if for no other reason than some measures may more adequately represent exposure to poor socioeconomic conditions at different stages of the lifecourse than others (Davey Smith et al. 1998a,b).

The area-based measures in Table 2–1 can be seen largely as aggregate correlates of the individual measures. In practice, however, it is important to distinguish whether a particular measure is meant as a proxy for individual characteristics or whether it is meant to actually characterize a certain quality of the area itself (Geronimus and Bound 1998; Diez-Roux 1998). For instance, in studies at the individual level when information is not available about a characteristic of interest (such as income) geocoding can be used to assign average aggregate levels of that characteristic to individuals, because the average income at a particular level of aggregation such as the block group or census tract is known from Census data. In this case, area measures are used as proxies for missing information on individuals. Area measures can also be used to assess "contextual" socioeconomic effects. In this case, the area measure actually represents an important aspect of exposure to certain socioeconomic conditions (Haan et al. 1987; Davey Smith and Dorling 1996). In other words, the percentage of unemployment in an area not only indicates something about the individuals who live there (the composition of the area); it may also provide other information about the area that conditions the health risks of all those who live in the area—not just the unemployed individuals: That is, the area characteristics may have a contextual effect on individual health.

One other issue related to measurement concerns how the relationship between a particular indicator of socioeconomic position and a health outcome is expressed. In other words, once a measure of socioeconomic position has been chosen, how should the "size" of the socioeconomic

health inequality be assessed? The most common approach in social epidemiology has been to express socioeconomic health differences as rate ratios of extreme socioeconomic groups. Results of studies are usually reported like this—compared to those with a university degree people with less than primary education had threefold increased risk of some health outcome. This approach is useful in expressing the relative health disadvantage in one particular socioeconomic group compared to another but it ignores the relationship in the rest of the population. In addition, rate ratios do not necessarily elucidate the public health importance of the socioeconomic health inequality in terms of the size of the exposed population, or the absolute level of risk (Pamuk 1985). These issues are very important for research that compares the size of socioeconomic health inequalities over time and among populations. Discussions of these issues have been presented by Wagstaff et al. (1991) and Mackenbach and Kunst (1997).

SOCIOECONOMIC POSITION AND HEALTH—THE ELEMENTS OF A FRAMEWORK

Our purpose has not been to adjudicate the relative worth of any particular sociological approach to understanding socioeconomic position. Rather, we think this overview suggests some important themes that can provide a general framework for understanding and measuring the association between socioeconomic position and health. Our view of how to understand socioeconomic position in the context of its relationship to health is what Wright (1996) has described as a "hybrid" Marxian-Weberian view. Its elements are:

1. The social and structural relations between groups in any particular society have a broadly defined material basis that is determined by productive relations to the economy. These relations are characterized by the effective control of resources and exercise of this control exploits, dominates,

alienates, and excludes other less advantaged groups.

2. The inevitable realities of exploitative production relations impose a set of systemic priorities and characteristics independent of the individuals who fill those roles. Thus, socioeconomic position, while observable in individuals, should also be conceptualized as extraindividual.

3. It is also clear that productive relations are important in determining lifestyles and are reflected in the socioeconomic patterning of risk factors, health behaviors, and psychosocial attributes (Lynch et al. 1997b). Far from being a surprise to Marx, Weber, and others in these sociological traditions, evidence that socioeconomic position is related to behavior, psychological states, and lifestyle would be a corollary. These individual behavioral and psychosocial characteristics can be considered the embodiments of particular structural locations in society. Bourdieu (1984) has demonstrated in exquisite detail how position in the social hierarchy is consistently related to almost every aspect of life from home decor, to taste in music and food, to opinions on art and desirable vacations, let alone dietary, exercise, and other behaviors. The imperatives and constraints of the structural dimensions of life are compelling and have important implications for how members of social groups are able to conduct their lives in other contexts.

4. It follows from this general formulation that the effective control of material, economic, social, political, symbolic, and cultural resources is differentially distributed within any society, so those who are exploited, dominated, or excluded have less resources and less control over them. Similarly, if exploitation, exclusion, and domination are basic facts of life in modern economies, then the negative exposures and demands which these exploited, excluded, and dominated groups face may be accompanied by inadequate resources which can be brought to bear. We think that this type of general framework of health damaging exposures, demands and health protective resources is useful in understanding relationships between socioeconomic position and health (Kaplan et al. 1987; Haan et al. 1989). The ways in which exposures and resources act, interact and are manifested in different contexts and at different stages of the lifecourse are important determinants of population health. An exposure-resources framework that is grounded in understanding how powerful economic and social forces are important determinants of position in the social structure may afford us some fresh interpretations of the already-voluminous literature on the association between socioeconomic position and health. More importantly for the present chapter, it suggests how we might advance our concepts and measures of socioeconomic position to include a broader range of exposures and resources that operate across the lifecourse. We severely limit our understanding of the socioeconomic patterns in adult health if we ignore consideration of how exposures and resources may cascade and accumulate over the lifecourse to effect adult health status (Geronimus 1992; Vågerö and Illsley 1995; Lundberg 1997; Lynch et al. 1997b; Davey Smith et al. 1997, 1998a; Kuh and Ben-Shlomo 1997).

BEYOND EDUCATION, OCCUPATION, AND INCOME

Interpretation of sociological theory implies that the stratification of society into classes or groups can be conceived as involving materially related economic, political, symbolic, psychosocial, and behavioral factors. These factors are related to the exercise of power in alienating, excluding, exploiting, and subordinating others. In regard to this theoretical conceptualization, the traditional individual measures of socioeconomic position—education, income, and occupation—perhaps can be seen as relatively limited indicators of the social and economic forces that dominate the social structure. It is striking that even with these limited indicators, the large amount of epidemiologic evidence showing the importance of these factors as health determinants should be so strong and consistent. In this section we will briefly discuss some of the strengths and weaknesses of the traditional educational, income, and occupational measures of socioeconomic position and suggest some directions for future research. It is worth reiterating that these measures of socioeconomic position bear the Weberian signature, in that they are individually specified. In social epidemiology, this may have helped us lose focus on more structural determinants of these individual characteristics. Even as we use individual-level indicators we should keep in mind that they are derived from larger social and economic processes that shape the distribution of education, occupation, and income across the population.

Level of education is an important marker of socioeconomic position that is usually measured at one key point in the lifecourse—the transition from childhood and adolescence into adulthood and exposure to the world of work. In a lifecourse perspective, it represents the transition from a socioeconomic position largely received from parents to an achieved socioeconomic position as an adult, although educational opportunities may reflect parental socioeconomic position. It is a useful indicator if for no other reason than it is generally available for both sexes, excludes few members of the population, and is less subject to negative adult health selection, although it is possible that childhood afflictions associated with low socioeconomic position may impact later educational attainment. Education may be particularly salient in less economically developed countries. In these countries the educational levels of women have been consistently demonstrated to be important determinants of population health (Desai and Alva 1989). Exposure to formal education involves gathering facts, learning concepts, and finding out how to access information. It may provide a set of cognitive resources that have broad potential to influence health.

In addition, educational success also provides information about likelihood of future success. Higher levels of education generally are predictive of better jobs; higher incomes; and better housing, neighborhood, and working conditions. However, economic returns on education may differ markedly across racial, ethnic, and gender groups. Women and minorities realize lower economic returns for the same investment in their education than do white men (Oliver and Shapiro 1995). In addition to its strictly material value, educational success also has an important social dimension—it has socially symbolic as well as material value. A college degree granted from a prestigious university has different social and symbolic value than the same college degree gained from a less prestigious institution.

In using education as a measure of socioeconomic position we should also understand some of its potential limitations. Knowing the number of years of education tells us nothing about the quality of that education or how it is socially and economically valued. Measures of years of education also do not acknowledge the importance of the credentials that are achieved with the attainment of particular educational milestones. Educational achievement has had different social meanings and consequences at different time periods and in different cultures. Receiving less than a primary school education may have very different consequences in a society which is economically stagnant compared to one where the overall economy is booming and many opportunities exist for well-paid employment and upward social mobility. In the latter kind of society, level of education may be a poorer predictor of later material and economic well-being (Lynch et al. 1994).

Our point here is that information about the number of years or the achieved level of education fails to directly reveal much of what might be important about education in terms of its relationship with health. Without knowledge of the cognitive, material, social, and psychological resources gained through education, and accumulated over the lifecourse, we cannot hope to make much sense of the association between educational experience and health, nor address important intervention questions.

Another important measure of socioeconomic position is occupation. Concern about the health consequences of employment in particular working environments has had a long history. Work in mines, cotton mills, and the factories of the early Industrial Revolution was linked to a variety of poor health outcomes (Paracelsus 1567; Villerme 1840; Engels 1848; Farr 1864). Since then many studies have examined not just how poor working conditions in particular industries have affected health but also how systematic health differences exist between broadly classified occupational groups such as white and blue collar workers despite important heterogeneity in working conditions and income within these occupational groupings (Mackenbach et al. 1997). Understanding the association between work and health is crucial because it is the most obvious, intimate, and stable connection between humans and the productive processes that dominate much of our adult lives. Work is the major structural link between education and income. In broad terms, educational experiences are important in determining what sorts of employment are available, and this employment then determines the amount of economic return. We cannot understand socioeconomic stratification or its health consequences without understanding how work or the lack of work structures people's lives. This is not to say that understanding the structural positions of women not engaged in formal employment or individuals out of work should be ignored, but it is to say that we need more sophisticated occupational classification schemes that can include these groups. Such schemes should also allow consideration of the dual structural burden for women who are not only formally employed but also hold other structural social roles, such as caregiving (Arber 1987, 1991).

Perhaps more than is the case for educa-

tion and income, studies of occupation and health have explored the multiple pathways through which work affects health. Many occupations require working in hazardous environments where exposure to chemicals, radiation, biological hazards, physical stress, noise, heat, unsafe conditions, cold, dust, and other pollutants are an inherent feature of work. These sorts of working environments are more common for those with less education. In addition to this focus on the physical environment, there has been a good deal of attention paid to the psychosocial environment of work. The work of Karasek and Theorell (1990) has been very influential in demonstrating the impact of the psychosocial work environment on health, with a focus on hypertension and cardiovascular disease. They have suggested that psychological demands, decision latitude, and social support at work form the three major dimensions relevant to understanding how the psychosocial work environment affects health. Studies using this model have shown that conditions of high psychological demand with low decision latitude and low social support are often related to the poorest health outcomes (Schnall and Landsbergis 1994).

In some ways, the demand–control approach to understanding the association between work and health is similar to what we have proposed as a more generalized exposure-resources model. However, the generalized exposure-resources framework suggested here is grounded in an attempt to understand how structural factors determine the distribution of working conditions across the population. Particular jobs with high psychological demands, low decision latitude, and poor workplace social support have to be seen as arising from the economic, political, historical, and sociocultural imperatives that define processes of production. In contrast, while the demand–control model has been useful in improving understanding of the association between work and health, it has been limited by interpretation within an individualistic psychosocial framework (Muntaner and O'Campo

1993). This orientation has led many researchers to examine the effects of psychosocial work conditions on health adjusted for measures of socioeconomic position such as income, education, and occupation and to claims that the adverse health effects of high demands and low control are "independent" of socioeconomic position (Karasek and Theorell 1990; Schnall and Landsbergis 1994). For both methodological and conceptual reasons we do not believe that there is much to be gained from statistically partitioning the separate contributions of socioeconomic position and psychosocial working conditions (Lynch et al. 1997d,e; Marmot et al. 1997; Davey Smith and Harding 1997). In reality they are intimately related in complex ways that may be trivialized by the crude statistical adjustment of one for the other. "Explaining" social-level phenomena such as socioeconomic gradients in health cannot be reduced to "explaining away" these gradients by statistical adjustment for workplace demands and control at the individual level— the demand–control attributes assigned to individuals are in large part a result of the social-level phenomena being explained (Macintyre 1997). Furthermore, such explanations are not even relevant for understanding socioeconomic health gradients among those who are not working.

It seems likely that we must reintegrate studies of psychosocial workplace factors and health within the broader context of an understanding of how socioeconomic position, understood as an extraindividual social-level factor, influences health. Siegrist and colleagues have developed an effort-reward model of job stress that explicitly examines how high effort conditions (characterized by high job demands and psychological immersion in work) are balanced against the economic, social, and promotional rewards of work (Siegrist et al. 1990; Siegrist 1996). While largely conceptualized within an individualist psychosocial framework, this approach extends the demand–control model to include nonwork factors and consideration of the income and other rewards derived from work. Consistent with this model, we have shown that high levels of workplace demands combined with low economic returns from work are associated with greater progression of carotid atherosclerosis and higher rates of myocardial infarction and mortality (Lynch et al. 1997d,e).

Income is a useful measure of socioeconomic position because it relates directly to the material conditions that may influence health. It is likely that there is nothing about the possession of money per se that is likely to affect health; rather, income level has influences on health because of what money can buy. Adequate income has important implications for a range of material circumstances that have direct implications for health; quality, type, and location of housing; food; clothing; transportation; medical care; opportunities for cultural, recreational, and physical activities; child care; and exposure to an array of environmental toxins. While increasing income is likely to produce diminishing returns on the health impact of these material conditions, it is nevertheless important to remember that differences in health-related material conditions exist across all levels of income.

The influence of "material conditions" on health is usually understood within the framework of the sanitary approach to public health that arose in response to 19th-century industrial society. In this view, which was entirely appropriate for the times, improved material conditions involved adequate housing, avoidance of hunger, safe water supply, and the reduction of environmental hazards through waste removal and treatment. The focus was on changing the material conditions associated with poverty. There is no doubt that providing the most basic of decent material conditions remains salient in much of the world and within many industrial countries, especially the United States. In 1994, 38 million Americans lived in poverty, 15 million of whom were under 18 years of age, and 6 million were preschoolers under the age of 6 (Corcoran and Chaudry 1997). These depressing statistics serve to illustrate that the 19th-century understanding of adequate material conditions remains highly relevant to the modern world.

However, we must add a "neo-material" interpretation to this view. There is a graded relationship between income and health that is not limited to the wrenching problems of poverty. Supplying clean water, shelter, adequate calories, and waste removal were important for socioeconomic differences in life expectancy in the middle of the 19th century. These were the basic material conditions relevant to understanding health inequalities within a context of relatively low life expectancies of 45 years for professionals, 26 years for skilled manual workers, and 16 years for laborers (Antonovsky 1967). In the late 20th century, social epidemiologists are trying to understand socioeconomic differences in life expectancy in a context where the average length of life in 1995 has increased to 75.8 years (National Center for Health Statistics 1998). The material basis of these socioeconomic health differences has changed. We need to consider the neo-material conditions that might be relevant to understanding socioeconomic health differences within the context of the historical overall improvement in health. For instance, adequate nutrition in terms of calories is not the same as a having a balanced, low-fat diet, rich in fresh fruit, grains, and vegetables. Adequate housing is not the same as housing that can protect people from extremes of heat and cold and overcrowding. Even if the most basic material conditions are satisfied through a low but adequate level of income, each step up the income ladder may bring added neo-material benefits that can produce gains in health. Davey Smith et al. (1990), Macintyre et al. (1998), and Blane et al. (1997) provide evidence that health and mortality are sensitive to fine gradations of neo-material conditions, as evidenced through access to cars, home ownership, having a home with a garden, and healthier food. Furthermore, better neo-material conditions may have immediate and cumulative benefits over the lifecourse and may also influence the socioeconomic position and health status of future generations. Children who have access to a home computer may be improving the likelihood of later educational success and so influence their subsequent socioeconomic position and health.

Neo-material conditions are intimately tied to psychological states, health behaviors, and social circumstances that also influence health. In a study in Finland, we showed that men who worked in low-paid employment were the most materially disadvantaged, had higher job and financial insecurity, and experienced more unemployment and work injury. It is not coincidental that these were the same men who tended to smoke more, exercise less, eat less nutritious diets, get drunk more often, have a cynically hostile outlook, and not feel full of hope about the future (Lynch et al. 1997b; Lynch, in press). One approach has conceptualized the psychosocial and behavioral correlates of low income as maladaptive phenomena that are amenable to cognitive, emotional, and behavioral modification. While they may be maladaptive in terms of health and longevity, within the generalized framework of socioeconomic position that we have developed here, these psychosocial states and health behaviors must be viewed as responses to adverse conditions imposed by broader social and economic structures (Evans et al. 1994). These two approaches to understanding health behaviors and psychosocial attributes have vastly different implications for intervention.

Adequate income provides a generalized resource that provides access to a larger variety and better quality of neo-material goods and conditions. It also provides ready access to the skills and labor of others. Disposable income can provide a buffer from many of the stresses of daily life through, for example, just having the ability to easily fix something as random as a flat tire. However, most sources of social and environmental stress are not randomly allocated among the population. It is precisely those groups with the least disposable income who are subject to the largest cumulative burden of stressors (Mcleod and Kessler 1990; Ross and Wu 1996; Turner et al. 1995). Interestingly, this cumulative, over-the-lifecourse burden of stress may have far-reaching physiologic consequences (McEwen 1998).

One potential limitation of studies that have examined income and health is that almost all of them have measured income at one only point in adulthood. There is little doubt that this strategy fails to fully capture the health effects of sustained exposure to low income or to account for transitions into and out of low-income groups; nor does it allow for the dynamic interrelationship of health and income. There is considerable volatility in income over the lifecourse, with between 26% and 39% of individuals in the United States, aged 45 to 65 years experiencing income reductions of 50% or more at least once in an 11-year period (Duncan 1996). These rises and falls in income are more pronounced for those at the bottom of the income distribution because they are less likely to have stable employment (McDonough et al. 1997). The first step in improving our understanding of the relationship between income and health is to better assess the exposure to varying income conditions by measuring income at multiple points in time. The utility of this approach can be seen in our 29-year study of economic hardship and functioning (Lynch et al. 1997c). By measuring income in 1965, 1974, and 1983 we were then able to examine the cumulative effects of sustained economic hardship on physical, psychological, cognitive, and social functioning in 1994. The results of this study showed strong dose–response associations between the number of periods of economic hardship and physical, psychological, and cognitive functioning. In addition, because we had multiple measures of income, we were able to examine the potential for reverse causation to explain our results. Reverse causation, or the fact that illness may cause lower incomes instead of the other way round, has been proposed as an important competing hypothesis for studies that have related income to health (Smith 1999). The most powerful examinations of the direction of potential causation can only arise when income and health data are measured at multiple time points. In an analysis of administrative data from the Canadian Pension Plan, Wolfson and colleagues (1993) used 10–20-year earnings histories to show that men whose incomes had steadily increased but who still remained in the lowest income group had higher mortality than more economically advantaged men. This approach convincingly demonstrated how reverse causation could not explain their findings. Investigations like these, which use multiple measures of health and income, will expand our understanding of the complex relationship between income and health.

There is another aspect of the income–health relationship that should be mentioned in terms of moving this field forward and that concerns issues of wealth. As we have suggested, if income can be thought of as a generalized resource that provides access to better neo-material conditions and can be used to buffer the effects of social and environmental stress, then it is possible that accumulated assets or wealth could further expand this resource. Several studies have suggested that the strength of the relationship between income and health declines after age 65 (Kaplan et al. 1987; House et al. 1994). This could reflect a true underlying trend, or it may be that after age 65 income is a less sensitive measure of socioeconomic position. This issue can be examined as information on income, wealth, and health becomes available through such studies as the Health and Retirement Study (HRS), Asset and Health Dynamics Among the Oldest Old (AHEAD) and the Panel Study of Income Dynamics (PSID). These longitudinal studies have information, detailed in some cases, on income, wealth, job histories, and health that will allow examinations of the dynamic interplay of these factors. Cross-sectional analysis of the first wave of the HRS study suggests that both income and wealth may make statistically separate contributions to health status (Kington and Smith 1997; Muntaner et al. 1998).

Households that have equivalent income levels may differ markedly in terms of their accumulated assets. This is most evident for comparisons across racial and ethnic groups. Race differences in wealth are much larger than income differences. Using data from the HRS study, Smith (1995) has shown how African-American and Hispanic households have far less wealth at every level of income. On average, for every one dollar of wealth of a middle-aged white household, an African-American household has 27 cents. Even for households with incomes that are in the top quintile, African-American households have 56% less net worth, and Hispanics households 67% less net worth, than white households. In low-income households the picture is even more stark. In the lowest income quintile, African-American and Hispanic households have 85% and 63% less net worth, respectively. The information that is used to calculate these figures for net worth includes housing equity. If we understand the relationship between wealth and health as in part reflecting the ability to respond to and buffer social and economic stress by calling on savings, then the role of liquid assets might be even more important than nonliquid assets such as a house. Decomposing the HRS wealth data shows that the median level of financial assets in white households is $17,300, but it is $400 in African-American households and only $78 in Hispanic households (Smith 1995). For all intents and purposes the average African-American and Hispanic households have no liquid monetary reserves at their disposal.

These data highlight how much can be hidden by only examining income levels. If wealth has an important role to play, then using income as a measure of socioeconomic position may underestimate the true differences in health. Perhaps, more importantly, studies that are not interested in socioeconomic effects per se normally adjust the association of interest with measures like income. The residual effect can then be claimed to be "independent" of socioeconomic position. However, the data on the distribution of wealth suggest that adjustment for income may be an inadequate representation of the true underlying socioeconomic differences. This is especially crucial for studies that seek to examine racial health differences adjusted for socioeconomic position. Adjustment for income in a study of African-American vs. white health differences clearly underestimates the true effect of socioeconomic factors. In fact, there are multiple socioeconomic differences between African-Americans and whites that are not captured in simple variables like education or income (Krieger et al. 1993; Krieger 1994). Kaufman et al. have shown how inadequate adjustment for socioeconomic factors can produce spurious results that favor the interpretation of residual racial health differences. They argued that "The social distinction between blacks and whites is multidimensional and cannot be captured fully in a scalar such as education or reported income" (Kaufman et al. 1997, p. 627).

While these traditional measures of education, occupation, and income are powerful predictors of health, they are limited. We must transform our thinking and analysis from static to dynamic approaches to more fully understand how socioeconomic factors influence health. This means conceptualizing, gathering, and analyzing data within a lifecourse perspective (Lynch et al. 1997b; Kaplan and Lynch 1997; Davey Smith et al. 1997; Power et al. 1997; Kuh and Ben-Shlomo 1997; Davey Smith et al. 1998a).

From such a perspective, observations of income or occupational health differences in adulthood would be seen to be the result of intertwining chains of biological and social factors operating over the course of life to influence adult health status. Figure 2–1 illustrates how some selected aspects of socioeconomic position can influence health at various stages of the lifecourse. The particular outcome depicted here is cardiovas-

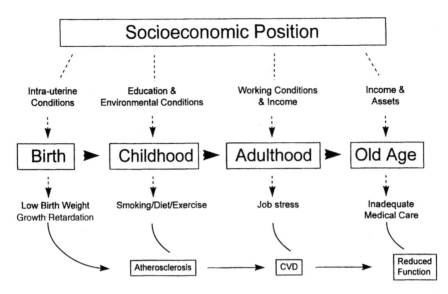

Figure 2–1. Socioeconomic influences on cardiovascular disease from a lifecourse perspective.

cular disease but similar links could be drawn for many conditions. From the very start of life the socioeconomic position of parents influences intrauterine conditions. This process can be understood as the intergenerational transmission of socioeconomic position through a stock of "health resources" that are passed on to the developing fetus. The later importance of these processes in regard to adult health is not entirely clear, but there has been a good deal of evidence relating low birth weight and other markers of suboptimal intrauterine environment and adult cardiovascular disease (Barker and Osmond 1986; Barker et al. 1989; Barker and Martyn 1992). During childhood, socioeconomic position of parents (such as income, type of housing, neighborhood) influences the types of environments in which children grow, learn, and begin to adopt a range of behaviors that can influence the early development of atherosclerosis. In adulthood, working conditions and income level affect job stress and have direct implications for the onset and progression of cardiovascular disease, while at older ages, income and assets impact the quality and availability of medical and

support care. All of these processes may contribute to what is observed as adult socioeconomic differences in cardiovascular disease (Lynch et al. 1997a). Future studies will need to examine the complex temporal interactions between the genetic and biological attributes that are endowed early in life, and the social, economic, and political environments which determine the accumulation and distribution of exposures and resources over the lifecourse and ultimately shape patterns of adult health.

SOCIOECONOMIC POSITION OF NEIGHBORHOODS AND COMMUNITIES

The previous discussion has focused on the socioeconomic position of individuals and groups. The focus on the individual is often seen as the logical place to start. After all, individuals have incomes and wealth, they acquire an education, and they practice particular jobs. Furthermore, the health effects of socioeconomic position on populations must ultimately be understandable in terms of biologic processes occurring at the individual level. Lacking individual measures of socioeconomic position, many studies have examined the association between area or community-based measures of socioeconomic position and the health of populations living in those areas (e.g. Townsend et al. 1988; Eames et al. 1993). The units of analyses have often been based on administrative definitions—for example, census blocks and tracts, postal codes, metropolitan statistical areas, states, and countries. The measures include median or per capita income, deprivation scores, percent in poverty, unemployment, median level of education, percent white collar occupations, and unemployment rate (Table 2–1). Generally, such analyses show strong, graded associations between these measures and most health outcomes, mimicking the associations seen at the individual or group level. These analyses have often proceeded as if the measurement of socioeconomic position at the ecologic or area level was simply a proxy for measurement at the individual level. An alternative view is that differences in the socioeconomic position of communities or areas reflect more than different distributions of individuals with specific characteristics in these areas (Haan et al. 1989; Kaplan 1996; Schwartz 1994). This view calls upon the exposure-resource model presented above, describing the distribution of resources and exposures at the community or area level. Thus, extraindividual socioeconomic factors closely related to the physical and social infrastructure of communities are thought to affect health above and beyond individual compositional aspects (Kaplan et al. 1987; Haan et al. 1989; Wing et al. 1988; Macintyre et al. 1993; Krieger 1991).

A growing amount of literature supports such a view (Kaplan 1996; Diez-Roux et al. 1997; Diez-Roux 1998; O'Campo et al. 1995, 1997; Robert 1998). One of the first studies to show an independent effect of community-level variables on health indicated that, in participants in the Alameda County Study, residence in a poverty area was associated with an approximately 50% increased nine-year risk of death, even when a large number of measures of individual status were taken into account statistically (Haan et al. 1987). The independent role of area effects is also shown in other studies which have used nationally representative samples (Anderson et al. 1997; Robert 1998). Finally, recent work indicating an association between mortality and life expectancy and the unequal distribution of income in areas, a variable which can only be measured at the community or aggregate level, lends further credence to the importance of extraindividual, aggregate measures of socioeconomic position (Kaplan et al. 1996; Kennedy et al. 1996; Wilkinson 1996; Lynch and Kaplan 1997; Daly et al. 1998; Lynch et al. 1998).

This emphasis on the importance of community or area characteristics that are by definition extraindividual is seen in a number of other areas of research. Criminologists (Sampson 1992; Sampson et al. 1997), researchers studying child development (Brooks-Gunn et al. 1997), and those interested in the plight of the disadvantaged (Wilson 1987) have all turned to a consideration of the structure, organization and function of communities. The exposure and demands model seems to characterize many of the factors within communities that may be associated with poorer health (Kaplan 1996).

CONCLUSIONS

There can be no doubt that the socioeconomic position of individuals, groups, and places is a defining characteristic of their levels of health and disease. While it is important to keep in mind the salience of socioeconomic position in determining the health status of individuals and populations, advancing our understanding of the reasons for these effects and their policy implications requires more than simply pointing to the association. We argue that several steps are necessary to advance epidemiologic studies in this area (Kaplan and Lynch 1997). In addition to an increased recognition of the intellectual foundations of measures of socioeconomic position, greater effort must be devoted to an attempt to understand what these measures are proxies for. This means, for example, a better specification of how exploitation, education, or income level could be related to health and health trajectories. Such a specification will, undoubtedly, be best informed by an analytic and conceptual view which incorporates a dynamic and life course perspective, in some cases one that is intergenerational. Within this perspective, new research should attempt to explicate what we have called the "epidemiology of everyday life." That is, how are daily experiences, and their cumulative trajectories, stratified according to socioeconomic position over the entire lifecourse? We are just beginning to see the critical nature and function of extraindividual factors such as institutions and communities as important agents in the socioeconomic stratification of the health of individuals and populations, and this work needs to be vigorously pursued. Finally, the role of macroeconomic factors cannot be ignored. Economic policy and social policy have much to do with the levels of resources and exposures that individuals and communities experience; they represent important loci for intervention and are the upstream determinants of public health.

The exposure and resources model, rooted in the intellectual traditions of the analysis of social class and stratification, is an overall organizing scheme for furthering the research agenda indicated above that may have heuristic value. At both the individual and community level it is possible to describe the levels, balance, determinants, and consequences of resources and exposures. What's more, such a conceptualization may relate well to recent work on the downstream, mediating pathways that link socioeconomic position to the health of individuals. This view may be useful in the evolution of a social epidemiologic approach to socioeconomic inequalities in health that strikes a balance between proximate and mechanistic approaches to disease causation in individuals and upstream,

global approaches to the health of populations.

ACKNOWLEDGMENTS

The authors would like to thank Carles Muntaner and George Davey Smith. Their insightful comments on an earlier draft made important contributions to the final version of this chapter.

REFERENCES

Anderson, R., Sorlie, P., Backlund, E., Johnson, N., and Kaplan, G.A. (1997). Mortality effects of community socioeconomic status. *Epidemiology*, 8:42–7.

Antonovsky, A. (1967). Social class, life expectancy and overall mortality. *Milbank Mem Fund Q*, 45:31–73.

Arber, S. (1987). Social class, non-employment and chronic illness: continuing the inequalities in health debate. *BMJ*, 294:1069–73.

Arber, S. (1991). Class, paid employment and family roles: making sense of structural disadvantage, gender and health status. *Soc Sci Med*, 32:425–36.

Armstrong, D.L., and Castorina, J. (1998). Community occupational structure, basic services and coronary mortality in Washington state, 1980–1994. *Ann Epidemiol*, 8:370–7.

Backlund, E., Sorlie, P.D., and Johnson, N.J. (1996). The shape of the relationship between income and mortality in the United States: evidence from the National Longitudinal Mortality Study. *Ann Epidemiol*, 6:1–9.

Barker, D.J., and Martyn, C.N. (1992). The maternal and fetal origins of cardiovascular disease. *J Epidemiol Community Health*, 46:8–11.

Barker, D.J., and Osmond, C. (1986). Infant mortality, childhood nutrition, and ischaemic heart disease in England and Wales. *Lancet*, 1:1077–81.

Barker, D.J., Osmond, C., Golding, J., Kuh, D., and Wadsworth, M.E. (1989). Growth in utero, blood pressure in childhood and adult life, and mortality from cardiovascular disease. *BMJ*, 298:564–7.

Bartley, M. (1994). Unemployment and ill health: understanding the relationship. *J Epidemiol Community Health*, 48:333–7.

Berkman, L.F., and Macintyre, S. (1997). The measurement of social class in health studies: old measures and new formulations. In Kogevinas, M., Pearce, N., Susser, M., and Boffeta, P. (eds.), *Social inequalities and cancer.*

Lyon, France: International Agency for Research on Cancer, pp. 51–64.

Blane, D., Bartley, M., and Davey Smith, G. (1997). Disease aetiology and materialist explanations of socioeconomic mortality differentials. *Eur J Public Health*, 7:385–91.

Boswell, T., and Dixon, W.J. (1993). Marx's theory of rebellion: a cross-national analysis of class exploitation, economic development, and violent revolt. *Am Soc Rev*, 58:681–702.

Bourdieu, P. (1984). *Distinction*. Cambridge, MA: Harvard University Press.

Brooks-Gunn, J., Duncan, G.J., and Aber, J.L. (eds.). (1997). *Neighborhood poverty*. New York: Russell Sage Foundation.

Carroll, D., Davey Smith, G., and Bennett, P. (1996). Some observations on health and socioeconomic status. *J Health Psychol*, 1:23–39.

Carstairs, V. (1995). Deprivation indices: their interpretation and use in relation to health. *J Epidemiol Community Health*, 49 Suppl 2:S3–8.

Corcoran, M.E., and Chaudry, A. (1997). The dynamics of children in poverty. In *The future of children—children in poverty*, vol. 7 (2). Los Altos, CA: Center for the Future of Children, pp. 40–54.

Daly, M., Duncan, G., Kaplan, G.A., and Lynch, J.W. (1998). Macro-to-micro linkages in the inequality-mortality relationship. *Milbank Mem Fund Q*. 76:315–339.

Davey Smith, G., and Dorling, D. (1996). "I'm all right, John": voting patterns and mortality in England and Wales, 1981–92. *BMJ*, 313:1573–7.

Davey Smith, G., and Harding, S. (1997). Is control at work the key to socioeconomic gradients in mortality? (letter). *Lancet*, 350: 1369–70.

Davey Smith, G., Shipley, M.J., and Rose, G. (1990). Magnitude and causes of socioeconomic differentials in mortality: further evidence from the Whitehall Study. *J Epidemiol Community Health*, 44:265–70.

Davey Smith, G., Neaton, J.D., Wentworth, D., Stamler, R., and Stamler, J. (1996). Socioeconomic differentials in mortality risk among men screened for the Multiple Risk Factor Intervention Trial: 1. White men. *Am J Public Health*, 86:486–96.

Davey Smith, G., Hart, C., Blane, D., Gillis C., and Hawthorne, V. (1997). Lifetime socioeconomic position and mortality: prospective observational study. *BMJ*, 314:547–52.

Davey Smith, G., Hart, C., Blane, D., and Hole, D. (1998a). Adverse socioeconomic conditions in childhood and cause specific adult mortality: prospective observational study. *BMJ*, 316:1631–51.

Davey Smith, G., Hart, C., Hole D., MacKinnon, P., Gillis, C., Watt, G., Blane, D., and Hawthorne, V. (1998b). Education and occupational social class: which is the more important indicator of mortality risk? *J Epidemiol Community Health*, 52:153–60.

Davis, K., and Moore, W. (1945). Some principles of social stratification. *Am Soc Rev*, 10: 242–9.

Desai, S., and Alva, S. (1989). Maternal education and child health: is there a strong causal relationship? *Demography*, 35:71–81.

Diez-Roux, A.V. (1998). Bringing context back into epidemiology: variables and fallacies in multilevel analysis. *Am J Public Health*, 88:216–22.

Diez-Roux, A.V., Nieto, F.J., Muntaner, C., Tyroler, H.A., Comstock, G.W., Shahar, E., Cooper, L.S., Watson, R.L., and Szklo, M. (1997). Neighborhood environments and coronary heart disease: a multilevel analysis. *Am J Epidemiol*, 146:48–63.

Duncan, G.J. (1996). Income dynamics and health. *Int J Health Services*, 26:419–44.

Duncan, O.D. (1961). A socioeconomic index for all occupations. In: Reiss, AJ. (ed.) *Occupations and Social Status*. New York: Free Press. 109–138.

Dye, T.D., and Lee, R.V. (1994). Socioeconomic status: developing a quantitative, community based index in rural Kashmir. *J Epidemiol Community Health*, 48:421–2.

Eames, M., Ben-Shlomo, Y., and Marmot, M.G. (1993). Social deprivation and premature mortality: regional comparison across England. *BMJ*, 307:1007–102.

Elo, I.T., and Preston, S.H. (1996). Educational differentials in mortality: United States, 1979–85. *Soc Sci Med*, 42:47–57.

Engels, F. (1848). *The condition of the working class in England* (tr. Henderson, O.W., and Chaloner, W.H., 1958). Stanford, CA: Stanford University Press.

Erikson, R., and Goldthorpe, J.H. (1992). *The constant flux*. Oxford: Clarendon Press.

Evans, R.G., Barer, M.L., and Marmor, T.R. (eds.). (1994). *Why are some people healthy and others not?* New York: Aldine de Gruyter.

Farr, W. (1864). Report of the evidence to the Royal Commission of Mines. In Buck, C., Llopis, A., Najera, E., and Terris, M. (eds.), *The challenge of epidemiology* (1989). Washington, DC: Pan American Health Organization, pp. 67–72.

Feinstein, J.S. (1993). The relationship between socioeconomic status and health: a review of the literature. *Milbank Mem Fund Q*, 71:279–322.

Feldman, J.J., Maroc, D.M., Kleinman, J.C., and

Cornoni-Huntley, J. (1989). National trends in educational differences in mortality. *Am J Epidemiol*, 129:919–33.

Geronimus, A.T. (1992). The weathering hypothesis and the health of African-American women and infants: evidence and speculations. *Ethnicity Dis*, 2:207–13.

Geronimus, A.T., and Bound, J. (1998). Use of census-based aggregate variables to proxy for socioeconomic group: evidence from national samples. *Am J Epidemiol*, 148:475–86.

Haan, M., Kaplan, G.A., and Camacho, T. (1987). Poverty and health: prospective evidence from the Alameda County Study. *Am J Epidemiol*, 125:989–98.

Haan, M.N., Kaplan, G.A., and Syme, S.L. (1989). Socioeconomic status and health: old observations and new thoughts. In Bunker, J.P., Gomby, D.S., and Kehrer, B.H. (eds.), *Pathways to health: the role of social factors*. Menlo Park, CA: HJ Kaiser Family Foundation, pp. 76–135

Haug, M.R. (1977). Measurement in social stratification. *Annu Rev Sociol*, 3:51–77.

Hollingshead, A.B., and Redlich, F.C. (1958). *Social class and mental illness: a community study*. New York: John Wiley.

House, J.S., Lepkowski, J.M., Kinney, A.M., Mero, R.P., Kessler, R.C., and Herzog, A.R. (1994). The social stratification of aging and health. *J Health Soc Behav*, 35:213–34.

Jargowsky, P.A. (1996). Take the money and run: economic segregation in U.S. metropolitan areas. *Am Sociol Rev*, 61:984–98.

Kaplan, G.A. (1996). People and places: contrasting perspectives on the association between social class and health. *Int J Health Services*, 26:507–19.

Kaplan, G.A., and Keil, J.E. (1993). Socioeconomic factors and cardiovascular disease: a review of the literature. *Circulation*, 88:1973–98.

Kaplan, G.A., and Lynch, J.W. (1997). Whither studies on the socioeconomic foundations of population health? (editorial). *Am J Public Health*, 87:1409–11.

Kaplan, G.A., Haan, M.N., Syme, S.L., Minkler, M., and Winkleby, M. (1987). Socioeconomic status and health. In Amler, R.W., and Dull, H.B. (eds.), *Closing the gap: the burden of unnecessary illness*. New York: Oxford University Press, pp. 125–129.

Kaplan, G.A., Pamuk, E., Lynch, J.W., Cohen, R.D., and Balfour, J. (1996). Inequality in income and mortality in the United States: analysis of mortality and potential pathways. *BMJ*, 312:999–1003.

Karasek, R., and Theorell, T. (1990). *Healthy work*. New York: Basic Books.

Kaufman, J.S., Cooper, R.S., and McGee, D.L.

(1997). Socioeconomic status and health in blacks and whites: the problem of residual confounding and the resiliency of race. *Epidemiology*, 8:621–8.

Kennedy, B.P., Kawachi, I., and Prothrow-Stith, D. (1996). Income distribution and mortality: cross-sectional ecologic study of the Robin Hood index in the United States. *BMJ*, 312:1004–7.

Kington, R.S., and Smith, J.P. (1997). Socioeconomic status and racial and ethnic differences in functional status associated with chronic diseases. *Am J Public Health*, 87:805–10.

Koopman, J.S., Prevots, D.R., Vaca-Marin, M.A., Gomez Dantes, H., Zarate Aquino, M.L., Longini, I.M.Jr, and Sepulveda Amor, J. (1991). Determinants and predictors of dengue infection in Mexico. *Am J Public Health*, 133:1168–78.

Krieger, N. (1991). Women and social class: a methodological study comparing individual, household, and census measures as predictors of black/white differences in reproductive history. *J Epidemiol Community Health*, 45:35–42.

Krieger, N. (1994). Epidemiology and the web of causation: has anyone seen the spider? *Soc Sci Med*, 39:887–903.

Krieger, N., Rowley, D., Hermann, A.A., Avery, B., and Phillips, M.T. (1993). Racism, sexism, and social class: implications for studies of health, disease, and well-being. *Am J Prev Med*, 9 Suppl 6:82–122.

Krieger, N., Williams, D.R., and Moss, N.E. (1997). Measuring social class in U.S. public health research: concepts, methodologies and guidelines. *Annu Rev Public Health*, 18:341–78.

Kuh, D., and Ben-Shlomo, Y. (eds.). (1997). *A lifecourse approach to chronic disease epidemiology*. Oxford: Oxford University Press.

Kunitz, S. (1994). *Disease and social diversity*. New York: Oxford University Press.

Kunst, A.E., and Mackenbach, J.P. (1994). The size of mortality differences associated with educational level in nine industrialized countries. *Am J Public Health*, 84:932–7.

Kunst, A.E., Groenhof, F., Mackenbach, J.P., and Heath, E.W. (1998). Occupational class and cause specific mortality in middle aged men in 11 European countries: comparison of population based studies. *BMJ*, 316:1636–42.

Liberatos, P., Link, B.G., and Kelsey, J.L. (1988). The measurement of social class in epidemiology. *Epidemiol Rev*, 10:87–121.

Link, B.G., and Phelan, J. (1995). Social conditions as fundamental causes of disease. *J Health Soc Behav*, Spec No:80–94.

Lord, W. (1955). *A Night to Remember*. New York: Henry Holt.

Lundberg, O. (1997). Childhood conditions, sense of coherence, social class and adult ill health: exploring their theoretical and empirical relations. *Soc Sci Med*, 44:821–31.

Lynch, J.W. (in press). Socioeconomic factors in the behavioral and psychosocial epidemiology of cardiovascular disease. In Schneiderman, N., Gentry, J., da Silva, J.M., Speers, M., and Tomes, H. (eds.), *Integrating behavioral and social sciences with public health.* Washington, DC: APA Press. (*in press*).

Lynch, J.W., and Kaplan, G.A. (1997). Understanding how inequality in the distribution of income affects health. *J Health Psychol,* 2:297–314.

Lynch, J.W., Kaplan, G.A., Cohen, R.D., Kauhanen, J., Wilson, T.W., Smith, N.L., and Salonen, J.T. (1994). Childhood and adult socioeconomic status as predictors of mortality in Finland. *Lancet,* 343:524–7.

Lynch, J.W., Kaplan, G.A., Cohen, R.D., Tuomilehto, J., and Salonen, J.T. (1996). Do cardiovascular risk factors explain the relation between socioeconomic status, risk of all-cause mortality, cardiovascular mortality and acute myocardial infarction? *Am J Epidemiol,* 144:934–42.

Lynch, J.W., Kaplan, G.A., Cohen, R.D., Salonen, R., and Salonen, J.T. (1997a). Socioeconomic status and progression of carotid atherosclerosis: prospective evidence from the Kuopio Ischemic Heart Disease Risk Factor Study. *Arterioscler Thromb Vasc Biol,* 17:513–9.

Lynch, J.W., Kaplan, G.A., and Salonen, J.T. (1997b). Why do poor people behave poorly? Variation in adult health behaviours and psychosocial characteristics by stage of the socioeconomic lifecourse. *Soc Sci Med,* 44:809–19.

Lynch, J.W., Kaplan, G.A., and Shema, S.J. (1997c). Cumulative impact of sustained economic hardship on physical, cognitive, psychological, and social functioning. *N Engl J Med,* 337:1889–95.

Lynch, J.W., Krause, N., Kaplan, G.A., Cohen, R.D., Salonen, R., and Salonen, J. T. (1997d). Workplace demands, economic reward and progression of carotid atherosclerosis. *Circulation,* 96:302–8.

Lynch, J.W., Krause, N., Kaplan, G.A., Tuomilehto, J., and Salonen, J.T. (1997e). Workplace conditions, socioeconomic status and the risk of mortality and acute myocardial infarction: the Kuopio Ischemic Heart Disease Risk Factor Study. *Am J Public Health,* 87: 619–24.

Lynch, J.W., Kaplan, G.A., Pamuk, E., Cohen, R.D., Heck, K., Balfour, J.L., Yen, I.H. (1998). Income inequality and mortality in metropolitan areas of the United States. *Am J Public Health.* 88:1074–1080.

Macintyre, S. (1997). The Black Report and beyond: what are the issues? *Soc Sci Med,* 44:723–46.

Macintyre, S., Maciver, S., and Sooman, A. (1993). Area, class and health: should we be focussing on places or people? *J Soc Pol,* 22:213–34.

Macintyre, S., Ellaway, A., Der, G., Ford, G., and Hunt, K. (1998). Do housing tenure and car access predict health because they are simply markers of income or self-esteem? a Scottish study. *J Epidemiol Community Health,* 52:657–64.

Mackenbach, J.P., and Kunst, A.E. (1997). Measuring the magnitude of socio-economic inequalities in health: an overview of available measures illustrated with two examples from Europe. *Soc Sci Med,* 44:757–71.

Mackenbach, J.P., Kunst, A.E., Cavelaars, A.E.J.M., Groenhof, F., and Geurts, J.J. (1997). Socioeconomic inequalities in morbidity and mortality in western Europe. *Lancet,* 349:1655–9.

Manuck, S.B., Kaplan, J.R., Adams, M.R., and Clarkson, T.B. (1988). Effects of stress and the sympathetic nervous system on coronary artery atherosclerosis in the cynomolgus macaque. *Am Heart J,* 116:328–33.

Marmot, M.G., Kogevinas, M., and Elston, M.A. (1987). Social/economic status and disease. *Annu Rev Public Health,* 8:111–37.

Marmot, M.G., Bosma, H., Hemingway, H., Brunner, E., and Stansfeld, S. (1997). Contribution of job control and other risk factors to social variations in coronary heart disease incidence. *Lancet,* 350:235–9.

Marx, K. (1894, 1991). *Capital: a critique of political economy,* vol. 3, ed. Engels, F. (tr. Fernbach, D., 1981). London: Penguin Classics, Chapter 47.

Mayer, S., and Jencks, C. (1989). Poverty and the distribution of material hardship. *J Hum Resour,* 24:88–113.

McDonough, P., Duncan, G.J., Williams, D., and House, J. (1997). Income dynamics and adult mortality in the United States, 1972 through 1989. *Am J Public Health,* 87:1–8.

McEwen, B.S. (1998). Protective and damaging effects of stress mediators. *N Engl J Med,* 338:171–9.

Mcleod, J.D., and Kessler, R.C. (1990). Socioeconomic status differences in vulnerability to undesirable life events. *J Health Soc Behav,* 31:162–72.

Miller, D.C. (1983). *Handbook of research design and social measurement.* New York: Longman.

Morris, J.N., Blane, D.B., and White, I.R.

(1996). Levels of mortality, education and social conditions in the 107 local education authority areas of England. *J Epidemiol Community Health*, 50:15–7.

Muntaner, C., and O'Campo, P.J. (1993). A critical appraisal of the demand/control model
of the psychosocial work environment: epistemological, social, behavioral and class considerations. *Soc Sci Med*, 36:1509–17.

Muntaner, C., and Parsons, P.E. (1996). Income,
social stratification, class, and private health
insurance: a study of the Baltimore area. *Int
J Health Serv*, 26:655–71.

Muntaner, C., Eaton, W.W., Diala, C., Kessler,
R.C., and Sorlie, P.D. (1998). Social class, assets, organizational control and the prevalence of common groups of psychiatric disorders. *Soc Sci Med*, 47:2043–53.

Nam, C.B., and Powers, M.G. (1983). *The socioeconomic approach to status measurement: with a guide to occupational and socioeconomic status scores*. Houston: Cap and
Gown Press.

Nam, C.B., and Terrie, E.W. (1986). *Comparing
the 1980 Nam-Powers and Duncan SEI occupational scores*. Tallahassee: Florida State University, Center for the Study of Population.

National Center for Health Statistics. (1998).
*Health, United States, 1998, with socioeco-
nomic status and health chartbook*. Hyattsville, MD: NCHS.

O'Campo, P., Gielen, A.C., Faden, R.R., Zue,
X., Kass, N., and Wang, M. (1995). Violence
by male partners against women during the
childbearing year: a contextual analysis. *Am
J Public Health*, 85:1092–7.

O'Campo, P., Xue, X., Wang, M., and O'Brien
Caughy, M. (1997). Neighborhood risk factors for low birthweight in Baltimore: a
multi-level analysis. *Am J Public Health*,
87:1113–8.

Oliver, M.L., and Shapiro, T.M. (1995). *Black
wealth/white wealth*. New York: Routledge.

Pamuk, E. (1985). Social class and inequality in
mortality from 1921–1972 in England and
Wales. *Population Studies*, 39:17–31.

Paracelsus. (1567). On the miner's sickness and
other miner's diseases. In Sigerist, H.E. (ed.),
*Four treatises of Theophrastus von Hohen-
heim called Paracelsus* (1941). Baltimore,
MD: Johns Hopkins University Press, pp.
56–61.

Parsons, T. (1970). Equality and inequality in
modern society. *Social Inquiry* (special issue):
13–72.

Poldenak, A.P. (1997). *Segregation, poverty, and
mortality in urban African Americans*. New
York: Oxford University Press.

Poulantzas, N. (1975). *Classes in contemporary
capitalism*. London: New Left Books.

Power, C., Hertzman, C., Mathews, S., and
Manor, O. (1997). Social differences in
health: life-cycle effects between ages 23 and
33 in the 1958 British birth cohort. *Am J
Public Health*, 87:1499–503.

Rather, L.J. (1988). Report on the typhus epidemic in Upper Silesia. In Rather, L.J. (ed.),
*Rudolph Virchow: collected essays on public
health and epidemiology*, vol. 1. Canton,
MA: Science History, pp. 205–20.

Robert, S.A. (1998). Community-level socioeconomic status effects on adult health. *J Health
Soc Behav*, 39:18–37.

Rose, G., and Marmot, M.G. (1981). Social class
and coronary heart disease. *Br Heart J*,
45:13–9.

Rosen, G. (1993). *A history of public health*. Baltimore: Md., Johns Hopkins University Press.

Ross, C.E., and Wu, C. (1996). Education, age,
and the cumulative advantage in health. *J
Health Soc Behav*, 37:104–20.

Sampson, R.J. (1992). Family management and
child development: insights from social dis-
organization theory. In McCord, J. (ed.),
Facts, frameworks, and forecasts, vol. 3 of
Advances in criminological theory. New
Brunswick, NJ: Transaction, pp. 63–93.

Sampson, R.J., Raudenbush, S.W., and Earls, F.
(1997). Neighborhoods and violent crime: a
multilevel study of collective efficacy. *Science*,
277:918–24.

Sapolsky, R.M. (1993). Endocrinology alfresco:
psychoendocrine studies of wild baboons.
Recent Prog Horm Res, 48:437–68.

Schnall, P.L., and Landbergis, P.A. (1994). Job
strain and cardiovascular disease. *Annu Rev
Public Health*, 15:381–411.

Schwartz, S. (1994). The fallacy of the ecological
fallacy: the potential misuse of a concept and
its consequences. *Am J Public Health*,
84:819–24.

Siegel, P.M. (1971). Prestige in the American occupational structure. University of Chicago
(doctoral dissertation).

Siegrist, J. (1996). Adverse health effects of high-
effort/low-reward conditions. *J Occ Health
Psychol*, 1:27–41.

Siegrist, J., Peter, R., Junge, A., Cremer, P., and
Seidel, D. (1990). Low status control, high effort at work and ischemic heart disease:
prospective evidence from blue-collar men.
Soc Sci Med, 31:1127–34.

Smith, J.P. (1995). Racial and ethnic differences
in wealth in the Health and Retirement Study.
J Hum Resources, 30 Suppl: S158–83.

Smith, J.P. (1999). Healthy bodies and thick wal-
lets: the dual relation between health and
economic status. *J Economic Perspectives*
13:145–66.

Smith, J.P., and Kington, R.S. (1997). Demographic and economic correlates of health in old age. *Demography*, 34:159–70.

Sorlie, P.D., Backlund, E., and Keller, J.B. (1995). U.S. mortality by economic, demographic, and social characteristics: the National Longitudinal Mortality Study. *Am J Public Health*, 85:949–56.

Susser, M., Watson, W., and Hopper, K. (1985). *Sociology in medicine.* New York: Oxford University Press.

Syme, S.L., and Berkman, L.F. (1976). Social class, susceptibility, and sickness. *Am J Epidemiol*, 104:1–8.

Szreter, S.R. (1984). The genesis of the Registrar General's social classification of occupations. *Br J Sociol*, 35:522–46.

Szreter, S.R. (1997). Economic growth, disruption, deprivation, disease, and death: on the importance of the politics of public health for development. *Popul Dev Rev*, 23:693–728.

Townsend, P., and Davidson, N. (eds.). (1982). *Inequalities in health: the Black Report.* Harmondsworth, UK: Penguin.

Townsend, P., Phillimore, P., and Beattie, A. (1988). *Health and deprivation: inequality in the North.* London: Croom Helm.

Treiman, D.J. (1977). *Occupational prestige in comparative perspective.* New York: Academic Press.

Troutt, D.D. (1993). *The thin red line: how the poor still pay more.* Oakland, CA: Consumers Union.

Turner, R.J., Wheaton, B., and Lloyd, D.A. (1995). The epidemiology of social stress. *Am Sociol Rev*, 60:104–25.

U.S. Census Bureau. (1963). *Methodology and scores of socioeconomic status.* (Working Paper No. 15.) Washington, DC: U.S. Government Printing Office.

Vågerö, D., and Illsley, R. (1995). Explaining health inequalities: beyond Black and Barker. *Eur Sociol Rev*, 11:219–41.

Villermé, L.R. (1840). *Tableau de l'etat physique et moral des ouvriers employés dans les manufactures de coton, de laine et de soie.* Paris: Jules Renouard.

Wagstaff, A., Paci, P., and van Doorslaer, E. (1991). On the measurement of inequalities in health. *Soc Sci Med*, 33:545–7.

Warner, W.L. (1960). *Social class in America.* New York: Harper and Row.

Weber, M. (1922). Class, status, party. In Gerth, H.H., and Mills, C.W. (eds.), *From Max Weber: essays in sociology* (1958). New York: Routledge and Kegan Paul, pp. 180–95.

Wilkinson, R.G. (1996). *Unhealthy societies.* London: Routledge.

Williams, D.R. (1990). Socioeconomic differentials in health: a review and redirection. *Soc Psychol Q*, 53:81–99.

Wilson, W.J. (1987). *The truly disadvantaged.* Chicago: University of Chicago Press.

Wing, S., Casper, M., Riggan, W., Hayes, C., and Tyroler, H.A. (1988). Socioenvironmental characteristics associated with the onset of decline of ischemic heart disease mortality in the United States. *Am J Public Health*, 78:923–6.

Wing, S., Barnett, E., Casper, M., and Tyroler, H.A. (1992). Geographic and socioeconomic variation in the onset of decline of coronary heart disease mortality in white women. *Am J Public Health*, 82:204–9.

Winkleby, M.A., Jatulis, D.E., and Fortmann, S.P. (1992). Socioeconomic status and health: how education, income and occupation contribute to risk factors for cardiovascular disease. *Am J Public Health*, 82:816–20.

Wohlfarth, T. (1997). Socioeconomic inequality and psychopathology: are socioeconomic status and social class interchangeable? *Soc Sci Med*, 45:339–410.

Wolfson, M., Rowe, G., Gentleman, J.F., and Tomiak, M. (1993). Career earnings and death: a longitudinal analysis of older Canadian men. *J Gerontol Soc Sci*, 48:S167–79.

Wright, E.O. (1985). *Classes.* London: Verso.

Wright, E.O. (1994). *Interrogating inequality.* London: Verso.

Wright, E.O. (1996). *Class counts: comparative studies in class analysis.* New York: Cambridge University Press.

3

Discrimination and Health

NANCY KRIEGER

Our future survival is predicated upon our ability to relate within equality.

Audre Lorde, 1980

Inequality hurts. Discrimination harms health. These seem like straightforward, even self-evident, statements. They are propositions that epidemiologists can test, just like any other proposition about health that we investigate.

Yet epidemiologic research explicitly focused on discrimination as a determinant of population health is in its infancy. At issue are both economic consequences of discrimination and accumulated insults arising from everyday and at times violent experiences of being treated as a second-class citizen, at each and every economic level. In asking whether discrimination harms health, this new work builds on a century and a half of research demonstrating that racial/ethnic economic disparities often—but not always—"explain" U.S. racial/ethnic inequalities in health (DuBois 1906; Tibbitts 1937; Krieger 1987; Krieger et al. 1993; Williams and Collins 1995; Lillie-Blanton et al. 1996). And it extends this work to address health consequences of other types of discrimination, based on gender, sexuality, disability, and age (Table 3-1).

Testing the hypothesis that discrimination harms health requires clear concepts, measures, and methods. This chapter will accordingly review definitions and patterns of discrimination within the United States, evaluate analytic strategies and instruments researchers have developed to study health effects of different kinds of discrimination, and conclude by delineating diverse pathways by which discrimination can harm health, both outright and by distorting production of epidemiologic knowledge about determinants of population health. Although the examples primarily are U.S.-based and pertain chiefly to racial discrimination and physical health, the broader issues raised should be relevant to other countries, to other types of discrimination, to mental health, and to overall well-being.

Throughout, the framework I use to conceptualize and operationalize relationships between discrimination, inequality, and health is ecosocial theory (Krieger 1994). Taking literally the notion of "embodiment," this theory asks how we incorporate biologically—from conception to death—

Table 3–1. Basic taxonomy of prevalent types of discrimination, United States, 1990s, by: type, constituent dominant and subordinate social groups, justifying ideology, material and social basis, and examples of embodiment as inequalities in health

Type of discrimination	Constituent social groups		Justifying ideology	Material and social basis	Examples of embodiment as inequalities in health
	Dominant	Subordinate			
Racial/ethnic	White, Euro-American	People of color*: Black Latino/a & Hispanic American Indian & Alaska Native Native Hawaiian and Pacific Islander Asian	Racism	Conquest, slavery, skin color, property	Higher infant mortality rates (per 1000 births; 1989–1991): Black: 17.1 American Indian: 12.6; American Indian: 12.6; Hispanic: 7.6; Asian/Pacific Islander: 6.6; White: 7.4 Age-adjusted mortality rates: 1.52 times higher among blacks vs whites (National Center for Health Statistics 1997; U.S Department of Health and Human Services 1991)
Gender**	Men and boys	Women and girls	Sexism	Property, gender roles, religion	Longer life expectancy of women (6.4 yrs) offset by higher rates of disability and illness, resulting in fewer years of disability-free life (National Center for Health Statistics 1997; Ruiz and Verbrugge 1997) Annually, 1 million women (vs 140,000 men) battered by spouse or partner, and 500,000 women raped or sexually assaulted (usually by a man they know) (Bachman and Saltzman 1995) By age 18, 1 in 3 or 4 girls and 1 in 10 boys sexually abused (Cosentino and Collins 1996)

(continued)

Table 3-1. Basic taxonomy of prevalent types of discrimination, United States, 1990s, by: type, constituent dominant and subordinate social groups, justifying ideology, material and social basis, and examples of embodiment as inequalities in health—Continued

Type of discrimination	Constituent social groups		Justifying ideology	Material and social basis	Examples of embodiment as inequalities in health
	Dominant	Subordinate			
Anti-gay/ anti-lesbian	Heterosexual	Lesbian, gay, bisexual, queer, transgender, transsexual	Heterosexism	Gender roles, religion	Elevated rates of: smoking, suicide, and substance abuse (Stevens 1992; Meyer 1995; Council on Scientific Affairs 1996)
Disability	Able-bodied	Disabled	Ableism	Costs of enabling access	Denial of health insurance; inadequate medical care (Gill 1996)
Age	Non-retired adults	Youth, elderly	Ageism	Family roles, property	Sexual abuse of children (see gender, above) Among elderly, poorer survival, due to less aggressive treatment (Minkler and Estes 1991)
Social class	Business owners, executives, professionals	Working class, poor	Class bias	Property, Education	Socioeconomic gradient in excess morbidity and mortality, especially among the poor (U.S. Department of Health and Human Services 1991; Williams and Collins 1995)

*Each of these groups is extremely heterogeneous; terminology employed categories employed is what will be used in the U.S. 2000 census. Examples (far from exhaustive) of sub-groups include: Black: African American, Afro-Caribbean, and Black African; Latino/a & Hispanic: Chicano, Mexican American, Cuban, Puerto Rican, Central and South American; Native Hawaiian and Pacific Islander: Native Hawaiian, Samoan, Guamanian; Asian: Chinese, Japanese, Filipino, Korean, Laotian, Hmong, Samoan; American Indian and Alaska Native: nearly 600 federally recognized and unrecognized American Indian tribes, Aleuts, and Eskimos.

**Also called "sex discrimination."

our social experiences and express this embodiment in population patterns of health, disease, and well-being. Bringing the metaphor of the body politic to life—a body "ruled" by a "head" and sustained by laboring "hands," a body that creates, consumes, excretes, reproduces, and evolves—this theory draws attention to why and how societal conditions daily produce population distributions of health. Critical causal components conjointly include: *(1)* societal arrangements of power and property and contingent patterns of production and consumption and *(2)* constraints and possibilities of our biology, as shaped by our species' evolutionary history, our ecologic context, and individual trajectories of biological and social development. These factors together structure inequalities in exposure and susceptibility to—and also options for resisting—pathogenic insults and processes across the life course (Krieger 1994; Kuh and Ben-Shlomo 1997). Ecosocial theory thus posits that how we develop, grow, age, ail, and die necessarily reflects a constant interplay, within our bodies, of our intertwined and inseparable social and biological history. Three additional assumptions, relevant to this chapter, are that we, as human beings, desire and are capable of living fully expressed lives replete with dignity and love, that epidemiologists are motivated to reduce human suffering, and that social justice is the foundation of public health.

Before considering how to conceptualize, measure, and quantify health consequences of discrimination, one caveat immediately is in order: The purpose of studying health effects of discrimination is not to prove that oppression is "bad" because it harms health. Unjustly denying people fair treatment, abrogating human rights, and constraining possibilities for living fully expressed, dignified, and loving lives is, by definition, wrong (United Nations General Assembly 1948; Tomasevski 1993)—*regardless* of effects on health. Rather, the rationale for studying health consequences of discrimination is to enable full accounting of what drives population patterns of health, disease, and well-being so as to produce knowledge useful for guiding policies and actions to reduce social inequalities in health and promote social well-being.

DISCRIMINATION IN THE UNITED STATES: DEFINITIONS AND PATTERNS

Definitions of Discrimination

According to the *Oxford English Dictionary*, the word "discriminate" derives from the Latin term *discriminare*, which means "to divide, separate, distinguish" (1971, p. 746). From this standpoint, "discrimination" simply means "a distinction (made with the mind, or in action)." Yet, when people are involved, as both agents and objects of discrimination, discrimination takes on a new meaning: "to discriminate against" is "to make an adverse distinction with regard to; to distinguish unfavorably from others" (p. 746). In other words, when people discriminate against each other, more than simple distinctions are at issue. Instead, those who discriminate restrict, by judgment and action, the lives of those whom they discriminate against.

The invidious meanings of adverse discrimination become readily apparent in the legal realm, where people have created and enforce laws both to uphold and to challenge discrimination. Legally, discrimination can be of two forms. One is *de jure*, meaning mandated by law; the other is *de facto*, without legal basis but sanctioned by custom or practice. Examples of *de jure* discrimination include Jim Crow laws, now overturned, that denied African Americans access to facilities and services used by white Americans (Jaynes and Williams 1989, pp. 57–111) and current laws prohibiting gay and lesbian marriage (Vaid 1995). By contrast, underrepresentation of people of color and white women in clinical trials constitutes a form of *de facto* discrimination (Sechzer et al. 1994; King 1996).

Whether *de jure* or *de facto*, discrimination can be perpetrated by a diverse array of actors. These include the state and its insti-

Table 3–2. Selected U.S. laws and international human rights instruments prohibiting discrimination

U.S. laws	International Human Rights Instruments
U.S. Constitution	Universal Declaration of Human Rights (1948)
13th Amendment (banned slavery)(1865)	Discrimination (Employment and Occupation Convention) (1958)
14th Amendment (guaranteed due process to all citizens, excepting American Indians) (1866)	Convention Against Discrimination (in Education) (1960) International Convention on the Elimination of All Forms of Racial Discrimination (1965)
15th Amendment (banned voting discrimination based on "race, color, or previous condition of servitude")(1870)	International Covenant on Civil and Political Rights (1966)
19th Amendment (banned voting discrimination "on account of sex")(1920)	International Covenant on Economic, Social, and Cultural Rights (1966) Declaration on the Elimination of Discrimination Against Women (1967)
Civil Rights Act (1875)(declared unconstitutional by US Supreme Court in 1883)	Declaration on Race and Racial Prejudice (1978)
Civil Rights Act (1964)	Convention on the Elimination of All Forms of Discrimination against Women (1979)
Voting Rights Act (1965)	Convention on the Rights of the Child (1989)
Fair Housing Act (1968)	
Equal Opportunity Act (1975)	
Americans with Disability Act (1990)	

Sources: Jaynes and Williams 1989, pp. 224–38; Tomasevski 1993; Gill 1996.

tutions (ranging from law courts to public schools), nonstate institutes (e.g., private sector employers, private schools, religious organizations), and individuals. From a legal or human rights perspective, however, it is the state that possesses critical agency and establishes the context—whether permissive or prohibitive—for discriminatory acts: It can enforce, enable, or condone discrimination, or, alternatively, it can outlaw and seek to redress its effects (Table 3–2) (Tomasevski 1993). A powerful example of the latter is the new post-apartheid South African constitution (de Vos 1997). This document mandates, in the most inclusive language of any national constitution in the world, that "The state may not unfairly discriminate directly or indirectly against anyone on one or more grounds, including

race, gender, sex, pregnancy, marital status, ethnic or social origin, colour, sexual orientation, age, disability, religion, conscience, belief, culture, language and birth"; discrimination by individuals on these terms is likewise prohibited.

Despite its legal dimensions, however, discrimination is never simply a legal affair. Conceptualized more broadly, it refers to all means of expressing and institutionalizing social relationships of dominance and oppression. At issue are practices of dominant groups to maintain privileges they accrue through subordinating the groups they oppress and ideologies they use to justify these practices; these ideologies revolve around notions of innate superiority and inferiority, difference, or deviance. Thus, the *Collins Dictionary of Sociology* defines "discrimination" as "the process by which a member, or members, of a socially defined group is, or are, treated differently (especially unfairly) because of his/her/their membership of that group" (Jary and Jary 1995, p. 169). Extending this definition, the *Concise Oxford Dictionary of Sociology* holds that discrimination involves not only "socially derived beliefs each [group] holds about the other" but also "patterns of dominance and oppression, viewed as expressions of a struggle for power and privilege" (Marshall 1994, pp. 125–126). In other words, random acts of unfair treatment do not constitute discrimination. Instead, discrimination is a socially structured and sanctioned phenomenon, justified by ideology and expressed in interactions, among and between individuals and institutions, intended to maintain privileges for members of dominant groups at the cost of deprivation for others.

Although sharing a common thread of systemic unfair treatment, discrimination nevertheless can vary in form and type, depending on how it is expressed, by whom, and against whom. As summarized in Table 3–3, diverse forms identified by social scientists include: *legal, illegal, overt* (or *blatant*), and *covert* (or *subtle*) discrimination, and also *institutional* (or *organizational*), *structural* (or *systemic*), and *interpersonal* (or *individual*) discrimination (Benokratis and Feagin 1986; Rothenberg 1988; Feagin 1989; Essed 1992). Although usage of these terms varies, *institutional discrimination* typically refers to discriminatory policies or practices carried out by state or nonstate institutions; *structural discrimination* refers to the totality of ways in which societies foster discrimination; and *interpersonal discrimination* refers to directly perceived discriminatory interactions between individuals—whether in their institutional roles (e.g., employer/employee) or as public or private individuals (e.g., shopkeeper/shopper). In all cases, perpetrators of discrimination act unfairly towards members of socially defined subordinate groups to reinforce relations of dominance and subordination,

thereby bolstering privileges conferred to them as members of a dominant group.

Patterns of Discrimination

A full accounting of discrimination in the United States today is beyond the scope of this chapter. Instead, to provide a reminder of its ubiquity as well as background to considering how it can harm health, I next review, briefly, five notable ways that discrimination can permeate people's lives.

First, as summarized in Table 3–1, many groups experience discrimination in the United States at present. Dominant types of discrimination are based on race/ethnicity, gender, sexuality (including sexual orientation and identity), disability, age, and, although not always recognized as such, social class (Rothenberg 1988; Jackman 1994; Essed 1996; Vaid 1995; Gill 1996; Minkler and Estes 1991; Sennett and Cobb 1972). Other types, more pronounced in the past, include discrimination based on religion and nationality (U.S. Equal Employment and Opportunity Commission 1992). These latter types are still highly relevant for American Indians and other indigenous people in the United States, for whom many governmental policies (e.g., restrictions on religious expression, abrogation of treaty rights, removal of children to non-Indian families) have been genocidal in effect, if not intent (Thorton 1987).

Second, as explicitly recognized by the South African constitution, people often can experience multiple forms of discrimination. Whereas white women may be subject, as women, to gender discrimination, women of color—whether black, Latina, Asian or Pacific Islander, or American Indian—may be subject to both gender and racial discrimination. Moreover, this experience of multiple subordination cannot simply be reduced to the "sum" of each type. Recent U.S. scholarship on gendered racism, for example, has begun to examine how, in a context of overall negative stereotypical portrayals of black Americans as lazy and unintelligent (Schuman et al. 1985; Kinder and Mendelberg 1995), black

Table 3–3. Conceptualizing discrimination as a determinant of population health

---

Aspects of Discrimination

Type: defined in reference to constituent dominant and subordinate groups, and justifying ideology
  (see Table 3–1)
Form: legal or illegal; institutional, structural, interpersonal; direct or indirect; overt or covert
Agency: perpetrated by state or by nonstate actors (institutional or individuals)
Expression: from verbal to violent; mental, physical, or sexual
Domain: e.g., at home; within family; at school; getting a job; at work; getting housing; getting credit or loans;
  getting medical care, purchasing other goods and services; by the media; from the police or in the courts; by
  other public agencies or social services; on the street or in a public setting
Level: individual, institutional, residential neighborhood, political jurisdiction, regional economy

Cumulative Exposure to Discrimination

Timing: conception; infancy; childhood; adolescence; adulthood
Intensity
Frequency (acute; chronic)
Duration

Pathways of Embodying Discrimination (Involving Exposure, Susceptibility, and Responses to)

#1 Economic and social deprivation: at home, in the neighborhood and other socioeconomic regions
#2 Toxic substances and hazardous conditions (pertaining to physical, chemical, and biological agents):
  at home, at work, and in the neighborhood
#3 Socially inflicted trauma (mental, physical, or sexual, ranging from verbal to violent): at home, at work,
  in the neighborhood, in society at large
#4 Targeted marketing of legal and illegal psychoactive and other substances (alcohol, smoking, other drugs,
  junk food)
#5 Inadequate health care, by health care facilities and by specific providers (including access to care,
  diagnosis, treatment)

Responses to Discrimination (Protective and Harmful)

Protective
Active resistance by individuals and communities (involving organizing, lawsuits, social networks,
  social support)
Creating safe spaces for self-affirmation (social, cultural, sexual)

Harmful
Internalized oppression and denial
Use of psychoactive substances (legal and illegal)

Effects of Discrimination on Scientific Knowledge

Theoretical frameworks
Specific hypotheses
Data collection
Data interpretation

---

women—as *black women*—are stereo-typed, as Patricia Collins has observed, as "mammies, matriarchs, welfare recipients and hot mammas" (1990, p. 67), while black men—as *black men*—are stereotyped as criminals and rapists (Rothenberg 1988; Collins 1990; Essed 1992). Understanding discrimination experienced by black women and men thus requires considering the salience of both their race/ethnicity and gender.

Third, singly or combined, different types of discrimination can occur in just about every facet of public and private life (Table 3–3). The full gamut extends from the grinding daily realities of what Philomena Essed has termed "everyday" discrimination (1992) to the less common yet terrifying and life-transforming events, such as being victim of a hate crime (Pierce 1995).

In a typical day experiences with discrimination accordingly can start—depending on type—in the morning, at home, continue with public encounters en route to or while at school or work or when shopping or eating at a restaurant or attending a public event, and extend on through the evening, whether in the news or entertainment or while engaging with family members (Rothenberg 1988; Jaynes and Williams 1989; Feagin 1989; Feagin and Sikes 1994; Essed 1992; Sennett and Cobb 1972; Jackman 1994; Gardner 1995; Vaid 1995; Minkler and Estes 1991; Gill 1996). Other common but not typically daily scenarios for experiencing discrimination include applying for a job (Benokratis and Feagin 1986; Turner et al. 1991; Vaid 1995), look-

ing for housing (Turner 1993), getting a mortgage or a loan (Oliver and Shapiro 1995), buying a car (Ayers 1991), getting health care (Stevens 1992; McKinlay 1996; Geiger 1996; Gill 1996), or interacting with the police or public agencies or the legal system (Rothenberg 1988; Jaynes and Williams 1989; Feagin 1989).

Fourth, while some experiences of discrimination may be interpersonal and obvious, they are also likely to be institutional and invisible. To know, for example, that you have been discriminated against in your salary, or that you have been denied a mortgage, or an apartment, or been steered away from certain neighborhoods when you are looking for a home, requires knowing how the employer, bank, landlord, or real estate agent treats other individuals (Fix and Stryck 1993; Feagin and Sikes 1994; Essed

Table 3–4. Selected racial/ethnic inequalities in socioeconomic position, United States, mid-1980s to mid-1990s

Outcome	Time period	Black	American Indian & Alaska Native	Asian & Pacific Islander	Hispanic	White
% below poverty	1990	29.5	31.6	14.1	25.3	9.8
Ratio compared to whites		3.0	3.2	1.4	2.6	[1.0]
Median household income	1989	$19,758	$19,897	$36,784	$24,156	$31,435
Ratio compared to whites		0.6	0.6	1.2	0.8	[1.0]
Median net worth in lowest income quintile	1991	$1	(na)	(na)	$645	$10,257
Ratio compared to whites		0.0			0.06	[1.0]
% unemployed (adults ≥ 16 years old):						
Men	1990	13.7	16.2	5.1	9.8	5.4
Ratio compared to whites		2.6	3.1	1.0	1.9	[1.0]
Women	1990	12.2	13.4	5.5	11.2	5.0
Ratio compared to whites		2.4	2.7	1.1	2.2	[1.0]
Educational attainment (adults ≥ 25 years old)						
Less than high school	1990	37.0	34.7	22.4	50.2	22.0
Ratio compared to whites		1.7	1.6	1.0	2.3	[1.0]
Bachelor's degree or higher	1990	11.4	8.9	36.6	9.2	21.5
Ratio compared to whites		0.5	0.4	1.7	0.4	[1.0]

Source: Indian Health Service 1997, p. 34; U.S. Department Census Bureau 1994.

1996). Typically, it is only when people file charges of discrimination in court that evidence of such patterns of inequality can be obtained. Other clues can be obtained by examining social patterning of economic inequality, since acts of discrimination—whether institutional or interpersonal, blatant or covert—usually harm economic as well as social well-being. Table 3–4 illustrates this point for racial/ethnic discrimination, depicting marked racial/ethnic inequalities in income, wealth, education, and unemployment.

Fifth and finally, attesting to some of the animosity that feeds and justifies discrimination are, to give but one example, numerous surveys of U.S. racial attitudes (Schuman et al. 1985; Jaynes and Williams 1989, pp. 115–160; Kinder and Mendelberg 1995). Despite declines in racial prejudice over time, reported levels remain high, even taking into account that (1) people underreport negative social attitudes (Schuman et al. 1985); (2) dominant groups typically deny discrimination exists, especially, as Essed has noted (1996), if it is no longer legal (see, for example, Herrnstein and Murray 1994; Thernstrom and Thernstrom 1997), and (3) as Jackman has argued (Jackman 1994), paternalism combined with (a) friendly feelings toward individual members of subordinate groups and (b) denial of any responsibility for institutional discrimination is as much a hallmark of contemporary discrimination as is outright conflict and negative attitudes. Strikingly, then, data from the 1990 General Social Survey reveal that fully 75% of white Americans agree that "black and Hispanic people are more likely than whites to prefer living on welfare" and a majority concur that "black and Hispanic people are more likely than whites to be lazy, violence-prone, less intelligent, and less patriotic" (Associated Press 1991; Kinder and Mendelberg 1995). These are ugly social facts, with profound implications for not only our body politic but also the very bodies in which we live, love, rejoice, suffer, and die.

MEASURING DISCRIMINATION TO ESTIMATE ITS EFFECTS ON POPULATION HEALTH

How, then, can epidemiologists study discrimination as a determinant of population health? Figure 3–1 summarizes three approaches to quantify health effects of discrimination: (1) indirectly, by inference, at the individual level; (2) directly, using measures of self-reported discrimination, at the individual level; and (3) in relation to institutional discrimination, at the population level. All three approaches are informative, complementary, and necessary. I review and provide examples for each method, below.

Indirectly Measuring Health Effects of Discrimination, Among Individuals

One of the more common approaches to studying health consequences of discrimination is indirect. Recognizing that discrimination may be difficult to measure, investigators instead compare health outcomes of subordinate and dominant groups (Fig. 3–1a). If distributions of these outcomes differ, then researchers determine if observed disparities can be explained by "known risk factors." If so, investigators interpret their findings in light of how discrimination may shape distribution of the relevant "risk factors." If, however, a residual difference persists, even after controlling for these other risk factors, then additional aspects of discrimination may be inferred as a possible explanation for the remaining disparities (assuming no unmeasured confounders).

Exemplifying this indirect method are U.S. studies examining whether socioeconomic factors "explain" black/white inequalities in health status (Krieger et al. 1993; Williams and Collins 1995; Lillie-Blanton et al. 1996; Lillie-Blanton and LaVeist 1996; Navarro 1990; U.S. Department of Health and Human Services 1991), exposure to occupational and environmental health hazards (Robinson 1987; Brown 1995; Northridge and Shepard 1997), or receipt of medical services (Council on Ethi-

a. *Indirect, at individual-level:* examine whether "known risk factors" explain differences in health outcomes between members of dominant and subordinate groups; if not, infer discrimination may contribute to residual difference

Discrimination by physician → Differences in treatment → Differences in outcome
(unobserved)   (observed)   (observed)

Possibly affected by:
—severity in illness
—comorbidity
—age
—insurance status
—economic resources
—family support
—patient "preference"
  (usually unobserved)
etc.

b. *Direct, at individual-level:* among subordinate group, examine whether self-reported experiences of discrimination are associated with specified health outcome

Discrimination → threat → fear → physiologic responses → health outcome
(self-reported)   anger   —cardiovascular   (observed)
                        denial   —endocrine
                        etc.   —neurologic
                                 —immune
                                 etc.

c. *Institutional, at population-level:* among subordinate group, examine whether group-level measures of discrimination are associated with population rates of health outcome

Discrimination → Residential segregation → Concentration of poverty, → elevated morbidity
(unobserved)   (observed)   poor housing quality,   and mortality rates
                                            increased population density, (observed)
                                            toxic exposures, lack of
                                            access to services and goods,
                                            political disempowerment, etc.

Figure 3–1. Three main epidemiologic approaches to studying health effects of discrimination.

cal and Judicial Affairs 1990; Gornick et al. 1996; Geiger 1996; King 1996; Peterson et al. 1997). In their earliest form, starting in the mid-1800s, these kinds of investigations compared health of enslaved and free blacks and also poorer and wealthier whites, thereby exposing how slavery and poverty, and not "race" per se, largely explained the poorer health of "the Negro" (Krieger 1987; Smith 1859; Reyburn 1866). The basic strategy, then and now, is to determine whether "adjusting" for socioeconomic position (along with relevant confounders) eliminates observed racial/ethnic disparities in the specified outcome. If so, economic consequences of racial discrimination are inferred to underlie the observed (unadjusted) disparities; in other words, both racism

and class matter (Krieger et al. 1993; Williams and Collins 1995; Lillie-Blanton and LaVeist 1996; Navarro 1990).

If, however, racial/ethnic differences persist, four alternative explanations can be offered. One is that inadequate measurement of socioeconomic position produces residual confounding (Krieger et al. 1993; Kaufman et al. 1997). Consider, for example, a disease whose incidence increases with poverty, with incidence rates identical among African Americans and white Americans at each income level. Under these circumstances, if African Americans below the poverty line were much poorer than white Americans below the poverty line, then analyses adjusting for being "above" vs. "below" poverty would fail to explain excess rates of disease among African Americans—even though black/white income disparities in fact fully explained black/white differences in disease incidence. A second hypothesis, discussed in the next section, is that the remaining difference reflects health consequences of unmeasured noneconomic aspects of racial discrimination, e.g., chronic psychologic stress (Krieger et al. 1993; Williams 1997a). A third explanation, unrelated to discrimination, posits that unexplained differences reflect unmeasured factors that are associated with both race/ethnicity and the specified outcome but are not related to either discrimination or socioeconomic position, e.g., culturally shaped patterns of food consumption. Finally, a fourth explanation—often invoked but rarely tested (Cooper and David 1986; Williams et al. 1994)—speculates that innate genetic differences are responsible. Whether and how investigators address these alternative explanations, when interpreting unexplained differences in health status between subordinate and dominant groups, varies considerably across studies.

Illustrating both the importance and ambiguity of research using indirect methodologies to study health effects of discrimination is research on a well-known public health problem: black/white disparities in risk of low birth weight (Institute of Medicine 1985; Rowley et al. 1993). Numerous investigations have demonstrated that poverty is associated with elevated risk of low birth weight among both African Americans and white Americans and also that "adjusting" for poverty substantially reduces—but does not eliminate—excess risk among African Americans (Institute of Medicine 1985; Rowley et al. 1993). Even so, not only is risk of low birth weight 1.5 to two times higher among African American compared to white and Hispanic infants born to poor or less educated parents (Rowley et al. 1993; National Center for Health Statistics 1997, p. 90), but it is also two times higher comparing black to white infants born of college-educated parents (Schoendorf et al. 1992), even after controlling for numerous covariates. Although additional noneconomic and economic dimensions of racial discrimination could account for these findings, so too could other unmeasured determinants or confounders. Absent data on these unmeasured factors, discrimination can be at best inferred, not demonstrated, as a determinant of health outcomes. These same caveats apply to the other major strand of research indirectly assessing effects of discrimination and health, which focuses on differentials in diagnosis and treatment of women and men with the same symptoms or diseases (Council on Ethical and Judicial Affairs 1991; McKinlay 1996).

The importance of discrimination in restricting economic resources, coupled with evidence of the profound impact of economic well-being on health (Townsend et al. 1990; Krieger et al. 1993; Evans et al. 1994; Williams and Collins 1995; Amick et al. 1995; see also Chapters 2, 4, and 6), accordingly suggests that one strategy for reducing ambiguity and improving epidemiologic research is employing appropriate measures of socioeconomic position (Krieger et al. 1997; Liberatos et al. 1988). Failing to take into account such issues as level of measurement (e.g., individual, household, neighborhood, or region) and time period (e.g., childhood, adult) can introduce bias and produce considerable residual confounding. Using individual-level—instead of household-level—measures of socioeconomic position for women, for example, will rarely be adequate for properly detecting socioeconomic gradients in women's health (Krieger et al. 1999; Arber 1990). Moreover, as illustrated by a study which found that childhood but not adult measures of socioeconomic position account for adult racial/ethnic disparities in infection by *Helicobacter pylori* (Malaty and Graham 1994)—presumably because most infection occurs in childhood—socioeconomic position should be measured at relevant points across the life span, in relation to both acute exposures and cumulative disadvantage (Krieger et al. 1997; Kuh and Ben-Shlomo 1997). For guidance on measuring socioeconomic position in epidemiologic studies, overall and with respect to time period and level of measurement, as well race/ethnicity, gender, and sexual orientation, readers are encouraged to consult the cited references (above) as well as Chapter 2 of this book.

Lastly, one further indirect approach to measuring health effects of discrimination on individuals—albeit relevant only to racial discrimination—addresses associations between skin color and health status. This approach has been employed in 17 U.S. epidemiologic studies focusing on health of African Americans (Boyle et al. 1967; Boyle 1970; Harburg et al. 1973, 1978; Keil et al. 1977, 1981, 1992; Coresh et al. 1991; Nelson et al. 1988, 1993; Garty et al. 1989; Klag et al. 1991; Dressler 1991a; Knapp et al. 1995; Gleiberman et al. 1995; Schwam et al. 1995; Churchill et al. 1996). Although most of these studies actually were attempting to use skin color as a biological marker for genetic admixture, several also conceptualized skin color as a marker for discrimination. The underlying presumption is that darker skin color increases risk of discrimination above and beyond a powerful "color line" markedly distinguishing people of color from white Americans.

Notably, among these 17 epidemiologic studies, 12 reported associations (all modest) between skin color and the specified outcomes (ranging from blood pressure to all-cause and cause-specific mortality) (Boyle et al. 1967; Boyle 1970; Harburg et al. 1973, 1978; Keil et al. 1977, 1981; Coresh et al. 1991; Klag et al. 1991; Dressler et al. 1991; Knapp et al. 1995; Gleiberman et al. 1995; Churchill et al. 1996). Of these 12, the ten collecting socioeconomic data (all but Boyle 1970 and Coresh et al. 1991) *all* found that socioeconomic position either typically explained or else substantially modified the observed association. Additionally, the single published U.S. study examining associations between skin color, socioeconomic position, and self-reported experiences of racial discrimination among African Americans documented that while darker skin color was moderately associated with socioeconomic deprivation (among men only), skin color and self-reported experiences of racial discrimination were largely unrelated (Krieger et al. 1998). Other sociologic research similarly has shown that while moderate associations exist between skin color and income among both African Americans and Mexican American (chiefly among men), income disparities are far greater comparing African Americans or Mexican Americans with light skin to white Euro-Americans than when comparing African Americans or Mexican Americans with dark vs. light skin (Telles and Murguia 1990; Keith and Herring 1991). The net implication is that while skin color may serve as a modest indirect marker for aspects of racial discrimination, it is not a direct marker for self-reported experiences of racial discrimination.

Taken together, then, existing research relying upon indirect strategies to measure health effects of discrimination provides precisely this: indirect evidence. They do not and cannot explicitly measure direct experiences of discrimination. Nor can they investigate effects related to intensity, duration, or time period of exposure to discrimination. What such studies *can* address, however, are *(1)* health effects of types of discrimination *not readily perceived by individuals* (e.g., treatment decisions of individuals' physicians), and *(2)* whether economic disparities or other factors presumed to be related to discrimination account for observed differences in health between dominant and subordinate groups. For these reasons, studies using indirect approaches to measuring health effects of discrimination can and do provide essential, powerful, and important evidence that discrimination shapes societal distributions of health and disease. To ask and answer the question of how directly perceived discrimination affects health accordingly requires a different set of questions and a different research strategy.

Measuring Self-Reported Experiences of Direct Discrimination and Its Health Effects, Among Individuals

To meet the challenge of explicitly measuring people's direct experiences of discrimination and relating this to their health status, a new generation of public health researchers is devising new methods and approaches. Indicating the novelty of this work, at the time of preparing this chapter I could identify only 20 studies in the public health literature employing instruments to measure self-reported experiences of discrimination (Table 3–5). Of these, 15 focused on racial discrimination (13 on African Americans, two on Hispanics and Mexican Americans), two of which additionally addressed gender discrimination; another solely examined gender discrimination; three investigated discrimination based on sexual orientation; and one concerned discrimination based on disability. I could find no published empirical studies on health effects of self-reported experiences of discrimination based on age.

In Table 3–5, I summarize measures of discrimination employed in, along with findings of, these 20 investigations. The most common outcome (ten studies) was mental health, e.g., depression, psychological distress; the second most common (five studies) was hypertension or blood pressure. Overall, studies consistently reported higher levels of self-reported experiences of discrimination were associated with poorer mental health; associations with somatic health, as discussed below, were more complex.

As indicated by the diversity of questions listed in Table 3–5, public health research presently lacks a standardized methodology to measure self-reported experiences of direct discrimination. Of particular note is variability in assessing: (1) time period of exposure (ever vs. recently), (2) domain of such exposures (globally or in specific situations), (3) intensity and frequency of exposure (major events or everyday types of discrimination), and (4) targets of discrimination (respondents only or also members of their family or their group overall). Only eight studies included additional questions asking respondents how much they were upset by and how they responded to experiences of discrimination. Less than half the studies reported psychometric measures regarding validity or reliability of their instruments.

At least two factors underlie proliferation of different measures of self-reported experiences of and responses to discrimination in epidemiologic research. One is the recent emergence of public health research on this topic. Thus, investigators are only now starting to develop, employ, and validate instruments appropriate for large-scale epidemiologic investigations. Methodologic research comparing associations of diverse measures of self-reported discrimination with selected health outcomes, within the same study population, has yet to be conducted. Without such validation research, choice of appropriate measures is likely to remain problematic.

Also contributing to eclectic use of questions about self-reported experiences of discrimination is an overall dearth of empirical studies on this topic, not just in public health but in research more broadly. Often, when epidemiologists decide to measure social phenomena to assess their impact on health, we look to social sciences for guidance. Yet, neither the sociologic nor psychologic literature currently offers well-characterized, "ready-to-use," validated instruments appropriate for large-scale empirical studies. Instead, most empirical sociologic studies on discrimination either have focused chiefly on racial attitudes of people who discriminate, rather than experiences of those who have endured discrimination (Schuman et al. 1985; Jackman 1994), or else, as is also the case in psychological research, they have employed in-depth interviews and qualitative approaches not readily transferable to epidemiologic research

Table 3-5. Measures of direct discrimination used in or designed for studies with health outcomes*

Type of discrimination	Study	Study Population**	Questions asked	Health outcome and association with self-reported experiences of discrimination***
Racial/ethnic	James et al. (1984)	112 African American men in N. Carolina	Occupational stressors: race as a hindrance to job success; unfair wages (not paid their worth) Response format: yes/no Psychometric evaluation: none	Blood pressure: ≈↑
	Amaro et al. (1987)	303 Hispanic women professionals (national sample)	Ever experienced discrimination at work Response format: yes/no Psychometric evaluation: none	Psychological distress: ↑
	Salgado de Snyder (1987)	140 Mexican immigrant women in Los Angeles	Ever been discriminated against as a Mexican, in the past 3 months (Note: question was one item in an acculturation scale) Response format: yes/no If yes: 4 point Likert scale on extent of related stress, ranging from "not very much" to "very stressful" Psychometric evaluation: Cronbach's α = 0.65	Depression: ≈ ↑
	Krieger (1990)	51 black and 50 white women in Oakland, CA	Ever discriminated against: at school; getting a job; at work; getting housing; getting medical care; from police or in the courts Response format: yes/no Psychometric evaluation: none Response to unfair treatment: accept as fact of life or take action; talk to others or keep to self Response format: select one of the 2 specified options Pyschometric evaluation: none	Hypertension (self-reported): ≈ ↑

(continued)

Table 3-5. Measures of direct discrimination used in or designed for studies with health outcomes*—Continued

Type of discrimination	Study	Study Population**	Questions asked	Health outcome and association with self-reported experiences of discrimination***
	Dressler (1990) (see also Dressler 1991b)	86 black women and 100 black men in Alabama	Chronic social role stressors: 4 questions on discrimination at work, regarding pay raises, promotion, job responsibilities, overall pay (Note: questions were items in a scale on chronic stressors) Response format: 4 point Likert scale on how often, ranging from "never" to "frequently" Psychometric evaluation: none	Blood pressure: Ø
	Murrell (1996)	165 African American women in N. California	Perceptions of Racism Scale (Green 1995): 20-item self-report inventory, of which 10 questions concern medical, 2 about lifetime experiences of discrimination Response format: 4-point Likert scale ranging from "strongly agree" to "strongly disagree" Psychometric evaluation: Cronbach's α = 0.91	Stress: ↑ Low birth weight: Ø
	Krieger and Sidney (1996)	4086 black and white women and men in a multicenter study (N = 1143 black women, 831 black men, 1106 white women, 1006 white men)	Discrimination questions: same as in Krieger (1990), plus one additional situation: ever discriminated against on the street or in a public setting Response format: yes/no Psychometric evaluation: none Response to unfair treatment: see Krieger (1990)	Blood pressure: ≈↑
	Jackson et al. (1996)	623 African Americans (national probability sample)	Respondent or family member treated badly because of race (in last 30 days) Response format: yes/no Psychometric evaluation: none Perception of whites' intentions: keep	Psychological distress: Ø Number of chronic conditions: Ø Disability: Ø Psychological distress: ↑

		blacks down, better break, don't care Response format: select one of the 3 specified options Psychometric evaluation: none	Number of chronic conditions: ↵ Disability: ∅
McNeilly et al. (1996)	165 African-American college students and 25 community members in N. Carolina ($N = 123$ women, 67 men)	Perceived Racism Scale (51 items): Frequency domain (items 1–43): Frequency of exposure to racist incidents (past year; lifetime) on the job, in academic settings, in public settings (overt and subtle), racist statements Response format: for each item, 6-point Likert-like scale, ranging from "almost never" to "several times a day" Psychometric evaluation: Cronbach's $\alpha = 0.96$ Test-retest reliability: range = 0.71–0.81 Response domain (items 44–51): emotional responses and behavioral coping responses to perceived racism Response format: Emotional response: —5-point Likert scale for each type of feeling (e.g., angry, sad), ranging from "not at all" to "extremely;" —rank importance (from most to least) of four responses to experiencing racism ("think Whites have a problem," "think that person being racist has a problem", "feel bad about being Black," "feel bad about myself") Behavioral responses: select one or more of 10 options (e.g., "speaking up," "forgetting it," "getting violent," "praying) Psychometric evaluation: Cronbach's $\alpha = 0.92$ Test-retest reliability: range = 0.50–0.78	[none; designed for use studies] in future public health

(continued)

Table 3–5. Measures of direct discrimination used in or designed for studies with health outcomes*—Continued

Type of discrimination	Study	Study Population**	Questions asked	Health outcome and association with self-reported experiences of discrimination***
	Broman (1996)	312 African-American adults in Detroit (N = 209 women, 103 men)	See Krieger 1990 study; rephrased to refer only to discrimination in the past three years	Hypertension (self-reported): Ø Heart disease (self-reported): Ø
	Ladrine and Klonoff (1996)	149 black students, staff and faculty at a university (location not specified) (N = 83 women, 66 men)	The Schedule of Racist Events: 18-item self-report inventory: frequency of racist events in past year and entire life and appraisal of related stress Response format: 6-point Likert scale Frequency: "never" to "almost all the time" Stress: "not at all" to "extremely" Psychometric evaluation: Recent discrimination (past year): Cronbach's α = 0.95 Split-half reliability: 0.93 Lifetime discrimination: Cronbach's α = 0.95 Split-half reliability: 0.91 Appraisal of stress: Cronbach's α = 0.92 Split-half reliability: 0.92	Psychiatric distress: ↑ Cigarette smoking: ↑
	Mays and Cochran (1997)	232 black women and 73 black men (heterosexual) in college, university, and junior college, in Los Angeles, CA	Frequency of discrimination: —based on race/ethnicity, gender, or both: in general; personally experienced —as perpetrated by three sources (black men, black women, white men): against black person of same gender as respondent; personally experienced —as perpetrated by other African Americans against blacks lacking economic resources: in general; personally experienced Response format: for each item, 7-point	Psychologic distress: ↑

Study	Sample	Measure	Findings
		Likert-like scale, ranging from "never" to "fairly often" Psychometric evaluation: not stated	
		Degree of upset and relation to perpetrator, for each type of personally experienced discrimination	
		Response format: 7-point Likert-like scale	
		Upset: ranging from "not at all" to "upset a great deal"	
		Relationship to perpetrator: "mostly by those I know well" to "mostly by complete strangers"	
		Psychometric evaluation: not stated	
Auslander et al. (1997)	55 African-American and 103 white children and their mothers or female guardians	Modified Perceptions of Racism Scale (Dressler 1991b): reduced to 6 questions about perception of unfair treatment on basis of race by city officials, restaurant workers, health care providers, school teachers	Satisfaction with medical care: ↓
		Response format: 4-point Likert scale, ranging from "strongly disagree" to "strongly agree"	
		Psychometric evaluation: Cronbach's $\alpha = 0.78$	
Williams and Chung (in press)	2107 African-Americans (national probability sample)	Respondent or family member treated badly because of race (in last 30 days); for ever-employed persons: own and awareness of others' experiences of racial discrimination at work	Psychological distress: ↑
		Response format: yes/no	
		Psychometric evaluation: none	
Williams et al. (1997b)	586 black and 520 white adults in Detroit	Discrimination:	Self-rated ill-health: ≈↑
		—Major events: ever unfairly fired or denied promotion; ever unfairly not hired; ever unfairly treated by police	Psychological distress: ↑
			Psychological well-being: ↑
		—Everyday discrimination: sum of ever experiencing 9 kinds	Bed-days: ↓
		Response format: yes/no	

(con inued)

Table 3–5. Measures of direct discrimination used in or designed for studies with health outcomes*—Continued

Type of discrimination	Study	Study Population**	Questions asked	Health outcome and association with self-reported experiences of discrimination***
Gender	Krieger (1990)	51 black and 50 white women in Oakland, CA	Psychometric evaluation: Everyday discrimination: Cronbach's α = 0.88 Ever discriminated against: at school; getting a job; at work; at home; getting medical care Response format: yes/no Psychometric evaluation: none Response to unfair treatment: same as Krieger (1990)	Hypertension: ≈↑
	Ladrine et al. (1995)	294 women students and staff at university; 337 women at an airport (403 white women, 117 Latinas, 38 black women, 25 Asian-American women, 46 women in other ethnic groups; location of study site not stated)	Schedule of Sexist Events (Klonoff and Ladrine 1995): 20-item self-report inventory: frequency of sexist events in past year and entire life Response format: 6-point Likert scale, ranging from "never" to "almost all the time" Psychometric evaluation: Recent discrimination (past year): Cronbach's α = 0.90 Split-half reliability: 0.83 Lifetime discrimination: Cronbach's α = 0.92 Split-half reliability: 0.87	Psychiatric distress: ↑ Premenstrual symptoms: ↑
	Mays and Cochran (1997)	232 black women and 73 black men (heterosexual) in college, university, and junior college, in Los Angeles, CA	Frequency of discrimination, perpetrator, degree of upset [see entry under "racial discrimination" for types of questions, format, psychometric evaluation]	Psychological distress: ↑
Sexual orientation	Bradford et al. (1994)	1925 lesbians (national survey; 88% white)	Experiences of discrimination: verbal attack, job loss, physical attack Response format: not stated Psychometric evaluation: none	Mental distress: high prevalence (compared to U.S. women overall; not analyzed in relation to reported discrimination)
	Meyer (1995)	741 Gay men in NYC not diagnosed with AIDS (89% white)	Prejudice: experienced antigay violence, experienced antigay discrimination, in past year Response format: yes/no Psychometric evaluation: none	Psychological distress: ↑

Category	Author (year)	Sample	Measure	Outcome
	Krieger and Sidney (1997)	204 black and white women and men with at least one same-sex sexual partner in a multicenter study (N= 27 black women, 13 black men, 87 white women, 77 white men)	Perceived stigma of being gay: 11-item scale about expectations of rejection and discrimination regarding homosexuality; Response format: 6 point Likert scale, ranging from "strongly agree" to "strongly disagree"; Psychometric evaluation: Cronbach's $\alpha = 0.86$	Psychological distress: ↑
			Internalized homophobia: 9-item scale about extent to which gay men are uneasy about their homosexuality and seek to avoid homosexual feelings; Response format: 4-point Likert scale, ranging from "often" to "never"; Psychometric evaluation: Cronbach's $\alpha = 0.79$	Psychological distress: ↑
			Ever discriminated against: in family; at home; at school; getting a job; at work; getting medical care; on the street or in a public setting; Response format: yes/no; Psychometric evaluation: none; Response to unfair treatment: see Krieger (1990)	Blood pressure: ≈↑
Disability	Li and Moore (1998)	1266 U.S. adults with disabilities (Ohio, Michigan, Illinois; 53% women; 78% white, 17% African American; 47% total annual family income < $10,000; 43% multiple disabilities; 23% congenital disabilities)	Perception of discrimination: 4-item scale about beliefs about treatment of disabled regarding friendship, intelligence, treatment in community, being hired for a job; Response format = yes/no; Psychometric evaluation: Cronbach's $\alpha = 0.72$	Acceptance of disability: ↓; Chronic pain: ↑

*I could find no empirical public health studies on health effects of self-reported age discrimination.

**Racial/ethnic categories as designated in each study.

***↑ = positive association (more discrimination associated with higher levels of outcome).

↓ = negative association (more discrimination associated with lower levels of outcome).

≈↑ = partial positive association (discrimination positively associated with outcome, but not in dose-response relationship).

≈↓ = partial negative association (discrimination negatively associated with outcome, but not in dose-response relationship).

∅ = no association (between discrimination and outcome).

(Essed 1992; Feagin and Sikes 1994; Mays 1995; Bobo et al. 1995; Parker et al. 1995). The net effect is an uncanny silence on empirical estimates of the prevalence (let alone the effects) of self-reported experiences of discrimination, even as this experience is widely recognized in many other avenues of discourse, e.g., law, political science, history, literature, film, other art forms, and the media, to name a few.

Fortunately, epidemiologic principles can nevertheless provide useful guidance in measuring and analyzing self-reported experiences of discrimination and its effects on health. At issue, as in any epidemiologic study, are (1) measurement of exposure, in relation to intensity, frequency, duration, and relevant etiologic period, i.e., time between exposure, onset of pathogenic processes, and occurrence of disease, (2) measurement of susceptibility, and (3) effect modification of associations between exposures and outcomes by relevant covariates. In the case of studies of discrimination and health, issues of susceptibility notably include responses to and ways of resisting discrimination, while those involving effect modification require considering how self-reported experiences of discrimination and ways of responding to such experiences may have different meaning or impact depending on a respondent's social position, as related to multiple subordination, degree of social and material deprivation, and historical cohort.

First, regarding measurement of exposure, extant research suggests questions should be direct and address multiple facets of discrimination for *each* type of discrimination being studied. Conversely, studies should avoid global questions about experiences or awareness of discrimination— whether for all types combined or even just for one type of discrimination—since global questions are likely to underestimate exposure and are of little use for guiding interventions and policies to reduce exposure. Recognizing the importance of assessing multiple domains of discrimination, the few

large-scale social science surveys investigating self-reported experiences of discrimination—whether racial discrimination (Campbell and Schuman 1968; Kerner Commission 1968; Sigelman and Welch 1991; Jackman 1994; Taylor et al. 1994), gender discrimination (Women's Bureau 1994; Jackman 1994), or antigay discrimination (Herek 1993)—accordingly have asked respondents questions about experiencing distinct types of discrimination or unfair treatment in a variety of policy-relevant situations. Multiple options for questions about responses to discrimination and unfair treatment are likewise advisable, since studies show reactions can span from "careful assessment to withdrawal, resigned acceptance, verbal confrontation, physical confrontation, or legal action" (Feagin and Sikes 1994, p. 274; see also: Lalonde and Cameron 1994; Ruggerio and Taylor 1995).

Studies listed in Table 3–5 support the recommendation to use specific, rather than global, questions about experiences of discrimination. Thus, rather than ask about experiencing, say, racial discrimination overall, it is likely to be more informative to inquire about experiencing a specific type of discrimination in several different situations, e.g., at school, at work, on the street. Even better would be asking separately about having experienced racial discrimination in work assignments, promotions, pay, layoffs, interactions with co-workers, and interactions with supervisors (Bobo et al. 1995; Feagin and Sikes 1994). The importance of considering multiple types of discrimination, moreover, is illustrated by one study of antigay discrimination which found that while white gay men reported chiefly antigay discrimination, white lesbians reported both antigay and gender discrimination, and black gay men and lesbians additionally reported racial discrimination (Krieger and Sidney 1997); another study notably found that lesbian and gay African Americans reported higher rates of depressive distress than would be predicted based on summing risk for their race/ethnicity, gender, and sexual orientation (Cochran and Mays 1994).

In addition to specifying domains in which different types of discrimination occur, questions should also address extent of exposure in relation to the presumed etiologic period. Depending on the health outcome(s) under study, both chronic and acute exposures may matter, as will intensity, duration, and frequency of exposure. Thus, in the case of asthma attacks or other outcomes with sudden onsets that can be triggered by adverse events, acute as well as cumulative exposure to discrimination may be relevant. By contrast, in the case of hypertension or other conditions with gradual onset, cumulative exposure, rather than recent or acute exposure, most likely will have greatest etiologic relevance (Krieger and Sidney 1996). Furthermore, just as "daily hassles" and "major life episodes" often differentially affect health (Cohen et al. 1995), daily wear-and-tear of everyday discrimination may pose health hazards distinct from those resulting from major episodes of discrimination (such as losing a job)(Williams et al. 1997b). Designing questions about exposure to discrimination accordingly requires careful development of a priori hypotheses about timing and intensity of exposure in relation to the outcome(s) under study.

Additionally, adequate measurement of exposure requires considering whether it is sufficient to ask individuals about only their own experiences of discrimination. Also of concern may be people's fears of experiencing discrimination and their awareness of or fears about discrimination directed against other members of their family or their social group. Notably, recent research on what has been termed "personal/group discrimination discrepancy" documents that people typically report perceiving greater discrimination directed toward their group than toward themselves personally (Crosby 1984; Taylor et al. 1990, 1994; Ruggerio and Taylor 1995; Mays and Cochran 1997). Possi-

ble explanations of this phenomenon range from overestimation of group experiences of discrimination to recognition of patterns of discrimination not readily discerned by personal experience (e.g., discriminatory hiring practices, as discussed earlier) to denial of personal experiences of discrimination, positive coping, optimism, and even illusions of invulnerability (Crosby 1984; Sigelman and Welch 1991; Taylor et al. 1994; Feagin and Sikes 1994). Fully measuring exposure to discrimination accordingly may entail asking individuals about their lifetime experiences and fears not only for themselves but for their family members and their appraisal of risk for their social group more generally. These estimates of individual and group exposure, moreover, may be influenced by period and cohort effects due to historical changes in legal status, intensity, and domains of discrimination, e.g., coming of age before, during, or after the heyday of the Civil Rights Movement in the 1960s.

Even assuming questions adequately address the breadth of individuals' experiences, awareness, and fears of discrimination, however, data on self-reported experiences of discrimination necessarily—and importantly—are inherently subjective. Issues of validity are thus the same as those with any epidemiologic data on self-reported exposures, particularly those about personal social experiences (Cohen et al. 1995).

In the case of discrimination, at least four factors may contribute to individuals reporting different experiences of discrimination even when subjected to the same "exposure" (e.g., a specific act). The first involves what has been termed "internalized oppression," whereby members of subordinated groups—especially those experiencing greater social and material deprivation—internalize negative views of the dominant culture and accept their subordinate status and related unfair treatment as "deserved" and hence nondiscriminatory (Fanon 1965; Krieger 1990; Krieger and Sidney 1996; Sigelman and Welch 1991;

Essed 1992; Crosby 1984; Taylor et al. 1994; Feagin and Sikes 1994; Meyer 1995). The second concerns ways members of subordinate groups relate to "positive" traits— if any—attributed to them by dominant groups, e.g., some women may interpret men looking them over sexually in public as evidence of their own sexual attractiveness and hence self-worth, whereas other women may perceive such staring as public harassment (Jackman 1994; Gardner 1995). Third, people consciously or unconsciously may shape answers to be "socially acceptable" (Schuman et al. 1985; Cohen et al. 1995) and may also vary in whether they find it helpful or distressing to speak about their problems (Ross and Mirowsky 1989). And fourth, individuals may exaggerate experiences of discrimination (system-blame) to avoid blaming themselves for failure (Neighbors et al. 1996).

If operative, any of these biases could potentially affect not only estimates of directly perceived discrimination but also its impact on health. It is important to emphasize, however, that existence of these potential biases does not render epidemiologic research on discrimination and health impossible or unfalsifiable. The logical inference, for example, of a study reporting comparable health status (controlling for relevant confounders) among, say, women reporting no, moderate, and high levels of discrimination within each and every specified sociodemographic stratum, e.g., class, race/ethnicity, age, sexual orientation, would be that discrimination is not causally related to the health outcome(s) under study. By contrast, if associations were, in some instances, a dose–response relationship (more discrimination associated with greater risk of poor health), or, in others, a J-shaped curve (since internalized oppression may affect meaning of a "no" reply), the data would offer suggestive evidence of links between self-reported experiences of discrimination and health.

The salience of these kinds of conceptual and methodological issues for studying self-reported experiences of discrimination in relation to health is illustrated by a recent investigation I conducted on racial discrimination and blood pressure (Krieger and Sidney 1996). Participants were members of the Coronary Artery Risk Development in Young Adults (CARDIA) study, a prospective multisite community-based investigation established in 1985–1986 that enrolled slightly over 5000 young black and white women and men, in fairly equal proportions, who were 18 to 27 years old at baseline. Questions on racial discrimination included in the Year 7 CARDIA examination are described in Table 3–5. To analyze data on exposure to discrimination, I set as referent group African Americans reporting moderate racial discrimination, defined as reporting racial discrimination in one or two of seven specified situations. I based this choice on the a priori logic that moderate exposure constitutes a normal experience for people subject to racial discrimination, and I further hypothesized—based on prior research—that this referent group would be at lower risk of elevated blood pressure than African Americans reporting no or extensive discrimination (Krieger 1990).

Key findings for the African American participants were that, first, 80% reported having ever experienced racial discrimination (28% in one or two, and 52% in three or more of seven specified situations); 20%, however, reported having never experienced racial discrimination. Second, systolic blood pressure (SBP) was independently associated with both self-reported experiences of racial discrimination and response to unfair treatment. Third, adjusting for relevant confounders, SBP was significantly elevated by 2 to 4 mmHg among *(1)* working class men and women and professional women reporting substantial compared to moderate discrimination, and *(2)* working class men and women reporting no compared to moderate discrimination; conversely, *(3)* among professional men, blood pressure was over 4 mmHg lower among those reporting no compared to moderate discrimination. Fourth, within economic strata, a net difference of 7 to 10 mmHg in average SBP existed comparing extremes of experience involving racial discrimination and responses to unfair treatment. Additional novel analyses, also adjusted for relevant confounders, showed that (1) black–white differences in SBP would be reduced by 33% among working class women and by 56% among working class men if SBP of all black working class women and men were equal to that of those reporting only moderate discrimination (whose SBP was the same as that of their white working class counterparts), and (2) no black–white differences in SBP occurred among professional black women and men reporting, respectively, moderate and no discrimination, as compared to their white professional counterparts.

One plausible interpretation of why a response of no compared to moderate racial discrimination was associated with *elevated* SBP among working class African American women and men but *lower* SBP among professional black men is that, as discussed above, the meaning of "no" may be related to social position, in this case, gender and class (Krieger and Sidney 1996). Thus, for people with relatively more power and resources, a "no" may truly mean "no." By contrast, among more disenfranchised persons, especially those subject to multiple forms of subordination or deprivation, a "no" may reflect internalized oppression. In such cases, a disjuncture between words and somatic evidence may be an instance of the body revealing experiences—translated into pathogenic processes—-that people cannot readily articulate with words. In my view, this is the interpretation that makes the most sense, which takes as real the patterns evinced by blood pressure levels in relation to self-reported experiences of racial discrimination. The body can teach us something here, together with our words. Adding plausibility to this interpretation are results of two additional smaller studies, both of which found higher blood pressure among members of groups subjected to discrimination (black women, in one; white

gay men, in the other) who said that they had experienced no vs. moderate discrimination (Krieger 1990; Krieger and Sidney 1997).

Resolving conceptual and methodologic questions raised by emerging research on self-reported discrimination and health will require conducting appropriate validation studies. I accordingly describe four complementary research strategies that could potentially be useful, involving smaller, in-depth studies as well as larger surveys.

One approach would be to employ qualitative interviews to assess respondents' perceptions of discrimination and to probe meanings of their answers to survey questions about experiences of discrimination. Along these lines, one small British study found that people who initially stated on the questionnaire that they had not experienced racial discrimination later said, in subsequent in-depth interviews, that they had experienced such discrimination but found it too hard—or too frightening or too pointless—to discuss (Parker et al. 1995). Were this finding to be replicated, and were discrepancies between survey responses and in-depth answers about experiencing discrimination found to be greatest among those most subject to subordination or deprivation, it would underscore the need to (1) develop more sensitive approaches to eliciting information on people's self-reported experiences of discrimination and to (2) take into account effect modification, by social position, of observed associations between self-reported experiences of discrimination and health status.

A second strategy could build on new research about people's physiologic responses to adverse stimuli pertaining to the type(s) of discrimination being studied. Several recent experimental studies, for example, have shown that blood pressure and heart rate among African Americans increase more quickly upon viewing movie scenes or imagining scenarios involving racist, as compared to nonracist but angry, or neutral, encounters (Armstead et al. 1989; Jones et al. 1996). These kinds of studies could be extended by also querying study participants about their self-reported experiences of discrimination and then analyzing associations between their responses to these questions and their experimentally induced physiologic responses to witnessing or imagining discrimination.

A third investigative technique, likewise addressing how self-reports of discrimination might be biased by self-presentational concerns or by impaired ability to engage in introspection (Greenwald and Banaji 1995), would be to use implicit measures designed to circumvent these biases. One such measure, recently developed by cognitive and social psychologists, is the Implicit Attitude Test (IAT) (Greenwald et al. 1998). This test involves a computer task that assesses the degree of association between two concepts, based on the assumption that people take less time to categorize two concepts at the same time when they are associated with each other than when they are not. Results indicate that white respondents more quickly associate typically "white" names with positively-valenced words (e.g., "heaven") and typically "black" names with negatively-valenced words (e.g., "cancer")—a result that held even among white respondents who did not display prejudice in their explicit self-reports of racial attitudes (Greenwald et al. 1998). Such implicit attitude tests could be adapted to measure beliefs about experiences of discrimination, thereby affording a measure of exposure less likely to be biased by cognitive distortion than explicit self-reports (Ruggiero et al., forthcoming).

A fourth approach, feasible for large-scale surveys, would be to include questions assessing identity formation, political consciousness, stigma, and internalized oppression (Bobo and Gilliam 1990; Waters and Eschbach 1995; Meyers 1995). The purpose would be to examine whether these expressions of self- and social-awareness modify associations between health status and self-reported experiences of discrimination. Notably, each of these constructs is distinct from—and cannot be reduced to—"self-esteem" and "self-efficacy." At least among African Americans, research indicates that awareness that discrimination hinders black people from getting a good education or good jobs is *not* associated with self-esteem and is only modestly associated with self-efficacy—presumably because people derive their self-esteem chiefly from relations with family and peers, and their sense of self-efficacy from how much they are able to influence their immediate conditions, even while understanding that societal discrimination exists (Neighbors et al. 1996).

Measuring Population-Level Experiences of Discrimination and Health Effects

Individual-level measures of exposures and responses to direct interpersonal discrimination, however, no matter how refined, can, by their very nature, describe only one of several levels of discrimination that affect people's lives. Also potentially relevant are population-level experiences of discrimination, such as residential segregation, and also population-level expressions of empowerment, such as representation in government. A small but growing body of research accordingly has begun to examine whether aspects of discrimination that can be measured only at the population level themselves determine population health. Thus far primarily focused on racial discrimination, studies employing this third strategy have examined associations of African American morbidity and mortality rates with residential segregation, racial/ethnic political clout, and racial attitudes (LaVeist 1992, 1993; Wallace and Wallace 1997; Polednak 1997; Kennedy et al. 1997).

A study on how infant postneonatal mortality (the death rate of infants 2 to 12 months old) may be related to black residential segregation and political empowerment exemplifies this third approach to quantifying health consequences of discrimination (LaVeist 1992). Following prior sociological research on residential segregation (Duncan and Duncan 1955; White 1986), this investigation used an index of dissimilarity to measure degree of residential segregation. This index ranges from 0 to 100 and essentially measures the percent of African Americans who would have to relocate so that the ratio of blacks to white in every neighborhood would be the same as that for the city as a whole. Black political empowerment (Bobo and Gilliam 1990) in turn was assessed with two measures: *(1)* relative black political power, defined as the ratio of the proportion of black representatives on the city council divided by the proportion of the voting age population that was black, and *(2)* absolute black political power, defined as the percentage of city council members who are black. This latter measures was conceptualized as reflecting "the level at which African-Americans are empowered to control the political and policy-making apparatus of the city" (LaVeist 1992, p. 1084). Analyses showed increased risk of black neonatal mortality was independently associated with higher levels of segregation, poverty, and lower levels of relative (but not absolute) black political power, even when controlling for intracity allocation of municipal resources (e.g., per capita spending, by neighborhood, on health, police, fires, streets, and sewers). One implication is that community organization, in addition to other community conditions, may affect population health, a finding likewise suggested by recent research on income inequality, community marginalization, and mortality (Wilkinson 1996; Wallace and Wallace 1997; see also Chapters 4 and 8).

As in the case of studies of self-reported discrimination, however, research on population health in relation to population-level measures of discrimination or empowerment is in its infancy. Potentially promising measures include population-level indicators of social inequality and discrimination created by the United Nations Development Programme (UNDP) (1996), none of which have been employed in epidemiologic studies. The UNDP's gender empowerment measure, for example, includes data pertaining to *(1)* "economic participation," operationalized as the percent of women and of men in administrative and managerial positions and in professional and technical jobs, *(2)* "political participation and decision-making power," measured as the percent of women and of men in parliamentary seats, and *(3)* "power over economic resources," operationalized as women's and men's proportional share of earned income (based on the proportion of women and men in the economically active workforce and their average wage) (UNDP 1996, p. 108). Similar measures of economic participation and political empowerment could be developed for other subordinate groups, e.g., the lesbian and gay or disabled populations. Also likely to be informative, though not yet incorporated in epidemiologic studies, are measures of *(1)* economic segregation of neighborhoods (Jargorskwy 1996); *(2)* occupational segregation of jobs by gender and race/ethnicity (Jaynes and Williams 1989; Rothenberg 1988); *(3)* voter registration and voting rates of subordinate and dominant groups; and *(4)* sociodemographic composition of additional branches of government, e.g., the judiciary.

A related strategy—also not yet employed in epidemiologic research—would be to examine population health in relation to government ratification and enforcement of diverse human rights instruments, including existence and enforcement of national laws prohibiting discrimination (e.g., in the United States, the Civil Rights Act and the Americans with Disability Act)(Table 3–2). For example, the United States has ratified the International Convenant on Civil and Political Rights (1966) and the International Convention on the Elimination of All Forms of Racial Discrimination (1965), but not the Universal Declaration of Human Rights (United Nations General Assembly 1948), the International Convenant on Economic, Social and Cultural Rights (1966), the Convention on the Rights of the Child (1989), nor the Convention on the Elimination of All Forms of Discrimination against Women (1979)(UNDP 1996, p. 216). Any or all of these human rights instruments could provide important benchmarks for assessing how discrimination relates to violation of these internationally stipulated rights affects population health. From a policy perspective, this could be particularly useful, since popular movements and professional organizations can hold governments, and sometimes even nonstate actors, accountable for stipulations in these human rights instruments (Tomasevski 1993). Epidemiologic research, for example, could analyze rates of domestic violence against women in relation to state funding for police training on domestic violence (a type of spending called for by the Convention on the Elimination of All Forms of Discrimination Against Women) or racial/ethnic disparities in infant mortality in relation to public expenditures to improve race relations (a type of spending called for by the International Convention on the Elimination of all Forms of Racial Discrimination).

Any studies investigating associations between population-level measures of determinants and outcomes, however, must address two concerns, regarding: *(1)* etiologic period and *(2)* ecologic fallacy. In the case of etiologic period, at issue—as in the case of studies using individual-level measures of discrimination—are distinctions between acute and cumulative exposures and between outcomes with short and longer latency periods. Thus, from a temporal standpoint, an association of higher levels of residential segregation or negative racial attitudes with, say, concurrent infant mortality rates or childhood morbidity rates or homicide rates would provide more compelling evidence of health effects of segregation or racial attitudes than would its association with all-cause mortality among adults, given the much longer latency period for most causes of death (e.g., cardiovascular disease, cancer). If, however, current levels of segregation reflected past levels and little bias were introduced by residential mobility, then inferences about links between segregation and adult mortality rates could be warranted. Comparable caveats about temporal plausibility have

been raised for studies examining current levels of income inequality in relation to adult mortality rates: These associations make sense only if current income inequality is a marker for systematic underinvestment in human resources over time (Davey Smith 1996).

The concern regarding ecologic fallacy centers on whether causal inferences at the population level are valid at the individual level. As discussed also in Chapters 14 and 15 of this book, ecologic fallacy chiefly results from confounding introduced through the grouping variable (e.g., census tract, city, state, nation) used to define the group-level dependent and independent variables (Robinson 1950; Alker 1969). In the classic case, reported by W.S. Robinson in 1950 (Robinson 1950), although state-level data showed strong associations between high illiteracy rates and the proportion of states' population that was black (Pearson correlation coefficient = 0.946), within these states the relationship between illiteracy and race/ethnicity was much weaker (Pearson correlation coefficient = 0.203).

A subsequent critique of Robinson's analyses demonstrated that grouping by state added an important confounding variable: state level of spending on public education (Langbein and Lichtman 1978). Because southern states—the ones with relatively high proportions of black residents—had a low tax base and spent relatively less on public education, illiteracy in these states was also high among their white residents. Had Robinson taken into account state per capita spending on education, a phenomenon that can only be measured at the group level, not only would the computed ecologic correlations have been less affected by aggregation bias but the study also would have identified how state funding for education determines literacy rates. In other words, had Robinson used relevant population-level data, his study would have avoided what has been termed the "individualistic fallacy": erroneous inferences about explanations of patterns observed at the individual level because they rely only upon individual-level data (Alker 1969; Krieger et al. 1993).

In addition to highlighting the importance of population-level determinants of outcomes measured among individuals, the critique of Robinson's study implies that population-level measures of discrimination could perhaps be meaningfully combined with individual-level measures to yield even more informative analyses of health consequences of discrimination (Krieger et al. 1993; Williams 1997a). Methodologically, this approach entails use of contextual or multilevel analyses, a technique first developed in the social sciences (Blalock 1984; DiPriete and Forristal 1994). Using such methods, U.S. epidemiologic studies have begun to show that health profiles of, say, poor people who live in poor neighborhoods generally are worse than those of equally poor people who live in more affluent neighborhoods (Haan et al. 1987; Diez-Roux et al. 1997; see also Chapters 2, 14, and 15). Residential segregation or community political empowerment could likewise conceivably modify experiences, perceptions, and effects of—as well as responses to—individually reported experiences of discrimination. The study design of contextual analysis, however, has yet to be used in epidemiologic research on health effects of discrimination.

HOW COULD DISCRIMINATION HARM HEALTH?

Prompting development of the kinds of research strategies I have been describing is the persistent question: Why does health status differ among subordinant and dominant groups? More than methodology, however, is required to conduct valid and informative analysis of health consequences of discrimination. Equally vital is systematic and explicit consideration of ways that discrimination can harm health. Theory matters. At issue is comprehending not only direct health consequences of discrimina-tion that we embody but also how discrimination can harm our very ability to understand—and provide knowledge useful for effectively intervening upon—the public's health.

Pathways to Embodying Discrimination

From an ecosocial standpoint, one useful concept for understanding links between discrimination and health is "biological expressions of discrimination," to extend a terminology I developed with Sally Zierler to discuss connections between gender and health. We defined biological expressions of gender (including gender discrimination) to mean "incorporation of social experiences of gender into the body and expressed biologically, in ways that may or may not be associated with biological sex" (Krieger and Zierler 1995). One example would be how girls' and women's body build and exercise patterns are affected by underfunding of girls' athletic programs. By the same logic, biological expressions of racial discrimination (or race relations, more broadly) refer to how people literally embody and biologically express experiences of racial oppression and resistance, from conception to death, thereby producing racial/ethnic disparities in morbidity and mortality across a wide spectrum of outcomes (Krieger 1998). Similar terminology could be used to discuss biological expressions of other types of discrimination, whether based on sexual identity or orientation, age, disability, social class, or other characteristics. For each type of discrimination, a key a priori assumption is that disparate social and economic conditions of subordinate and dominant groups will produce differences in their physiologic profiles and health status.

Conversely, constructs such as "gendered expressions of biology" (Krieger and Zierler 1995) or "racialized expressions of biology" (Krieger 1998) are useful for denoting how social relations of dominance and subordination affect expression of health outcomes linked to biological processes and traits invoked to define membership in subordinate and dominant groups. In the case of biological sex and gender, for example, women's ability to become pregnant has been used to define women's roles and to restrict women's employment in certain male and relatively well-paid occupations, even though other less well-paid and typically female occupations may be equally hazardous—with these gendered roles in turn shaping distributions of pregnancy outcomes (Krieger and Zierler 1995). Or, in the case of race/ethnicity, examples of racialized components of our biology include skin color, hair type, and facial features, and also such genetic disorders as sickle cell anemia, cystic fibrosis, and Tay-Sachs syndrome. Rather than being conceptualized as particular aspects of human diversity, with varying distributions among populations— distributions notably shaped by geography, conquest, and laws about who can have children with whom—these traits instead typically are construed, tautologically, as evidence of "racial types" (Krieger 1998). Particular biologic characteristics accordingly become imbued with meanings of "race," conjuring up notions of fundamental difference on a whole host of other characteristics, even though within-group differences far exceed those between groups (King 1981; Lewontin 1982; Cooper and David 1986; Krieger et al. 1993; Williams et al. 1994; Cavalli-Sforza et al. 1996).

From an ecosocial vantage, specific pathways potentially leading to embodiment of experiences of discrimination—whether perpetrated by institutions or individuals, in public or private domains—are legion, as are plausible health outcomes. This is because discrimination creates and structures exposures to noxious physical, chemical, biological, and psychosocial insults, all of which can affect biological integrity at numerous integrated and interacting levels, simultaneously comprised of genes, cells, tissues, organs, and organ systems. The net effect, as discussed in a growing literature on causal pathways leading to inequalities in health across the life course, is to create, using Eric Brunner's term, a "biology of in-

equality" (Brunner 1997; Breilh 1979; Townsend et al. 1990; Krieger et al. 1993; Doyal 1995; Evans et al. 1994; Amick et al. 1995; Williams and Collins 1995; Wilkinson 1996; Kuh and Ben-Shlomo 1997; see also Chapter 13).

Conceptually, however, the myriad socially structured trajectories—operative throughout the life course—by which discrimination can affect health can be coalesced into five clusters. As delineated in Table 3–3, these pathways involve exposure, susceptibility, and responses (both social and biologic) to:

1. Economic and social deprivation: at work, at home, in the neighborhood, and other relevant socioeconomic regions
2. Toxic substances and hazardous conditions (pertaining to physical, chemical, and biological agents): at work, at home, and in the neighborhood
3. Socially inflicted trauma (mental, physical, or sexual, ranging from verbal to violent): at work, at home, in the neighborhood, in society at large
4. Targeted marketing of legal and illegal psychoactive substances (alcohol, smoking, other drugs) and other commodities (e.g., junk food)
5. Inadequate health care, by health care facilities and by specific providers (including access to care, diagnosis, and treatment)

Also relevant are health consequences of people's varied responses to discrimination. These can range from internalized oppression and use of psychoactive substances to reflective coping, active resistance, and community organizing to end discrimination and promote social justice (Cooper et al. 1981; Anderson et al. 1989; Essed 1992; Krieger et al. 1993; Feagin and Sikes 1994).

From a theoretical standpoint, the utility of an ecosocial framework is that it encourages development of specific testable hypotheses by systematically tracing pathways between social experiences and their biologic expression. Applying these five pathways to the case of racial discrimination and population distributions of blood pressure among black and white Americans, an eco-social framework thus guides researchers to explore the following kinds of hypotheses.

Pathway #1

Residential segregation and occupational segregation lead to greater economic deprivation among African Americans and increased likelihood of living in neighborhoods without good supermarkets, thereby reducing access to affordable, nutritious diets; risk of hypertension is elevated by nutritional pathways involving high fat, high salt, and low vegetable diets (Anderson et al. 1989; Troutt 1993; Khaw 1993).

Pathway #2

Residential segregation increases risk of exposure to lead among African Americans via contaminated soil (related to proximity of neighborhoods to freeways) and lead paint (related to decreased resources for removing and replacing lead paint); lead elevates risk of hypertension by damaging renal physiology (Sorel et al. 1991; Lanphear et al. 1996; Northridge and Shepard 1997).

Pathway #3

Perceiving or anticipating racial discrimination provokes fear and anger; the physiology of fear ("flight-or-fight" response) mobilizes lipids and glucose to increase energy supplies and sensory vigilance and also produces transient elevations in blood pressure; chronic triggering of these physiologic pathways leads to sustained hypertension (Krieger 1990; Krieger and Sidney 1996; Harburg et al. 1973; Anderson et al. 1989; Armstead et al. 1989; James et al. 1984; Dressler 1991a; Jones et al. 1996; Williams 1997a; Williams et al., 1997b).

Pathway 4

Targeted marketing of high-alcohol content beverages to African-American communities increases likelihood of harmful use of alcohol to reduce feelings of distress; excess alcohol consumption elevates risk of high blood pressure (Anderson et al. 1989; Moore et al. 1996).

Pathway #5

Poorer detection and clinical management of hypertension among African Americans increases risk of uncontrolled hypertension due to insufficient or inappropriate medical care (Anderson et al. 1989; Ahluwalia et al. 1997).

By specifying these discrete pathways—however entangled in people's real lives—ecosocial theory thus provides a coherent way to integrate social and biologic reasoning about discrimination as a determinant of population health. Instead of cataloguing an eclectic list of risk factors—or presuming genetic explanations as sufficient or fundamental (e.g., Wilson and Grim 1991; for refutation, see Curtin 1992), ecosocial theory proposes that explanations of population health are incomplete—and their ability to guide healthy public policy crimped—unless they take into account interweaving of social and biological determinants of well-being.

Effects of Discrimination Upon Epidemiologic Knowledge

Discussion of how theory directs generation of hypotheses in turn points to one important additional way discrimination can affect population health: its impact on epidemiologic knowledge and public health practice. At issue are the kinds of questions epidemiologists do and do not ask, the studies we conduct, and ways we analyze and interpret our data and consider their likely flaws.

That scientists' ideas are shaped, in part, by dominant social beliefs of their times is well documented by historians of public health, medicine, and science (Haller 1971; Rose and Rose 1979; Fee 1987; Haraway 1989; Rosenberg and Golden 1992). Relevant to epidemiology, during the last 20 years a substantial body of literature has begun to document how scientific knowledge and, more importantly, real people, have been harmed by scientific racism, sexism, and other related ideologies, including eugenics, that justify discrimination in relation to class, age, sexual orientation, and disability (Krieger et al. 1993; Krieger 1987, 1992; Haller 1971; Jones 1981; Navarro 1986; Gamble 1989, Hubbard 1990; Leslie 1990; Minkler and Estes 1991; Stevens 1992; Williams et al. 1994; Fee and Krieger 1994; Gill 1996; Muntaner et al. 1996).

At issue are both acts of omission and commission. These range from the virtual invisibility of lesbians and gay men in major public health databases (Stevens 1992; Council on Scientific Affairs 1996), to distortions of etiologic and therapeutic knowledge due to underrepresentation of people of color and women in epidemiologic studies, clinical trials, and even medical textbooks (Sechzer et al. 1994; Mendelsohn et al. 1994; King 1996; Ruiz and Verbrugge 1997), to the conduct of research premised on the view that innate differences underlie poorer health of subordinate groups, absent consideration of how subordination might affect health. Vividly illustrating detrimental effects of discrimination upon generation and application of scientific knowledge, to choose but one example, is the pernicious and longstanding legacy of "race" epidemiology; comparable accounts exist for eugenic constructions of class-based differences in health (Sydenstricker 1933; Kevles 1985), for sexist analyses of women's health (Hubbard 1990; Fee and Krieger 1994; Doyal 1995), and, to a lesser extent, for heterosexist research on lesbian and gay health (Stevens 1992; Erwin 1993; Council on Scientific Affairs 1996).

Historically, "race" first attained prominence in U.S. medical research in the early 1700s (Stanton 1960; Krieger 1987; Gamble 1989). Appearance of "race" as category relevant to health followed institutionalization of the "one drop rule" in various slave codes established in the mid-to-late 1600s (Stanton 1960; Davis 1991). This rule specified that if someone had only "one drop" of African "blood," she or he was deemed "black." Embedded in this alleged-ly biologic and innate definition of "race" was the notion of intrinsic "racial" superiority and inferiority. Based on this belief, leading scientists and physicians conducted studies to document—and occasionally fabricate (Jarvis 1844; Deutsch 1944)—racial/ethnic differences in every physical feature imaginable and then use these data both to explain observed racial/ethnic disparities in health and to prove the "black race" was innately inferior to the "white race" and "fit" only for slavery (Krieger 1987; Gamble 1989; Haller 1971; Cartwright 1850; Nott and Gliddon 1857).

During the mid-1800s, however, the first generation of U.S. black physicians—along with abolitionists—challenged the very category of "race." Arguing that people were more alike than different, they instead conducted studies showing diversity of health outcomes among free and enslaved blacks and similarity of health outcomes among blacks and poor whites (Krieger 1987; Smith 1859; Reyburn 1866). Based on these studies, they accordingly argued that slavery and economic duress—not innate constitution—were the principal reasons that black Americans had worse or different health than white Americans. This alternative viewpoint flourished briefly during and after the Civil War. After the destruction of Reconstruction, however, leading medical and scientific researchers again conducted studies and proffered explanations based on the premise that "race"—not racial subordination—was the root cause of racial inequalities in health (Krieger 1987; Gamble 1989; Haller 1971).

The next serious challenge to biologic definitions of "race" in biomedical literature emerged in the aftermath of World War II, in part in reaction to Nazi racial science, especially its fusion of eugenics and anti-Semitism to justify both "Aryan" supremacy and the Holocaust (Kevles 1985; Proctor 1988). In 1951, UNESCO released its first statement on race, rebutting its validity as a biologic category; subsequent revisions, amplifying this point, were issued in 1964, 1969, and, most recently, 1997 (Kupper 1975; Katz 1998). All editions emphasize that although distributions of specific genetic traits may vary across geographic regions, no ensemble of linked characteristics exists that delineates distinct "races." Empirical evidence supporting this view is now so well established that the dominant view among contemporary population geneticists, other biologists, anthropologists, and social scientists is that racial categories reflect social and ideological conventions, not meaningful natural distinctions (King 1981; Lewontin 1982; Jary and Jary 1995; Cavalli-Sforza et al. 1996; Williams 1997a; Katz 1998). Or, as stated in the 1997 revision of the UNESCO statement: "Pure races, in the sense of genetically homogenous populations, do not exist in the human species today, nor is there any evidence that they have ever existed in the past" (Katz 1998).

Yet, despite this scientific consensus, the 1995 third edition of the *Dictionary of Epidemiology* (sponsored by the International Epidemiological Association) continues to defines "race" as "persons who are relatively homogeneous with respect to biological inheritance" (Last 1995, p. 139). Worse, flouting contemporary scientific knowledge, it baldly asserts that "In a time of political correctness, classifying by race is done cautiously," as if only ideology, and not scientific evidence, were at issue. The net effect of such views has been an overemphasis in epidemiologic research on allegedly genetic explanations of racial/ethnic inequalities in health and a disregard for how racism, rather than "race," drives these disparities (Krieger and Bassett 1986; Cooper and David 1986; Jones et al. 1991; Krieger et al. 1993; Ahmad 1993; Williams et al. 1994; Williams and Collins 1995; Muntaner et al. 1996; Lillie-Blanton and LaVeist 1996; Williams 1997a; Freeman 1998; President's Cancer Panel 1998). Tellingly, whereas the keyword "race" identifies 33,921 articles indexed in Medline since 1966, only about 2,600 (7%) are additionally indexed by the keyword "socioeco-nomic" and only the 16 studies (0.0005%) listed in Table 3–5 have attempted to study self-reported experiences of racial discrimination in relation to health. Correcting this imbalance requires explicit attention to theories guiding research to explain population patterns of health, disease, and well-being.

INTIMATE CONNECTIONS: EPIDEMIOLOGY AND THE TRUTHS OF OUR BODY AND BODY POLITIC

In summary, epidemiologists can draw on a variety of study designs (Fig. 3–1) and concepts (Table 3–3) to develop and test epidemiologic hypotheses about health consequences of discrimination. Arguably the most fruitful approaches will systematically address discrimination in relation to *(1)* its varied aspects (type; form; agency; expression; domain; level); *(2)* cumulative exposure (timing; intensity; frequency; duration); *(3)* likely pathways of embodiment; *(4)* likely forms of responses and resistance and their health consequences; and *(5)* effects upon scientific knowledge.

Stated simply, the epidemiology of health consequences of discrimination is, at heart, the investigation of intimate connections between our social and biological existence. It is about how truths of our body and body politic engage and enmesh, thereby producing population patterns of health, disease, and well-being.

To research how discrimination harms health, we accordingly must draw on not only a nuanced understanding of the likely biological pathways of embodying discrimination, from conception to death, but also a finely tuned historical, social, and political sensibility, situating both the people we study and ourselves in the larger context of our times. Out of the epidemiologic commitment to reduce human suffering, we can extend our discipline's scope to elucidate how oppression, exploitation, and degradation of human dignity harm health—and, simultaneously, further knowledge and inspire action illuminating how social justice is the foundation of public health. Embodying equality should be our goal for all.

ACKNOWLEDGMENTS

Thanks to Lisa Berkman, David Williams, Sal Zierler, Karen Ruggiero, Sofia Gruskin, Hortensia Amaro, Donna Sullivan, and Gillian Steele for their helpful suggestions; to Hannah Cooper, Melissa Abraham, and Shannon Brome for locating references; and to the many study participants and researchers, including my mentors, Ruth Hubbard, Noel Weiss, and Len Syme, for the sharing of lives and work that inform this text.

REFERENCES

Ahluwalia, J.S., McNagny, S.E., and Rask, K.J. (1997). Correlates of controlled hypertension in indigent, inner-city hypertensive patients. *J Gen Intern Med*, 12:7–14.

Ahmad, W.I.U. (ed.). (1993). *"Race" and health in contemporary Britain*. Buckingham, UK: Open University Press.

Alker, H.R. Jr. (1969). A typology of ecological fallacies. In Doggan, M., and Rokkan, S. (eds.), *Social ecology*. Cambridge, MA: MIT Press, pp. 69–86.

Amaro, H., Russo, N.F., and Johnson, J. (1987). Family and work predictors of psychological well-being among Hispanic women professionals. *Psychol Women Q*, 11:505–21.

Amick, B.C. III, Levine, S., Tarlov, S., and Walsh, D.C. (eds.).(1995). *Society and health*. New York: Oxford University Press.

Anderson, N.B, Myers, H.F., Pickering, T., and Jackson, J.S. (1989). Hypertension in blacks: psychosocial and biological perspectives. *J Hypertens*, 7:161–72.

Arber, S. (1990). Revealing women's health: reanalysing the General Household Survey. In Roberts, H. (ed.), *Women's health counts*. London: Routledge, pp. 63–92.

Armstead, C.A., Lawler, K.A., Gorden, G., Cross, J., and Gibbons J. (1989). Relationship of racial stressors to blood pressure responses and anger expression in black college students. *Health Psychol*, 8:541–56.

Associated Press. (1991). Whites retain negative view of minorities, survey finds. *New York Times*, Jan. 10, 1991, p. A15.

Auslander, W.F., Thompson, S.J., Dreitzer, D., and Santiago, J.V. (1997). Mothers' satisfaction with medical care: perceptions of racism, family stress, and medical outcomes in children with diabetes. *Health Soc Work*, 22:190–9.

Ayers, I. (1991). Fair driving: gender and race discrimination in retail car negotiations. *Harvard Law Rev*, 104:817–72.

Bachman, R., and Saltzman, L.E. (1995). *Violence against women: estimates from the redesigned survey*. (NCJ-154348.) Washington, DC: U.S. Department of Justice.

Benokratis, N.V., and Feagin, J.R. (1986). *Modern sexism: blatant, subtle, and covert discrimination*. Englewood Cliffs, NJ: Prentice Hall.

Blalock, H.M. Jr. (1984). Contextual-effects models: theoretic and methodologic issues. *Annu Rev Sociol*, 10:353–72.

Bobo, L., and Gilliam, F.D. (1990). Race, sociopolitical participation and black empowerment. *Am Polit Sci Rev*, 84:377–93.

Bobo, L., Zubrinsky, C.L., Johnson, J.H. Jr., and Oliver, M.L. (1995). Work orientation, job discrimination, and ethnicity: a focus group perspective. *Res Soc Work*, 5:45–85.

Boyle, E. Jr. (1970). Biological patterns in hypertension by race, sex, body weight, and skin color. *JAMA*, 213:1637–43.

Boyle, E. Jr., Griffey, W.P. Jr., Nichaman, M.Z., and Talbert, C.F. Jr. (1967). An epidemiologic study of hypertension among racial groups of Charleston County, South Carolina. The Charleston Heart Study, Phase II. In Stamler, J., Stamler, R., and Pullman, T. (eds.), *The epidemiology of hypertension*. New York: Grune & Stratton, pp. 193–203.

Bradford, J., Ryan, C., and Rothblum, E.D. (1994). National lesbian health care survey: implications for mental health care. *J Consulting Clin Psychol*, 62:228-42.

Breilh, J. (1979). *Epidemiologia economia medicina y politica*. Mexico City: Distribuciones Fontamara.

Broman, C.L. (1996). The health consequences of discrimination: a study of African Americans. *Ethn Dis*, 6:148–52.

Brown, P. (1995). Race, class, and environmental health: a review and systematization of the literature. *Environ Res*, 69:15–30.

Brunner, E. (1997). Stress and the biology of inequality. *BMJ*, 314:1472–6.

Campbell, A., and Schuman, H. (1968). *Racial attitudes in fifteen American cities*. Ann Arbor: Survey Research Center, Institute for Social Research, University of Michigan.

Cartwright, S.A. (1850). The diseases and physical pecularities of the Negro race. *N Orleans Med Surg J*, 7:691–715.

Cavalli-Sforza, L.L., Menozzi, P., and Piazza, A. (1996). *The history and geography of human genes*. Princeton, NJ: Princeton University Press.

Churchill, J.E., Bild, D.E., Wallace, D., Kiefe, C.,

Lewis, C.E., and Roseman, J. (1996). Skin color, blood pressure and body mass in young adult blacks: the CARDIA study. Paper presented at the 11th International Interdisciplinary Conference on Hypertension in Blacks, New Orleans, LA, July 14–17, 1996.

Cochran, S.D., and Mays, V.M. (1994). Levels of depression in homosexually active African-American men and women. *Am J Psychol,* 151:524–9.

Cohen, S., Kessler, R.C., and Gordon, L.U. (eds.). (1995). *Measuring stress: a guide for health and social scientists.* New York: Oxford University Press.

Collins, P.H. (1990). *Black feminist thought: knowledge, consciousness, and the politics of empowerment.* London: HarperCollins Academic Press.

Cooper, R.S., and David, R. (1986). The biological concept of race and its application to public health and epidemiology. *J Health Polit Policy Law,* 11:97–116.

Cooper, R., Steinhauer, M., Schatzkin, A., and Miller, W. (1981). Improved mortality among U.S. blacks, 1968–1978: the role of antiracist struggle. *Int J Health Serv,* 11: 511–22.

Coresh, J., Klag, M.J., Whelton, P.K., and Kuller, L.H. (1991). Left ventricular hypertrophy and skin color among American blacks. *Am J Epidemiol,* 134:129–36.

Cosentino, C.E., and Collins, M. (1996). Sexual abuse of children: prevalence, effects, and treatment. *Ann N Y Acad Sci,* 789:45–65.

Council on Ethical and Judicial Affairs, American Medical Association. (1990). Black-white disparities in health care. *JAMA,* 263:2344–6.

Council on Ethical and Judicial Affairs, American Medical Association. (1991). Gender disparities in clinical decision making. *JAMA,* 266:559–62.

Council on Scientific Affairs, American Medical Association. (1996). Health care needs of gay men and lesbians in the United States. *JAMA,* 275:1354–9.

Crosby, F. (1984). The denial of personal discrimination. *Am Behav Scientist,* 27:371–86.

Curtin, P.D. (1992). The slavery hypothesis for hypertension among African Americans: the historical evidence. *Am J Public Health,* 82: 1681–6.

Davey Smith, G. (1996). Income inequality and mortality: why are they related? *BMJ,* 312: 987–8.

Davis F. (1991). *Who is black? One nation's definition.* University Park: Pennsylvania State University Press.

De Vos, P. (1997). Appendix I: introduction to South Africa's 1996 Bill of Rights. *Neth Q J Human Rights,* 15:225–52.

Deutsch, A. (1944). The first U.S. census of the insane (1840) and its use as pro-slavery propaganda. *Bull Hist Med,* 15:469–82.

Diez-Roux, A.V., Nieto, F.J., Muntaner, C., Tyroler, H.A., Comstock, G.W., Shahar, E., Cooper, L.S., Watson, R.L., and Szklo, M. (1997). Neighborhood environments and coronary heart disease: a multilevel analysis. *Am J Epidemiol,* 146:48–63.

DiPriete, T.A., and Forristal, J.D. (1994). Multilevel models: methods and substance. *Annu Rev Sociol,* 20:331–57.

Doyal, L. (1995). *What makes women sick? Gender and the political economy of health.* New Brunswick, NJ: Rutgers University Press.

Dressler, W.W. (1990). Lifestyle, stress, and blood pressure in a southern black community. *Psychosom Med,* 52:182–98.

Dressler, W.W. (1991a). Social class, skin color, and arterial blood pressure in two societies. *Ethn Dis,* 1:60–77.

Dressler, W.W. (1991b). *Stress and adaptation in the context of culture: depression in a southern black community.* Albany: State University of New York Press.

Dubois, W.E.B. (ed.). (1906). *The health and physique of the Negro American.* Atlanta, GA: Atlanta University Press.

Duncan, O.D., and Duncan, B. (1955). A methodological analysis of segregation indexes. *Am Sociol Rev,* 20:210–7.

Erwin, K. (1993). Interpreting the evidence: competing paradigms and the emergence of lesbian and gay suicide as a "social fact." *Int J Health Serv,* 23:437–53.

Essed, P. (1992). *Understanding everyday racism: an interdisciplinary theory.* London: Sage.

Essed, P. (1996). *Diversity: gender, color, and culture.* Amherst: University of Massachusetts Press.

Evans, R.G., Barer, M.L., and Marmor, T.R. (eds.). (1994). *Why are some people healthy and others not? The determinants of health of populations.* New York: Aldine de Gruyter.

Fanon, F. (1965). *The wretched of the earth* (tr. Farrington, C.). New York: Grove Press.

Feagin, J.R. (1989). *Racial and ethnic relations* (3rd ed.). Englewood Cliffs, NJ: Prentice Hall.

Feagin, J.R., and Sikes, M.P. (1994). *Living with racism: the black middle class experience.* Boston: Beacon Press.

Fee, E. (1987). *Disease and discovery: a history of the Johns Hopkins School of Hygiene and*

Public Health, 1916–1936. Baltimore, MD: Johns Hopkins University Press.

Fee, E., and Krieger, N. (eds.). (1994). *Women's health, politics, and power: essays on sex/gender, medicine, and public health*. Amityville, NY: Baywood Publications.

Fix, M., and Struyk, R. (eds.). (1993). *Clear and convincing evidence: measurement of discrimination in America*. Washington, DC: Urban Institute Press.

Freeman, H.P. (1998). The meaning of race in science—considerations for cancer research: concerns of special populations in the National Cancer Program. *Cancer*, 82:219–25.

Gamble, V.N. (ed.). (1989). *Germs have no color lines: blacks and American medicine, 1900–1940*. New York: Garland.

Gardner, C.B. (1995). *Passing by: gender and public harassment*. Berkeley: University of California Press.

Garty, M., Stull, R., Kopin, I.J., and Goldstein, D.S. (1989). Skin color, aging, and plasma L-dopa levels. *J Auton Nerv Syst*, 26:261–3.

Geiger, H.J. (1996). Race and health care—an American dilemma? *N Engl J Med*, 335:815–6.

Gill, C.J. (1996). Cultivating common ground: women with disabilities. In Moss, K.L. (ed.), *Man-made medicine: women's health, public policy, and reform*. Durham, NC: Duke University Press, pp. 183–93.

Gleiberman, L., Harburg, E., Frone, M.R., Russel, M., and Cooper, M.L. (1995). Skin color, measures of socioeconomic status, and blood pressure among blacks in Erie County, NY. *Ann Hum Biol*, 22:69–73.

Gornick, M.E., Eggers, P.W., Reilly, T.W., Mentnech, R.M., Filterman, L.K., Kucken, L.E., and Vladek, B.C. (1996). Effects of race and income on mortality and use of services among Medicare beneficiaries. *N Engl J Med*, 335:791–9.

Green, N.L. (1995). Development of a perceptions of racism scale. *Image J Nurs Sch*, 27:141–6.

Greenwald, A.G., and Banaji, M.R. (1995). Implicit social cognition: attitudes, self-esteem, and stereotypes. *Psychological Rev*, 102:4–27.

Greenwald, A.G., McGhee, D.E., and Schwartz, J.K.L. (1998). Measuring individual differences in implicit cognition: the implicit association test. *J Personality Social Psychol*, 74:1464–80.

Haan, M., Kaplan, G.A., and Camacho, T. (1987). Poverty and health: prospective evidence from the Alameda County Study. *Am J Epidemiol*, 125:989–98.

Haller, J.S. Jr. (1971). *Outcasts from evolution:*

scientific attitudes of racial inferiority, 1859–1900. Urbana: University of Illinois Press.

Haraway, D. (1989). *Primate visions: gender, race, and nature in the world of modern science*. New York: Routledge.

Harburg, E., Erfrut, J.C., Hauenstein, L.S., Chape, C., Schull, W.J., and Schork, M.A. (1973). Socio-ecological stress, suppressed hostility, skin color, and black–white male blood pressure: Detroit. *Psychosom Med*, 35:276–95.

Harburg, E., Gleibermann, L., Roeper, P., Schork, M.A., and Schull, W. (1978). Skin color, ethnicity and blood pressure. I: Detroit blacks. *Am J Public Health*, 68:1177–83.

Herek, G.M. (1993). Documenting prejudice against lesbians and gay men on campus: the Yale Sexual Orientation Survey. *J Homosex*, 25:15–30.

Herrnstein, R.J., and Murray, C. (1994). *The bell curve: intelligence and class structure in American life*. New York: Free Press.

Hubbard, R. (1990). *The politics of women's biology*. New Brunswick, NJ: Rutgers University Press.

Indian Health Services. (1997). *Trends in Indian health—1996*. Rockville, MD: U.S. Department of Health and Human Services.

Institute of Medicine (U.S.), Committee to Study the Prevention of Low Birthweight. (1985). *Preventing low birthweight*. Washington, DC: National Academy Press.

Jackman, M.R. (1994). *The velvet glove: paternalism and conflict in gender, class, and race relations*. Berkeley: University of California Press.

Jackson, J.S., Brown, T.N., Williams, D.R., Torres, M., Sellers, S.L., and Brown, K. (1996). Racism and the physical and mental health status of African Americans: a thirteen year national panel study. *Ethn Dis*, 6:132–47.

James, S.A., LaCroix, A.Z., Kleinbaum, D.G., and Strogatz, D.S. (1984). John Henryism and blood pressure differences among black men. II. The role of occupational stressors. *J Behav Med*, 7:259–75.

Jargowsky, P.A. (1996). Take the money and run: economic segregation in U.S. metropolitan areas. *Am Sociol Rev*, 61:984–98.

Jarvis, E. (1844). Insanity among the coloured population of the free states. *Am J Med Sci*, 7:71–83.

Jary, D., and Jary, J. (eds.). (1995). *Collins dictionary of sociology* (2nd ed.). Glasgow, UK: HarperCollins.

Jaynes, G.D., and Williams, R.M. Jr. (eds.). (1989). *A common destiny: blacks and American society*. Washington, DC: National Academy Press.

Jones, C.P., LaVeist, T.A., and Lillie-Blanton, M. (1991). "Race" in the epidemiologic literature: an examination of the *American Journal of Epidemiology*, 1921–1990. *Am J Epidemiol*, 134:1079–84.

Jones, D.R., Harrell, J.P., Morris-Prather, C.E., Thomas, J., and Omowale, N. (1996). Affective and physiological responses to racism: the roles of afrocentrism and mode of presentation. *Ethn Dis*, 6:109–22.

Jones, J.H. (1981). *Bad blood: the Tuskegee syphilis experiment*. New York: Free Press.

Katz, S. (1998). The biological anthropology of race. In *Report of the President's Cancer Panel. The meaning of race in science—considerations for cancer research*. (April 9, 1997). Bethesda, MD: National Institutes of Health, National Cancer Institute, pp. A32–A35.

Kaufman, J.S., Cooper, R.S., and McGee, D.L. (1997). Socioeconomic status and health in blacks and whites: the problem of residual confounding and the resiliency of race. *Epidemiology*, 8:621–28.

Keil, J.E., Tyroler, H.A., Sandifer, S.H., and Boyle, E. Jr. (1977). Hypertension: effects of social class and racial admixture: the results of a cohort study of the black population of Charleston, South Carolina. *Am J Public Health*, 67:634–9.

Keil, J.E., Sandifer, S.H., Loadholt, C.B., and Boyle, E. Jr. (1981). Skin color and education effects on blood pressure. *Am J Public Health*, 71:532–4.

Keil, J.E., Sutherland, S.E., Knapp, R.G., Tyroler, H.A., and Pollitzer, W.S. (1992). Skin color and mortality. *Am J Epidemiol*, 136:1295–302.

Keith, V.M., and Herring, C. (1991). Skin tone and stratification in the black community. *Am J Sociol*, 97:760–78.

Kennedy, B.P., Kawachi, I., Lochner, K., Jones, C., and Prothrow-Stith, D. (1997). (Dis)respect and black mortality. *Ethn Dis*, 7:207–14.

Kerner Commission (US). (1968). *Report of the National Advisory Commission on Civil Disorders*. New York: Bantam Books.

Kevles, D.J. (1985). *In the name of eugenics: genetics and the uses of human heredity*. New York: Knopf.

Khaw, K.T. (1993). Sodium and potassium: blood pressure and stroke. In Poulter, N., Sever, P., and Thom, S. (eds.), *Cardiovascular disease: risk factors and intervention*. Oxford: Radcliffe Medical Press, pp. 145–51.

Kinder, D., and Mendelberg, C. (1995). Cracks in American apartheid: the political impact of prejudice among desegregated whites. *J Politics*, 57:402–24.

King, G. (1996). Institutional racism and the medical/health complex: a conceptual analysis. *Ethn Dis*, 6:30–46.

King, J.D. (1981). *The biology of race*. Berkeley: University of California Press.

Klag, M.J., Whelton, P.K., Coresh, J., Grim, C.E., and Kuller, L.H. (1991). The association of skin color with blood pressure in U.S. blacks with low socioeconomic status. *JAMA*, 265:599–602.

Klonoff, E.A., and Landrine, H. (1995). The schedule of sexist events: a measure of lifetime and recent sexist discrimination in women's lives. *Psychol Women Q*, 19:439–72.

Knapp, R.G., Keil, J.E., Sutherland, S.E., Rust, P.F., Hames, C., and Tyroler, H.A. (1995). Skin color and cancer mortality among black men in the Charleston Heart Study. *Clin Genet*, 47:200–6.

Krieger, N. (1987). Shades of difference: theoretical underpinnings of the medical controversy on black–white differences, 1830–1870. *Int J Health Serv*, 7:258–79.

Krieger, N. (1990). Racial and gender discrimination: risk factors for high blood pressure? *Soc Sci Med*, 30:1273–81.

Krieger, N. (1992). The making of public health data: paradigms, politics, and policy. *J Public Health Policy*, 13:412–27.

Krieger, N. (1994). Epidemiology and the web of causation: has anyone seen the spider? *Soc Sci Med*, 39:887–903.

Krieger, N. (1998). Racial discrimination and health: an epidemiologist's perspective. In *Report of the President's Cancer Panel. The meaning of race in science—considerations for cancer research*. (April 9, 1997). Bethesda, MD: National Institutes of Health, National Cancer Institute, pp. A32–A35.

Krieger, N., and Bassett, M. (1986). The health of black folk: disease, class, and ideology in science. *Monthly Rev*, 38:74–85.

Krieger, N, and Sidney, S. (1996). Racial discrimination and blood pressure: the CARDIA study of young black and white adults. *Am J Public Health*, 86:1370–78.

Krieger, N., and Sidney, S. (1997). Prevalence and health implications of anti-gay discrimination: a study of black and white women and men in the CARDIA cohort. *Int J Health Serv*, 27:157–76.

Krieger, N., and Zierler, S. (1995). Accounting for health of women. *Curr Issues Public Health*, 1:251–56.

Krieger, N., Rowley, D., Hermann, A.A., Avery, B., and Phillips, M.T. (1993). Racism, sexism, and social class: implications for studies of health, disease, and well-being. *Am J Prev Med*, 9 Suppl 6:82–122.

Krieger, N., Williams, D.R., and Moss, N.E. (1997). Measuring social class in U.S. public health research: concepts, methodologies, and guidelines. *Annu Rev Public Health*, 18:341–78.

Krieger, N., Sidney, S., and Coakley, E. (1998). Racial discrimination and skin color in the CARDIA study: implications for public health research. *Am J Public Health*, 88:1308–13.

Krieger, N., Chen, J.T., and Selby, J.V. (1999). Comparing individual-based and household-based measures of social class to assess class inequalities in women's health: a methodological study of 684 US women. *J Epidemiol Community Health*, 53:612–23.

Kuh, D., and Ben-Shlomo, Y. (eds.). (1997). *A lifecourse approach to chronic disease epidemiology: tracing the origins of ill-health from early to adult life*. Oxford: Oxford University Press.

Kupper, L. (ed.). (1975). *Race, science, and society*. Paris: UNESCO Press.

Ladrine, H., and Klonoff, E.A. (1996). The schedule of racist events: a measure of racial discrimination and study of its negative physical and mental health consequences. *J Black Psychol*, 22:144–68.

Ladrine, H., Klonoff, E.A., Gibbs, J., Manning, V., and Lund, M. (1995). Physical and psychiatric correlates of gender discrimination: an application of the schedule of sexist events. *Psychol Women Q*, 19:473–92.

Lalonde, R.N., and Cameron, J.E. (1994). Behavioral responses to discrimination: a focus on action. In Zanna, M.P., and Olson, J.M. (eds.), *The psychology of prejudice: the Ontario Symposium*, vol. 7. Hillsdale, NJ: Lawrence Erlbaum, pp. 257–88.

Langbein, L.I., and Lichtman, A.J. (1978). *Ecological inference*. Sage University series on quantitative applications in the social sciences. Beverly Hills, CA: Sage.

Lanphear, B.P., Weitzman, M., and Eberly, S. (1996). Racial differences in urban children's environmental exposures to lead. *Am J Public Health*, 86:1460–63.

Last, J.M. (ed.). (1995). *A dictionary of epidemiology* (3rd ed.). New York: Oxford University Press.

LaVeist, T.A. (1992). The political empowerment and health status of African-Americans: mapping a new territory. *Am J Sociol*, 97:1080–95.

LaVeist, T.A. (1993). Segregation, poverty, and empowerment: health consequences for African Americans. *Milbank Q*, 71:41–64.

Leslie, C. (1990). Scientific racism: reflections on peer review, science, and ideology. *Soc Sci Med*, 32:891–905.

Lewontin, R. (1982). *Human diversity*. New York: Scientific American Books.

Li, L., and Moore, D. (1998). Acceptance of disability and its barriers. *J Soc Psychol*, 138:13–25.

Liberatos, P., Link, B.G., and Kelsey, J.L. (1988). The measurement of social class in epidemiology. *Epidemiol Rev*, 10:87–121.

Lillie-Blanton, M., and LaVeist, T. (1996). Race/ethnicity, the social environment, and health. *Soc Sci Med*, 43:83–92.

Lillie-Blanton, M., Parsons, P.E., Galye, H., and Dievler, A. (1996). Racial differences in health: not just black and white, but shades of gray. *Annu Rev Public Health*, 17:441–8.

Lorde, A. (1980). Age, race, class, and sex: women redefining difference. In Rothenberg, P.S. (ed.), *Racism and sexism: an integrated study* (1988). New York: St. Martin's Press, pp. 352–59 (opening quote, p. 358).

Malaty, H.M., and Graham, D.Y. (1994). Importance of childhood socioeconomic status on the current prevalence of *Helicobacter pylori* infection. *Gut*, 35:742–5.

Marshall, G. (ed.). (1994). *The concise Oxford dictionary of sociology*. Oxford: Oxford University Press.

Mays, V.M. (1995). Black women, women, stress, and perceived discrimination: the focused support group model as an intervention for stress reduction. *Cult Divers Ment Health*, 1:53–65.

Mays, V.M., and Cochran, S.D. (1997). Racial discrimination and health outcomes in African Americans. Paper presented at the National Center for Health Statistics 1997 Joint Meeting of the Public Health Conference on Records and Statistics and the Data Users Conference, Washington, DC, July 28–31, 1997.

McKinlay, J.G. (1996). Some contributions from the social system to gender inequalities in heart disease. *J Health Soc Behav*, 37:1–26.

McNeilly, M.D., Anderson, N.B., Armstead, C.A., Clark, R., Corbett, M., Robinson, E.L., Pieper, C.F., and Lepisto, E.M. (1996). The perceived racism scale: a multidimensional assessment of the experience of white racism among African Americans. *Ethn Dis*, 6:154–66.

Mendelsohn, K.D., Nieman, L.Z., Isaacs, K., Lee, S., and Levison, S.P. (1994). Sex and gender bias in anatomy and physical diagnosis text illustrations. *JAMA*, 272:1267–70.

Meyer, I.H. (1995). Minority stress and mental health in gay men. *J Health Soc Behav*, 36:38–56.

Minkler, M., and Estes, C.L. (eds.). (1991). *Critical perspectives on aging: the political and moral economy of growing old.* Amityville, NY: Baywood.

Moore, D.J., Williams, J.D., and Qualls, W.J. (1996). Target marketing of tobacco and alcohol-related products to ethnic minority groups in the United States. *Ethn Dis,* 6: 83–98.

Muntaner, C., Nieto, F.J., and O'Campo, P. (1996). The bell curve: on race, social class, and epidemiological research. *Am J Epidemiol,* 144:531–6.

Murrell, N.L. (1996). Stress, self-esteem, and racism: relationships with low birth weight and preterm delivery in African American women. *J Natl Black Nurses Assoc,* 8:45–53.

National Center for Health Statistics. (1997). *Health, United States, 1996–97, and injury chartbook.* Hyattsville, MD: National Center for Health Statistics.

Navarro, V. (1986). *Crisis, health, and medicine: a social critique.* New York: Tavistock.

Navarro, V. (1990). Race or class versus race and class: mortality differentials in the United States. *Lancet,* 336:1238–1240.

Neighbors, H.W., Jackson, J.S., Broman, C., and Thompson, E. (1996). Racism and the mental health of African Americans: the role of self and system blame. *Ethn Dis,* 6:167–75.

Nelson, D.A., Kleerekoper, M., and Parfitt, A.M. (1988). Bone mass, skin color, and body size among black and white women. *Bone Miner,* 4:257–64.

Nelson, D.A., Kleerekoper, M., Peterson, E., and Parfitt, A.M. (1993). Skin color and body size as risk factors for osteoporosis. *Osteoporos Int,* 3:18–23.

Northridge, M.E., and Shepard, P.M. (1997). Environmental racism and public health. *Am J Public Health,* 87:730–2.

Nott, J.C., and Gliddon, G. (eds.). (1857). *Indigenous races of the Earth; or new chapters of ethnological enquiry.* Philadelphia: Lippincott.

Oliver, M.L., and Shapiro, T.M. (1995). *Black wealth/white wealth.* New York: Routledge.

Oxford English Dictionary. (1971). *The compact Oxford English dictionary.* New York: Oxford University Press.

Parker, H., Botha, J.L., and Haslam, C. (1995). "Racism" as a variable in health research—can it be measured? (abstract). *J Epidemiol Community Health,* 48:522.

Peterson, E.D., Shaw, K.L., DeLong, E.R., Pryro, D.B., Califf, R.M., and Mark, D.B. (1997). Racial variations in the use of coronary-revascularization procedures: are the differences real? do they matter? *N Engl J Med,* 336:480–6.

Pierce, C.M. (1995). Stress analogs of racism and sexism: terrorism, torture, and disaster. In Willie, C.V., Rieker, P.P., Kramer, B.M., and Brown, B.S. (eds.), *Mental health, racism, and sexism.* Pittsburgh, PA: University of Pittsburgh Press, pp. 277–93.

Polednak, A.P. (1997). *Segregation, poverty, and mortality in urban African Americans.* New York: Oxford University Press.

President's Cancer Panel. (1998). *Report of the President's Cancer Panel. The meaning of race in science—considerations for cancer research.* (April 9, 1997). Bethesda, MD: National Institutes of Health, National Cancer Institute.

Proctor, R. (1988). *Racial hygiene: medicine under the Nazis.* Cambridge, MA: Harvard University Press.

Reyburn, R. (1866). Remarks concerning some of the diseases prevailing among the freed-people in the District of Columbia (Bureau of Refugees, Freedman, and Abandoned Lands). *Am J Med Sci,* n.s. 51:364–9.

Robinson, J.C. (1987). Trends in racial inequality and exposure to work-related hazards, 1968–1986. *Milbank Q,* 65 Suppl 2: 404–20.

Robinson, W.S. (1950). Ecological correlations and the behavior of individuals. *Am Sociol Rev,* 15:351–7.

Rose, H., and Rose, S. (eds.). (1979). *Ideology of/in the natural sciences.* Cambridge, MA: Schenkman.

Rosenberg, C.D., and Golden, J. (eds.). (1992). *Framing disease: studies in cultural history.* New Brunswick, NJ: Rutgers University Press.

Ross, C.E., and Mirowsky, J. (1989). Explaining the social patterns of depression: control and problem solving—or support and talking? *J Health Soc Behav,* 30:206–19.

Rothenberg, P.S. (1988). *Racism and sexism: an integrated study.* New York: St. Martin's Press.

Rowley, D.L., Hogue, C.J.R., Blackmore, C.A., Ferre, C.D., Hatfield-Timajchy, K., Branch, P., and Atrash, H.K. (1993). Preterm delivery among African-American women: a research strategy. *Am J Prev Med,* 9 Suppl 6:1–6.

Ruggerio, K.M., and Taylor, D.M. (1995). Coping with discrimination: how disadvantaged group members perceive the discrimination that confronts them. *J Personal Soc Psychol,* 68:826–38.

Ruggiero, K.M., Mitchell, J.P., and Krieger, N. (forthcoming) Now you see it, now you don't: explicit versus implicit measures of the personal/group discrimination discrepancy. *Psychological Science*

Ruiz, M.T., and Verbrugge, L.M. (1997). A two

way view of gender bias in medicine. *J Epidemiol Community Health*, 51:106–9.

Salgado de Snyder, V.N. (1987). Factors associated with acculturative stress and depressive symptomatology among married Mexican immigrant women. *Psychol Women Q*, 11:475–88.

Schoendorf, K.C., Hogue, C.J., Kleinman, J.C., and Rowley, D. (1992). Mortality among infants of black as compared with white college-educated parents. *N Engl J Medicine*, 326:1522–6.

Schuman, H., Steehm, C., and Bobo, L. (1985). *Racial attitudes in America: trends and interpretations*. Cambridge, MA: Harvard University Press.

Schwam, B.L., Kalenak, J.W., Meyers, S.J., and Kansupada, K.B. (1995). Association between skin color and intraocular pressure in African Americans. *J Clin Epidemiol*, 38:491–6.

Sechzer, J.A., Rabinowitz, V.C., Denmark, F.L., McGinn, M.F., Weeks, B.M., and Wilkens, C.L. (1994). Sex and gender bias in animal research and in clinical studies of cancer, cardiovascular disease, and depression. *Ann N Y Acad Sci*, 736:21–48.

Sennett, R., and Cobb, J. (1972). *The hidden injuries of class*. New York: Knopf.

Sigelman, L., and Welch, S. (1991). *Black Americans' views of racial inequality: the dream deferred*. Cambridge, UK: Cambridge University Press.

Smith, J.M. (1859). On the fourteenth query of Thomas Jefferson's notes on Virginia. *Anglo-African Magazine*, 1:225–38.

Sorel, J.E., Heiss, G., Tyroler, H.A., Davis, W.B., Wing, S.B., and Ragland, D.R. (1991). Black–white differences in blood pressure among participants in NHANES II: the contribution of blood lead. *Epidemiology*, 2:348–52.

Stanton, W. (1960). *The leopard's spots: scientific attitudes towards race in America, 1815–1859*. Chicago: University of Chicago Press.

Stevens, P.E. (1992). Lesbian health care research: a review of the literature from 1970 to 1990. *Health Care Women Int*, 13:91–120.

Sydenstricker, E. (1933). *Health and environment*. New York: McGraw Hill.

Taylor, D.M., Wright, S.C., Moghaddam, F.M., and Lalonde, R.N. (1990). The personal/group discrepancy: perceiving my group, but not myself, to be a target of discrimination. *Pers Soc Psychol Bull*, 16:254–62.

Taylor, D.M., Wright, S.C., and Porter, L.E. (1994). Dimensions of perceived discrimination: the personal/group discrimination discrepancy. In Zanna, M.P., and Olson, J.M. (eds.), *The psychology of prejudice: the Ontario Symposium*, vol. 7. Hillsdale, NJ: Lawrence Erlbaum, pp. 233–55.

Telles, E.E., and Murguia, E. (1990). Phenotypic discrimination and income differences among Mexican Americans. *Soc Sci Q*, 71:682–96.

Thernstrom, S., and Thernstrom, A. (1997). *American in black and white: one nation, indivisible*. New York: Simon & Schuster.

Thorton, R. (1987). *American Indian Holocaust and survival: a population history since 1492*. Norman: University of Oklahoma Press.

Tibbitts, C. (1937). The socio-economic background of Negro health status. *J Negro Educ*, 6:413–28.

Tomasevski, K. (1993). *Women and human rights*. London: Zed Books.

Townsend, P., Davidson, N., and Whitehead, M. (1990). *Inequalities in health: the Black Report and the health divide*. London: Penguin.

Troutt, D.D. (1993). *The thin red line: how the poor still pay more*. Oakland, CA: Consumers Union.

Turner, M.A. (1993). Limits on neighborhood choice: evidence of racial and ethnic steering in urban housing markets. In Fix, M., and Struyk, R. (eds.), *Clear and convincing evidence: measurement of discrimination in America*. Washington, DC: Urban Institute Press, pp. 118–147.

Turner, M.A., Fix, M., and Struyk, R.J. (1991). *Opportunities denied, opportunities diminished: racial discrimination in hiring*. (Urban Institute Report No. 91–9.) Washington, DC: Urban Institute Press.

U.S. Census Bureau. (1994). *Household wealth and asset ownership, 1991*. (Current Population Reports, Series P70, No. 34.) Washington, DC: U.S. Government Printing Office.

U.S. Department of Health and Human Services. (1991). *Health status of minorities and low-income groups* (3rd ed.). Washington, DC: U.S. Government Printing Office.

U.S. Equal Employment and Opportunity Commission. (1992). *Facts about religious discrimination*. Washington, DC: U.S. Government Printing Office.

United Nations Development Programme (UNDP). (1996). *Human development report 1996*. New York: Oxford University Press.

United Nations General Assembly. (1948). *Universal declaration of human rights*. Resolution 217A (III). Adopted and proclaimed December 10, 1948.

Vaid, U. (1995). *Virtual equality: the main-*

streaming of gay and lesbian liberation. New York: Anchor Books.

Wallace, R., and Wallace, D. (1997). Community marginalisation and the diffusion of disease and disorder in the United States. *BMJ,* 314:1341–5.

Waters, M.C., and Eschbach, K. (1995). Immigration and ethnic and racial inequality in the United States. *Annu Rev Sociol,* 21:419–46.

White, M.J. (1986). Segregation and diversity measures of population distributions. *Popul Index,* 52:198–221.

Wilkinson, R.G. (1996). *Unhealthy societies: from inequality to well-being.* London: Routledge.

Williams, D.R. (1997a). Race and health: basic questions, emerging directions. *Ann Epidemiol,* 7:322–33.

Williams, D.R., Yu, Y., Jackson, J., and Anderson, N. (1997b). Racial differences in physical and mental health: socioeconomic status, stress, and discrimination. *J Health Psychol,* 2:335–51.

Williams, D.R., and Chung, A-M. (in press). Racism and health. In Gibston, R.C., and Jackson, J.S. (eds.), *Health in black America.* Thousand Oaks, CA: Sage.

Williams, D.R., and Collins, C. (1995). U.S. socioeconomic and racial differences in health: patterns and explanations. *Annu Rev Sociol,* 21:349–86.

Williams, D.R., Lavizzo-Mourey, R., and Warren, R.C. (1994). The concept of race and health status in America. *Public Health Rep,* 109:26–41.

Wilson, T.W., and Grim, C.E. (1991). Biohistory of slavery and blood pressure differences in blacks today: a hypothesis. *Hypertension,* 17 Suppl 1:I122–8.

Women's Bureau, U.S. Department of Labor (1994). *Working women count: a report to the nation.* Washington, DC: U.S. Government Printing Office.

4

Income Inequality and Health

ICHIRO KAWACHI

The world's wealth is becoming concentrated in fewer hands. According to the 1996 Human Development Report (United Nations Development Program—UNDP) (1996), the world's 358 richest individuals controlled assets equivalent to the combined annual incomes of countries where 45 percent of the world's people live. Of the $23 trillion global gross domestic product (GDP) in 1993, $18 trillion accrued to the industrialized countries and only $5 trillion to the developing countries, home to 80% of the world's people. The poorest 20% of the world's population saw their share of global income decline from 2.3% to 1.4% in the past 30 years. Meanwhile the share of the richest 20% increased from 70% to 85%. That doubled the ratio of the shares of the richest to the poorest, from 30:1 to 61:1 (UNDP 1996). Polarization of assets has worsened within individual countries as well.

The United States is one of the richest countries in the world, yet it is also one of the most unequal in terms of how that wealth is shared (Atkinson et al. 1995). In 1967, the first year the U.S. Census Bureau began collecting data on the incomes of households, the poorest 20% of households shared just 4% of the aggregate income earned by all households. By contrast, the highest 20% of households accounted for 43.8% of aggregate income. Thirty years later, in 1996, the share of the bottom 20% of households had shrunk to 3.7%, while the share of the top 20% of households increased to 49.0%. The mean household income in the bottom 20% was $8596 (1996 dollars), compared to $115,514 in the top 20% (U.S. Census Bureau 1997). Between 1991 and 1995, the median annual pay of the chief executive officers of America's 100 largest companies was $2.8 million (plus an additional $8.4 million in stock options), which amounted to 112 times the median earnings of full-time wage and salary workers in the rest of America ($24,908) (Hacker 1997). Inequalities in the distribution of wealth (defined as the total value of one's assets minus debts or liabilities) are even more severe: The best-off 1% of the American population owns between 40% and 50% of the nation's wealth (Wolff 1995; Hacker 1997). In contrast, at the bottom of the economic hierarchy, the poverty rate (13.7% in 1996) has remained virtually unchanged during the last 30 years, and currently some 36.5 million Americans are officially poor (U.S. Census Bureau 1997).

What are the public health consequences, if any, of these trends in the polarization of incomes? Do widening inequalities matter if everyone's standard of living is rising? A variety of emerging evidence suggests that the size of the gap between the rich and poor—as distinct from the absolute standard of living enjoyed by the poor—matters in its own right for population health.

LINKING INCOME INEQUALITY TO HEALTH: THEORY AND EVIDENCE

There is a well-established relationship between income and health (see Chapter 2). As we descend down the hierarchy of income, rates of ill health increase, and the resulting gradient in health status extends well into the middle-class range of incomes (Adler et al. 1994; Pappas et al. 1993; Macintyre 1996). Although the following discussion will focus on mortality and life expectancy, the income gradient itself has been replicated using virtually every measure of health outcome, including morbidity, disability, and perceived health status (Dutton and Levine 1989). One of the universally observed characteristics of the income/life expectancy (or income/mortality) curve is that its slope declines with increasing income, i.e., there are diminishing returns to rising income. In other words, the income/life expectancy curve is steep in the regions of absolute income deprivation; but it levels off beyond a certain standard of living. This characteristic nonlinear relationship appears to hold not only for data within a single country but also for data across different countries (Kawachi et al. 1994; Wilkinson 1996). Thus, the relationship between income and life expectancy is steeply linear up to a level of about $5000 Gross National Product per capita (GNPpc). Be-

yond this point (that is to say, among developed countries), further increments to GNP make little difference to life expectancy, and the curve appears to plateau (Wilkinson 1996).

An important consequence of the shape of the income/life expectancy curve is that the *distribution* of income must influence the average life expectancy of a society. The tendency for greater dispersion of income to be associated with lower mean life expectancy can be illustrated by considering a hypothetical society with mean income x (Fig. 4–1). In this society, income is steeply related to life expectancy on the left-hand side of x, but the curve levels off toward the right. If the income dispersion is between x_1 and x_4, mean life expectancy would be y_1 (assuming equal numbers of people on either side of mean income). Now if income dispersion in this society is reduced via a policy that takes the amount x_4 minus x_3 from the rich and transfers that amount to raise the incomes of the less well-off from x_1 to x_2, then, other things being equal, mean life expectancy in this society would rise to y_2. In other words, redistributing income to the poor will raise life expectancy even if the average level of income remains the same. This prediction is a consequence of the downwardly concave relation between income and life expectancy; i.e., the rise in life expectancy among the poor as a result of the redistribution more than offsets any loss in life expectancy among the affluent (Rodgers 1979). Following the same line of reasoning, we might expect that two countries with the same average income but different income distributions would experience different levels of health, with the country with the more equitable income distribution exhibiting higher life expectancy. In fact, a number of cross-country studies have reported such a relationship.

Income Inequality and Health: Cross-Country Evidence

Rodgers (1979) examined cross-sectional data from 56 rich and poor countries to test the relationship between income distribu-

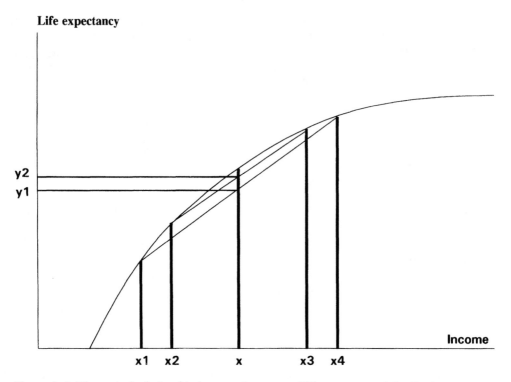

Figure 4–1. Theoretical relationship between income and life expectancy (after Rodgers, 1979).

tion and three measures of health—life expectancy at birth, life expectancy at age five, and infant mortality. Both per capita GNP and income distribution (measured by the Gini coefficient—see below for explanation) were highly correlated with life expectancy at birth, with r^2 exceeding 0.75. The correlations were less strong for life expectancy at age five and infant mortality; nonetheless, income distribution remained a significant predictor. Rodgers (1979) estimated that the difference between a relatively egalitarian and relatively inegalitarian country amounted to about 5 to 10 years in average life expectancy.

The cross-national evidence on the health effects of income inequality gained renewed prominence through the work of Richard Wilkinson (1986, 1992). In a cross-sectional examination of 11 countries belonging to the Organisation for Economic Cooperation and Development (OECD), Wilkinson found a strong inverse correlation ($r =$

-0.81, $P < 0.0001$) between income inequality—as measured by Gini coefficients of post-tax income standardized for differences in household size—and life expectancy (1986). Similarly, a close correlation ($r = 0.86, P < 0.001$) was found between the life expectancy of nine OECD countries and the proportion of income accruing to the least well-off 70% of the population (1992). The proportion of income earned by the least well off 70%, combined with GNP per capita, explained about three quarters of the variation in life expectancy between these countries. By itself, GNP per capita could explain less than 10% of the variance in life expectancy (Wilkinson 1992).

Flegg (1982) examined predictors of infant mortality rates in 46 developing countries. A regression model that included just GDP per capita and the Gini coefficient explained 55% of the variance in infant mortality across countries. Both variables were highly statistically significant predictors.

Further addition to the models of maternal illiteracy rates and the number of nurses and physicians per 1000 persons only modestly increased (by 15%) the amount of variance explained. Flegg then estimated the policy implications of income redistribution. A 1% reduction in the coefficient of variation of incomes (i.e., a measure of the extent to which incomes diverge from their mean) was estimated to decrease the infant mortality rate by 0.471% (95% confidence interval, CI: 0.169% to 0.773%). In absolute terms, if the coefficient of variation for a hypothetical country were to be reduced from 1.2 (the geometric mean for the 46 countries studied) to 0.7 (a figure characteristic of relatively egalitarian countries at that time, such as Bangladesh, Pakistan, and Taiwan), infant mortality rates would be predicted to decline by 20 deaths per 1000 live births. Conversely, an increase in the coefficient of variation from 1.2 to 1.9 (a figure that characterized highly unequal countries, such as Ecuador, Gabon, and Kenya) would raise the infant mortality rate by 25 deaths per 1000 live births.

LeGrand (1987) examined the relationship between average age-at-death for 17 developed countries and GDP per capita, per capita expenditure on medical care, and the proportion of national income earned by the least well-off 20% of the population. Age-at-death was found to be most closely correlated with income distribution ($P <$ 0.01), but not to GDP or medical expenditure per capita.

Waldman (1992) analyzed data from 70 rich and poor countries and found that infant mortality is positively related to the income share of the rich (the top 5% of the income distribution) when the incomes of the poor (the bottom 20%) are equalized among countries. Also working on infant mortality in 18 industrialized countries between 1950 and 1985, Wennemo (1993) found a close association between it and the extent of relative poverty in society.

In summary, then, a number of cross-national studies have suggested an association between income inequality and population longevity. One of the limitations of the above-cited studies, however, is that data from different countries—especially on income distribution—may not be comparable in terms of their quality or reliability (McIsaac and Wilkinson 1997). This problem has led investigators to turn to the study of within-country variations in income distribution.

Income Inequality and Health: Within-Country Evidence

For some time, criminologists have accepted that there is a relationship between income inequality and rates of crime within society. For example, Merva and Fowles (1993) examined the relationship between wage inequality and crime rates in 30 metropolitan areas within the United States. Using multivariate techniques, the authors reported that a 5% increase in wage inequality (measured by the Gini coefficient) between successive business cycle peaks in 1977 and 1988 was associated with the following increases in criminal activity: violent crime up 2.05%, murder/non-negligent man-slaughter by 4.21%, robbery by 1.79%, aggravated assault 3.10%, larceny/theft 1.95%, and motor vehicle theft 2.21%. Hsieh and Pugh (1993) conducted a meta-analysis of the 34 aggregate data studies that had been published up to 1993 on poverty, income inequality, and rates of violent crime. Despite differences in methodology, the vast majority of studies agreed that violent crime is related to poverty ($r =$ 0.44) as well as to income inequality ($r =$ 0.44). Interestingly, poverty was more consistently positively related to violent crime in studies utilizing smaller units of geographical aggregation (e.g., cities). The opposite was true for income inequality, which yielded more consistent effects sizes in studies using data aggregated to the state or national level.

Income inequality within a country was linked to broader health outcomes for the first time in two American studies published simultaneously in 1996. Kaplan et al. (1996) and Kennedy et al. (1996) indepen-

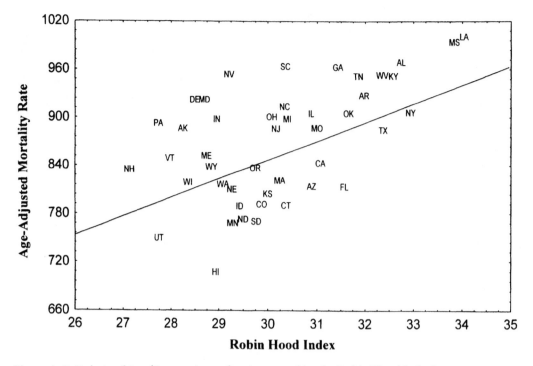

Figure 4–2. Relationship of income inequality (measured by the Robin Hood Index) to age-adjusted total mortality rates in the 50 U.S. states (from Kennedy et al. 1996).

dently examined the relationship between the degree of household income inequality across the 50 U.S. states and state-level variation in all-cause and cause-specific mortality. Kaplan et al. (1996) used as their measure of income distribution the share of total income earned by the bottom 50% of households in each state: If incomes were perfectly equally shared, the bottom half of households should account for exactly half of the aggregate income. In reality, the U.S. states ranged from a minimum of 17.5% (Louisiana, the most unequal) to a high of 23.6% (New Hampshire, the most egalitarian). A strong correlation ($r = -0.62$, $P < 0.001$) was found between this measure of inequality and age-standardized mortality rates; it was present in both men and women and in whites as well as African Americans. Kennedy et al. (1996) in turn examined two measures of income distribution: the Gini coefficient and the Robin Hood Index. The Gini index is perhaps the most widely used measure of income distri-

bution; it theoretically ranges from 0.0 (perfect equality) to 1.0 (perfect inequality). The Robin Hood Index can be interpreted as the proportion of aggregate income that must be redistributed from rich to poor households in order to attain perfect equality of incomes.[1] Both measures were strongly correlated with age-adjusted total and cause-specific mortality rates. In regression models adjusting for poverty rates and median income, a 1% increase in the Robin Hood Index (an increase in inequality) was associated with an excess mortality of 21.7 deaths per 100,000 (95% CI: 6.6 to 36.7), which suggests that even a modest reduction in inequality could have an important impact on public health. Income inequality was associated with not only higher rates of total mortality (Fig. 4–2) but also with higher rates of death from coronary heart disease, malignant neoplasms, homicide, and infant mortality. Income inequality and poverty together could account for about one quarter of the state variations in total

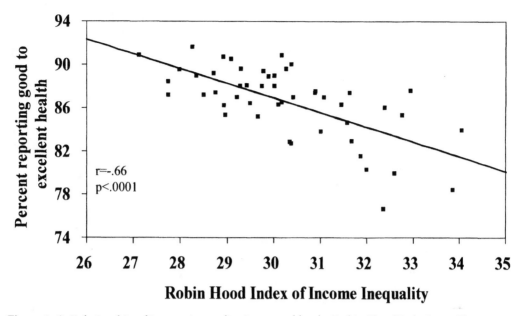

Figure 4–3. Relationship of income inequality (measured by the Robin Hood Index) to self-rated health in the 50 U.S. states (from Kawachi et al. 1997b).

mortality, as well as just over half of the variation in homicide rates. The findings persisted after controlling for urban/rural mix as well as health behaviors such as rates of cigarette smoking. Finally, the Robin Hood Index has been linked to cross-sectional state variations in self-reported health, as assessed in the Behavioral Risk Factor Surveillance System, a representative survey of over 205,000 Americans. In response to the question "How would you rate your overall health?" the proportion of residents in each state who answered "Excellent" or "Very Good" (as opposed to "Fair" or "Poor") was strongly inversely correlated ($r = -0.66$) with the Robin Hood Index (Kawachi et al. 1997b) (Fig. 4–3).

In England, Ben-Shlomo et al. (1996) examined the relationship between the extent of material and social deprivation (as measured by the Townsend Index) in 369 local authorities (geographic areas administered by local government), and their average mortality rates. Mortality was strongly positively associated with levels of deprivation.

The average trend in death rates was 26 per 100,000 per quartile of deprivation ($P < 0.001$). Mortality was also positively associated with the degree of socioeconomic variability in the area units that made up the local authorities. The more variable the extent of deprivation within an area (as indicated by the interquartile range of Townsend scores), the higher was the death rate, with an average trend of seven per 100,000 ($P < 0.001$) across quartiles of variation.

More recently, Lynch et al. (1998) have extended their finding of a relationship between income inequality and mortality down to the level of metropolitan areas within the United States. Income inequality measures were calculated for 282 U.S. greater metropolitan areas, ranging in population size from 56,735 for Enid, Oklahoma, to 18,087,251 for New York. In weighted linear regressions, metropolitan areas with high income inequality and low per capita income had excess mortality of 149.8 deaths per 100,000 compared to areas with low inequality and high per capita income. This mortality difference was estimated to be equivalent to eliminating all deaths from heart disease.

In summary, within-country studies support the findings of cross-national studies in demonstrating a link between income distribution and health. But the robustness of the evidence has been questioned by some (Judge 1995; Saunders 1996), and we turn now to the critique of income distribution studies.

CRITIQUE OF STUDIES LINKING INCOME DISTRIBUTION TO HEALTH

Four lines of criticism attack the empirical evidence linking income distribution to health (Judge 1995; Saunders 1996): *(1)* Different studies used different indicators to measure income inequality, and the choice often appears to have been arbitrarily made; *(2)* the household income data used to derive the income distribution measures were not adjusted for taxes and transfer payments; *(3)* the household income data were not adjusted for household size and composition; and *(4)* studies have not taken adequate account of sources of confounding. Each of these is discussed in turn.

Does the Choice of Indicator Matter?

With regard to the selection of income inequality indicator, researchers have had a wide pool to choose from. Some studies have used the Gini coefficient (Wilkinson 1986), while others have used the share of aggregate income earned by the bottom 50% (Kaplan et al. 1996) and 70% (Wilkinson 1992) of households; still others have used the Robin Hood Index (Kennedy et al. 1996) or the ratio of the income shares of the 90th percentile of households to the shares of the 10th percentile (Lynch et al. 1998). Repeated corroboration of the same hypothesis using different indicators of income distribution provides some reassurance about the robust nature of the association. The apparent lack of theoretical justification for the use of different indicators, however, has prompted some critics to suggest that the choice was "data driven"

(Judge 1995). In particular, "It is important that any . . . attempt to investigate the income inequality hypothesis should specify *a priori* what measures of income distribution might be expected to be associated with life expectancy and why" (Judge 1995, p. 1284).

To be sure, there is an established tradition in economics concerning the theory and measurement of income inequality (Sen 1973; Cowell 1977; Atkinson 1983). The choice of indicator matters in social policy because the various indicators may give rise to different conclusions depending on the type of redistributive policies. For example, the Gini coefficient is much less sensitive to an income transfer from a better-off household to a less well-off household if the two households lie near the middle of the income distribution than at either tail (Cowell 1977). The Robin Hood Index is insensitive to income transfers from a well-off household to a less well-off household if both lie on the same side of the mean income (Sen 1973; Cowell 1977). Virtually none of the conventionally used indicators incorporates societal values about equity, which is unfortunate given that judgments about inequality are undeniably normative. The Atkinson Index is alone among measures in incorporating explicit normative judgments about the social aversion to inequality (Atkinson 1970).

In response to the valid criticisms of Judge (1995) and Saunders (1996), Kawachi and Kennedy (1997a) reanalyzed the U.S. data on income inequality and mortality using a comprehensive range of indicators including the Gini coefficient, the decile ratio (ratio of the share of the 90th percentile to that of the 10th), the shares of the bottom 50%, 60%, and 70% of households, the Robin Hood Index, Theil's entropy measure, and the Atkinson Index, under two alternative assumptions of inequality aversion.[2] Despite differences in their theoretical meaning and method of derivation, all measures were in fact highly correlated with each other. The lowest pairwise correlation was between the decile ratio and the Theil index ($r = 0.86$); most other measures were correlated between 0.95 to 0.99. In turn, each indicator was about equally strongly correlated with age-adjusted mortality rates. Of note, the strongest correlation with mortality was found for the Atkinson Index ($r = 0.66$), which is the only indicator to assign an explicit weight to the societal aversion for inequality. In conclusion, there was little evidence to suggest that a choice of any particular indicator would have unduly influenced the conclusion reached about the relationship between income inequality and longevity.

Adjustment of Household Incomes for Taxes, Transfer Payments, and Household Size

A further criticism of studies on the income inequality hypothesis relates to their failure to adjust household incomes for taxes and transfer payments. To the extent that taxes and transfer payments redistribute incomes, failure to adjust for them will overstate the extent of income inequality between households (Judge 1996). Adjusting for taxes and transfer payments is especially important in cross-national comparisons, since countries vary a great deal in their redistributive policies. However, in the context of within-country studies (such as a comparison of states across America), evidence suggests that the major part of income inequality arises as a result of disparities in *pretax* incomes and that taxes and transfers have a relatively modest impact on income distribution (Krugman 1994). Moreover, if the unit of analysis is the state, the same federal income taxes apply to all households.

A second, related, criticism of existing studies is that they failed to adjust household incomes for differences in household size and composition. In a small ($N = 9$) cross-national study, Judge (1995) was able to demonstrate a correlation between average life expectancy and the Gini coefficient unadjusted for family size ($r = -0.77$). However, when the income data were adjusted for household size, the correlation disappeared ($r = -0.19$).

While it is a truism that two households with the same annual income of $13,000 will have very different needs depending on their size (two adults vs. a single parent) and composition (no children vs. several), in practice there is no universally agreed upon method to adjust for such differences (Atkinson et al. 1995). For example, some studies have used household income *per member* to adjust total incomes according to the number of persons in the household. But this approach ignores economies of scale in household consumption relating to size and other differences in needs among household members (e.g., the costs of running a TV, refrigerator, lighting, and heating are about the same whether there are one or two persons in the house). Economists have used equivalence scales to adjust household incomes for size and composition, where economic well-being (W) (or "adjusted income") is related to disposable income (D) and household size (S) in the following manner:

$$W = D/S^E$$

where E is the equivalence elasticity, which varies between 0.0 and 1.0. The value $E = 0.0$ corresponds to no adjustment for household size, while for $E > 0$, economies of scale are assumed, which reduce as E is increased, giving more generous "equivalents" for additional family members (Buhmann et al. 1988).

Whether adjusting for household size would alter the income inequality/mortality relationship was tested by Kawachi and Kennedy (1997a) using household microdata provided by the Luxembourg Income Study (Timothy Smeeding, project director: personal communication). Household incomes in the 50 U.S. states were equivalized with the elasticity set to 0.5, which provides a useful contrast between per capita income ($E = 1.0$) and no adjustment for household size ($E = 0.0$). In the same analysis, disposable (as opposed to gross) household income was used, which meant adjusting for federal and state income and payroll taxes,

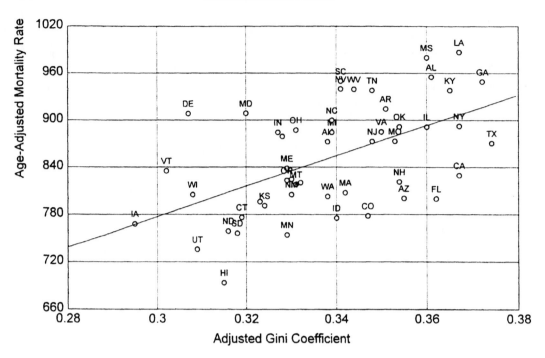

Figure 4–4. Relationship of income inequality (adjusted for taxes, transfer payments, and household size) and age-adjusted mortality rates in the 50 U.S. states (from Kawachi and Kennedy 1997a).

as well as cash or near-cash benefits, including food stamps, the Earned Income Tax Credit, and school lunches. The results of simultaneously adjusting for taxes, transfer payments, and household size demonstrated that the relationship between income inequality and mortality rates was virtually unchanged ($r = 0.54$ using the adjusted Gini coefficient, compared to $r = 0.51$ using the unadjusted Gini) (Kawachi and Kennedy 1997a) (Fig. 4–4). In summary, the income inequality/mortality link cannot be explained away by failure to use disposable income or to adjust for differences in household size.

Confounding

Much work remains to be carried out in identifying and taking account of the potential confounding factors that underlie the income inequality/mortality relationship. Skeptics are likely to remain unconvinced until all reasonable alternative explanations have been eliminated. A crucial task in this

process is sorting out confounding factors from mediating variables, i.e., factors that lie in the pathway between income inequality and adverse health outcomes. For example, is poverty a confounding or mediating variable? What about race, unemployment, educational attainment, or access to health care?

To give one example, state-level income inequality is strongly correlated with the level of poverty ($r = 0.73$). In other words, states may exhibit greater inequality in the distribution of incomes *because* a greater number of impoverished households tend to be concentrated in these areas. (This is referred to as the "compositional" effect of income inequality.) However, if income inequality is simply a reflection of the extent of underlying poverty, there would be no need to study income distribution as a predictor of health. Social policy would accordingly need to focus more on alleviating poverty rather than addressing the entire income gradient.

A recent study by Fiscella and Franks (1997) made exactly this suggestion. Based on prospective follow-up data from a nationally representative cohort of 14,407 Americans aged 25–74 (the First National Health and Nutrition Examination Survey, NHANES I), the authors examined the relationship between income inequality and mortality in two ways: firstly, at the ecologic level, and secondly, taking into account individual household income. Income inequality was calculated from the share of total income earned by the bottom 50% of residents in 105 areas (primary sampling units) of the United States.[3] In the ecologic analysis, income inequality was statistically significantly related to mortality rates ($r = -0.34$, $P < 0.004$). But when adjustment was made for individual household income in multivariate proportional hazards models, the relative risk (RR) of mortality was no longer statistically significant for income inequality (RR = 0.81, 95% CI: 0.22 to 2.92), while remaining significant for individual household income (in thousands of dollars) (RR = 0.97, 95% CI: 0.96 to 0.98). The authors concluded that "the effect of income inequality reported in ecological studies may result from confounding by income at the individual level" (Fiscella and Franks 1997, p. 1725).

One negative study is rarely sufficient to reject a hypothesis. Meanwhile, the Fiscella and Franks (1997) study raises several questions. For example, income distribution in this study was estimated just once at baseline, in 1971–1975, before the major trends in income inequality commenced. Most observers date the beginning of the spiral of income disparity in America to the mid-1970s (Krugman 1994). The income distribution estimates of the Fiscella and Franks study may have correspondingly suffered from significant misclassification during the 20-year follow-up period. The study may have also lacked sufficient power to detect an effect of income inequality, as evidenced by the width of the confidence interval of the point estimate, as well as the evident lack of variability in their income distribution mea-

sure (mean = 28% for total sample, S.D. = 3%). No information was provided on the actual numbers of deaths occurring in the cohort sample.

Following the study by Fiscella and Franks (1997), other studies have appeared utilizing similar multilevel approaches, i.e., examining the effects of income distribution on individual health outcomes while simultaneously adjusting for individual household income. The results of these studies appear to overturn the conclusions of the earlier study. Kennedy et al. (1998) carried out a multilevel analysis examining the effects of income inequality on individual self-rated health, adjusting for household income as well as a range of other individual-level characteristics. The study was based on the Behavioral Risk Factor Surveillance System (BRFSS) surveys, which is a state-representative telephone survey of U.S. residents. The total sample size of the study was 205,245 individuals living in the 50 states. In 1993, the BRFSS began asking a question about self-rated health: "Would you say that in general your health is: Excellent, Very Good, Good, Fair, or Poor?" A review of 27 community studies concluded that even such a simple global assessment appears to have high predictive validity for subsequent risk of mortality, even after taking account of other medical, behavioral, or psychosocial risk factors (Idler and Benyamini 1997). Controlling for individual household income, educational attainment, cigarette smoking, overweight, and access to health care, an individual residing in the states with the highest levels of income inequality was 1.25 times (95% CI: 1.17 to 1.33) as likely to report being in only fair or poor health compared to an individual living in the most equal states. Although low household income was more strongly linked with poor self-rated health (for example, individuals from households earning < $10,000 annually were 3.4 times more likely to report fair/poor health compared to those earning >$35,000), the effect of income inequality was statistically significant, and independent of absolute income. An interaction was found between level of household income and income inequality: The deleterious effects of income inequality were most marked for individuals from households earning less than $20,000 per year. This study and other forthcoming reports using different datasets (Soobader and LeClere 1999; Lochner 1999) suggest that there is in fact an environmental effect (sometimes referred to as a "contextual" effect) of income inequality on individual health status.

In summary, the effect of income inequality on health does not appear to be entirely explained by a *compositional* effect (i.e., a greater concentration of poor people who have higher risk of mortality dwelling in areas of high income inequality). There is some evidence to support a *contextual* effect of income inequality on individual health. (For an excellent discussion of the two types of effects, see Chapter 14.) Success at excluding confounders will ultimately rest on the ability of researchers to refine the theories about the mechanisms by which income inequality affects health—to which we now turn.

MECHANISMS LINKING INCOME INEQUALITY TO MORTALITY: TOWARD A THEORY OF INCOME DISTRIBUTION AND HEALTH

At least three distinct pathways have been proposed through which income inequality may affect health: *(1)* Income inequality leads to underinvestment in human capital (Kaplan et al. 1996); *(2)* income disparities disrupt the social fabric and lead to disinvestment in "social capital" (Kawachi et al. 1997a; Kawachi and Kennedy 1997b); *(3)* disparities in income result in poor health through direct psychological pathways, e.g., frustration engendered by invidious social comparisons (Kawachi et al. 1994; Wilkinson 1996).

Kaplan and colleagues (1996) reported striking correlations between the degree of income inequality and indicators of human capital investment (Table 4–1). States with

high income inequality (as measured by the proportion of total household income received by the less well of 50%) spent a smaller proportion of the state budget on education and showed poorer educational outcomes, ranging from worse reading and math proficiency to higher high school dropout rates. One reason why high income disparity translates into lower social spending is that in societies with rising inequalities, the interests of the rich begin to diverge from those of the typical family. As Paul Krugman put it: "A family at the 95th percentile pays a lot more in taxes than a family at the 50th, but it does not receive a correspondingly higher benefit from public services, such as education. The greater the income gap, the greater the disparity in interests. This translates, because of the clout of the elite, into a constant pressure for lower taxes and reduced public services" (Krugman 1996, p. 48). Reduced social spending, in turn, translates into truncated life opportunities and thence to poorer population health.

A second pathway through which income inequality may affect health is via the disruption of the social fabric (Kawachi and Kennedy 1997b). Wilkinson (1996) offers several case studies of societies that at certain points in history underwent either a rapid compression of the income distribution (e.g., Britain during the two world wars) or a rapid widening of income differentials (e.g., the Italian-American community of Roseto in Pennsylvania during the 1960s). In wartime Britain, narrowing of income differentials was accompanied by a greater sense of solidarity and social cohesion as well as dramatic improvements in life expectancy. For over 25 years, the rural town of Roseto has served as a population laboratory for researchers like Stewart Wolf and colleagues (Wolf and Bruhn 1992). The town originally came to the attention of medical researchers because the people who lived there had half the death rate from heart attack of people in neighboring towns despite similar profiles of risk factors such as smoking, obesity, and fat intake. Wolf

Table 4–1. Correlations between state-level income inequality (proportion of total household income received by less well of 50% of households) and indicators of human capital investment, adjusted for median income: United States, 1989–1991

Human capital indicator	Correlation coefficient (r)	P value
No high school (%)	−0.71	0.001
High school dropout (%)	−0.50	0.001
Reading proficiency (4th grade)	0.58	0.001
Math proficiency (4th grade)	0.64	0.001
Education spending/total spending	0.32	0.02
Library books per capita	0.42	0.002

Source: From Kaplan et al. 1996, p. 1001. Reproduced with permission.

and colleagues eventually came to the conclusion that the protective factor was the close-knit social relationships among inhabitants in the town. Beginning in the mid-1960s, however, the town experienced rapid economic growth, which opened a gap between rich people and poor people. The resulting breakdown of community solidarity was followed by a sharp increase in deaths from coronary disease such that Roseto "caught up" with neighboring towns. Most recently, my colleagues and I (Kawachi et al. 1997a) have tested the association between income inequality and social cohesion at the ecological level. Using indicators of "social capital" developed by political scientists (Putnam 1993, 1995), we demonstrated that citizens living in states characterized by high income disparities tend to be more mistrustful of each other ($r = 0.71$) and to belong to fewer civic associations ($r = −0.41$). In turn, both indicators of social capital were strongly correlated with rates of age-adjusted mortality ($r = 0.79$ for social mistrust, and $r = −0.49$ for membership of civic associations; $P < 0.05$ for both). Collectively, these examples lend support to the notion that income inequality erodes social cohesion and that public health is threatened when the social glue becomes unstuck. (These studies, together with a more detailed exegesis of the notion of social capital, can be found in Chapter 8 of this book).

Yet a third pathway by which income inequality might produce ill health is through psychologically mediated effects of relative deprivation (Kawachi et al. 1994; Wilkinson 1996). According to the theory of relative deprivation, so long as there is stability and predictability in material conditions, people are apt to feel that they are in the same boat. However, when there is rapid improvement in conditions, those of some improve more rapidly than those of others. Those for whom conditions are not improving very rapidly see others, perhaps no more deserving, doing much better than they are. The perceived widening of the gap leads to frustration, with potential health consequences. This theory gained credibility from empirical findings of earlier studies on the U.S. military (Stouffer et al. 1949; Merton and Rossi 1950): Morale was higher among officers in the military police, where promotion was very slow, than among officers in the Air Force, where promotion was very rapid. Researchers attributed this difference to frustration engendered by social comparisons in the Air Force.

Epidemiological studies that directly connect frustrated expectations to health outcomes are still relatively sparse. The anthropologist William Dressler has conducted a series of anthropological and epidemiological investigations addressing the association between status inconsistency and health outcomes (elevated blood pressure) (Dressler 1996, 1998; Dressler et al. in press). Using a technique in anthropology called *cultural consensus analysis* which involves interviewing key informants,

Dressler has established that many communities have a single, shared cultural model of what is the acceptable standard of living in such communities (1996). For example, the acceptable standard of living in a rural U.S. black community is defined by a set of lifestyle items such as ownership of a house and car, access to media via TV and newspapers, and socially specific items such as holding a position of leadership within the local church. According to Dressler, individuals strive to adopt material styles of life that are considered customary for their community. Moreover, the "customary" standard of living turns out not to be one characterized by "conspicuous consumption" but one more defined by what Veblen termed a "community defined standard of decency" (Veblen 1899). Dressler has coined the term "cultural consonance in lifestyle" to refer to the degree to which individuals succeed in achieving the cultural model of lifestyle. To the extent that individuals strive and fail to meet the cultural ideal, adverse health consequences follow. In studies conducted in Brazil (in press) and the United States (1996), Dressler has demonstrated that the extent of departure from cultural consonance is the strongest predictor of systolic blood pressure (SBP), even after adjusting for other established risk factors for elevated blood pressure including age, sex, skin color, body mass index, occupation, education, and income.[4]

Of course, the adverse consequences of relative deprivation need not be confined to the psychological realm. As society becomes more prosperous, material needs increase not just because people *think* they need more when their neighbors have more, but also for *very practical reasons.* Christopher Jencks elaborates on this theme:

In 1900, for example, America was organized on the assumption that city residents would get around on foot or by streetcar. Outside the cities, Americans traveled by foot or horse. In such a world an automobile was clearly a luxury. Over the course of the twentieth century, however, most Americans acquired cars. This had two effects. First, public transportation atrophied. Second, most employers and shops moved to areas that were accessible only by car, and most families did the same. Outside a few major cities, therefore, not having a car meant not being able to get to work, to shops, or to friends' homes, making a car a necessity for most Americans.

Many other consumer goods have followed the same trajectory, starting as luxuries but gradually becoming necessities. Telephones were a luxury in 1900, when hardly anyone had one. Today, when almost everyone has a telephone, those without service are cut off from family and friends. . . . Indeed, those without telephones often have trouble even keeping a job, both because employers now expect workers to call in if they are sick and because workers without telephones cannot make hasty changes in their childcare or transportation arrangements. (Jencks 1992, p. 7)

AN AGENDA FOR RESEARCH

Much work remains to be carried out beyond elucidating the mechanisms that potentially link societal income distribution to health. In this section, we begin to outline an agenda for further research. In other words, what do we need to know in order to begin to apply knowledge of the effects of income inequality on health in order to achieve practical policy and intervention goals?

At What Level of Geographic Aggregation Does Income Inequality Affect Health?

Much of the work to date has been carried out at the level of very large geographic aggregates—either whole countries (Wilkinson 1986, 1992) or states within countries (Kaplan et al. 1996; Kennedy et al. 1996). An important question that needs to be addressed when we use more refined data is: At what level of geographic aggregation does income inequality affect health? Answering this question calls for the simultaneous collection of data at multiple levels— at the state level, county level, census tract level, neighborhood level, and individual level. Pinpointing the level of aggregation at which income distribution affects health outcomes will provide important clues about the etiological mechanisms involved and clarify the options for policy interventions. For example, if income inequality acts on health via reductions in social spending, then we might expect to detect health effects only at politically meaningful units of aggregation, such as states or entire nations. Alternatively, if income inequality harms health through effects at the neighborhood level (e.g., via reduction in social cohesion), then one would expect to detect links to health at smaller units of aggregation. Recent work has begun to address these issues. For example, Soobader and LeClere (1999) found that while income inequality affects the health of individuals at the county level, it did not seem to have an effect at the census tract level. At the level of census tracts, individual socioeconomic status (measured by poverty status and absolute income) appeared to be the dominant predictor of health status. Thus, income inequality appears to have different effects on health, depending on the unit of geographical aggregation. One possible explanation for this finding is that processes of social comparison (which partly account for the harmful effects of relative deprivation) occur across areas that are larger than neighborhoods. In other words, residents of impoverished neighborhoods may feel deprived not in comparison with their immediate neighbors (who are likely to be equally poor) but in relation to members of society at large (Wilkinson 1997). Unfortunately, very little is known about the reference groups people use in making social comparisons, i.e., whether they primarily compare themselves to their immediate neighbors, the rest of the country, or something in between.

Time Series Analysis

Little is also understood about time trends in income inequality in relation to population health status. Kaplan and colleagues (1996) reported that state-level income inequality in 1980 was strongly predictive of percent change in age-adjusted mortality rates between 1980 and 1990 ($r = 0.62$, $P < 0.0001$). Although mortality rates de-

clined in all states over the decade, states that were more unequal in income distribution experienced smaller declines in mortality. Income inequality appeared thus to introduce a drag effect on secular declines in mortality rates. However, Kaplan et al. (1996) found no relationship between 1980–1990 *changes* in income distribution and 1980–1990 trends in mortality ($r = 0.12$, $P > 0.05$). These findings have yet to be tested in more extended time series analyses. Additionally, work remains to be carried out on the effects of trends in inequality on the health of different population subgroups (for example, declining *average* mortality might obscure stagnant or even rising mortality rates among vulnerable subgroups); similarly little is known about the differential timing of the effects of inequality on specific causes of death. (For example, do the lag times and induction periods vary for different causes of mortality?)

Gender and Race Effects

Researchers need to understand more about the ways in which vertical hierarchy (along a dimension like income) expresses itself through inequalities along horizontal, or ascriptive, dimensions like race and gender. It is a truism that the severity of income deprivation varies by race and gender. African Americans are overrepresented among households in poverty. Poverty has also become feminized with the rise in single female-headed households (Danziger and Gottschalk 1995). Preliminary work has begun to map out the effects of income maldistribution on the health of African Americans and women. Kennedy and colleagues (1997) examined the relationship between income inequality and racial prejudice in the United States. States that tolerate high income inequalities also turn out to have high levels of racial prejudice, as revealed in public opinion polls. The General Social Survey, a nationally representative survey of American adults conducted by the National Opinions Research Center, asked citizens in 39 states to respond to the question: "On the average blacks have worse

Table 4–2. Indicators of women's status at the state level and their correlations with female mortality rates and activity limitations

Indicators of women's status	Mortality rates	Mean days of activity limitations
Women in elected office	−0.38*	−0.34*
Women who voted in 1992/1994 (%)	−0.54*	−0.49*
Median earnings for full-time women	0.02	−0.23
Earnings ratio between women and men	−0.30*	−0.31*
Women in labor force (%)	−0.55*	−0.55*
Percent businesses owned by women	−0.31*	−0.21

*$P < 0.05$.

Source: From Kawachi et al., 1999.

jobs, income, and housing than white people. Do you think the differences are: (a) Mainly due to discrimination? (yes/no); (b) Because most black have less in-born ability to learn? (yes/no); (c) Because most blacks don't have the chance for education that it takes to rise out of poverty? (yes/no); and (d) Because most blacks just don't have the motivation or will power to pull themselves up out of poverty? (yes/no)." The proportion of the population who believed that blacks have less in-born ability was correlated −0.44 with the Robin Hood Index. In turn, the extent of racial prejudice was strongly correlated with black mortality rates ($r = 0.56$).

The status of women also tends to be the least advanced in areas with the widest income disparities. Kawachi et al. (1999) examined the relationships between income inequality and various composite indices of women's status developed by the Institute for Women's Policy Research (1996). Indices of women's status—including women's political participation and women's economic autonomy—were negatively correlated with the Gini coefficient of income inequality ($r = −0.49$ and −0.36, respectively; $P < 0.05$). Indicators of women's status were, in turn, correlated with female age-adjusted mortality rates as well as mean days of activity limitations (Table 4–2). These studies suggest ways in which the concepts of racism and sexism, which have been hitherto examined at the individual level (Krieger et al. 1993), can be fruitfully extended to the ecological level. It makes sense to attempt to measure racism and sexism as collective properties of society and to begin to document their effects on population health.

Inequality of What?

Last but not least, any discussion of inequality begs the question: inequality of *what*? Although the present chapter has focused on income inequality, the distribution of wealth in society is even more polarized and may in fact turn out to be a more potent predictor of health at certain stages of the lifecourse, such as after retirement. More importantly, the process of social stratification takes place along a vast array of dimensions, including (but not limited to) political power (household authority, workplace control, legislative authority), cultural assets (privileged lifestyles, high-status consumption practices), social assets (access to social networks, ties, associations), honorific status (prestige, respect, "good reputation"), and human resources (skills, expertise, training) (Grusky 1994). A major objective of social epidemiology is to elucidate the patterning of health through differential access to the diverse forms of capital—not just economic capital but also social, human, political, cultural, and symbolic capital.

To give an example of how concepts discussed in the present chapter might be translated into other domains of social stratification, consider the unequal distribution of autonomy and control in workplaces. The maldistribution of control, expressed in the degree of hierarchy in the workplace, has been postulated to influence the health status of workers independent of the absolute level of job stress (Kawachi et al. 1994). (For a detailed discussion of the evidence linking job autonomy to health outcomes, see Chapter 5). If perceptions of autonomy and control are *relative*, then a more democratic workplace—consisting of shared authority and decision making—might be more conducive to worker health. Karasek and Theorell advocate exactly such a strategy in their vision of how to go about creating healthy workplaces:

The inequitable distribution of creative opportunities and decision-making opportunities can be resolved by alternative decision structures within existing institutions, by changing responsibilities between occupational groups. The jobs of the professional and manager do not need job enrichment, job enlargement, or additional social interaction. . . . [T]he appropriate health intervention might be to diminish their demands by reducing their decision latitude . . . rather than increasing them. This strategy would offload some of the ever-increasing decision responsibilities and qualification requirements of those at the top of public and private bureaucracies to lower-level occupations such as our bureaucratized and commercial service workers, and even the technicians and administrators. Such a policy could diminish the enormous disparities in decision-making opportunity between blue-collar and professional workers from both ends of the occupational spectrum, reducing overload decision demands at the top of the hierarchy and increasing decision opportunities and skill discretion at the bottom end. The result might be a health-promoting double-attack on psychosocial health risk at work. (Karasek and Theorell 1990, pp. 293–294)

CONCLUSION

As various commentators have remarked (Pearce 1996; Macintyre and Ellaway, Chapter 14), the emerging focus of social epidemiology on variables like income inequality marks a renaissance of interest in the broadest societal determinants of health. Following decades of comparative neglect, epidemiologists seem willing to bring back a consideration of social forces into their causal models. Although far from well understood, growing evidence points to the size of the economic gap as an important predictor of health, independent of the absolute standard of living. Consideration of income inequality forces researchers to ask, "Why are some societies healthier than others?" in contrast to the more traditional epidemiological concerns about understanding why some individuals get sick while others stay healthy. In doing so, social epidemiology rises to the challenge posed by the late Geoffrey Rose (1992): Uncover the foundations of good health instead of only identifying the causes of individual illness.

NOTES

1. An important distinction should be drawn between "equal" vs. "equitable" distribution of incomes. Virtually all measures of income distributions express the degree of inequality against a hypothetical state of perfect equality in the distribution of income.
2. For a detailed description of the derivation and meaning of each measure, see Kawachi and Kennedy (1997a).
3. The paper did not provide details as to how the income distribution measure was calculated. Based on a personal communication with the authors, it appears they were estimated directly from the survey respondents (ranging from 48 to 323 individuals in the 105 areas), rather than from Census-derived information.
4. An interesting side note: Cultural consonance appears to be strongly related to SBP but not to the diastolic blood pressure (DBP). For example, in a study in Brazil (1996), the actual spread of SBP across 3 S.D. of cultural consonance was as much as 16 mmHg among middle-aged subjects. The differential effect of cultural consonance on SBP and DBP begin to suggest a biological mechanism by which cultural consonance "gets under the skin." Blood pressure can be elevated by either increased cardiac output (mediated by beta-adrenergic mechanisms) or by increased total peripheral resistance (mediated by alpha-adrenergic mechanisms). Since DBP is considered to reflect the influence of total peripheral resistance, the effect of cultural consonance on SBP may reflect effects on increased cardiac output (Dressler 1996).

REFERENCES

Adler, N.E., Boyce, T., Chesney, M.A., Cohen, S., Follman, S., Kahn, R.L., and Syme, S.L. (1994). Socioeconomic status and health: the challenge of the gradient. *Am Psychol,* 49:15–24.

Atkinson, A.B. (1970). On the measurement of inequality. *J Econ Theory,* 2:244–63.

Atkinson, A.B. (1983). *The economics of inequality* (2nd ed.). Oxford: Oxford University Press.

Atkinson, A.B., Rainwater, L., and Smeeding, T.M. (1995). *Income distribution in OECD countries: evidence from the Luxembourg Income Study.* Paris: Organisation for Economic Co-operation and Development.

Ben-Shlomo, Y., White, I.R., and Marmot. M. (1996). Does the variation in the socioeconomic characteristics of an area affect mortality? *BMJ,* 312:1013–4.

Buhmann, B., Rainwater, L., Schmauss, G., and Smeeding, T. (1988). Equivalence scales, well-being, inequality and poverty: sensitivity estimates across 10 countries using the LIS database. *R Income Wealth,* 34:115–42.

Cowell, F.A. (1977). *Measuring inequality.* Oxford: Philip Allan.

Danziger, S., and Gottschalk, P. (1995). *America unequal.* Cambridge, MA: Harvard University Press.

Dressler, W.W. (1996). Culture and blood pressure: using consensus analysis to create a measurement. *Cult Anthropol Methods,* 8:6–8.

Dressler, W.W. (1998). Stress and hypertension in the African-American community. Proceedings of the Conference on Public Health in the 21st Century: Behavioral and Social Science Contributions, Atlanta, GA, May 7–9, 1998.

Dressler, W.W., Balieiro, M.C., and Dos Santos, J.E. (in press). Culture, skin color, and arterial blood pressure in Brazil. *Am J Hum Biol.*

Dutton, D.B., and Levine, S. (1989). Overview, methodological critique, and reformulation. In Bunker, J.P., Gomby, D.S., and Kehrer, B.H. (eds.), *Pathways to health: the role of social factors.* Menlo Park, CA: Henry J. Kaiser Foundation, pp. 29–69.

Fiscella, K., and Franks, P. (1997). Poverty or income inequality as predictor of mortality: longitudinal cohort study. *BMJ,* 314:1724–8.

Flegg, A.T. (1982). Inequality of income, illiteracy and medical care as determinants of infant mortality in underdeveloped countries. *Popul Stud,* 36:441–58.

Grusky, D.B. (1994). The contours of social stratification. In Grusky, D.B. (ed.), *Social stratification in sociological perspective.* Boulder, CO: Westview Press, pp. 3–35.

Hacker, A. (1997). *Money: who has how much and why.* New York: Scribner.

Hsieh, C.C., and Pugh, M.D. (1993). Poverty, income inequality, and violent crime: a meta-analysis of recent aggregate data studies. *Crim Just Rev,* 18:182–202.

Idler, E.L., and Benyamini, Y. (1997). Self-rated health and mortality: a review of twenty-seven community studies. *J Health Soc Behav,* 38:21–37.

Institute for Women's Policy Research. (1996). *The status of women in the states.* Washington, DC: Institute for Women's Policy Research.

Jencks, C. (1992). *Rethinking social policy: race, poverty, and the underclass.* Cambridge, MA: Harvard University Press.

Judge, K. (1995). Income distribution and life expectancy: a critical appraisal. *BMJ,* 311:1282–5.

Judge, K. (1996). Income and mortality in the United States (letter). *BMJ,* 313:1206.

Kaplan, G.A., Pamuk, E., Lynch, J.W., Cohen, R.D., and Balfour, J.L. (1996). Income inequality and mortality in the United States: analysis of mortality and potential pathways. *BMJ,* 312:999–1003.

Karasek, R., and Thoerell, T. (1990). *Healthy work: stress, productivity and the reconstruction of working life.* New York: Basic Books.

Kawachi, I., and Kennedy, B.P. (1997a). The relationship of income inequality to mortality: does the choice of indicator matter? *Soc Sci Med,* 45:1121–7.

Kawachi, I., and Kennedy, B.P. (1997b). Health and social cohesion: why care about income inequality? *BMJ,* 314:1037–40.

Kawachi, I., Levine, S., Miller, S.M., Lasch, K., and Amick, B.C. III (1994). Income inequality and life expectancy: theory, research, and policy. Boston: The Health Institute, New England Medical Center.

Kawachi, I., Kennedy, B.P., Lochner, K., and Prothrow-Stith, D. (1997a). Social capital, income inequality, and mortality. *Am J Public Health,* 87:1491–8.

Kawachi, I., Kennedy, B.P., and Lochner, K. (1997b). Long live community: social capital as public health. *Am Prospect,* November/December: 56–9.

Kawachi, I., Kennedy, B.P., Gupta, V., and Prothrow-Stith, D. (1999). Women's status and the health of men and women: a view from the states. *Soc Sci Med.* 48:21–32.

Kennedy, B.P., Kawachi, I., and Prothrow-Stith, D. (1996). Income distribution and mortality: cross-sectional ecological study of the

Robin Hood Index in the United States. *BMJ*, 312:1004–7. [See also Important Correction, *BMJ*, 312:1194.]

Kennedy, B.P., Kawachi, I., Lochner, K., Jones, C.P., and Prothrow-Stith, D. (1997). (Dis)respect and black mortality. *Ethn Dis*, 7: 207–14.

Kennedy, B.P., Kawachi, I., Glass, R., and Prothrow-Stith, D. (1998). Income distribution, socioeconomic status, and self-rated health: a U.S. multi-level analysis. *BMJ*, 317:917–21.

Krieger, N., Rowley, D.L., Herman, A.A., Avery, B., and Phillips, M.T. (1993). Racism, sexism, and social class: implications for studies of health, disease, and well-being. *Am J Prev Med*, 9:82–122.

Krugman, P. (1994). *Peddling prosperity*. New York: Norton.

Krugman, P. (1996). The spiral of inequality. *Mother Jones*, November/December: 44–9.

LeGrand, J. (1987). Inequalities in health: some international comparisons. *Eur Econ Rev*, 31:182–91.

Lochner, K. (1999). Income inequality, residential segregation and mortality differentials by SES and race. Harvard University (doctoral dissertation).

Lynch, J.W., Kaplan, G.A., Pamuk, E.R., Cohen, R.D., Balfour, J.L., and Yen, I.H. (1998). Income inequality and mortality in metropolitan areas of the United States. *Am J Public Health*, 88:1074–80.

Macintyre, S. (1996). Socioeconomic inequalities in health: some key contemporary issues. (Society & Health Working Paper Series, No. 96-6.) Boston: The Health Institute, New England Medical Center.

McIsaac, S.J., and Wilkinson, R.G. (1997). Income distribution and cause-specific mortality. *Eur J Public Health* 7:45–53.

Merton, R.K., and Rossi, A.S. (1950). Contributions to the theory of reference group behavior. In Merton, R.K., and Lazarsfield, P.F. (eds.), *Continuities in social research*. New York: Free Press, pp. 40–105.

Merva, M., and Fowles, R. (1993). *Effects of diminished economic opportunities in social stress: heart attacks, strokes, and crime*. Washington, DC: Economic Policy Institute.

Pappas, G., Queen, S., Hadden, W., and Fisher, G. (1993). The increasing disparity in mortality between socioeconomic groups in the United States, 1960 and 1986. *N Engl J Med*, 329:103–9.

Pearce, N. (1996). Traditional epidemiology, modern epidemiology and public health. *Am J Public Health*, 86:678–83.

Putnam, R.D. (1993). *Making democracy work: civic traditions in modern Italy*. Princeton, NJ: Princeton University Press.

Putnam, R.D. (1995). Bowling alone: America's declining social capital. *J Democracy*, 6: 65–78.

Rodgers, G.B. (1979). Income and inequality as determinants of mortality: an international cross-section analysis. *Popul Stud*, 33: 343–51.

Rose, G.A. (1992). *The strategy of preventive medicine*. Oxford: Oxford University Press.

Saunders, P. (1996). *Poverty, income distribution and health: an Australian study*. (SPRC Reports and Proceedings No. 128.) Sydney: Social Policy Research Center, University of New South Wales.

Schwartz, S. (1994). The fallacy of the ecological fallacy: the potential misuse of a concept and the consequences. *Am J Public Health*, 84:819–24.

Sen, A.K. (1973). *On economic inequality*. Oxford: Clarendon Press.

Soobader, M.J., and LeClere, F.B. (1999). Aggregation and the measurement of income inequality: effects on morbidity. *Soc Sci Med*, 48:733–44.

Stouffer, S.A., Suchman, E.A., DeVinney, L.C. Starr, S.A., and Williams, Jr., R.M. (1949). The American Soldier, adjustment during army life. Vol. 1. Princeton, NJ: Princeton University Press.

Stouffer, S.A., Lumsdaine, A.A., Parker-Lumsdaine, M., Williams, Jr. R.M., Smith, M.B., Janis, I.L., and Starr, S.A. (1949). The American Soldier, combat and its aftermath. Vol. 2, Princeton, NJ: Princeton University Press.

U.S. Census Bureau (1997). *Income inequality*. (March Current Population Survey.) Washington, DC: Government Printing Office.

United Nations Development Program (UNDP). (1996). *Human development report 1996*. New York: Oxford University Press.

Veblen, T. (1899). *The theory of the leisure class*. New York: B.W. Huebsch, 1922 edition.

Waldman, R.J. (1992). Income distribution and infant mortality. *Q J Econ*, 107:1283–302.

Wennemo, I. (1993). Infant mortality, public policy, and inequality: a comparison of 18 industrialised countries, 1950–85. *Sociol Health Illness*, 15: 429–46.

Wilkinson, R.G. (1986). Income and mortality. In Wilkinson, R.G. (ed.), *Class and health: research and longitudinal data*. London: Tavistock, pp. 88–114.

Wilkinson, R.G. (1990). Income distribution and mortality: a "natural" experiment. *Sociol Health Illness*, 12:391–412.

Wilkinson, R.G. (1992). Income distribution and life expectancy. *BMJ*, 304:165–8.

Wilkinson, R.G. (1996). *Unhealthy societies: the afflictions of inequality*. London: Routledge.

Wilkinson, R.G. (1997). Income inequality sum-marises the health burden of individual relative deprivation (commentary). *BMJ*, 314: 1727–8.

Wolf S., and Bruhn, J. (1992). *The power of clan: a 25-year prospective study of Roseto, PA.* New Brunswick, NJ: Transaction.

Wolff, E. (1995). *Top heavy: a study of the increasing inequality of wealth in America.* New York: 20th Century Fund.

5

Working Conditions and Health

TÖRES THEORELL

We are living in a rapidly changing world, and this includes working conditions. In order to understand the association between health and working conditions, we need multiple, sensitive systems that can record these conditions.

This chapter presents a theoretical framework for measuring working conditions as we study how they relate to health. It focuses on cardiovascular disease but also refers to other health outcomes. First, the historical background of current theoretical models is reviewed. Second, the chapter describes alternative measures of work conditions, including their advantages and disadvantages. Two major models of demand–control–support and effort–reward then are discussed. In the last section, evidence from studies based on these models is evaluated, as well as potential pathways and mechanisms underlying the relationship between work environments and health outcomes.

CONCEPTUAL AND THEORETICAL DEVELOPMENT OF MODELS—HISTORICAL BACKGROUND

The relationship between the psychosocial work environment and health has attracted considerable attention. In modern western societies, this focus seems logical because of the dramatic changes in the workplace. Physical job demands are diminishing for many workers, and the growing complexity of modern society increases work-related psychosocial demands. For instance, analyses of the living conditions of randomly selected working Swedes (Statistics Sweden 1996), have shown that noise and heavy lifting are physical conditions of work that have become less frequent during the past 20 years. Psychological demands, however, have increased in intensity, according to self-reported data from other studies. In several countries, an increasing number of employees' unions and trade unions, as well

as employers, have realized that a functioning psychosocial work environment depends heavily on how work is organized
and that health-promoting factors in the
work organization can also improve productivity. In occupational medicine as
well, psychosocial working conditions have
gained recognition in recent years. Where
once this field was focused exclusively on
physically noxious exposures, researchers
and clinicians have now turned some attention to behavioral and social workplace issues.

Cardiovascular disease has been regarded
as an important outcome in the study of the
relationship between working conditions
and health. Furthermore, it is theoretically
interesting as a model in the study of social
conditions and health since many factors,
social as well as biological, contribute to its
development. For these reasons, much of
this chapter is devoted to a discussion of
work conditions and heart disease.

Historical Perspective on "Work Stress"

In the 1960s there were several systematic
studies of how working conditions relate to
myocardial infarction risk. Many were
cross-sectional in nature (Biörck et al. 1958;
Buell and Breslow 1960; Russek and Zohman 1958; Kasanen et al. 1963). They indicated that there may be a relationship
between excessive overtime work and cardiovascular illness risk. Hinkle's study of
"night college" men in the Bell Telephone
Company was the first prospectively designed study that confirmed an association
between excessive demands and myocardial
infarction risk (Hinkle et al. 1968). Kornitzer and colleagues (1982) later observed
in a retrospective study of two bank groups
in Belgium, one private and one state-
owned, that employees in the private banks
had a higher incidence of myocardial infarction than employees in the state owned
banks. This difference could not be explained by biomedical risk factors (Kittel et
al. 1980). The Belgian bank study was one
of the first to indicate a possible relationship
between a certain element of working con-

ditions, *work demands* (which were higher
in the private banks), and risk of myocardial
infarction.

During the 1960s, an important prospective study revealed a higher incidence of myocardial infarction among lower-level as
compared to higher-level employees in large
companies (Pell and d'Alonzo 1963). This
evidence raised suspicion for the first time
that psychosocial stress might not be primarily a problem for people with a lot of responsibility, as researchers had tended to
believe previously, and paved the way for a
more complex understanding of the relationship between occupational status and
work stress. In this phase of research, there
were still few explicit or compelling theoretical models.

The Demand–Control Model

As research progressed in this area, social
scientists began to develop more theoretically grounded models. Organizational
phsychologists began describing potentially
stressful aspects of the work environment
(Katz and Kahn 1966), and by the mid-
1970s, review articles appeared describing
occupational sources of stress (Cooper and
Marshall 1976). Among the most important
of these investigators was Karasek, an ar-
chitect by training, who described initially a
two-dimensional model of occupational
stress. It was comprised of job demands and
job control.

In this model, job demands were related
to earlier psychological stress models having to do with pressure and heavy demands.
In generating the concept "lack of control,"
or "lack of decision latitude," Karasek had
been following earlier sociological traditions related to alienation and the work
process. These traditions assumed that the
possibility for the employee to utilize and
develop skills (*skill utilization*) was closely
related to his or her *authority over decisions*. It was posited that skill utilization
had to do with the employee's control over
the use and development of his/her skills
whereas authority over decisions had to do
with the employee's control over decision

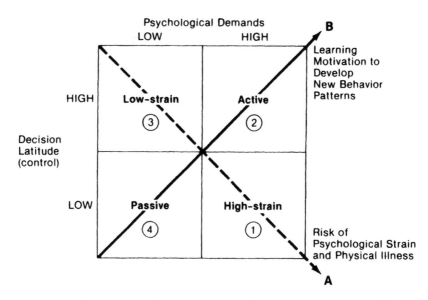

Figure 5–1. Psychological demand–decision latitude model. Source: Karasek (1979).

making relevant to his work tasks. Statistical analysis of the way in which responses to questions about work content are clustered (such as factor analysis) shows that these two factors go together. Accordingly, they have been added together to constitute a measure of *decision latitude* (see Karasek 1979; Karasek and Theorell 1990).

The other dimension in the original demand–control model, *psychological demands*, includes *qualitative* emotional (Soderfeldt et al. 1997) as well as *quantitative* demands. These are grouped as one factor in many of the studies of representative working populations in the Western hemisphere. Quantitative demands may be easier to study than emotional demands since number of performances per time unit, for instance, could be recorded objectively. Such demands may also be easier to record in a self-administered questionnaire since they are objective assessments. That does not mean that quantitative demands are more important than emotional ones. In work involving patients, clients, and customers, for instance, emotional demands may be crucial. In the study of such work, it has been shown that it is meaningful to sep-

arate the two components of psychological demands (Söderfeldt et al. 1997).

It should be emphasized that the demand–control model was never intended to explain all work-related illnesses. For instance, no element of fit with an individual's abilities to accomplish work-related tasks was introduced into its original construction. On the contrary, the model dealt with the way in which work is organized and the way in which this structure relates to illness. This simplicity has made the model useful in organizational work.

According to Karasek, there is an interaction between high psychological demands and low decision latitude. If demands are regarded as the x-axis and decision latitude as the y-axis in a two-dimensional system, four combinations are recognized (Fig. 5–1). The high-demand–low-decision latitude quadrant, *job strain*, is regarded as the most relevant to illness development. Karasek uses a powerful analogy to describe the combination of high-demand–low-decision latitude: If a person is crossing a street and sees a truck approaching, he may speculate that he will be able to cross the street without being hit by the truck if he regulates his

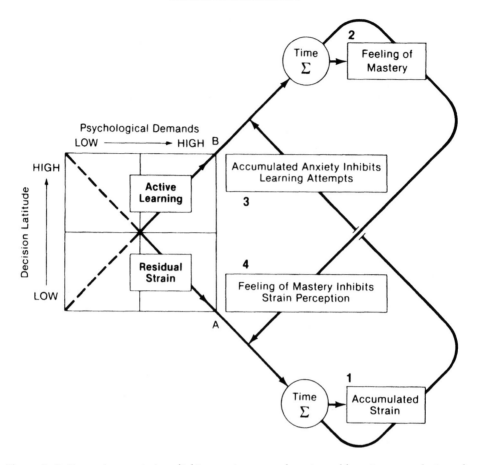

Figure 5–2. Dynamic associations linking environmental strain and learning to evolution of personality. Source: Karasek (1979).

speed appropriately. However, if his foot gets stuck in the street his decision latitude diminishes dramatically and he is now in an extremely stressful situation. According to the theory, if prolonged and repeated for a long time, this kind of situation, characterized by low latitude and high demand, increases sympathoadrenal arousal and at the same time decreases anabolism, the body's ability to restore and repair tissues.

The combination of high psychological demands and high decision latitude is defined as the *active* situation. In this situation, the worker has been given more resources to cope with high psychological demands because he/she can make relevant decisions, such as planning working hours

according to his/her own biological rhythm. In addition he/she has greater possibilities to improve coping strategies—facilitating feeling of mastery and control in unforeseen situations. This situation corresponds to psychological growth.

The low-demand–high-decision latitude quadrant—the *relaxed* one—is theoretically the ideal one, whereas the low-demand–low-decision latitude quadrant, which is labeled *passive,* may be associated with risk of loss of skills and to some extent psychological atrophy (Karasek and Theorell 1990). Figure 5–2 shows the dynamic version of the demand–control model. Active learning in the active situation may stimulate feelings of mastery whereas accumulated tension in the strain situation may lead to accumulated anxiety which inhibits active learning.

Addition of Social Support—The Demand–Control–Support Model Becomes Three-Dimensional

There is a third dimension to work characterictics that was neglected in earlier models. This dimension relates to characteristics of job-related social support. Johnson has discussed this component extensively (Johnson et al. 1996). His research supports the idea that social support at work may affect the relationship between job strain and heart disease. He supports previous research that shows social support may modify the impact of psychosocial demands. In particular, Johnson's study suggests that people experiencing low social support in conjunction with high psychosocial demands and low control (isostrain) experience the highest relative risk for cardiovascular disease as compared to the people experiencing other combinations of demand–control and social support.

The Effort–Reward Imbalance Model

In the past few years, another model of the work environment has emerged. According to Siegrist (1996), a crucial factor in terms of health consequences is the degree to which workers are rewarded for their efforts. When a high degree of effort does not meet a high degree of reward, emotional tensions arise and illness risk increases. Effort is the individual's response to the demands made upon him or her. These responses may be divided into *extrinsic* effort, which refers to the individual's effort to cope with external demands, and *intrinsic* effort, which correspond to the his/her own drive to fulfil his/her goals. According to Siegrist and colleagues (Siegrist et al. 1988; Siegrist 1996), the development of intrinsic effort follows a long-term course in the individual. For example, young employees without extensive work experience with a high degree of "vigor" get involved in more and more commitments. Due to the increasing numbers of commitments, there

may be an increasing number of conflicts. If the individual is unable to decrease the number of commitments, "immersion" will be the result as the employee ages, causing feelings of frustration and irritation. A corporate culture that includes a high level of psychological demands may force employees to internalize extrinsic demands.

Although there is overlap between the effort–reward imbalance and the demand–control–support models, they are differently focused. While the demand–control–support model is entirely focused on the organization's structure, the effort–reward model examines the individual's fit in the environment and includes not only *extrinsic* but also *intrinsic* effort. The latter is closely related to coping—the individual's way of handling difficulties. Reward is a composite measure of financial rewards, self-esteem, and social control. According to the theory, a "healthy state" occurs when reward is increased as effort increases. This state may be achieved by means of external work-related changes such as increased salary and improved social status or increased possibilities for promotion. But it may also be obtained by means of changes in internal effort. Changes in the employees' internal effort can come about only as a result of changes in coping strategies among the employees, not by changing work conditions per se.

Integration of Effort–Reward Imbalance and Demand–Control

There is already evidence (Bosma et al. 1998) that the decision latitude component of the demand–control model and the effort–reward imbalance model contribute independently of one another to the prediction of episodes of coronary heart disease. This finding confirms that the models are related to different psychosocial mechanisms linking work conditions to health outcomes. The models share psychological demands (extrinsic effort) in common but control (decision latitude) and reward are clearly different. A logical step would be to combine the models. Even if resources (control and support) are optimal for the development of good coping strategies in a highly demanding situation, the employees will need reward for high effort and hence balance between the components is needed

Having described two theoretical models widely used in epidemiological research it is necessary to discuss how to measure the components in the models.

Measurement—How to Record the Psychosocial Work Environment

First of all it is necessary to discuss some general techniques, with related problems and benefits for the measurement of the psychosocial work environment.

Self-administered questionnaires
Self-administered questionnaires have been used extensively in the study of the psychosocial working environment, mainly because they enable the researcher to do studies of large samples efficiently. The assessment of demand–control–support and effort–reward imbalance by means of self-administered questionnaires will be discussed more in detail below. Work-stress questionnaires based upon Cooper-Marshall's model are very commonly used in many countries and they give immediate guidance to those who are exploring work environments and trying to improve conditions. Similarly, measurements of person–environment fit have frequently been made by means of standardized questionnaires (Katz and Kahn 1966).

Self-administered questionnaires may be grouped according to two different dimensions: *(1)* a dimension of response categories: those with fixed response categories in one end and open-ended questions in the other end, and *(2)* along a dimension from general use to specific work site use: e.g., those intended to be used for "general use" (everybody in the work force or at least very large segments of working men and/or women) in one end and those for "local use" (specified questions for those working in one specific work site) in the other end (see Fig. 5-3).

A very useful kind of questionnaire in

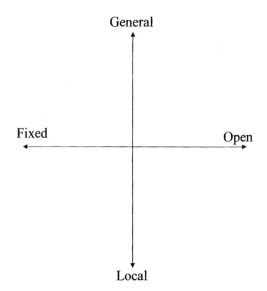

Figure 5–3. Relationship between age group and decision latitude in male and female workers.

studying many situations is the *diary*. A diary could be prepared as a booklet that the subjects are asked to fill out at regular intervals several times a day or week. It differs from conventional questionnaires in the sense that it does not require global judgments but rather immediately catches the impressions and observations that the subjects themselves make in a given moment or short period. Diaries could also be divided according to the fixed–open and general–local dimensions. Diaries have been used extensively in the study of sleepiness and alertness at work (Åkerstedt 1988).

It may be possible to incorporate nontraditional and highly specialized kinds of written material that may have been stored such as letters and other documents. This method could be regarded as an "open" and "local" source of information.

Interviews
Interviews in which a trained interviewer asks questions of employees is a second way of assessing work conditions. Interviews may also be divided according to the fixed–open and general–local dimensions. For instance, an interview with fixed response cat-

egories for general use is one that has been formatted, tested, and standardized according to a general theory. Sometimes it may be necessary to define two or three components of the work tasks normally present in an employee's workday. After an interview each one of the components could be assessed with regard to creativity, routine use of skills, and monotony without skill requirement, respectively. After assessment of percentage time in each one of the components, a weighted measure of each one of them for total working time could be calculated (Waldenström et al. 1998).

The group interview may be useful in many situations. This is mostly semi-structured. The goal of the group interview is to uncover group phenomena—for instance, ways of communicating—that are not identifiable in individual interviews. One important aspect of the psychosocial job environment that could be studied in this way is *group coping*—the way in which employees try to handle difficult situations as a group rather than as individuals.

Observations in work sites
Many kinds of observations may be used in the exploration of work environments. They range from recording the physiological reactions in employees (which could be summarized on a group level)—as has been done in studies of urinary excretion of catecholamines as an indicator of sympathoadrenal arousal—to number of specified operations performed per time unit in a work site. As with questionnaires and interviews, observations can be divided according to the fixed–open and general–local dimensions, respectively. As an example of observations with fixed categories that build upon a general theory (fixed–general), a whole system of standardized observations of work organization for general use in industry and office work, respectively, has been constructed (Hacker 1978; Volpert 1989). It includes numbers and kinds of hindrances, degree of monotony, time pressure, qualitative demands, and several other dimensions. Social anthropology typically uses measurement

techniques that are in the opposite quadrant. They are open (make no assumptions about relevant factors to be observed) and focus on local conditions (open–local). The technique is usually based on participant observation where the researcher participates in regular work in the studied site for several weeks to months and records everything that occurs. Afterwards observations are categorized and systematized.

With so many methods to choose from, there are many potential pitfalls in epidemiological studies in this field. It is accordingly important to choose measurement tools and realted methodology with care. The following general dimensions have to be considered in the choice of methodology:

The subjects' own distortion of the description. Subjects may distort the description of the environment for several reasons. The most important ones are listed below:

1. *Social pressure.* This may result in overestimation as well as underestimation of environmental risks. Underestimation will be the result when an employer/supervisor puts pressure on the employees not to report problems—"If you report adverse conditions I will not promote you in the future." Overestimation would be the result if there were a collective decision among employees to obtain specific results by overreporting a specific adverse condition.

2. *Psychological defense mechanisms.* If many of the employees are prone to use denial or similar defense mechanisms when they are faced with difficulties, there will be an underestimation of adverse conditions. This may be more common in certain groups than in others—a "macho oriented" climate, for instance, may enforce denial. If there is a large proportion of subjects who have weak defense mechanisms and who tend to develop anxiety easily, these may overreport adverse conditions and cause overestimation.

3. *Individual ability to describe and analyse conditions.* There is both a cognitive and an emotional side to this ability. In certain groups, employees are trained and

encouraged to analyze their own conditions. This may result in improved cognitive
ability with regard to reporting job strain.
In such groups, subjects may be able to report conditions in a balanced way. This may
be true, for instance, of workers in health
care who have become used to analyzing the
conditions of their patients: The process
stimulates them to analyze their own conditions more often. In groups with less training there will be less cognitive ability to analyze the condition, and this may result in
either overestimation or underestimation of
the true prevalence of adverse as well as
beneficial conditions. On the emotional
side, the inability to differentiate and analyze one's own feelings may also influence
the results. If subjects have alexithymia, for
instance, there may be no identified emotional reactions to the environment. This
circumstance will result in underestimation
of adverse as well as beneficial conditions.

The investigators' distortion. The investigators may have preconceptions that influence their way of exploring the conditions.
Sometimes they may not be aware of them.
Preconceptions may influence the choice
and formulation of questions, as well as the
way of asking questions in personal interviews and the way of making observations.
Finally, such preconceptions may also influence the interpretation and analysis of responses.

Long-term goals of the exploration—tension between neutral and engaged. If the
long-term research goal is merely to describe the prevalence of concrete conditions,
this may not require strong engagement
among the employees themselves. A neutral,
relatively detached attitude may even be ad-
vantageous from the scientific descriptive
point of view. But if the long-term goal of
the study is to initiate changes in the studied work sites and if complicated psychosocial processes are to explored, employees
need to participate actively in the analytical
process. There is tension between these two
kinds of strategies, the strictly scientific/

standardized and the action-oriented. For
instance, if the goal is pure scientific measurement of blood pressure reactions to the
working environment, fully automated
equipment is preferable. If the goal is educational and action-oriented, it may be better to instruct the participants to record
their own blood pressure by means of simple equipment and have subjects record activities and conditions for each measurement occasion. In this way the participants
gain active knowledge regarding physiological reactions to their working conditions—
which may initiate action. However, some
of the participants may record blood pressure in a biased way, which is disadvante-
gous for the researcher. The investigator
needs to be aware of such tensions between
the methods that he/she chooses.

Financial costs. The choice of research
methodology has to take the costs into consideration. It is important for the group in
charge of the exploration to convince the
employer of the importance of the research.
Moreover, they should not start without
knowing that there will be adequate financial resources to complete study of high
quality and to follow it up adequately.

General Rules

When the investigators have evaluated
available techniques and information related to the four dimensions outlined above, a
choice can be made. A few rules may be formulated.

1. If the investigator is dealing with a situation which is unexplored and contains
novel circumstances, which is certainly the
case in the new working-world scenario, the
first analyses should preferably be of the
"open" character. This will be true regardless of whether questionnaires, interviews,
or observations are used.

2. If the most important long-term goal of
the exploration is to improve the work situation, it is important to choose a methodology that engages the employees in this
process from the beginning. Questions with
open-ended response catgories—in particu-

lar, asking for suggestions for improvements—are to be preferred. Interviews should be preferred to questionnaires as well.

3. If the most important goal is to provide information needed for resource allocation and a neutral description is required for this process or if the goal is to explore a basic scientific relationship between a psychosocial phenomenon and a physiological or medical outcome, standardized general methods which allow comparisons between a wide range of groups may be preferable.

4. If there is reason to believe that there is low motivation among employees to participate in the exploration and hence low quality of questionnaire responses and low participation rates could be expected, interviews and observations may be preferable. In the interview, it is possible for the interviewer to motivate the participant and to make sure that the meaning of the questions is clear to him/her. This process could be difficult with questionnaires unless special precautions are taken.

5. If there is a high degree of suspicion among the employees, anonymously distributed questionnaires may be the only possible choice.

6. If it is difficult to recruit interviewers or observers who are independent and not involved in the work at the work site, a serious investigator's distortion may arise. Anonymous questionnaires may be preferable in such a situation.

7. Combinations of several methods in the same exploration are often preferable. For instance, standardized questions with fixed response categories could be combined with more locally focused questions which the participants are asked to answer in their own words.

8. The use of questionnaires is of course less expensive than that of interviews or observations. However, in some situations where low-quality information could be expected from a questionnaire exploration, a high-quality interview study of a relatively small number of representative employees may be less expensive in the long-term perspective.

9. Regardless of choice of methodology, the definitive exploration has to be preceded by pilot tests of the methodology. Furthermore, the exploration has to be preceded by discussions with representatives of the study population, management, local unions, and safety representatives.

Specific Measures of the Demand–Control–Support Model

Three different methods have dominated in the assessment of the demand and control dimensions, and they are discussed below.

Self-administered questionnaires

The American Job Content Questionnaire (JCQ) and the Swedish version of the demand–control questions have been the most common questionnaires. JCQ (available from Karasek) is a development of the American demand–control–support questionnaire presented in the book *Healthy Work* (Karasek and Theorell 1990). It is presently used in many countries, whereas the Swedish version is used mainly in Sweden and other Scandinavian countries. The Swedish version has five questions about demands and six about decision latitude. The demand questions deal mainly with quantitative aspects of demands, such as "Do you have time enough to do your work?" and "Do you have to work fast?" but there is also one question that is more qualitative: "Are there conflicting demands in your job?" The decision latitude questions deal both with intellectual discretion (use and development of skills) and authority over decisions. The questions about intellectual discretion are for instance: "Do you learn new things in your job?", "Is your job monotonous?", and "Does your job require creativity?" The questions about authority over decisions are: "Can you influence how to do your job?" and "Can you influence how your work is to be performed?" The internal consistency of the two dimensions for both men and women in the general working population has proved satisfactory, and factor analysis has confirmed that it is meaningful to group the questions in this way (Theorell 1996b). In the American version, there are more questions both about demands and about decision latitude, and there are also several other relevant work dimensions. Its internal consistency has been shown to be satisfactory in several countries. The two versions (which have the same origin—Karasek's initial factor analyses of the American quality of employment surveys in 1968, 1974, and 1977) differ slightly in format since the Swedish version is based upon frequency grading (four grades, from Never to Always) of responses to direct questions, and the American one is based upon intensity grading (five grades, from Not at all to Very much) of rejection or acceptance of a number of statements.

The operationalization of job strain in these questionnaires has varied. The most frequently used option has been to require demands to be high and decision latitude low at the same time (above/below median or upper/lower quartile or tertile). Another frequently used alternative has been to calculate the ratio between demands and decision latitude and define exposure to job strain equal to those in the upper quartile of this ratio.

Work stress defined on the basis of job category

Another approach to assessing job stress is achieved by classifying job on the basis of questionnaire data and then looking at the relationship between the jobs and health status. The classification systems are called job exposure matrices (JEMs). JEMs are based on national surveys of the working population. Initially the job exposure matrices were constructed to serve as a proxy for work environment assessments in epidmiological studies that were missing such data. The only requirement for the use of JEMs was that there should be a three-digit occupational code for the person. By means of computations of means or distributions of answers to relevant questions about the psychosocial work environment, the three-digit code could be translated into a crude estimate of the typical level for this particular variable in that occupational group. It

was reasoned that typical responses would vary between men and women, between older and younger workers, and between those who had been employed in the occupation for a long or a short period. In the American JEM, corrections for such differences were made by means of knowledge regarding the typical responses in such subgroups (older/younger, etc.) of the total working population, whereas the Swedish JEM (which included larger samples) was based on specific information about subgroups of the population—for instance, typical responses in older male carpenters who had been working for less than 5 years as carpenters. This may seem to be a small difference. However, since the differences between age groups may be specific to the occupation group, corrections based upon the total working population may be erroneous. But some subgroups are very small in the total working population. Thus, a detailed system could only be constructed for the largest occupation groups in the population.

Two JEM databases have been presented and utilized: the U.S. quality of employment suveys (Schwartz et al. 1988) and the Swedish Level of Living Surveys (Johnson and Stewart 1993). There was a precursor to the Swedish system according to Alfredsson and Theorell (1983). It was based on a number of single questions that were related to the main dimensions of psychological demands and decision latitude. The older version provides tables indicating which quartile a given subgroup belongs to in a given stratum (a stratum is defined by means of gender and age below/above 45). Male workers in occupation X who are above age 45 and who have been working for at least 20 years in this occupation may, for instance, belong to the lowest quartile for hectic work and the highest quartile for influence over working hours. In the new version, this particular subgroup is presented with a mean and a standard deviation for control and demand, respectively. Furthermore, strata are also defined with regard to duration of work in the occupation (below 5, between 5 and 20, and finally above 20 years). In the Swedish JEM, social support is one factor that is derived from the survey of level of living conditions.

The American JEM was constructed on the basis of exactly the same questions as the original version of the JCQ. The Swedish one was based on questions available in the Level of Living Surveys and these questions are not the same as the ones in the Swedish demand–control–support questionnaire.

The JEM is not the best choice if it is possible to make more direct assessments. However, it can provide useful information. For decision latitude, similar results have been found for the JEM and the self-reported assessments in relation to coronary heart disease risk (Theorell et al. 1998).

When considering whether or not to use self-administered questionnaires or a JEM, one must consider the methodological issue of whether self-reports correspond to more objective measures. In other words, do subjects who have recently suffered an acute illness describe their work situation in a way that is systematically different from subjects in the normal working population? In the SHEEP study (Stockholm Heart Epidemiology Program) in Stockholm, "objective" (obtained by means of the Swedish JEM, see above) and "subjective" (self reports) job descriptions were compared (Theorell et al. 1998). For decision latitude, the cases and the referents were very similar with regard to job reporting behaviour (the way in which self-reports and JEM assessments related to one another), although as expected there was only a moderate correlation between the two sources of information. The conclusion was that (in this case male) subjects who had had a recent myocardial infarction (interviewed within 1 month after the event) did not show "differential recall bias" (memory distortion that is systematically different in the two groups) in relation to decision latitude. This means that systematic "recall bias" on the part of the patient ("My infarction was caused by too little say at work") is an unlikely explanation of the relationship between low decision latitude and elevated risk of myocardial infarction in case-referent studies of this kind. The same was found for psychological demands although in this instance the findings were weaker since the aggregated measure for demands was methodologically poor. Controlling for chest pain preceding the first myocardial infarction did not change the conclusions in this study either, which is further support for the conclusion that differential recall bias is not a significant problem. However, if subjects had had a *long-lasting*, serious, debilitating coronary heart disease preceding the examination the situation might be markedly different (see above) with resulting distortion of self-reports.

Expert assessments

These assessments are based upon knowledge about the work that is performed in different occupations. Sometimes such measurements are used as an "objective" measure. In the British Whitehall study, for instance, independent experts assessed the individual work sites and these assessments were later compared with self-ratings. For work control, the agreement (measured as a correlation coefficient) was on the order of 0.3, which indicates only moderate agreement. Despite this, the associations between psychosocial work environment measured by means of expert ratings and coronary heart disease as outcome measure were of the same order of magnitude as the associations between self-rated psychosocial factors and work and coronary heart disease risk. Such findings may strengthen the conclusion that there are true associations (Bosma et al. 1997).

Measuring the Effort–Reward Imbalance Model

Siegrist's group has developed a self-administered questionnaire that includes all the relevant dimensions for the effort–reward imbalance model. It includes external and internal effort as well as three groups of reward: financial, self-esteem, and social. Furthermore the group has established and tested a questionnaire measuring "need for control" (Siegrist et al. 1988). In recently published epidemiological studies (Bosma et al. 1998; Peter et al. 1998) the recommended questionnaire has not been available, and for some of the variables proxy measures have been used. Accordingly, the formula for adding the dimensions and the summary scores has varied among studies. Furthermore, the imbalance between total effort and total reward scores has not always been consistently calculated and operationalized. The measurement of effort–reward imbalance that is rapidly becoming popular in epidemiology has not been completely tested in its final form.

Evaluation of the Evidence

Empirical tests of the demand–control model

Karasek's original hypothesis, that the combination of excessive psychological demands and lack of decision latitude is associated with increased risk of cardiovascular disease, has been tested in a large number of epidemiological studies (Karasek and Theorell 1990; Alfredsson 1983; Johnson and Hall 1988; Alfredsson and Theorell 1983; La Croix 1984; Reed et al. 1989; Haan 1985; Karasek et al. 1981). Many prospective and cross-sectional studies have now been published, although often the methodology has varied considerably among studies. The most important distinction between the methodologic approaches is that some studies have used the subjects' own descriptions of their work situations, whereas others have used aggregated job descriptive data, such as the JEM, based on representative workers in the occupations in the population. As we have discussed, both methods have advantages and problems. For example, individual traits may be associated with systematically distorted work descriptions, and this systematic distortion may be related to illness risk—with both overestimation and underestimation of the relative risk as possible result. The use of aggregated data gives an opportunity to avoid individual distortion (although of course collective distortion may still take place). The use of aggregated data does not allow for variations between work sites. This may

lead to substantial misclassification (Alfredsson 1983). The underestimation problem in the use of aggregated data is probably most pronounced in estimating the importance of psychological demands, since this variable shows relatively small variance between occupations. Decision latitude shows considerable variance between occupations (Karasek and Theorell 1990). Even the aggregated methodology has varied across studies. In some studies, the classifications have been based on means for each one of the dimensions from employees in the different occupations in the working population. In others, single questions have represented the dimensions, and several combinations (demand/skill utilization and skill/authority over decisions) have been tested. Finally, in a third group of studies, expert ratings have been used as way of assessing working conditions objectively.

An epidemiological study in Sweden (Hammar et al. 1994) using one of the aggregated methodologies merits some attention as it serves as an example of standard results. In this study, a large number of cases of myocardial infarction were identified by means of the nationwide Swedish death registry and by means of county registers that included hospitalizations. Referents stratified with regard to gender, age, and geographical area were selected randomly from the population. Analyses were confined to "occupationally stable" subjects who stayed in the same occupation during the two most recent censuses (which were 5 years apart) and to those who had a first myocardial infarction (in contrast to subsequent infarctions). The expected pattern of finding the strongest relative risk in the strain quadrant and the lowest risk in the relaxed quadrant was observed, with intermediately low risk in the active and intermediately high risk in the passive quadrant, respectively. The strongest excess risk of developing myocardial infarction was found in occupations that had a high prevalence of hectic work as well as work in which there was little influence over planning, the relative risk being 1.6 in the age group below 55 for this combination. The results were typical for this kind of study, with stronger age-adjusted relative risks among the younger men (below age 55).

One of the most recent studies of civil servants in Great Britain was prospective. Self-reports of degree of decision latitude at work were obtained on two occasions 3 years apart. Those who described a low decision latitude on both occasions had a relative risk of developing coronary heart disease during follow-up of 1.9 compared to other participants. The relationship was significant both for men and women, even after adjustment for negative affectivity, social class, and all the known biomedical risk factors (Bosma et al. 1997).

Studies that have used the two dimensions together have for the most part provided better predictions than studies using either one of them alone. At the same time, decision latitude has been of greater significance empirically in most studies than has psychological demands. In several studies during recent years it has turned out that it is difficult to operationalize and conceptualize psychological demands for epidemiological studies. This may be the main reason why studies have shown inconsistent results with regard to the association between psychological demands and heart disease risk.

The summary of relative risks indicates, as expected, that studies utilizing self-reported work descriptions have shown higher and more statistically consistent relative risks (1.3–4.0 vs. 1.2–2.0) than those using occupational codes as indicators of job strain. Some of the studies have incorporated other risk factors as well, including personality factors. In general, the adjustment for standard risk factors for cardiovascular disease does not eliminate the association between the high-demand–low-decision latitude combination and cardiovascular disease risk. In most studies, the cardiovascular disease risk was clinically verified myocardial infarction, and in three studies it was coronary heart disease (CHD). In fact, in one case, the Framingham study (La Croix 1984), the adjustment for other risk factors strengthened the association. In other words, it actually masked associations.

Studies of participants younger than 55 years of age in general have typically shown stronger associations than those including older subjects (see review, Theorell and Karasek 1996). Psychosocial job conditions may be of less importance during the 10 later years of the working career than before that period. The patterns are probably different for men and women. Another observation is that the high-demand–low-decision latitude has proven to be a more powerful predictor of cardiovascular illness risk in blue collar than in white collar men. For instance, a Finnish study (Haan 1985) included mainly blue collar workers and showed a strong association. The study by Johnson and Hall (1988) includes separate analyses of blue collar and white collar men which illustrate this point. The SHEEP study has shown that the job strain factor has better predictive value for blue collar than for white collar workers (Theorell et al. 1998; for further discussion, see Marmot and Theorell 1988).

So far, fewer studies have been performed on women than on men. There is no indication, however, that job strain is less important to women than to men (Reuterwall et al. 1998). Hall (1990), in a study of random samples of Swedish working men and women, showed that the interaction between activities outside work (unpaid work) and work activities was more important in relation to psychosomatic symptoms than it was for men. As a consequence, the pattern of associations between psychosocial factors and health was different in men and women. Hall furthermore pointed out that men and women in general work in different kinds of occupations. This may also be a reason why the patterns of association are gender specific.

Shift Work: A Special Psychological Demand

Shift work is a special example of psychological and physical demands. Such demands may have an effect of their own, outside the theoretical models discussed above. Adverse working hours could be psychologically demanding. Accordingly it is important to study the relationship between working hours and coronary heart disease risk. Constant rotation between night and day work, mostly labeled shift work, is associated with increased risk of developing a myocardial infarction in people of working age (Knutsson 1989). Relative risks of the same order as those found for job strain have been found, particularly after many years of exposure to shift work. Knutsson et al. (1998) have recently discussed whether shift work exerts its effect over and above that of job strain on myocardial infarction risk. On the basis of an extended SHEEP study which includes not only cases of a first myocardial infarction and their referents in Stockholm but also cases and referents in northern Sweden (Västernorrland), they showed that job strain and shift work were both independently associated with increased myocardial infarction risk after adjustment for accepted biomedical risk factors.

There have also been several studies with no findings for both demands and decision latitude. The following characteristics seem to be common in such negative studies:

1. Long follow-up periods. A single measure of job conditions at one point of time is not likely to be predictive for periods longer than 5 years. Workers may change jobs and conditions may change, too.

2. Indirect "aggregated" measures of job conditions. In particular, aggregated measures based upon working populations in the 1960s and 1970s may not be relevant. Such aggregated measures have to be reconstructed as the labour market changes.

3. Older study populations, in particular when participants are older than 55 years from the start. In this type of study, many of the participants retire during follow-up.

4. Study populations with little variation in decision latitude, such as groups which have only one type of white collar worker. In such a study, the only "available variance" is in *perception* of working conditions, which the study is not designed to test.

5. Case samples with coronary heart disease of varying duration preceding the examination. This factor may lead to adaptation to the illness, which may cause those subjects who have the most pronounced symptoms of illness to select easier jobs and improved conditions. This could cause serious underestimation of the causal role of job conditions.

In one negative study (Hlatky et al. 1995), there were at least three factors which made interpretations difficult. First of all, the study population (referrals to coronary angiography at a university hospital) was not representative of the general working population. Moreover, those people who complain very much of symptoms and have good financial resources are more likely to be referred to coronary angiography. This means that sensitive persons (who may also complain about working conditions) without coronary atherosclerosis are likely to be overrepresented, which may disturb the analysis. Finally, participants in the study had had (or did not have at all) coronary heart disease for varying periods of time. Thus, they may have had systematically different adaptations to work, different reactions to disease, and may even have shifted between job tasks in response to these factors and the disease itself.

One of the important theoretical questions in this field is whether the psychological demands variable interacts with decision latitude in generating increased risk; that is, are they more than additive (Kasl 1996)? A few attempts at elucidating this question have been made (for instance, Alfredsson and Theorell 1983; Johnson and Hall 1988; Reed et al. 1989), but most studies have not addressed this question specifically. On the basis of the SHEEP study, Hallquist et al. (1998) showed that there may be a strong interaction between psychological demands and decision latitude in relation to myocardial infarction risk but that this interaction depends upon the cutoffs for demands and decision latitude, respectively. When the cutoff for demands was set in such a way that 37% of the studied men were considered exposed to high demands and in a corresponding way 7% to low decision latitude the synergy index was particularly strong and statistically significant even after adjustment for social class and all accepted biomedical risk factors. In this study it was also shown that men in blue collar occupations are particularly vulnerable to the effects of job strain. Thus, although many studies have not specifically tested the interaction between psychological demands and decision latitude in relation to myocardial infarction risk, recent research indicates that this is a subject that should be explored in future research.

Empirical test when social support is added to the demand–control model
Several studies have explored the three-dimensional model of job strain which incorporates social support at work as an important domain. Good social support at work could be a protective factor for myocardial infarction. A study of cardiovascular disease prevalence in a large random sample of Swedish men and women indicated that the joint action of high demands and lack of control (decision latitude) was of particular importance to blue collar men whereas the combined action of lack of control and lack of support is more important for women and white collar men (Johnson and Hall 1988). The relative importance of these three components may accordingly be different in different strata of the population. The effect of the interaction between all the three of them (isostrain) was tested in a 9-year prospective study of 7000 randomly selected Swedish working men (Johnson et al. 1989). For the most favored 20% of men (low demands, good support, good decision latitude) the progression of cardiovascular mortality with increasing age was slow and equally so in the upper and lower social classes. In blue collar workers, however, the age progression was much steeper in the worst isostrain group than it was in the cor-responding isostrain group in white collar workers.

Career trajectories: an adult lifecourse model
Researchers have pointed out (House et al. 1986) that an estimate of work conditions only at one point in time may provide a very imprecise estimation of the total exposure to adverse conditions. Attempts are being made to use the occupational classification systems in order to describe the "psychosocial work career." Three-digit job titles are obtained for each year during the whole work career for the participants. Occupational scores derived from national samples of other subjects are subsequently used for a calculation of an indirect measure of "total lifetime exposure" that would facilitate the study of cumulative effect. The "total job control exposure" in relation to 9-year age-adjusted cardiovascular mortality in working Swedes was studied in this way. It was observed for both men and women that the cardiovascular mortality differences between the lowest and highest quartiles were almost twofold even after adjustment for age, smoking habits, and physical exercise (Johnson et al. 1996).

The direction and amount of variation in job control may also be important in the development of disease. A recent study (Theorell et al. 1998) has shown that changes in the level of control inferred from the job title may have an important impact on the risk of myocardial infarction. Thus, decreasing levels of control were more common in the group of men developing the first myocardial infarction, particularly during the 5 years preceding the illness. This observation may illustrate that the timing of a first myocardial infarction may be related to decreases in control level at work. An important observation, however, was that decrease in control was much more important for men below age 55 than in older men. The finding in men is in line with the observation in several studies that the *level* of decision latitude is also more important for men below age 55 than for older men. For

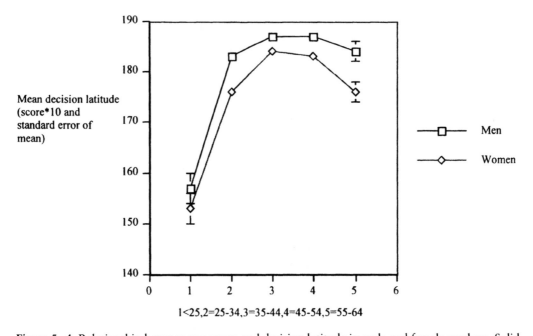

Figure 5–4. Relationship between age group and decision latitude in male and female workers. Solid line with standing squares, men; dotted line with tilted squares, women; Y axis, mean decision latitude. (questionnaire score * 10 and corresponding standard error of mean) for men and women in different age groups; X axis, age groups from left to right: 1, below 25; 2, 25–34; 3, 35–44; 4, 45–54; 5, 55–64.

women decreased decision latitude was not a significant risk factor.

The decrease in the importance of changes in decision latitude to the risk of developing myocardial infarction after age 55 may be explained by the progression of decision latitude with age. Figure 5–4 illustrates the association between age and decision latitude in Swedish men and women. The means are based upon the WOLF (work, lipids, fibrinogen) study in Stockholm (Alfredsson et al. 1997). It includes nearly 6000 working men and women. As can be seen in the diagram, decision latitude increases rapidly during the first years of a person's career. In middle age (around 55 in men and around 45 in women) the peak is reached and during later years of the career, a slight decrease is observed. Accordingly, in future studies it will be important also to relate stages in the life career to the effect of decision latitude and of change in decision latitude.

Effort–reward imbalance results

Siegrist's group has analyzed the association between effort–reward imbalance and coronary heart disease risk in several epidemiological studies. In a study of blue collar workers in Germany (Siegrist et al. 1988), a very clear relationship was found between effort–reward imbalance and an atherogenic blood lipid pattern. Effort–reward imbalance was also shown to be associated with myocardial infarction risk even after adjusting for accepted biological risk factors (Siegrist et al. 1990). Siegrist has summarized findings from several epidemiological studies (1996). A recently published study of men and women in the Whitehall study showed that decision latitude and effort–reward imbalance both contributed independently of one another to the prediction of new events of coronary heart disease in men and women, even after adjustment for a number of biological risk factors and social class (Bosma et al. 1998). Effort–reward imbalance thus seems to be a factor that should be studied along with demand–control–support.

Pathways Linking Work Conditions to Health Status

The question now arises, how is the relationship between isostrain and risk of cardiovascular illness mediated? One pathway might be related to the fact that there is a relationship between accepted behavioral risk factors such as cigarette smoking and job strain (Karasek and Theorell 1990; Green and Johnson 1990). Part of it could also be direct effects of an adverse job environment on biochemical and endocrinological factors.

Interesting results have been found with regard to the association between job strain and blood pressure. According to the results, job strain is relevant primarily to the blood pressure levels during working hours but not to blood pressure during other parts of the day and night. However, after longlasting exposure to an adverse job environment, the effect may also spread to the whole day and night, including during sleep. Most researchers have found a positive relationship between job strain and ambulatory blood pressure measurements, particularly during working hours. In the study of women, a clear association was also observed between job strain and plasma prolactin level when the subject arrived at work in the morning; plasma prolactin was also significantly associated with blood pressure levels at work. Schnall et al. (1992) found very clear relationships between job strain and hypertension, and for the younger participants in their study sample between job strain and ventricular hypertrophy (increased thickness of the myocardium), even after adjustment for a number of potential confounders.

Blood lipid levels have not been studied extensively in relation to the demand–control–support model, but there are several studies that have started to add research to this area. One study (Stjernström et al. 1993) has shown a relationship between job strain and low levels of high density lipoprotein in blood in farmers, however. A recent study of nearly 6000 working men and women in Stockholm (Alfredsson et al. 1997) showed a relationship between a high ratio between low- and high-density lipoprotein (LDL and HDL) cholesterol (which is known to be an "atherogenic" index) on one hand and job strain on the other hand, particularly in young men. Recently a clear relationship was observed between low decision latitude and suppression of HDL cholesterol in a random sample of Swedish working women (Wamala et al. 1997). A study by Siegrist et al. (1988) of industry workers has shown a relationship between chronic job stressors (such as threat of unemployment, lack of promotion possibility, and shift work) and a high LDL/HDL ratio. A recent study has shown similar findings with regard to hypertension and atherogenic lipids in a large sample of Swedish workers (Peter et al. 1998), with different patterns for men and women, respectively.

Thus, there may be a relationship between some aspects of the theoretical job stress models and suppression of the blood concentration of high density lipoprotein which is protective against atherosclerosis as well as an elevation of atherogenic lipoproteins.

Blood coagulation has also been discussed in relation to psychosocial job conditions. Markowe (1985) found relationships between low control and high fibrinogen in the Whitehall study, and this finding has been verified in later studies of the same cohort (Brunner et al. 1997).

A Concrete Example—The Bus Driver

One area which has developed more specifically than other research endeavors in this field is the study of bus drivers. There is now overwhelming evidence that bus drivers, particularly those driving in inner-city areas, have an excess risk of developing myocardial infarction (Alfredsson et al. 1992; Rosengren et al. 1991; Belkic et al. 1994) at an early age as compared to other types of workers.

Several hypotheses about why bus drivers are at excess risk exists relate to biochemical and job stress interactions. It has been shown that standard risk factors cannot explain all of the excess risk. It has previously been suspected that exposure to carbon monoxide may be of importance but this seems unlikely (Söndergård-Kristensen and Damsgaard 1987). Other toxicological exposures may be of importance, such as combustion products (Gustavsson 1989).

More recently, there has been an exploration of social contributors. In particular, it has been emphasized in recent research that job strain may be a very important factor (Hedberg et al. 1991), and some researchers have subsequently explored physiological consequences of job strain in bus drivers. Research suggests that catecholamines (Evans and Carrere 1991) are elevated in bus drivers who experience a high degree of job strain, for instance. However, more specific hypotheses have also been developed. Belkic and her colleagues (1992) have found that bus drivers seem to develop an aroused electrophysiological response to "the glare pressor test" more rapidly than others, particularly when instructions simulate a traffic situation (1992). It is possible that professional drivers have an accumulated experience of dangerous situations associated with sudden "glares" particularly at night and that this may be a potent factor explaining why bus drivers develop an excess risk for myocardical infarction after some years of driving; they become constantly hyperalert during driving.

Other Illnesses Than Cardiovascular Disease

Job conditions have been related to illnesses aside from cardiovascular disease. It has been found, for instance, that functional gastrointestinal disorders are particularly common among male and female workers who report low authority over decisions (Westerberg and Theorell 1997) and that those men who report good social support at work are more likely than other men to recover spontaneously from their symp-toms. Psychological demands, decision latitude, and social support at work have been shown to be associated with musculoskeletal disorder. The important components of work stress vary among studies. The most important factor may change according to the outcome—low back pain, for example—and the population studied: white males, for example (Kilbom et al. 1996; Theorell 1996a). There is growing evidence that both psychosocial and ergonomic (such as awkward positions and heavy) working conditions may be important causal factors in relation to acute episodes of musculoskeletal disorder. Psychosocial factors may be particularly important in the prediction of duration of illness after the acute onset. For example, in a large recent case referent study of first episodes of low back pain in a mixed suburban and rural population, the Musculoskeletal Intervention Center (MUSIC) Norrtälje study, exposure to forward bending (for at least 60 minutes a day) and holding a job which comprised mostly routine work without the possibility of learning new skills were shown to be independent risk factors for low back pain in men after adjustment for age, body mass index, job strain, social support at work and outside work, physical exercise, low back pain episodes previously, and negative life events during the past year. In this case the psychosocial job factor was measured by means of a special interview (Waldenström et al. 1998). The questionnaire based job strain measure was not a significant predictor of low back pain (Vingård et al. 1998). But for women the combination of high physical load (forward bending, manual materials handling, and high energy consumption during a typical working day) in combination with job strain (according to the Swedish demand–control questionnaire—high demands *and* low control) was associated with markedly elevated risk (RR = 3.6, with 95% confidence limits 1.3–10.9) of developing low back pain.

Psychiatric conditions have also been studied in relation to working conditions. In Karasek's early work (1979), depression and exhaustion were particularly common conditions in workers who reported high psychological demands and low decision latitude. Similar findings have been made in Japanese (Kawakami et al. 1992) and British studies (Stansfeld et al. 1995).

Research has also examined sick leave. The patterning of psychosocial job effects on sick leave is more complicated than that of psychosocial job effects on other health outcomes. The reason for this is that sick leave rates are more culturally and financially determined than other outcomes. North et al. (1996) have shown strong relationships in the expected direction between low decision latitude and sick leave among state employees in England, even after adjustment for a number of confounders. The effects of psychological demands were different in different social strata, although in general, high psychological demands did predict increased sick leave when they were combined with low decision latitude. In this study, expert ratings and self-reports were associated with similar excess risks. Peter and Siegrist (1997) have shown strong relationships between the effort–reward model and sick leave in middle managers.

The future

The workplace is undergoing major changes in almost all parts of the world as economies develop and as different societies adapt to the emerging markets. This dynamic environment makes it an exciting time to study the influences of the workplace on health outcomes. Moreover, it suggests that this may be a time when people can make fundamental changes in the workplace to influence the lives of workers in the future. Some of the studies we have discussed in this chapter become especially relevant with this end in sight. For example, the demand–control model research has shed light on elements of the workplace environment that are particularly amenable to organizational change. Thus, conclusions that we derive from the research might be used to benefit people very dramatically.

In order to work toward such goals, we need to do research in some previously un-derdeveloped areas. For example, the effect of workplace environments on women's health is not well researched. It is important to consider the fact that men and women differ in psychosocial correlates of cardiovascular illness (Theorell 1991; Hall 1990). Similarly, there is room for more comprehensive study of ethnic and social subgroups in populations, as these groups may have different health-related responses to workplace environments.

In these changing times, it will also be important to examine larger social forces that may shape work environments of all people. With this lens, we may better understand how the new work environments will effect health. For example, in many of the industrialized nations, we may expect some of the following changes to influence our workplace:

1. Increasing financial competition, which may place greater demands to produce more with limited resources and time.
2. Changing communication strategies, which may alter the way we do business and where we do business.
3. Increasing risks of becoming unemployed or being required to change jobs, which may create new types of strains for workers in new functions and for those who remain in their old positions.

Research that takes such factors into consideration will be well positioned to help make changes in the work environment and to ensure that new work environments are designed to enhance health from the start.

REFERENCES

Åkerstedt, T. (1988). Sleepiness as a consequence of shift work. *Sleep,* 11:17–34.

Alfredsson, L. (1983). Myocardial infarction and environment: use of registers in epidemiology. Karolinska Institute, Stockholm (doctoral dissertation).

Alfredsson, L., and Theorell, T. (1983). Job characteristics of occupations and myocardial infarction risk: effects of possible confounding factors. *Soc Sci Med,* 17:1497–503.

Alfredsson, L., Hammar, N., and Hogstedt, C. (1992). Incidence of myocardial infarction and mortality from specific causes among bus drivers. *Int J Epidemiol,* 22:57–61.

Alfredsson, L., Hammar, N., de Faire, U., Hallqvist, J., Theorell, T., and Westerholm, P. (1997). Self-reported job strain, blood lipids and fibrinogen baseline results from the WOLF study (abstract). *Can J Cardiol*, 13 Suppl B: 153B.

Arbetsmiljölag. (1976). Swedish law on work environment. SOU 1976:1.

Belkic, K., Ercegovac, D., Savic, C., Panic, B., Djordjevic, M., and Savic, S. (1992). EEG and cardiovascular reactivity in professional drivers: the glare pressor test. *Eur Heart J*, 13:304–9.

Belkic, K., Savic, C., Theorell, T., Rakic, L., Ercegovac, D., and Djordjevic, M. (1994). Mechanisms of cardiac risk in professional drivers. *Scand J Work Environ Health*, 20:73–86.

Biörck, G., Blomqvist, G., and Sievers, J. (1958). Studies on myocardial infarction in Malmö 1935–1954. II. infarction rate by occupational group. *Acta Med Scand*, 161:21–29.

Bosma, H.,. Marmot, M.G., Hemingway, H., Nicholson, A.C., Brunner, E., and Stansfeld, S.A. (1997). Low job control and risk of coronary heart disease in Whitehall II (prospective cohort study). *BMJ*, 314:558–65.

Bosma, H., Peter, R., Siegrist, J., and Marmot, M. (1998). Two alternative job stress models and the risk of coronary heart disease. *Am J Public Health*, 88:68–74.

Brenner, M.H. (1983). Unemployment and health in the context of economic change. *Soc Sci Med*, 17:1125–38.

Brunner, E., Davey Smith, G., Marmot, M., Canner, R., Beksinska, M. and O'Brien, J. (1996). Childhood social circumstances and psychosocial and behavioral factors as determinants of plasma fibrinogen. *Lancet*, 347: 1008–13.

Buell, P., and Breslow, L. (1960). Mortality from coronary heart disease in California men who work long hours. *J Chron Dis*, 11: 615–26.

Cooper, C.L., and Marshall, J. (1976). Occupational sources of stress: a review of the literature relating to coronary heart disease and mental ill health *J Occ Psychol*, 49:11–28.

Evans, G., and Carrere, S. (1991). Traffic congestion, perceived control and psychophysiological stress among urban bus drivers. *J Applied Psychol*, 76:658–63.

Green, K.L., and Johnson, J.V. (1990). The effects of psychosocial work organization on patterns of cigarette smoking among male chemical plant employees. *Am J Public Health*, 80:1368–71.

Gustavsson, P. (1989). Cancer and ischemic heart disease in occupational groups exposed to combustion products. *Arbete och Hälsa*, 1989:21. Solna, Sweden: National Institute of Occupational Health.

Haan, M. (1985). Job strain and cardiovascular disease: a ten-year prospective study. *Am J Epidemiol*, 122:532–40.

Hacker, W. (1978). *Allgemeine arbeits- und ingenieurpsychologie (General psychology of work and engineering)*. Bern: Huber.

Hall, E. M. (1990). Women's work: an inquiry into the health effects of invisible and visible labor. Karolinska Institute, Stockholm (doctoral dissertation).

Hall, E.M. (1992). Double exposure: the combined impact of the home and work environments on psychosomatic strain in Swedish women and men. *Int J Health Serv*, 22:239–60.

Hallquist, J., Diderichsen, F., Therorell, T., Reuterwall, C., Ahlbom, A. and the SHEEP study group. (1998). Is the effect of job strain on myocardial infarction risk due to interaction between high psychological demands and low decision latitude? Results from Stockholm Heart Epidemiology Program (SHEEP). *Soc Sci Med*, 46:1405– 15.

Hammar, N., Alfredsson, L., and Theorell, T. (1994). Job characteristics and incidence of myocardial infarction: a study of men and women in Sweden, with particular reference to job strain. *Int J Epidemiol*. 23:277–84.

Hammarström, A. (1994). Unemployment and change of tobacco habits: a study of young people from 16 to 21 years of age. *Addiction*, 89:1691–96.

Hedberg, G., Jacobsson, K. A., Janlert, U., and Langendoen, S. (1991). Riskindikatorer för ischemisk hjärtsjukdom i en kohort av manliga yrkesförare. *Arbete och hälsa*, 1991:48, Solna: National Institute of Occupational Health.

Hinkle, L.E., Whitney, L.H., Lehman, E.W., Dunn, J., Benjamin, B., King, R., Plakun, A., and Flehinger, B. (1968). Occupation, education and coronary heart disease. *Science*, 161:238–48.

Hlatky, M.A., Lam, L.C., Clapp-Channing, N.E., Williams, R.B., Pryor, D.B., Califf, R.M., and Mark, D.B. (1995). Job strain and the prevalence of and outcome of coronary artery disease. *Circulation*, 92:327–33.

House, J.S., Strecher, V., Metzner, H.L., and Robbins, C. (1986). Occupational stress and health among men and women in the Tecumseh Community Health Study. *J Health Soc Behav*, 27:62–77.

Janlert, U. (1992). Unemployment and blood pressure in Swedish building labourers. *J Intern Med*, 231:241–6.

Johnson, J.V., and Hall, E.M. (1988). Job strain, workplace social support and cardiovascular disease: a cross-sectional study of a random sample of the Swedish working population. *Am J Public Health*, 78:1336–42.

Johnson, J.V., and Stewart, E.M. (1993). Measuring life course exposure to the psychosocial work environment with a job exposure matrix. *Scand. J. Work Environ Health,* 19:21–28.

Johnson, J.V., Hall, E.M., and Theorell, T. (1989). Combined effects of job strain and social isolation on cardiovascular disease morbidity and mortality in a random sample of the Swedish male working population. *Scand J Work Environ Health,* 15:271–9.

Johnson, J., Stewart, W., Hall, E.M., Fredlund, P., and Theorell, T. (1996). Long-term psychosocial work environment and cardiovascular mortality among Swedish men. *Am J Publ Health,* 86:324–31.

Karasek, R.A. (1979). Job demands, job decision latitude, and mental strain: implications for job redesign. *Admin Sci Q,* 24:285–307.

Karasek, R.A., and Theorell, T. (1990). *Healthy work.* New York: Basic Books.

Karasek, R.A., Baker, D., Marxer, F., Ahlbom, A., and Theorell, T. (1981). Job decision latitude, job demands, and cardiovascular disease: a prospective study of Swedish men. *Am J Public Health,* 71:694–705.

Kasanen, A., Kallio, V., and Forsström, J. (1963). The significance of psychic and socioeconomic stress and other modes of life in the etiology of myocardial infarction. *Ann Med Intern Fenn,* 52 Suppl 43.

Kasl, S.V. (1996). The influence of the work environment on cardiovascular health: a historical, conceptual and methodological perspective. *J Occup Health Psychol,* 1:42–56.

Katz, D., and Kahn, R. (1966). *Social psychology of organizations.* New York: John Wiley.

Kawakami, N., Haratani, T., and Araki, S. (1992). Effects of perceived job stress on depressive symptoms in blue-collar workers of an electrical factory in Japan. *Scand J Work Environ Health,* 18:195–200.

Kilbom, Å., Armstrong, T., Buckle, P., Fine, L., Hagberg, M., Haring-Sweeney, M., Martin, B., Punnett, L., Silverstein, B., Sjögaard, G., Theorell, T., and Viikari-Juntura, E. (1996). Musculoskeletal disorders: work-related risk factors and prevention. *Int J Occup Environ Health,* 2:239–46.

Kittel, F., Kornitzer, M., and Dramaix, M. (1980). Coronary heart disease and job stress in two cohorts of bank clerks. *Psychother Psychosom,* 34:110–23.

Knutsson, A. (1989). Shift work and coronary heart disease. *Scand J Soc Med,* 44 Suppl: 1–36.

Knutsson, A., Hallquist, J., Reuterwall, C., Theorell, T., and Åkerstedt, T. (1999). Shiftwork and myocardial infarction: a case-control study. *Occup Environ Med,* 56:46–50.

Kornitzer, M., and Kittel, F. (1986). How does stress exert its effects—smoking, diet and obesity, physical activity. *Postgrad Med J,* 62:695–6.

Kornitzer, M., Kittel, F., Dramaix, M., and de Backer, G. (1982). Job stress and coronary heart disease. *Adv Cardiol,* 19:56–61.

La Croix, A.Z. (1984). Occupational exposure to high demand/low control work and coronary heart disease incidence in the Framingham cohort. University of North Carolina (doctoral dissertation).

Lennernäs, M. A.C. (1993). *Nutrition and shift work.* Karolinska Institute, Stockholm (doctoral dissertation).

Markowe, H.L., Marmot, M.G., Shipley, M.J., Bulpitt, C.J., Meade, T.W., Stirling, Y., Vickers, M.V., and Semmence, A. (1985). Fibrinogen: a possible link between social class and coronary heart disease. *BMJ,* 291: 1312–4.

Marmot, M., and Theorell, T. (1988). Social class and cardiovascular disease: the contribution of work. *Int J Health Serv,* 18:659–74.

Mattiasson, I., Lindgärde, F., Nilsson, J.Å., and Theorell, T. (1990). Threat of unemployment and cardiovascular risk factors: longitudinal study of quality of sleep and serum cholesterol concentrations in men threatened with redundancy. *BMJ,* 301:461–6.

Nirkko, O., Lauramaa, M., Siltanen, P., Tuominen, P., and Vanhala, K. (1982). Psychological risk factors related to coronary heart disease: prospective studies among policemen in Helsinki. *Acta Med Scand,* 660 Suppl: 137–45.

North, F.M., Syme, S.L., Feeney, A., Shipley, M., and Marmot, M.G. (1996). Psychosocial work environment and sickness absence: the Whitehall II Study. *Am J Public Health,* 86:332–40.

Ostfeld, A.M., Lebovits, B.Z., Shekelle, R.B., and Paul, O. (1964). A prospective study of the relationship between personality and coronary heart disease. *J Chron Dis,* 17: 265–73.

Pell, S., and d'Alonzo, C.A. (1963). Acute myocardial infarction in a large employed population: report of six-year study of 1,356 cases. *JAMA,* 185:831–41.

Peter, R., Alfredsson, L., Hammar, N., Siegrist, J., Theorell, T. and Westerholm, P. (1998). High effort, low reward, and cardiovascular risk factors in Swedish employed men and women: baseline results from the WOLF study. *J Epidemiol Community Health,* 52:540–7.

Peter, R., and Siegrist, J. (1997). Chronic work stress, sickness absence and hypertension in middle-managers: general or specific sociological explanations. *Soc Sci Med,* 45: 1111–20.

Public health report, County of Stockholm. (1994).

Reed, D.M., La Croix, A.Z., Karasek, R.A., Miller, D., and McLean, C.A. (1989). Occupational strain and the incidence of coronary heart disease. *Am J Epidemiol,* 129:495–502.

Reuterwall, C., Hallquist, J., Ahlbom, A., de Faire, U., Diderichsen, F., Hogstedt, C., Pershagen, G., Theorell, T., Wiman, B., Wolk, A., and the SHEEP study group. (1999). Higher relative but lower absolute risks of myocardial infarction in women than in men for some major risk factors in the SHEEP study. *J Internal Med,* in press.

Rosengren, A., Anderson, K., and Wilhelmsen, L. (1991). Risk of coronary heart disease in middle-aged bus and tram drivers compared to men in other occupations: a prospecitve study. *Int Epidemiol,* 20:82–7.

Rosengren, A., Eriksson, H., Larsson, B., Svärdsudd, K., Welin, L., Wilhelmsen, L., and Tibblin, G. (1997). CVD risk factors over three decades in 50-year-old men in Göteborg, Sweden. Paper presented at the International Congress on Preventive Cardiology, Montreal, Canada, June 29–July 3, 1997.

Russek, H.I., and Zohman, B.L. (1958). Relative significance of heredity, diet and occupational stress in coronary heart disease among young adults. *Am J Med Sci,* 235:266–75.

Schnall, P.L., Schwartz, J.E., Landsbergis, P.A., Warren, K., and Pickering, T.G. (1992). Relation between job strain, alcohol, and ambulatory blood pressure. *Hypertension,* 19:488–94.

Schnorr, T.M., Thun, M.J., and Halperin, W.E. (1987). Chest pain in users of video display terminals. *JAMA,* 257:627–40.

Schwartz, J., Pieper, C., and Karasek, R (1988). A procedure for linking job characteristics to health surveys. *Am J Public Health,* 78:904–9.

Siegrist, J. (1996). Adverse health effects of high effort/low reward conditions. *J Occ Health Psychol,* 1:27–41.

Siegrist, J., Matschinger, M., Cremer, P., and Seidel, D. (1988). Atherogenic risk in men suffering from occupational stress. *Atherosclerosis,* 69:211–8.

Siegrist, J., Peter, J., Junge, A., Cremer, A., and Seidel, D. (1990). Low status control, high effort at work and ischemic heart disease: prospective evidence from blue-collar men. *Soc Sc. Med,* 31:1127–34.

Stansfeld, S.A., North, F.M., White, I., and Marmot, M.G. (1995). Work characteristics and psychiatric disorder in civil servants in London. *J Epidemiol Comm Health,* 49:48–53.

Stjernström, E.L., Thelin, A., Holmberg, S., and

Svärdsudd, K. (1993). The occurrence of risk factors for CHD in farmers and non-farming controls in Sweden. Paper presented at the World Congress on Occupational Health, Nice, France, September 27, 1993.

Statistics Sweden. (1996). Appendix 16: The Swedish survey of living conditions. Stockholm: Statistics Sweden.

Söderfeldt, B., Söderfeldt, M., Jones, K., O'Campo, P., Muntaner, C., Ohlson, C.G., and Warg, LE. (1997). Does organization matter? A multilevel analysis of the demand–control model applied to human services. *Soc Sci Med,* 44:527–34.

Söndergård-Kristensen, T., and Damsgaard, M.T. (1987). *Hjerte-kar-sygdomme og arbejdsmiljö* [Cardiovascular disease and work environment]. Copenhagen: Arbejdsmiljöfondet.

Theorell, T. (1991). On cardiovascular health in women: results from epidemiological and psychosocial studies in Sweden. In Frankenhaeuser, M., Chesney, M., and Lundberg, U. (eds.), *Women, work and health.* Chicago: Plenum Press, pp. 187–204.

Theorell, T. (1996a). Possible mechanisms behind the relationship between the demand–control–support model and disorders of the locomotor system. In Moon, S.D., and Sauter, S.L. (eds.). *Beyond biomechanics: psychosocial aspects of musculoskeletal disorders in office work.* Bristol, PA: Taylor & Francis, 65–73.

Theorell, T. (1996b). The demand–control–support model for studying health in relation to the work environment: an interactive model. In Orth-Gomér, K. and Schneiderman, N. (eds.), Behavioral Medicine Approaches to Cardiovascular Disease Prevention. Mahwak, New Jersey: Lawrence Erlbaum, pp. 69–85.

Theorell, T., and Karasek, R.A. (1996). Current issues relating to psychosocial job strain and cardiovascular disease research. *J Occup Health Psychol,* 1:9–26.

Theorell, T., Nordemar, R., Michélsen, H., and the Stockholm Music I Study Group. (1993). Pain thresholds during standardized psychological stress in relation to perceived psychosocial work situation. *J Psychosom Res,* 37:299–305.

Theorell, T, Tsutsumi, A., Hallquist, J., Reuterwall, C., Hogstedt, C., Fredlund, P., Emlund, N., Johnson, J.V., and the SHEEP Study Group. (1998). Decision latitude, job strain and myocardial infarction: a study of working men in Stockholm. *Am J Public Health,* 88:382–8.

Vingård, E., Alfredsson, L., Hagberg, M., Kilbom, Å., Theorell, T., Waldenström, M.,

Wigéus Hjelm, E., Wiktorin, C., Hogstedt, C., and the MUSIC-Norrtälje Study Group. (1999). How much do current and past occupational physical and psychosocial factors explain of low back pain in a working population? in press *Spine*.

Volpert, W. (1989). Work and personality development from the viewpoint of the action regulation theory. In Leymann, H., and Kornbluh, F. (eds.), *Socialization at work: a new approach to the learning process in the workplace and society.* London: Glower.

Waldenström, M., Josephson, M., Persson, C. and Theorell, T. (1998). Interview reliability for assessing mental work demands. *J Occup Health Psychol*, 3:209–16.

Wamala, S.P., Wolk, A., Schenck-Gustafsson, K. and Orth-Gomér, K. (1997). Lipid profile and socio-economic status in healthy middle-aged women. *J Epidemiol Community Health*, 51:400–7.

Westerberg, L., and Theorell, T. (1997). Working conditions and family situation in relation to functional gastrointestinal disorders. The Swedish Dyspepsia Project. *Scand J Prim Health Care*,15:76–81.

6

The Impact of Job Loss and Retirement on Health

STANISLAV V. KASL AND BETH A. JONES

The evidence about the impact of work on health can be divided, artificially and arbitrarily, into the impact of the *chronic* (steady-state) work environment and the impact of *changes* in the work environment or in aspects of the work role. This is a distinction of convenience only. Consider some of the following possible scenarios: *(1)* Individuals cope with and adapt to enduring conditions so that the impact over time changes rather than remaining constant. *(2)* An expected and desired promotion that does not materialize becomes a changing situation of increasing failure and frustration while the objective work conditions remain the same. *(3)* An acute threat of downsizing becomes a chronic situation of indeterminate duration. *(4)* The acute event of retirement is preceded by decades of planning and rehearsing for the coming event. In short, while this chapter focuses only on changes in work, ideally the coverage should be of acute changes against the background of specific enduring work conditions.

A number of changes in one's work set-

ting and work role can be studied for their impact. Some are broad transitions from a life-cycle perspective while others may be specific changes in some aspect of one's work. Among the major transitions are those from schooling to initial job, from working to becoming unemployed, and from working to retiring. Other permutations are possible, from schooling to unemployment, from working to schooling, from unemployment to retirement, and from retirement to working again. Recognizing other states, such as working fewer hours than desired (underemployment), experiencing downward mobility after job loss, and working under the threat of losing one's job, increases the number of possible transitions of interest. Changes in specific aspects of work are too numerous to list here. Some major ones would include change in shift time, increases and decreases in workload, changes in supervision, changes in coworker relations, and increased mechanization and fractionation of tasks.

In this chapter we begin with studies of the impact of job loss on health and well-being and also consider studies of threat of job loss and of job insecurity. The second topic of this chapter, the impact of retirement, receives much less detailed coverage, primarily because the story here is less complicated and the evidence converges much more clearly: Most studies do not demonstrate a negative impact, except in very narrow domains of functioning or in very special subgroups.

In our review we wish not only to summarize some of the evidence but also to pay attention to issues of study design and conceptualization/measurement of exposure variables. While raised in the context of examining studies of the health impact of unemployment and retirement, these issues are generic for other domains of research in social epidemiology.

CONCEPTUAL AND METHODOLOGICAL ISSUES IN STUDIES OF JOB LOSS

In classical occupational epidemiology, it is generally a straightforward task to define and operationalize the exposure variable, its dose and duration, the pathways of exposure, and so on. In unemployment studies, the exposure variable is potentially more complex than can be captured by a simple dichotomy, employed vs. unemployed. One issue centers on the meaning of work and the impact work can have on individuals and their families. Jahoda (1992) suggests that a job, aside from meeting economic needs, has additional "latent functions": It (1) imposes time structure on the day, (2) implies regularly shared experiences and contacts with others, (3) links an individual to goals and purposes which transcend his/her own, (4) defines aspects of personal status and identity, and (5) enforces activity. Warr (1987) discusses a number of environmental features of work which he postulates are responsible for psychological well-being: opportunity for control, skill use, interpersonal contact, external goal and task demands, variety, environmental clarity, availability of money, physical security, and

valued social position. In addition, for some individuals, job loss may represent the termination of exposures, such as work stress or specific work hazards, which themselves may be adverse influences on health.

The implication of such formulations is that the experience of job loss and unemployment is likely to be multifaceted and involve different intervening processes, moderating influences, and outcomes. At a minimum, one should try to separate the effects of economic hardships from the other effects of unemployment (Jahoda 1992), a distinction that many studies do not address.

The unemployment experience may also affect subgroups of individuals differently. For example, age (and stage of the life cycle) is an important consideration: The unemployment experience is likely to be different for (1) a young person completing his/her education and unable to find a job vs. (2) a young worker with unclear career goals, and in his/her first job which s/he finds unsatisfying vs. (3) a middle-aged head of household, with dependents at home, losing a long-held job made obsolete by new technology vs. (4) an elderly worker, in poor health and close to retirement, in a job which is physically demanding.

A labor economic perspective on unemployment introduces additional issues. For example, Burchell (1992) argues for the need to understand the broader context of the labor market when studying the psychological health of unemployed individuals. In particular, he points to the inappropriate neglect of other labor market phenomena such as job insecurity, promotions and demotions, and stagnated careers. Cahill (1983) argues from a broader macroeconomic perspective and argues for the need to attend to five characteristics of the current economic system: instability in the business cycle, unemployment, inequality in income distribution, capital mobility, and fragmentation of the work process.

The most dominant methodological issue in unemployment research centers on the distinction between causation and selection: Does the observation of poorer physical and mental health reflect the impact of unemployment or does it, instead, denote the influence of prior characteristics of the individuals who later become unemployed? The latter alternative, biased selection into exposure status, could reflect either *(1)* the direct influence of health, i.e., persons with poorer health are more likely to become unemployed, or *(2)* indirect influence of characteristics, such as disadvantaged social status and unstable occupational career, which lead to greater likelihood of both unemployment and poorer health. The interpretive dilemma, causation vs. selection, also applies to studies in which the independent (exposure) variable is either length of unemployment or the contrast between reemployment vs. continued unemployment: the poorer health of those with prolonged unemployment could again be either because this reflects a higher dose of the exposure variable or because those with prior poorer health have a lower chance of being reemployed.

The evidence on unemployment and health supports both the causation and the selection interpretations (Schwefel 1986; Miles 1987; Bartley 1988; Jahoda 1992; Wilson and Walker 1993; Hammarstrom 1994a and 1994b; Jin et al. 1995; Arrow 1996; Dooley et al. 1996; Shortt 1996). The two interpretations are not incompatible, even within a single study. We note that this broad conclusion is actually based on a variety of types of evidence: *(1)* ambiguous results where either or both interpretations are tenable, *(2)* evidence for selection but not causation, *(3)* evidence for causation (usually after statistical adjustments for some set of prior characteristics) but not selection, and *(4)* evidence for both within the same study. Studies which show no difference in health or well-being between the employed and the unemployed are relatively rare since selection reflects the broader effects of social disadvantage on health. Thus, studies likely to show no difference are generally those where the two groups (of employed and unemployed) are selected to be

highly comparable on most background variables.

Many different study designs have been used to examine the impact of unemployment on health and well-being (e.g., Kasl 1982; Stern 1983; Cook 1985). One primary distinction made among designs (e.g., Cook 1985; Catalano 1991) is whether the data are aggregated (also referred to as ecological or macroeconomic) or are based on individuals. The ecological studies are briefly evaluated in the next section, while below we comment on epidemiological designs using data on individuals.

With the exception of some controlled randomized intervention programs (Caplan et al. 1989; Vinokur et al. 1991; Price 1992; Proudfoot et al. 1997) designed to promote job search skills and thereby prevent adverse mental health consequences of prolonged unemployment, the usual design in studies of unemployment and health is an observational (nonexperimental) study, both longitudinal and cross-sectional. Retrospective case–control designs are relatively rare in unemployment research with the possible exception of suicide studies (Platt 1984).

Longitudinal studies of unemployment use three kinds of designs:

1. Natural experiments: The typical study is one of a plant or factory closure in which all employees lose their jobs and are then followed for health status changes. Morris and Cook (1991) have discussed the advantages and disadvantages of such an approach. The primary advantages are the absence of self-selection and the possibility of collecting baseline data before the plant closes. Possible disadvantages include: *(a)* There may be difficulty in finding a sufficiently comparable control group of stably employed workers; *(b)* generally, small numbers of subjects are studied; *(c)* high specificity of the setting and the circumstances of the plant closing may reduce generalizability; *(d)* "baseline" data may be collected when subjects are already aware of the impending event and many variables

may show anticipatory effects (Kasl et al. 1968; Kasl and Cobb 1970).

2. Longitudinal comparisons of the employed and unemployed: This design is rather weak when no baseline data are available on health and social characteristics of the two cohorts. This weakness is aggravated if the "exposed" cohort has been unemployed for a long time (thus allowing further self-selection to take place since healthier subjects may become reemployed sooner) and if no retrospective data are available on the circumstances of the original job loss. If the unemployed cohort has already experienced adverse health changes by the start of the follow-up, adjustments for initial differences will overcorrect in analyses intended to only adjust for self-selection.

3. Follow-up of the unemployed to detect benefits of reemployment: This design can offer highly suggestive results if the unemployed show an improvement in health or well-being after becoming reemployed, if this improvement brings them up to par with the continuously employed, and if the continuously unemployed do not show such an improvement. The reasonable inference is that the variable showing improvement had declined earlier due to the impact of the unemployment. Two caveats are in order here: (a) If the unemployment experience has already produced irreversible changes on some outcome by the start of follow-up (but this cannot be detected, given the design), the failure to show improvement after reemployment should not lead to the interpretation that this outcome had not been affected by unemployment. (b) The usual monitoring of a cohort may not be sufficiently frequent to identify correctly the underlying temporal sequence. For example, recovery from depression among the unemployed may precede finding a new job, while failure to recover from depression may interfere with job search. Thus self-selection is at work in the observed association of depression with reemployment. And this could be the case even if there is a true initial impact of unemployment on depression.

Cross-sectional designs showing an association between unemployment and poor health normally cannot disentangle the causation vs. selection interpretations. Statistical adjustments can be made for the influence of stable social characteristics, such as education, but these can control, at best, for indirect selection only. However, there may be additional variables which allow for stratified analyses or more extensive statistical controls, and thus somewhat stronger inferences. For example, retrospective information regarding original circumstances of the job loss might identify a subgroup of unemployed to whom self-selection processes are unlikely to apply.

We should also note the existence of a *hybrid* design in which data on individuals are supplemented with ecological information on economic indicators for the community or the region (e.g., Dooley et al. 1988; Turner 1995). This is a strong design, particularly when longitudinal data are collected. Specifically, it enables one to answer two additional questions: *(1)* Do changes in community level of unemployment impact on the health and well-being of those who remain employed? *(2)* Do the levels of community unemployment moderate the impact on the unemployed—e.g., is the impact on the individual unemployed person greater when the community level of unemployment is high vs. low?

Overall, this discussion of conceptual and methodological issues permits the conclusion that job loss as an acute event and unemployment as a potentially enduring exposure are both richly embedded in a social matrix involving the interdependence of the individual, the family, the network of friends and relatives, the immediate community, the regional economy, and the society as a whole. This leaves ample room for variability of impact, linked to variations in the meaning of the experience and to the role of diverse moderators which can affect the process and the outcomes. All this represents a formidable challenge to investigators trying to meet the two major goals: *(1)* to isolate one broad cause–effect relationship, from unemployment to health and well-being, from a larger matrix of causal and reciprocal influences, and *(2)* to capture the richness of the phenomenon of unemployment and the diversity of the underlying etiological dynamics.

A NOTE ON ECOLOGICAL AND BUSINESS CYCLE ANALYSES

Studies that use cross-sectional ecological data with some geopolitical entity as the unit of aggregation (e.g., Charlton et al. 1987; Robinson and Pinch 1987; Mackenbach and Looman 1994; Borrell and Arias 1995) cannot really go much beyond noting the coexistence of high unemployment with high mortality (or some other outcome). Statistical adjustments for potential confounders can reduce somewhat the ambiguity of such associations but disentangling causal pathways remains quite difficult.

Of greater interest are ecological analyses of time series data in which annual fluctuations in some economic indicator, often the nationwide percent of the labor force that is unemployed, are related to annual changes in some outcome, such as total mortality, cause-specific mortality, alcohol consumption, and acts of domestic violence. There is no doubt that the foremost practitioner of the aggregate time series approach during the last 20 years has been M.H. Brenner (Brenner 1983, 1987a–c; Brenner and Monney 1983). While his approach has become more sophisticated over the years and his statistical models have included a longer list of potential confounders and control variables, his fundamental strategy has remained the same: to demonstrate that fluctuations in some economic indicator, such as unemployment and business failures, are causally associated with fluctuations in some adverse outcome, particularly total or cause-specific mortality. Adjustments are made for various short- and long-term trends, and time lags of varying lengths are explored. The unvarying conclusion in

Brenner's reports is that, indeed, unemployment adversely impacts a nation's health.

Brenner's work has been aptly characterized as "controversial but ground-breaking" (Shortt 1996, p. 570). Some early critics (e.g., Eyer 1977a,b) didn't object to the overall macroeconomic strategy as much as to the broad conclusions; i.e., they saw an association of mortality rates with business booms, not economic depressions. Other critics (e.g., Cohen and Felson 1979) were disturbed by the strong inferences for public policy drawn from such difficult-to-interpret data analytic strategies. The last 10 to 15 years have produced numerous critical examinations of this methodology and of the results it has yielded (Kasl 1979, 1982; Gravelle et al. 1981; Colledge 1982; Spruit 1982; Wagstaff 1985; Forbes and McGregor 1987; Starrin et al. 1990; Morris and Cook 1991; Sogaard 1992). The net effect of such scrutiny has been to provide a basis for considerable skepticism about the data and the conclusions. At the same time, there is no consensus about just what exactly is wrong with the methodology, how exactly it may bias the findings, and what are the correct analytic strategies. Dooley and Catalano, themselves quite sophisticated researchers, arrive at an indeterminate conclusion that "the field is uncertain how to interpret the findings from the aggregate time series approach" (1988, p. 6).

Briefly, some of the criticisms of Brenner's work and of the aggregate time series approach have been: *(1)* inability to understand and follow the actual methods used, based on information provided; *(2)* inability to replicate the findings using the *same* data; *(3)* inability to obtain similar results when carrying out attempted cross-validation with comparable data; *(4)* apparent arbitrariness of selected time lags; *(5)* insufficient justification for detrending strategies which often drastically alter the findings; *(6)* difficulty in estimating the magnitude of effects attributable to economic variables; and *(7)* inappropriateness of units of analysis (e.g., total country) when there is substantial variation in the independent and dependent variables at levels of smaller geopolitical units, suggesting the need for a finer grained analysis. It might also be noted that all analyses so far have been of past trends; no investigator seems to have attempted to develop a model from past data to forecast future trends or to use one segment of past data to develop a model to "forecast" trends in a later segment of past data. Developing successful models which predict future trends would address the criticism that the analyses are tailor-made and distorted in order to obtain the expected results.

THE IMPACT OF UNEMPLOYMENT ON MORTALITY

There are a number of epidemiologic studies which have examined the relationship between unemployment and mortality. Three British reports are based on a 10-year follow-up of men in the Office of Population Censuses and Survey (OPCS) longitudinal study (Moser et al. 1984, 1986, 1987). Men who were seeking work during the week before the 1971 survey had a higher age-adjusted mortality than would be expected from the rates in the total OPCS; after adjustment for social class, the obtained Standardized Mortality Ratio (SMR) was 121. Particularly high mortality was observed for suicide (SMR = 169). Statistical adjustments for possible prior health status differences were not possible. A shorter follow-up of men after the 1981 census confirmed the earlier findings but obtained a somewhat lower adjusted SMR of 112. Analyses by regions of the country suggested that the region with the highest mortality and unemployment rates had higher SMRs due to unemployment.

A recent report by Morris et al. (1994) is based on a prospective cohort study (British Regional Heart Study). All men (ages 40–59) had been continuously employed for at least 5 years before initial screening. On a postal questionnaire 5 years later, they indicated changes in employment during the previous 5 years. Then they were followed

for 5.5 years (after the questionnaire) for mortality. Compared to the continuously employed men, those who had some unemployment (but not due to illness, according to self reports) showed an elevated age-adjusted relative risk (RR) of 1.59. This was reduced only slightly to RR = 1.47 with further adjustment for social class, smoking, alcohol intake, and preexisting disease at screening. Two additional groups are of interest: those "retired not due to illness" had an RR of 1.86 and those "unemployed or retired due to illness" had an RR of 3.14. Both values are adjusted for the full set of covariates. The RR for retirement suggests that it is a more adverse experience than unemployment—an improbable conclusion, given the uniform evidence that retirement per se doesn't have a negative impact on mortality (see below). The high value of an RR of 3.14 for those citing illness as reason for not working reveals the inadequacy of baseline health status adjustments which used data from the time when they all were still continuously employed. This suggests that baseline health status needs to be updated in such studies and/or supplemented with adjustments for reports of illness reasons for not working.

A number of additional reports are available for Sweden (Stefansson 1991), Finland (Martikainen 1990), Denmark (Iversen et al. 1987), and Italy (Costa and Segnan 1987); they all use designs similar to the British OPCS analyses. Several conclusions are suggested: (1) Excess mortality associated with unemployment is observed in all studies, with the magnitude of effect generally between SMRs of 150 and 200, adjusted for age and socioeconomic status. (2) Gender differences were examined in two studies, with the Danish data showing no gender difference in magnitude of effect attributable to unemployment, while the Swedish data showed a much weaker impact on women (SMR = 114). (3) Adjustments for sociodemographics generally reduce the magnitude of effect, while additional adjustments for various (imperfect) indicators of health status make much less of a difference. *(4)* Younger subjects tend to show stronger effects of unemployment, but these effects do not vary consistently by subgroups of occupational status. *(5)* Cause-specific analyses suggest that suicides, accidents, violent deaths, and alcohol-related deaths tend to be especially elevated, but do not explain all of the excess mortality. *(6)* Analyses by regional unemployment rates were possible in the Danish data. These showed that in regions of higher unemployment, the impact attributable to the unemployed status of individuals was weaker, thus contradicting the British OPCS results (Moser et al. 1986). A recent Finnish study (Martikainen and Valkonen 1996) found that the association between unemployment and mortality weakened as the general unemployment rate increased over time.

These results from Europe are contradicted by a U.S. study which matched U.S. Census Bureau Current Population Surveys to the National Death Index (Sorlie and Rogot 1990). After adjusting for age, education, and income, the SMRs due to unemployment, among those 45–64 years of age, were 107 for men and 81 for women; neither was significantly different from an SMR of 100. There was some hint of an effect among younger men (35–44), but the numbers were too small to yield a reliable conclusion. This discrepancy with the European data is not easily explained, particularly since it is believed that the "social net" protecting the unemployed is stronger in these European countries than in the United States.

It is worth emphasizing that strong causal inferences are seldom justified from these observational studies. Even apparently good evidence, such as the unemployment suicide association, is neither so consistent nor so compelling as to allow the conclusion that the causal issue has been settled (Platt 1984; Dooley et al. 1989; Platt et al. 1992; Johansson and Sundquist 1997). Platt points out that the prior role of psychiatric illness in both the unemployment and the (later) suicide has not been satisfactorily ruled out.

THE IMPACT OF UNEMPLOYMENT ON PHYSICAL MORBIDITY

Studies of unemployment and physical morbidity introduce a new concern not applicable to mortality studies: the measurement of health status outcomes. There are at least two concerns: *(1)* The influence of psychological distress on measurement: physical symptoms and complaints could be due to the distress rather than some underlying physical condition or distress could lower the threshold for reporting existing physical symptoms. *(2)* Measures based on seeking and/or receiving care could indicate differences in illness behavior rather than underlying illness.

Morris and Cook (1991) review about ten studies which represent longitudinal investigations of factory closures. In some of these studies, the measures of outcomes are difficult to interpret. Thus in a nicely designed prospective study of closure of a sardine factory in Norway (Westin et al. 1988, 1989; Westin 1990a,b), the rates of disability pension observed over a 10-year follow-up period were higher compared to rates at a nearby "sister factory" which didn't close. While these pensions are "granted for medical conditions only," it is still difficult to know what exactly is being assessed and what health status differences would have been observed with other types of measurements. In another study, the outcome was rates of medical consultation, which are difficult to interpret, particularly in the absence of a control group (Yuen and Balarajan 1986).

There is reasonable agreement in the several longitudinal studies that the job loss experience has some negative impact on health, though the precise nature of this impact is difficult to pinpoint. For example, in a Canadian study of factory closure (Grayson 1989), former employees reported about 2.5 times more ailments during a 27-month follow-up than the expected average. What these results mean is difficult to determine. The higher prevalence was for a wide range of conditions, e.g., headaches, acute respiratory ailments, ulcers, arthritis, sight and hearing disorders, and dental troubles. Only heart disease, asthma, and endocrine diseases showed no significant differences. The authors offer the interpretation that these data indicate higher levels of stress, which produce "a series of symptoms that people mistake for illness itself."

In an earlier Michigan study of two plants that shut down and of several control plants (Cobb and Kasl 1977), the number of men studied was rather small, with resultant low power to detect differences in disease conditions. However, there were two suggestive findings involving higher rates among the unemployed: *(1)* dyspepsia (ulcer activity) among those with no ulcer history and *(2)* observed joint swellings suggestive of rheumatoid arthritis. Measures based on administrations of a 2-week health diary, including *days complaint* ("did not feel as well as usual") and *days disability* ("did not carry out usual activities") showed significant fluctuations over time, but not those which could be linked to employment–unemployment status changes (Kasl et al. 1975). For example, *the measure days complaint* was elevated when they were interviewed 6 weeks before the plant closing, when all men were still working but fully aware of the coming event. Some 6 weeks after closure when many of the men were unemployed, levels of *days complaint* were significantly below average, and this was true irrespective of work status. At 6–8 months after the plant closing the levels were elevated again, and equally so for men still unemployed as for those recently reemployed or those who were stabilizing their employment.

A British study of factory closure examined the impact on general practice consultation rates (Beale and Nethercott 1987, 1988a,b). The closure was clearly associated with increased rates of consultations, referrals, and visits to the hospital. Consultations for very common illnesses did not show the impact; rather, the increase was for "chronic" illnesses, those conditions which had required in the past four or more consultations per year. It is not clear if these conditions were exacerbated by the factory closure or if there was simply a higher rate of consulting without any underlying clinical changes.

A Danish study of shipyard workers (Iversen et al. 1989) obtained somewhat different results from those noted above: The relative risk of admission to hospital in the study group, compared to controls, declined from 1.29 some 4–5 years before closure to 0.74 for the 3 years thereafter. Cause-specific analyses revealed strong declines for accidents and diseases of the digestive system. Increases were observed for circulatory and cardiovascular diseases (0.8 to 1.6 and 1.0 to 2.6, respectively). The authors suggest that two processes are at work: the workers are removed from workplace hazards, on the one hand, and exposed to stresses of unemployment, on the other.

There are many reports of cross-sectional associations between unemployment and poor health. Some are based on excellent datasets, such as the Canada Health Survey (D'Arcy and Siddique 1985; D'Arcy 1986), the British General Household Survey (Arber 1987), and the British Regional Heart Study (Cook et al. 1982). In general, such studies provide very poor control of prior health status, creating potential for selection bias. In the Heart Study, the authors separated the unemployed into those who did and did not regard their unemployment as being due to ill-health. The latter group, which is more appropriate for examining the impact of unemployment, were quite comparable to the employed men on self-reported history of chronic conditions. On four major illnesses diagnosed from the screening information, the two groups were comparable on bronchitis, hypertension, and obstructive lung disease; only on ischemic heart disease were the unemployed men significantly higher.

THE IMPACT OF UNEMPLOYMENT ON BIOLOGICAL AND BEHAVIORAL RISK FACTORS

The biological variables which have been examined in relation to unemployment include *(1)* indicators of "stress" reactivity, such as neuroendocrine changes, which do not have a well-documented relationship to specific diseases; (2) a very diverse set of indicators of immune functioning which are linked to possible disease outcomes theoretically rather than empirically; and (3) risk factors for specific diseases, typically cardiovascular disease, where the presumption is that a chronic impact on these due to unemployment translates into higher risk for clinical disease.

Studies which have examined *neuroendocrine* variables (Cobb 1974; Cobb and Kasl 1977; Fleming et al. 1984; Arnetz et al. 1987; Brenner and Levi 1987; Brenner and Starrin 1988) show a range of findings which do not allow any simple conclusion: (1) no effects; (2) large fluctuations within the continuously unemployed, and thus not easily linked to work status changes; (3) inconsistent effects of duration of unemployment; and (4) well-replicated strong anticipation effects. One interesting observation was that a greater magnitude of the anticipatory reaction was associated with shorter length of subsequent unemployment (Cobb and Kasl 1977). Overall, it is likely that neuroendocrine parameters are better suited for describing acute phases of reactivity rather than chronic stress effects suggestive of increased risk of future disease.

There appears to be only one study which has examined *immune functioning* in relation to unemployment. (Arnetz et al. 1987; Brenner and Levi 1987). The results suggested that unemployment lasting more than 9 months is accompanied by a significant decrease in immune function; after 24 months of unemployment, normal reactivity was restored. There were no benefits of a psychosocial intervention administered to some of the unemployed. These findings apply to some, but by no means all, indicators of immune functioning used in the study.

The impact of employment–unemployment on *cardiovascular risk factors* has also been examined. Analyses of blood pressure and serum cholesterol changes from the Michigan study of a plant closure (Kasl and Cobb 1982) revealed a substantial sensitivity of these variables to the experience of an-

ticipating the closing of the plant, losing the job and going through a period of unemployment, and finding a new job. However, these were acute effects reflecting specific transitions. Men who continued to be unemployed did not continue to show elevated levels; their levels declined even in the absence of finding a new job. Two years after the event, the study cohort had "normal" blood pressure levels and somewhat below normal cholesterol levels.

Janlert et al. (1992) have reported on cross-sectional results from a population survey (ages 25–64) conducted in northern Sweden. Data on lifetime history of unemployment were used to create two contrasting groups: unemployed for 1 year or more vs. never unemployed or unemployed for less than 1 year. Men with a more serious history of unemployment were higher on systolic blood pressure, serum cholesterol levels, and cigarettes smoked daily, and lower on high density lipoproteins (HDL) and physical activity. However, the authors were unable to rule out selection as an alternative explanation.

An Irish study (Cullen et al. 1987) reported cross-sectional results from the pilot phase of a study of young men and women (ages 16–23) who were either unemployed, or blue collar trainees, or in white collar jobs. Data on blood pressure, heart rate, height, weight, and percent body fat were examined. While a few significant differences were obtained in comparisons of the three groups, none were supportive of the notion that the unemployed youth would be higher on the risk variables.

There are several reports which are concerned with the impact of unemployment on *health habits* and *behavioral risk factors*. The typical variables examined include cigarette smoking, alcohol consumption, body weight, and physical exercise. Longitudinal data from the British Regional Heart Study (Morris et al. 1992, 1994) showed only an increase in weight attributable to unemployment; there was no evidence for such impact on cigarette or alcohol consumption. Because of the longitudinal nature of the data, the study was able to show that higher levels of smoking and heavy drinking were predictive of greater likelihood of subsequent unemployment. The Michigan data (Kasl and Cobb 1980) showed that cigarette smoking remained quite stable and was not sensitive to the job loss experience. Data on body weight did suggest an impact; however, the effect was a decrease following reemployment rather than an increase due to job loss. While those who lost their jobs did not show long-term trends different from controls, they did show greater temporal instability in phase-to-phase weight changes over the 2 years of observation.

Cross-sectional data generally do show an association between unemployment and adverse health behaviors (e.g., Raitakari et al. 1995; Rasky et al. 1996). However, the U.S. national cross-sectional data on unemployment and behavioral risk factors (Schoenborn and National Center for Health Statistics 1988) show a mixed and confusing picture: For some health habits the unemployed showed adverse effects; for other habits, beneficial effects; and for still others, no effects.

Alcohol consumption has been of particular interest to unemployment investigators, but it is difficult to arrive at a coherent picture. Longitudinal data on alcohol consumption yield a somewhat mixed picture. In a Norwegian study of young people (ages 17–20), results showed that unemployment did not increase consumption of alcohol (Hammer 1992); in fact, in a high-consumption subgroup, unemployment led to a decrease. But an analysis of panel data from a psychiatric epidemiologic study (Catalano et al. 1993) suggested that the incidence of clinically significant alcohol abuse was greater among those who had been laid off than among those who had not been laid off. Interestingly, employed persons in communities with higher unemployment were at reduced risk of becoming alcohol abusers. This study shows the strength of the hybrid design in which both individual-level and community-level data are collected. Two recent reports based on cross-sectional data

(Lahelma et al. 1995; Ettner 1997) suggest the possibility of no effects or even reduced alcohol consumption as a result of unemployment. In general, reviews of the alcohol consumption and unemployment literature (e.g., Forcier 1988; Hammarstrom 1994a and 1994b) point to many difficulties in arriving at a coherent picture regarding documented impact. For example, losing a job may increase the need for alcohol consumption but also reduce the ability of the unemployed to afford such expenditures. The conclusion that both causation and selection ("drift") dynamics are supported by the evidence is perhaps the most suitable one (Dooley et al. 1992).

THE IMPACT OF UNEMPLOYMENT ON MENTAL HEALTH AND WELL-BEING

There is little doubt that unemployment has a negative impact on mental health and well-being. Longitudinal studies strongly support the expectation that unemployment has an adverse impact on subclinical symptomatology or symptoms of poor mental health (e.g., Frese and Mohr 1987; Kaplan et al. 1987; Brenner and Starrin 1988; Warr et al. 1988); it is unlikely that the impact is also on overt diagnosable clinical disorders, but only one study is available for this conclusion (Dew et al. 1987). Longitudinal studies also generally demonstrate that becoming reemployed is associated with a reduction in symptomatology (Kessler et al. 1987a, 1988; Ensminger and Celentano 1988; Iversen and Sabroe 1988; Warr et al. 1988). One striking exception is a report (Dooley et al. 1988) which found that the transition from unemployment to reemployment was accompanied by an increase in symptoms. The longitudinal reemployment studies also allow for an examination of selection processes which might be involved in influencing chances of reemployment. By and large, the evidence (e.g., Kessler et al. 1987a, 1988, 1991; Warr et al. 1988) suggests that levels of symptoms do not significantly predict reemployment, but

SOCIAL EPIDEMIOLOGY

this is not always the case, (e.g., Beiser et al. 1993).

Among different domains of distress, the evidence suggests that depression is more likely to be affected by unemployment than other dimensions, such as anxiety or psychophysiological symptoms. Impact on other outcomes has also been documented, such as lower self-confidence and higher externality (one's life is beyond one's control); self-esteem may be affected only on items which reflect self-criticism (Warr et al. 1988).

A number of studies have concerned themselves with the impact of unemployment on *young adults* (Cullen et al. 1987; Broomhall and Winefield 1990; Graetz 1993; Winefield et al. 1993; Hammarstrom 1994a,b; Morrell et al. 1994; Fryer 1997; Patterson 1997; Schaufeli 1997). The experience being investigated may be different than for older adults since *(1)* the transition is often from school to unemployment rather than from employment to unemployment, *(2)* the employed respondents can also experience adaptation stress because of new work role demands, and *(3)* other significant changes may be taking place for all of them, such as leaving home, which could attenuate the impact of the specific employed–unemployed contrast.

Several of the reports are based on Australian longitudinal studies. The Adelaide study (Winefield et al. 1993) showed that *(1)* the difference between the employed and the unemployed was due to the fact that getting a job was associated with improved well-being rather than a decline in well-being due to becoming unemployed; *(2)* those who were dissatisfied on their jobs (a minority) had low levels of well-being comparable to the unemployed; *(3)* leaving school was associated with greater impact than that due to employment status differences. A second Australian study (Graetz 1993) obtained similar results. Specifically, symptoms were highest among dissatisfied workers and lowest among satisfied workers, with the unemployed at intermediate levels. Furthermore, *(1)* increases in symptoms were comparable whether the transition

was from employment to unemployment or from studying to unemployment, and *(2)* decreases in symptoms were comparable whether the transition was from unemployment to employment or from studying to employment. A third Australian study (Morrell et al. 1994) showed that the negative psychological impact of the employment-to-unemployment transition was fully reversed among those who then became reemployed; among those continuing to remain unemployed, there was no further negative impact.

A report based on the British national child development study (Montgomery et al. 1996) is a very important reminder that factors in childhood may represent precursors of unemployment in young adulthood. For example, men with short stature and poor social adjustment in childhood were at greater risk of unemployment, even after controlling for socioeconomic background, education, and parental height.

Some studies have been concerned with the impact of unemployment on *women* and with possible gender differences in impact. One study (Dew et al. 1992) showed higher depressive symptoms but only among women with longer unemployment; becoming reemployed was not associated with a decrease in such symptoms. The same research team (Penkower et al. 1988) also examined the impact of a husband's layoff on the wife. Elevated symptoms were observed, but only during the second year of follow-up, and this was true whether or not the husbands had become reemployed. Reports of cross-sectional results suggest either no gender differences in impact of unemployment (e.g., Ensminger and Celentano 1990; Schaufeli and Van Yperen 1992), or somewhat stronger effects on women, particularly in the health care seeking area (D'Arcy 1986), or somewhat weaker effects for women (Harding and Sewel 1992).

Rural–urban differences in impact are also of interest. One study (Dooley et al. 1981) failed to replicate in a nonmetropolitan community the effect of unemployment on depressed mood previously described for a metropolitan community. Harding and Sewel (1992), in their study of a Scottish island community, also suggest that the impact of unemployment in the rural setting may be weaker. Results from the Michigan study (Kasl and Cobb 1982) revealed the expected impact on mental health indicators in the urban setting, while in the rural setting, the impact was on work role deprivation scales (i.e., missing aspects of work and work-related activities). A Dutch study (Leeflang et al. 1992), however, did not find rural–urban differences in mental health impact.

Some studies have attempted to identify possible *mediators* of the impact of unemployment on mental health and well-being. Financial strain is one strong candidate for mediating the effects (e.g., Frese and Mohr 1987; Kessler et al. 1987b; Whelan 1992). If one separates primary deprivation (e.g., food, heat, clothing) from secondary (e.g., holidays, telephone, car), one finds a more important mediating role for the former (Whelan 1992). Dooley and Catalano (1984) identified "undesirable economic life events" as a mediator between the community unemployment rate and psychological symptoms.

Studies of possible *moderators* or *modifiers* of the impact of unemployment are more common inasmuch as there has been a growing interest in this issue (Fryer 1992). One frequently examined moderator is social support. There is reasonable evidence about the benefits of social support (e.g., Brenner and Starrin 1988; Kessler et al. 1988; Broomhall and Winefield 1990; Turner et al. 1991; Mallinckrodt and Bennett 1992; Winefield et al. 1993; Hammarstrom 1994a), though the findings are not straightforward. For example, preexisting levels of support did not act as a moderator (Dew et al. 1987, 1992), but *after* layoff, spousal levels of support ("crisis support") did moderate the impact. Findings from the Michigan study (Kasl and Cobb 1982) suggest that the role of social support may change depending on the phases of adaptation to the experience: *(1)* in the early phases, men who found prompt reemployment showed a greater decrease in anxiety-tension (from the time of anticipation) if they were low on support rather than high; *(2)* in the later phases, however, men who failed to find stable employment increased in anxiety-tension under conditions of low support and decreased under conditions of high support.

Among preexisting psychological characteristics acting as modifiers, absence of psychiatric history (Penkower et al. 1988), sense of mastery (Brenner and Starrin 1988), and positive self-concept (Kessler et al. 1988) have been identified. Additional analyses revealed that the self-concept variable operates primarily by attenuating vulnerability to other stressful life events (Turner et al. 1991). This is an important moderating process since the unemployment experience itself leaves the individual more vulnerable to the impact of other, unrelated life events (Kessler et al. 1987b).

The moderators listed above have applicability to a variety of stressful life events and their mental health impact. One moderator, however, which is specific to the unemployment situation is (nonfinancial) work commitment. There is reasonable consensus on its moderating role (Warr et al. 1988; Hammarstrom 1994a and b; for an exception, see Winefield et al. 1993); high work commitment aggravates the negative impact of becoming unemployed, but among those going from unemployment to reemployment, high work commitment enhances the degree of recovery.

THE IMPACT OF JOB INSECURITY AND THREATENED JOB LOSS

There are a few studies dealing with the health consequences of job insecurity. Foremost among these is the Whitehall II study (Ferrie et al. 1995, 1998), which showed that white collar workers under threat of major organizational change (elimination or transfer to the private sector) showed adverse changes in self-rated health, longstanding illness, sleep patterns, number of physical symptoms, and minor psychiatric morbidity. Only health-related behaviors did not show an adverse change. Longitudinal data on male Swedish shipyard workers threatened with closure and on stably employed controls (Mattiasson et al. 1990) showed that serum cholesterol concentrations increased significantly among those threatened with job loss. The increase was greater among those with higher levels of sleep disturbance as well as those with increases in cardiovascular risk factors, particularly weight and blood pressure. However, no significant differential trends over time were seen for weight, blood pressure, or glucose. In a study of Finnish local government workers (Vahtera et al. 1997), downsizing was associated with increases in medically certified sick leave. Among American automobile workers (Heaney et al. 1994) extended periods of job insecurity were associated with a decrease in job satisfaction and an increase in physical symptomatology. However, workers who remain in an organization after a downsizing do not experience a decline in well-being despite an increase in work demands (Parker et al. 1997).

Cross-sectional data on German blue collar workers in steel and metal plants, some of which were undergoing reductions in work force (Siegerist et al. 1988), showed that "atherogenic risk" was higher among those threatened with job loss, especially those who were also high on subjectively perceived job insecurity. Atherogenic risk was defined as the ratio of low- to high-density lipoproteins, and this was adjusted for potential confounders, such as body weight, smoking, and alcohol consumption. In a recent theoretical formulation, Siegrist (1996) argues that several consequences of threatened downsizing—overtime work, reduction in personnel, fear of job loss, job instability—all contribute to a negative effort/reward imbalance which increases cardiovascular risk.

A NOTE ON THE IMPACT OF RETIREMENT

Older reviews of the evidence (e.g., Kasl 1980; Minkler 1981) have concluded that a negative impact of retirement on physical and mental health of retirees has not been demonstrated. Furthermore, this conclusion is based on rather convergent evidence showing an absence of an adverse impact rather than confusing evidence that might show a variety of results but would not permit any broad generalizations. More recent assessments of the evidence (e.g., McGoldrick 1989; Moen 1996) do not alter this fundamental conclusion.

The older studies (e.g., Palmore et al. 1984) tended to show neither adverse effects nor benefits. Some specific variables, such as subjective global evaluations of one's health, might show improvement, but this was seen as a function of reinterpreting one's health in the absence of physical demands on the job. More recent studies (e.g., Salokangas and Jowkamaa 1991; Ostberg and Samuelsson 1994; Midanik et al. 1995; Gall et al. 1997) have tended to show some benefits of retirement, primarily in the psychological domain and in health behaviors. One longitudinal study did show modest adverse effects on blood pressure and serum cholesterol (Ekerdt et al. 1984) but these were deemed clinically insignificant. Retirement could lead to a higher propensity to seek care (Roberts et al. 1997), which might be misinterpreted as more illness. It is interesting to note that a study of older steelworkers who were forced to retire early because of downsizing (Gillanders et al. 1991) did not show any adverse effects on their health. Thus loss of a job close to normal retirement age may have only small negative effects, if any.

In addition to the broad conclusion of no adverse impact, on the average, on health and functioning, the following points can be made on the basis of accumulated evidence (Kasl 1980):

1. Variations in postretirement outcomes are most convincingly seen as reflecting continuities of preretirement status, particularly in the areas of physical health, social and leisure activities, and general well-being and satisfaction.

2. Certain predictors of outcome, such as prior attitudes toward the process of retire-

ment and expectations about postretirement outcomes, appear to make their contribution primarily via their association with underlying variables, such as prior health status and financial aspects of retirement. Consequently, they do not indicate the differential impact of retirement but rather reflect, once again, the continuities noted in the previous point.

3. Variables reflecting aspects of the work role (such as job satisfaction, work commitment) do not appear to be powerful or consistent predictors of outcomes. This conclusion may be viewed as somewhat of a surprise, and those who do not wish to accept it can rightfully argue that the cumulative evidence is not yet very compelling.

There is no question that poor health leads to "early" or "involuntary" retirement (McGoldrick 1989; Moen 1996). This makes it difficult to test the proposition that while planned and "on schedule" retirement does not have a negative impact, it is the unplanned, involuntary, "off schedule" retirement which should have adverse effects since the downward health status trajectory which precipitated the retirement will manifest itself as poor health status after retirement.

Men who choose to continue labor force participation well beyond conventional retirement age are an unusual group who are in good health and have a strong commitment to work (Parnes and Sommers 1994). It is in this group that we should study effects of "mandatory" retirement, not among blue collar workers who usually prefer to retire early (and do so if retirement benefits are adequate). But such doctors, judges, farmers, and others, who continue working beyond normal retirement, cannot be easily recruited into a study of "mandatory" retirement.

Moen (1996) has argued that the relationship between retirement and health is a very complex one and that most designs do not capture such complexity. She develops a lifecourse model which should lead to a more sophisticated research agenda for the future. Our brief commentary and summarizing generalizations set aside this complexity. However, our main purpose was to highlight the striking difference in the evidence of impact of unemployment vs. retirement.

CONCLUDING COMMENTS ON IMPACT OF UNEMPLOYMENT

This review has revealed that there is an extensive research literature on the impact of unemployment on health and well-being. Unemployment is a complex, multifaceted experience, richly embedded in a large matrix of other psychosocial variables and processes, and the usual observational designs seldom fully capture the underlying processes. The evidence can be summarized as follows:

1. Unemployment appears to be associated with a 20%–30% excess all cause mortality in most studies.

2. The impact of unemployment on physical morbidity is also evident, but the results are more variable and more difficult to interpret.

3. Biological indicators of stress reactivity and disease risk provide rather good evidence of their acute sensitivity to some aspects of the unemployment experience (including anticipation) but chronic elevations in relation to enduring unemployment are infrequently documented.

4. Behavioral and lifestyle risk factors, such as smoking or exercise, show sporadic evidence of impact as well as considerable complexity of findings: some of these variables seem implicated in selection rather than causation.

5. Unemployment clearly increases psychological distress, particularly symptoms of depression, but overt diagnosable disorders are probably not elevated. The increases in distress seem reversible upon reemployment.

6. The impact of threatened job loss is less adequately documented but the topic is gaining increasing attention. A variety of indicators of physical and psychological morbidity and cardiovascular risk are likely to show adverse effects under conditions of heightened job insecurity. High community

levels of unemployment have a negative impact on depressive symptoms of employed individuals (urban setting), an effect which can be interpreted as due to threatened job loss.

REFERENCES

Arber, S. (1987). Social class, non-employment, and chronic illness: continuing the inequalities in health debate. *BMJ*, 294:1069–73.

Arnetz, B.B., Wasserman, J., Petrini, B., Brenner, S.O., Levi, L., Eneroth, P., Salovaara, H., Hjelm, R., Salovaara, L., Theorell, T., and Petterson, I.L. (1987). Immune function in unemployed women. *Psychosom Med*, 49:3–12.

Arrow, J.O. (1996). Estimating the influence of health as a risk factor on unemployment: a survival analysis of employment durations for workers surveyed in the German Socio-Economic Panel (1984–1990). *Soc Sci Med*, 42:1651–9.

Bartley, M. (1988). Unemployment and health: selection or causation—a false antithesis. *Sociol Health Illness*, 19:41–67.

Beale, N., and Nethercott, S. (1987). The health of industrial employees from years after compulsory redundancy. *J R Coll Gen Pract*, 37:390–4.

Beale, N., and Nethercott, S. (1988a). The nature of unemployment morbidity. 1. Recognition. *J R Coll Gen Pract*, 38:197–9.

Beale, N., and Nethercott, S. (1988b). The nature of unemployment morbidity. 2. Description. *J R Coll Gen Pract*, 38:200–2.

Beiser, M., Johnson, P.J., and Turner, R.J. (1993). Unemployment, underemployment and depressive affect among Southeast Asian refugees. *Psychol Med*, 23: 731–43.

Borrell, C., and Arias, A. (1995). Socioeconomic factors and mortality in urban settings: the case of Barcelona, Spain. *J Epidemiol Community Health*, 49:460–5.

Brenner, M.H. (1983). Mortality and economic instability: detailed analyses for Britain and comparative analyses for selected industrialized countries. *Int J Health Serv*, 13:563–619.

Brenner, M.H. (1987a). Economic change, alcohol consumption, and heart disease mortality in nine industrialized countries. *Soc Sci Med*, 25:119–32.

Brenner, M.H. (1987b). Economic instability, unemployment rates, behavioral risk, and mortality rates in Scotland, 1952–1983. *Int J Health Serv*, 17:475–87.

Brenner, M.H. (1987c). Relation of economic change to Swedish health and social well-being, 1950–1980. *Soc Sci Med*, 25:183–95.

Brenner, M.H., and Monney, A. (1983). Unemployment and health in the context of economic change. *Soc Sci Med*, 17:1125–38.

Brenner, S.O., and Levi, L. (1987). Long-term unemployment among women in Sweden. *Soc Sci Med*, 25:153–61.

Brenner, S.O., and Starrin, B. (1988). Unemployment and health in Sweden: public issues and private troubles. *J Soc Issues*, 44: 125–40.

Broomhall, H.S., and Winefield, A.H. (1990). A comparison of the affective well-being of young and middle-aged unemployed men matched for length of unemployment. *Br J Med Psychol*, 63:43–52.

Burchell, B. (1992). Towards a social psychology of the labour market: or why we need to understand the labour market before we can understand unemployment. *J Occup Organiz Psychol*, 65:345–4.

Cahill, J. (1983). Structural characteristics of the macroeconomy and mental health: implications for primary prevention research. *Am J Community Psychol*, 11:553–71.

Caplan, R.D., Vinokur, A.D., Price, R.H., and van Ryn, M. (1989). Job seeking, reemployment, and mental health: a randomized field experiment in coping with job loss. *J Appl Psychol*, 74:739–69.

Catalano, R. (1991). The health effects of economic insecurity. *Am J Public Health*, 81: 1148–52.

Catalano, R., Dooley, D., Wilson, G., and Hough, R. (1993). Job loss and alcohol abuse: a test using data from the Epidemiologic Catchment Area Project. *J Health Soc Behav*, 34:215–25.

Charlton, J.R.H., Bauer, R., Thakhore, A., Silver, R., and Aristidou, M. (1987). Unemployment and mortality: a small area analysis. *J Epidemiol Community Health*, 41:107–13.

Cobb, S. (1974). Physiologic changes in men whose jobs were abolished. *J Psychosom Res*, 18:245–58.

Cobb, S., and Kasl, S.V. (1977). *Termination: the consequences of job loss.* (National Institute for Occupationl Safety and Health research report. DHEW (NIOSH) Pub. No. 76-1261.) Cincinnati, OH: U.S. Department of Health, Education, and Welfare.

Cohen, L.E., and Felson, M. (1979). On estimating the social costs of national economic policy: a critical examination of the Brenner study. *Soc Indicators Res*, 6:251–9.

Colledge, M. (1982). Economic cycles and health: towards a sociological understanding of the impact of the recession on health and illness. *Soc Sci Med*, 16:1919–27.

Cook, D.G. (1985). A critical view of the unemployment and health debate. *Statistician*, 34:73–82.

Cook, D.G., Cummins, R.O., Bartley, M.J., and Shaper, A.G. (1982). Health of unemployed middle-aged men in Great Britain. *Lancet,* 1:1290–4.

Costa, G., and Segnan, N. (1987). Unemployed and mortality. *Lancet,* 1:1550–1.

Cullen, J.H., Ryan, G.M., Cullen, K.M., Ronayne, T., and Wynne, R.F. (1987). Unemployed youth and health: findings from the pilot phase of a longitudinal study. *Soc Sci Med,* 25:133–46.

D'Arcy, C. (1986). Unemployment and health: data and implications. *Can J Public Health,* 77: 124–31.

D'Arcy, C., and Siddique, C.M. (1985). Unemployment and health: an analysis of Canada Health Survey data. *Int J Health Serv,* 15:609–35.

Dew, M.A., Bromet, E.J., and Schulberg, H.C. (1987). A comparative analysis of two community stressors' long-term mental health effects. *Am J Community Psychol,* 15:167–84.

Dew, M.A., Bromet, E.J., and Penkower, L. (1992). Mental health effects of job loss in women. *Psychol Med,* 22:751–64.

Dooley, D., and Catalano, R. (1984). The epidemiology of economic stress. *Am J Community Psychol,* 12:387–409.

Dooley, D., and Catalano, R. (1988). Recent research on psychological effects of unemployment. *J Soc Issues,* 44:1–12.

Dooley, D., Catalano, R., Jackson, R., and Brownell, A. (1981). Economic, life and symptom changes in a nonmetropolitan community. *J Health Soc Behav,* 22:144–54.

Dooley, D., Catalano, R., and Rook, K.S. (1988). Personal and aggregate unemployment and psychological symptoms. *J Soc Issues,* 44:107–23.

Dooley, D., Catalano, R., Rook, K., and Serxner, S. (1989). Economic stress and suicide: multilevel analyses. Part I: aggregate time series analyses of economic stress and suicide. *Suicide Life Threat Behav,* 19:321–36.

Dooley, D., Catalano, R., and Hough, R. (1992). Unemployment and alcohol disorder in 1910 and 1990: drift versus social causation. *J Occup Organ Psychol,* 65:277–90.

Dooley, D., Fielding, J., and Levi, L. (1996). Health and unemployment. *Annu Rev Public Health,* 17:449–65.

Ekerdt, D.J., Sparrow, D., Glynn, R.J., and Bosse, R. (1984). Change in blood pressure and total cholesterol with retirement. *Am J Epidemiol,* 120:64–71.

Ensminger, M., and Celentano, D.O. (1988). Unemployment and psychiatric distress: social resources and coping. *Soc Sci Med,* 27: 239–47.

Ensminger, M.E., and Celentano, D.O. (1990). Gender differences in the effects of unemployment on psychological distress. *Soc Sci Med,* 30:469–77.

Ettner, S.L. (1997). Measuring the human cost of a weak economy: does unemployment lead to alcohol abuse? *Soc Sci Med,* 44:251–60.

Eyer, J. (1977a). Does unemployment cause the death rate peak in each business cycle? a multifactor model of death rate change. *Int J Health Serv,* 7:625–62.

Eyer, J. (1977b). Prosperity as a cause of death. *Int J Health Serv,* 7:125–50.

Ferrie, J.E., Shipley, M.J., Marmot, M.G., Stansfeld, S., and Smith, G.D. (1995). Health effects of anticipation of job change and nonemployment: longitudinal data from the Whitehall II study. *BMJ,* 311:1264–9.

Ferrie, J.E., Shipley, M.J., Marmot, M.G., Stansfeld, S., and Smith, G.D. (1998). The health effects of major organisational change and job insecurity. *Soc Sci Med,* 46:243–54.

Fleming, R., Baum, A., and Reddy, D. (1984). Behavioral and biochemical effects of job loss and unemployment stress. *J Hum Stress,* 10:12–7.

Forbes, J.F., and McGregor, A. (1987). Male unemployment and cause-specific mortality in postwar Scotland. *Int J Health Serv,* 249: 233–49.

Forcier, M.W. (1988). Unemployment and alcohol abuse: a review. *J Occup Med,* 30: 246–51.

Frese, M., and Mohr, G. (1987). Prolonged unemployment and depression in older workers: a longitudinal study of intervening variables. *Soc Sci Med,* 25:173–8.

Fryer, D. (1992). Introduction to marienthal and beyond (editorial). *J Occup Organ Psychol,* 65:257–68.

Fryer, D. (1997). International perspectives on youth unemployment and mental health: some central issues. *J Adolesc,* 20:333–42.

Gall, T.L., Evans, D.R., and Howard, J. (1997). The retirement adjustment process: changes in the well-being of male retirees across time. *J Gerontol B Psychol Sci Soc Sci,* 52:P110–7.

Gillanders, W.R., Buss, T.F., Wingard, E., and Gemmel, D. (1991). Long-term health impacts of forced early retirement among steelworkers. *J Fam Pract,* 32:401–5.

Graetz, B. (1993). Health consequences of employment and unemployment. *Soc Sci Med,* 36:715–24.

Gravelle, H.S., Hutchinson, G., and Stern, J. (1981). Mortality and unemployment: a critique of Brenner's time-series analysis (editorial). *Lancet,* 2:675–9.

Grayson, J.P. (1989). Reported illness after CGE closure. *Can J Public Health,* 80:16–9.

Hammarstrom, A. (1994a). Health consequences of youth unemployment. *Public Health*, 108:403–12.

Hammarstrom, A. (1994b). Health consequences of youth unemployment: review from a gender perspective. *Soc Sci Med*, 38:699–709.

Hammer, T. (1992). Unemployment and use of drugs and alcohol among young people: a longitudinal study in a general population. *Br J Addict*, 87:1571–81.

Harding, L., and Sewel, J. (1992). Psychological health and employment status in an island community. *J Occup Organ Psychol*, 65:269–75.

Heaney, C.A., Israel, B.A., and House, J.S. (1994). Chronic job insecurity among automobile workers: effects on job satisfaction and health. *Soc Sci Med*, 38:1431–7.

Iversen, L., and Sabroe, S. (1988). Psychological well-being among unemployed and employed people after a company closedown: a longitudinal study. *J Soc Issues*, 44:141–52.

Iversen, L., Anderson, O., Andersen, P.K., Christoffersen, K., and Keiding, N. (1987). Unemployment and mortality in Denmark. *BMJ*, 295:879–84.

Iversen, L., Sabroe, S., and Damsgaard, M.T. (1989). Hospital admissions before and after shipyard closure. *BMJ*, 299:1073–6.

Jahoda, M. (1992). Reflections on Marienthal and after. *J Occup Organ Psychol*, 65:355–8.

Janlert, U., Asplund, K., and Weinehall, L. (1992). Unemployment and cardiovascular risk indicators. *Scand J Soc Med*, 20:14–8.

Jin, R.L., Shah, C.P., and Svoboda, T.J. (1995). The impact of unemployment on health: a review of the evidence. *CMAJ*, 153:529–40.

Johansson, S.-E., and Sundquist, J. (1997). Unemployment is an important risk factor for suicide in contemporary Sweden: an 11-year follow-up study of a cross-sectional sample of 37,789 people. *Public Health*, 111:41–5.

Kaplan, G.A., Roberts, R.E., Camacho, T.C., and Coyne, J.C. (1987). Psychosocial predictors of depression. *Am J Epidemiol*, 125:206–20.

Kasl, S.V. (1979). Mortality and the business cycle: some questions about research strategies when utilizing macrosocial and ecological data. *Am J Public Health*, 69:784–8.

Kasl, S.V. (1980). The impact of retirement. In Cooper, C.L., and Payne, R. (eds.). *Current Concerns in Occupational Stress*. Chichester: J. Wiley, pp. 137–86.

Kasl, S.V. (1982). Strategies of research on economic instability and health. *Psychol Med*, 12:637–49.

Kasl, S.V., and Cobb, S. (1970). Blood pressure changes in men undergoing job loss: a preliminary report. *Psychosom Med*, 32:19–38.

Kasl, S.V., and Cobb, S. (1980). The experience of losing a job: some effects on cardiovascular functioning. *Psychother Psychosom*, 34:88–109.

Kasl, S.V., and Cobb, S. (1982). Variability of stress effects among men experiencing job loss. In Goldberger, L., and Breznitz, S. (eds.), *Handbook of stress*. New York: Free Press, pp. 445–65.

Kasl, S.V., Cobb, S., and Brooks, G.W. (1968). Changes in serum uric acid and serum cholesterol in men undergoing job loss. *JAMA*, 206:1500–7.

Kasl, S.V., Gore, S., and Cobb, S. (1975). The experience of losing a job: reported changes in health, symptoms, and illness behavior. *Psychosom Med*, 37:106–22.

Kessler, R.C., House, J.S., and Turner, J.B. (1987a). Unemployment and health in a community sample. *J Health Soc Behav*, 28:51–9.

Kessler, R.C., Turner, J.B., and House, J.S. (1987b). Intervening processes in the relationship between unemployment and health. *Psychol Med*, 17:949–61.

Kessler, R.C., Turner, J.B., and House, J.S. (1988). Effects of unemployment on health in a community survey: main, modifying, and mediating effects. *J Soc Issues*, 44:69–85.

Kessler, R.C., Turner, J.B., and House, J.S. (1991). Unemployment, reemployment, and emotional functioning in a community sample. *Am Sociol Rev*, 54:648–57.

Lahelma, E., Kangas, R., and Manderbacka, K. (1995). Drinking and unemployment: contrasting patterns among men and women. *Drug Alcohol Depend*, 37:71–82.

Leeflang, R.L.I., Klein-Hesrelink, D.J., and Spruit, I.P. (1992). Health effects of unemployment: I. Long-term unemployed men in a rural and urban setting. *Soc Sci Med*, 34:341–50.

Mackenbach, J.P., and Looman, C.W.N. (1994). Living standards and mortality in the European community. *J Epidemiol Community Health*, 48:140–5.

Mallinckrodt, B., and Bennett, J. (1992). Social support and the impact of job loss in dislocated blue-collar workers. *J Couns Psychol*, 39:482–9.

Martikainen, P.T. (1990). Unemployment and mortality among Finnish men, 1981–5. *BMJ*, 301:407–11.

Martikainen, P.T., and Valkonen, T. (1996). Excess mortality of unemployed men and women during a period of rapidly increasing unemployment. *Lancet*, 348:909–12.

Mattiasson, I., Lindgarde, F., Nilsson, J.A., and Theorell, T. (1990). Threat of unemployment and cardiovascular risk factors: longitudinal study of quality of sleep and serum cholesterol concentrations in men threatened with redundancy. *BMJ*, 301:461–5.

McGoldrick, A.E. (1989). Stress, early retirement and health. In Markides, K.S., and Cooper, C.L. (eds.), *Aging, stress and health*. Chichester: John Wiley, pp. 91–118.

Midanik, L.T., Soghikian, K., Ransom, L.J., and Tekawa, I.S. (1995). The effect of retirement on mental health and health behaviors: the Kaiser Permanente Retirement Study. *J Gerontol B Psychol Soc Sci*, 50:S59–61.

Miles, I. (1987). Some observations on "unemployment and health" research. *Soc Sci Med*, 25:223–5.

Minkler, M. (1981). Research on the health effects of retirement: an uncertain legacy. *J Health Soc Behav*, 22:117–30.

Moen, P. (1996). A lifecourse perspective on retirement, gender, and well-being. *J Occup Health Psychol*, 1:131–44.

Montgomery, S.M., Bartley, M.J., Cook, D.G., and Wadsworth, M.E.J. (1996). Health and social precursors of unemployment in young men in Great Britain. *J Epidemiol Community Health*, 50:415–22.

Morrell, S., Taylor, R., Quine, S., Kerr, C., and Western, J. (1994). A cohort study of unemployment as a cause of psychological disturbance in Australian youth. *Soc Sci Med*, 38:1553–64.

Morris, J.K., and Cook, D.G. (1991). A critical review of the effect of factory closures on health. *Br J Ind Med*, 48:1–8.

Morris, J.K., Cook, D.G., and Shaper, A.G. (1992). Non-employment and changes in smoking, drinking, and body weight. *BMJ*, 304:536–41.

Morris, J.K., Cook, D.G., and Shaper, A.G. (1994). Loss of employment and mortality. *BMJ*, 308:1135–9.

Moser, K.A., Fox, A.J., and Jones, D.R. (1984). Unemployment and mortality in the OPCS Longitudinal Study. *Lancet*, 2:1324–8.

Moser, K.A., Fox, A.J., Jones, D.R., ., and Goldblatt, P.O. (1986). Unemployment and mortality: further evidence from the OPCS Longitudinal Study 1971–81. *Lancet*, 1:365–7.

Moser, K.A., Goldblatt, P.O., Fox, A.J., and Jones, D.R. (1987). Unemployment and mortality: comparison of the 1971 and 1981 longitudinal study census samples. *BMJ*, 294:86–90.

Ostberg, H., and Samuelsson, S.M. (1994). Occupational retirement in women due to age: health aspects. *Scand J Soc Med*, 22:90–6.

Palmore, E.G., Fillenbaum, G.G., and George, L.K. (1984). Consequences of retirement. *J Gerontol*, 39:109–16.

Parker, S.K., Chmiel, N., and Wall, T.D. (1997). Work characteristics and employee well-being within a context of strategic downsizing. *J Occup Health Psychol*, 2:289–303.

Parnes, H.S., and Sommers, D.G. (1994). Shunning retirement: work experience of men in their seventies and early eighties. *J Gerontol*, 49:S117–24.

Patterson, L.J.M. (1997). Long-term unemployment among adolescents: a longitudinal study. *J Adolesc*, 20:261–80.

Penkower, L., Bromet, E.J., and Dew, M.A. (1988). Husbands' layoff and wives' mental health. *Arch Gen Psychiatry*, 45:994–1000.

Platt, S. (1984). Unemployment and suicidal behavior: review of the literature. *Soc Sci Med*, 19:93–115.

Platt, S., Micciolo, R., and Tansella, M. (1992). Suicide and unemployment in Italy: description, analysis and interpretation of recent trends. *Soc Sci Med*, 34:1191–201.

Price, R.H. (1992). Impact of preventive job search intervention on likelihood of depression among unemployed. *J Health Soc Behav*, 33:158–67.

Proudfoot, J., Guest, D., Carson, J., Dunn, G., and Gray, J. (1997). Effect of cognitive-behavioural training on job-finding among long-term unemployed people. *Lancet*, 350:96–100.

Raitakari, O.T., Leino, M., Raikkonen, K., Porkka, K.V.K., Taimela, S., Rasanen, L., and Viikari, J.S.A. (1995). Clustering of risk habits in young adults. *Am J Epidemiol*, 142:36–44.

Rasky, E., Stronegger, W.J., and Freidl, W. (1996). Employment status and its health-related effects in rural Styria, Austria. *Prev Med*, 25:757–63.

Roberts, R.O., Rhodes, T., Girman, C.J., Guess, H.A., Osterling, J.E., Lieber, M.M., and Jacobsen, S.J. (1997). The decision to seek care. *Arch Fam Med*, 6:218–22.

Robinson, D., and Pinch, S. (1987). A geographical analysis of the relationship between early childhood death and socio-economic environment in an English city. *Soc Sci Med*, 25:9–18.

Salokangas, R.K.R., and Jowkamaa, M. (1991). Physical and mental health changes in retirement age. *Psychother Psychosom*, 55:100–7.

Schaufeli, W.B. (1997). Youth unemployment and mental health: some Dutch findings. *J Adolesc*, 20:281–92.

Schaufeli, W.B., and Van Yperen, N.W. (1992). Unemployment and psychological distress among graduates: a longitudinal study. *J Occup Organ Psych*, 65:291–305.

Schwefel, D. (1986). Unemployment, health and health services in German-speaking countries. *Soc Sci Med*, 22:409–30.

Schoenborn, C.A., and National Center for Health Statistics (1988). *Health promotion and disease prevention, United States 1985.* (DHHS Pub. No. (PHS) 88–1591.) Hyattsville, MD: U.S. Department of Health and Human Services.

Shortt, S.E.D. (1996). Is unemployment pathogenic? A review of current concepts with lessons for policy planners. *Int J Health Serv*, 26:569–89.

Siegrist, J. (1996). Adverse health effects of high-effort/low-reward conditions. *J Occup Health Psychol*, 1:27–41.

Siegerist, J., Matschinger, H., Cremer, P., and Seidel, D. (1988). Atherogenic risk in men suffering from occupational stress. *Atherosclerosis*, 69:211–8.

Sogaard, J. (1992). Econometric critique of the economic change model of mortality. *Soc Sci Med*, 34:927–57.

Sorlie, P.D., and Rogot, E. (1990). Mortality by employment status in the National Longitudinal Mortality Study. *Am J Epidemiol*, 132:983–92.

Spruit, I.P. (1982). Unemployment and health in macro-social analysis. *Soc Sci Med*, 16:1903–17.

Starrin, B., Larsson, G., Brenner, S.O., Levi, L., and Petterson, I.L. (1990). Structural changes, ill health, and mortality in Sweden, 1963–1983: a macroaggregated study. *Int J Health Serv*, 20:27–42.

Stefansson, C.G. (1991). Long-term unemployment and mortality in Sweden, 1980–1986. *Soc Sci Med*, 32:419–23.

Stern, J. (1983). The relationship between unemployment, morbidity, and mortality in Britain. *Popul Stud*, 37:61–74.

Turner, J.B. (1995). Economic context and the health effects of unemployment. *J Health Soc Behav*, 36:213–29.

Turner, J.B., Kessler, R.C., and House, J.S. (1991). Factors facilitating adjustment to unemployment: mplications for intervention. *Am J Community Psychol*, 19:521–42.

Vahtera, J., Kivimaki, M., and Pentti, J. (1997). Effect of organizational downsizing on health of employees. *Lancet*, 350:1124–28.

Vinokur, A., van Ryn, N., Gramlich, E.M., and Price, R.H. (1991). Long-term follow-up benefit-cost analysis of the jobs program: a preventive intervention for the unemployed. *J Appl Psychol*, 76:213–9.

Wagstaff, A. (1985). Time series analysis of the relationship between unemployment and mortality: a survey of econometric critiques and replications of Brenner's studies. *Soc Sci Med*, 21:985–66.

Warr, P.B. (1987). *Unemployment and mental health*. Oxford: Clarendon Press.

Warr, P.B., Jackson, P., and Banks, M. (1988). Unemployment and mental health: some British studies. *J Soc Issues*, 44:47–68.

Westin, S. (1990a). The structure of a factory closure: individual responses to job-loss and unemployment in a 10-year controlled follow-up study. *Soc Sci Med*, 31:1301–11.

Westin, S. (1990b). Unemployment and health: medical and social consequences of a factory closure in a ten-year controlled follow-up study. University of Trondheim, Faculty of Medicine, Norway (doctoral dissertation).

Westin, S., Norum, D., and Schlesselman, J.J. (1988). Medical consequences of a factory closure: illness and disability in a four-year follow-up study. *Int J Epidemiol*, 17:153–61.

Westin, S., Schlesselman, J.J., and Korper, M. (1989). Long-term effects of a factory closure: unemployment and disability during ten years' follow-up. *J Clin Epidemiol*, 42:435–41.

Whelan, C.T. (1992). The role of income, lifestyle deprivation and financial strain in mediating the impact of unemployment on psychological distress: evidence from the Republic of Ireland. *J Occup Organ Psychol*, 65:331–44.

Wilson, S.H., and Walker, G.M. (1993). Unemployment and health: a review. *Public Health*, 107:153–62.

Winefield, A.H., Tiggemann, M., Winefield, H.R., and Goldney, R.D. (1993). *Growing up with unemployment: a longitudinal study of its psychological impact*. London: Routledge.

Yuen, P., and Balarajan, R. (1986). Unemployment and patterns of consultation with the general practitioner. *BMJ*, 298:1212–4.

7

Social Integration, Social Networks, Social Support, and Health

LISA F. BERKMAN AND THOMAS GLASS

It is difficult now to reconstruct the logic that led us to believe that the nature of human relationships—the degree to which an individual is interconnected and embedded in a community—is vital to an individual's health and well-being as well as to the health and vitality of entire populations. In retrospect, a combination of observations and reading the rich theoretical literature on social integration, attachment, and social networks led us to test these ideas empirically. Now, almost 25 years after John Cassel (1976), Sidney Cobb (1976), and other seminal thinkers in social epidemiology suggested that this was a critical area of investigation, and 20 years after the earliest studies in Alameda County, California; Tecumseh, Michigan; and North Carolina revealed the influence of social relationships on mortality (Berkman and Syme 1979; Blazer 1982; House et al. 1982), it is time to take stock of the vast literature on this topic. Our aim is to revisit some of the seminal theories that have guided empirical work, revise and reformulate some of those ideas, and point the

way toward productive lines of inquiry for the future.

When investigators write about the impact of social relationships on health, many terms are used loosely and interchangeably, including social networks, social support, social ties, and social integration. A major aim of this chapter is to clarify these terms under a single framework. We discuss *(1)* theoretical orientations from diverse disciplines that we believe are fundamental to advancing research in this area, *(2)* an overarching model that integrates multilevel phenomena, *(3)* a set of definitions accompanied by major assessment tools, *(4)* some of the strongest findings linking social networks or support to morbidity, mortality, or functioning, and finally, *(5)* a series of recommendations for future work. Since there are now numerous books and literature reviews on networks, support, and health (Cohen and Syme 1985; Broadhead et al. 1983; House et al. 1988; Sarason et al. 1990; Thoits 1995; Berkman 1985, 1995; Seeman 1996), our aim is not to be all-inclusive but rather to highlight work that has substantially advanced our thinking in this area and to give the reader a sense of the range and depth of this literature, now a body several decades in the making.

THEORETICAL ORIENTATIONS

Several sets of theories form the bedrock for the empirical investigation of social relationships and their influence on health. The earliest theories came from sociologists such as Émile Durkheim as well as from psychoanalysts such as John Bowlby, who first formulated attachment theory. A major wave of conceptual development came from anthropologists, including Elizabeth Bott, John Barnes, and Clyde Mitchell, and quantitative sociologists such as Claude Fischer, Edward Laumann, Barry Wellman, and Peter Marsden, who, along with others, developed social network analysis. This eclectic mix of theoretical approaches, coupled with the work on stress by Cannon and Selye (see Chapter 13), addresses the protective roles of social resources and support within the context of research on stress. The contributions of the epidemiologists John Cassel and Sidney Cobb, combined with this earlier work, together form the foundation of research on social ties and health.

Émile Durkheim: Social Integration, Alienation, and Anomie

Suicide varies inversely with degree of integration of the social groups of which the individual forms a part.

Durkheim 1897, 1951, p. 209

Émile Durkheim, a French sociologist working late in the 19th century, was one of the founding fathers of sociology. Durkheim's contribution to the study of the relationship between society and health is immeasurable. Perhaps most important is the contribution he has made to the understanding of how social integration and cohesion influence mortality. Durkheim's primary aim was to explain individual pathology as a function of social dynamics. In light of recent attention to "upstream" determinants

of health (Link and Phelan 1995), Durkheim was indeed ahead of his time.

While a professor at the University of Bordeaux, Durkheim wrote three of his four most important books: *The Division of Labor in Society* (1893), *The Rules of Sociological Method* (1895), and *Suicide* (1897). It is *Suicide* that lays the framework for understanding the role of social integration in health. Building on *The Rules of Sociological Method*, Durkheim challenges himself to understand how the patterning of one of the most psychological, intimate, and, on the surface, individual acts rests on the patterning of "social facts." As noted by Bierstedt (1966), it is as if Durkheim chooses for himself the hardest of challenges to prove the power of social phenomena to influence what seem to be individual acts.

In *Suicide*, Durkheim shows how "social facts" can be used to explain changing patterns of aggregate tendency toward suicide. He argues that individuals are bonded to society by two forms of integration: attachment and regulation. Attachment is the extent to which an individual maintains ties with members of society. Regulation involves the extent to which an individual is held in the fabric of society by its values, beliefs, and norms (Turner et al. 1989). Because Durkheim's logic and language are so elegant, in the following paragraphs we try to give the reader the flavor of his thinking as it relates to social integration and suicide.

Durkheim starts his work with the observation that countries and other geographic units and social groups have very stable rates of suicide year after year. Thus:

individuals making up a society change from year to year, yet the number of suicides itself does not change . . . the population of Paris renews itself very rapidly, yet the share of Paris in the total number of French suicides remains practically the same . . . the rate of military suicides varies only very slowly in a given nation. . . . Likewise, regardless of the diversity of individual temperaments, the relation between aptitude for suicide of married persons and that of widowers and widows is identically the same in widely differing social groups. The causes which thus fix the contingent of voluntary deaths for a given society or one part of it must then be independent of individuals, since they retain the same intensity no matter what particular persons they operate on. (Durkheim 1897, 1951, p. 307)

Once armed with the evidence of social patterning of suicide, Durkheim goes on to theorize that the underlying explanation for suicide relates, for the most part, to the level of social integration of the group. Thus, with regard to differences in suicide by religion, Durkheim notes that while both Protestant and Catholic doctrines forbid suicide, Protestantism is much less integrated in its social organization than Catholicism. This differential level of attachment and regulation reinforces authoritarian thought and provides less room for individual inquiry. Thus, Catholic countries had lower suicide rates according to Durkheim's theory because the bonds that tie the individual to the group are comparatively stronger. The advantage of the married compared to unmarried is also related to the attachment of the individual to the family, and Durkheim further notes (and statistically supports) that intergenerational ties linking families together are stronger and more protective than the "conjugal" tie linking a husband and wife, two individuals, together.

Anomic suicide, a special type of suicide defined by Durkheim, is related to large-scale societal crises of an economic or political nature often occurring during times of rapid social change and turbulence. In these situations, social control and norms are weakened (e.g., the regulatory function of integration). Such rapid change serves to deregulate values, beliefs, and general norms and fails to rein in or guide individual aspirations (Turner et al. 1989). The current crises in Russia and eastern Europe might be regarded as classical situations leading to anomic suicide. Both egoistic and anomic suicide are triggered by the erosion of a society's capacity for integration.

Durkheim's contribution to our understanding of how social structure, particularly levels of integration based on religious, family, and occupational organization, is

unparalleled. He paved the way for much of the work in this area through the development and testing of basic sociological theories that have largely survived the test of time. He saw suicide not as an "isolated tragedy" in the life of an individual but as a reflection of conditions of society as a whole (LaCapra 1972).

John Bowlby: The Architect of Attachment Theory

All of us from the cradle to the grave are happiest when life is organized as a series of excursions, long or short, from the secure base provided by our attachment figures.

Bowlby 1988

John Bowlby has been described as one of the three or four most important psychiatrists in the 20th century (Storr 1991). He qualified as a psychoanalyst in 1937, and soon thereafter he was proposing theories to the British Psychoanalytic society suggesting that the environment, especially in early childhood, plays a critical role in the genesis of neurosis. Early in his career, he believed that the separation of infants from their mothers was unhealthy. He saw loss and separation as key issues for psychotherapy. Bowlby proposed that there is a universal human need to form close affectional bonds (Fonagy 1996). Between 1964 and 1979, Bowlby wrote a major trilogy, *Attachment* (1969), *Separation* (1973), and *Loss* (1980), in which he lays out his theory of attachment and how it relates to both childhood and adult development.

Attachment theory contends that the attached figure, most often but not necessarily the mother, creates a secure base from which an infant or toddler can explore and venture forth. Bowlby argued with many psychoanalysts that attachment is a "primary motivational system" (e.g., not secondary to feeding or warmth) (1969). "Secure attachment," he wrote, "provides an external ring of psychological protection which maintains the child's metabolism in a stable state, similar to the internal homeostasis mechanisms of blood pressure and temperature control" (1969). These inti-

mate bonds created in childhood form a secure base for solid attachment in adulthood
and provide prototypes for later social relations (Fonagy 1996). Secure attachment, as
opposed to avoidant, ambivalent, or disorganized attachment, allows the maintenance of affectional bonds and security in a
larger system.

In adulthood, Bowlby saw marriage as
the adult equivalent of attachment between
infant and mother during childhood. If secure, marriage would provide a solid base
from which to work and explore the world
enmeshed in a "protective shell in times of
need" (Holmes 1993, p. 81).

The strength of Bowlby's theory lies in its
articulation of an individual's need for secure attachment for its own sake, for the
love and reliability it provides, and for its
own "safe haven." Primary attachment promotes a sense of security and self-esteem
that ultimately provides the basis upon
which the individual will form lasting and
loving relationships in adult life. The psychosocial environment in infancy and childhood paves the way for successful development that continues through adulthood. For
Bowlby, the capacity for intimacy in adult
life is not given; it is instead the result of
complex dynamic forces involving attachment, loss, and reattachment. Throughout
this volume, we have seen the growing importance of bringing such a lifecourse and
dynamic perspective to understanding social determinants of disease.

Social Network Theory: A New Way of Looking at Social Structure and Community

During the mid-1950s, a number of British
anthropologists found it increasingly difficult to understand the behavior of either individuals or groups on the basis of traditional categories such as kin groups, tribes,
and villages. Barnes (1954) and Bott (1957)
developed the concept of "social networks"
to analyze ties that cut across traditional
kinship, residential, and class groups to explain features they observed such as access
to jobs, political activity, and marital roles.

The development of social network models
provided a way to view the structural properties of relationships among people with
no constraints or expectations that these relationships occurred only among bounded
groups defined a priori.

As this work and the work of other European post-WWII sociologists (i.e., Sim-
mel) became known in the United States,
American sociologists extended the concept
of social network analysis, incorporating
into it their more quantitative orientation.
Wellman (1993), in several historical reviews of the development of social network
analysis, has described "the network" of
network analysis. A strong center started at
Harvard under Harrison White and Charles
Tilly and extended to their graduate students: Edward Laumann (1973) went to the
midwest; Barry Wellman (Wellman and
Leighton 1979) went to Toronto; Mark
Granovetter (1973) and Claude Fischer
(Fischer et al. 1977; Fischer 1982) went to
the University of California, Berkeley. These
sociologists developed what has come to be
known as an egocentric network approach
to social network analysis in which the
structure and function of networks are assessed from the perspective of an individual.
Network analysis "focuses on the characteristic patterns of ties between actors in a
social system rather than on characteristics
of the individual actors themselves. Analysts search for the structure of ties underlying what often appears to be incoherent
surface appearances and use their descriptions to study how these social structures
constrain network member's behavior"
(Hall and Wellman 1985, p. 26). Network
analysis addresses the structure and composition of the network and the contents or
specific resources that flow through those
networks. Social network analysis includes
analyses of both egocentric networks with
an individual at the center and entire sets of
networks at the level of communities or
workplaces.

The strength of social network theory
rests on the testable assumption that the social structure of the network itself is largely

responsible for determining individual behavior and attitudes by shaping the flow of resources which determine access to opportunities and constraints on behavior. Network theorists share many of the central assumptions of Durkheim and the structure functionalists. The central similarity is the view that the structural arrangement of social institutions shapes the resources available to the individual and hence that person's behavioral and emotional responses. Another contribution of network theory is the observation, initially made by Barnes and Bott, that the structure of networks may not always conform to preconceived notions of what constitutes "community" defined on the basis of geographic or kinship criteria. Thus, Wellman argues that the essence of community is its social structure, not its spatial structure (1988, p. 86). By assessing actual ties between network members, one can empirically test whether community exists and whether that community is defined on the basis of neighborhood, kinships, friendship, institutional affiliation, or other characteristics. This emphasis is shared by Durkheim, who describes a shift from mechanical solidarity (based on kinship ties) to organic solidarity (based on rational exchange-based ties) as the basis of social organization.

Weaving the Threads Together

How do these three theories from very different perspectives come together to help us develop a conceptual framework with which to examine the ways social relationships influence health? How can we hope to integrate a set of ideas proposed by sociologists, anthropologists, and psychiatrists writing over the last century, none of whom was interested primarily in the broad array of health outcomes falling under the purview of the epidemiologist? To begin with, we will draw from these theorists the greatest contributions (as we see them) to the development of a comprehensive framework of use to social epidemiology. For instance, a singular contribution of Durkheim's was his anchoring of an individual's death in the social experience of the group. His steadfast orientation toward population patterns of mortality permitted him to identify social integration as a critical contributor to the social patterning of suicide. Without denying that the characteristics of the individual or proximate and precipitating factors could influence *who* among many in a particular group might commit suicide, his constant orientation to population patterns allowed him to uncover collective, societal characteristics related to suicide.

Bowlby's view of attachment as a "primary motivational system" is critical not because attachment provides food, warmth, or other material resources but because it provides love, security, and other nonmaterial resources. This theory is also central to our thinking of the way in which social relationships may be health-promoting. Bowlby tried to identify critical periods in development when bonds of attachment are made. This lifecourse perspective is gaining strength in social epidemiology now.

Finally, much of our framework builds directly upon the work of social network theorists. Critical contributions center on the network approach itself, in which the structure and function of ties are assessed without the assuming they are defined by specific kinds of "bounded" affiliations such as kin, neighborhood, and work. This orientation permitted social network analysts from Bott (1957) to Wellman (1988) to identify the social structure underlying behaviors when a traditional focus on either family or neighborhood was incapable of explaining behavioral patterns. An example of this approach is illustrated by Wellman's study of East York, a community in Toronto. He writes:

Rather than study communities, defined by neighborhoods, we have examined communities defined by networks. The network approach has enabled us to see which attributes of ties and networks best foster sociable relations, interpersonal support, informal social control and a sense of personal identity—the traditional output of variables of community studies. For, if neighborhood and kinship ties make up only a portion of community ties, then studies restricted to neighborhood and kinship groups give a distorted picture of community. (Wellman et al. 1988, p. 131)

Two other strengths of network theories deserve mention. We are struck by the flexibility of social network models in spanning assessment of intimate as well as extended ties, permitting a deep understanding and appreciation of the critical roles many kinds of relationships play in everyday life. Perhaps most important is that network theories virtually force researchers to identify characteristics of the network (at the social level) rather than characteristics of the individual as explanatory variables. Thus we see structural network characteristics explaining support, access to jobs (Granovetter 1973, 1982), social influence (Marsden and Friedkin 1994), health behaviors, and disease transmission (Morris 1994). By integrating these diverse theories and weaving them together, we derive powerful theories and models. We use them to build a more comprehensive framework, and use it to examine how social relations and networks influence a broad array of health outcomes.

A CONCEPTUAL MODEL LINKING SOCIAL NETWORKS TO HEALTH

An Overview

Beginning with seminal work in epidemiology by Cassel (1976) and Cobb (1976), who first suggested a link between social resources, support, and disease risk, epidemiologists began to investigate the role of social relationships on health. Throughout the 1970s and 1980s a series of studies appeared which consistently showed that the lack of social ties or social networks predicted mortality from almost every cause of death (see reviews by Berkman 1995; House et al. 1988; Cohen 1988). These studies most often captured numbers of close friends and relatives, marital status, and affiliation or membership in religious and voluntary associations. These measures were conceptualized in any number of ways as assessments of social networks or ties, social

connectedness, integration, activity, or embeddedness. Whatever they were named, they uniformly defined embeddedness or integration as involvement with ties spanning the range from intimate to extended. Most studies included measures of both "strong" and "weak" ties. As defined by Mark Granovetter (1973), weak ties involve contacts with extended nonintimate ties who he found to be central to occupational mobility.

Although the power of these measures to predict health outcomes is indisputable, the interpretation of what the measures actually measure has been open to much debate. Hall and Wellman (1985) have appropriately commented that much of the work in social epidemiology has used the term social networks metaphorically since rarely have investigators conformed to more standard assessments used in network analysis. For instance, the existence of "weak ties" is not assessed directly but inferred from membership in voluntary and religious organizations. This criticism has been duly noted and several calls have gone out to develop a second generation of network measures (Berkman 1986; Antonucci and Jackson 1990; House et al. 1988).

A second wave of research developed in reaction to this early work and as an outgrowth of work in health psychology that changed the orientation of the field in several ways. Major contributors to this second wave include Antonucci (Antonucci 1986; Antonucci and Akiyama 1987b), Kahn (1979), Lin (Dean and Lin 1977; Lin and Dean 1984; Lin et al. 1981, 1985), House (1981; House and Kahn 1985; LaRocca et al. 1980), and Barbara and Irwin Sarason (Sarason et al. 1990; Schaefer et al. 1981). These social scientists focused on the provision of social support rather than on the elaboration of the structural aspects of social networks. Especially important among these contributions was Kahn and Antonucci's formulation of the *convoy model,* in which the individual is seen in a lifecourse perspective as traveling through life surrounded by members of his/her cohort who share experiences and life histories and who

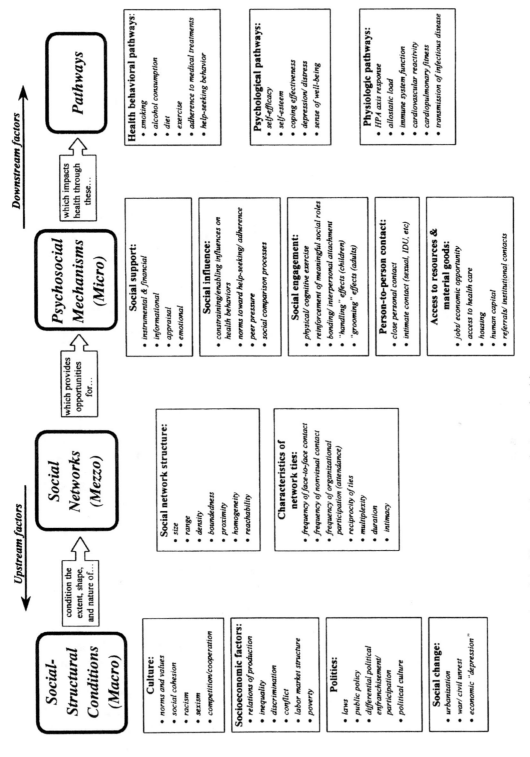

Figure 7-1. Conceptual models of how social networks impact health.

provide support to one another reciprocally over time (Antonucci and Akiyama 1987a,b; Kahn and Antonucci 1980).

Our understanding of the richness and complexity of social support has been advanced immeasurably by:

- Lin and colleagues' social resource theory (1986)
- Rigorous attempts to define the critical domains of support by House (1981)
- Sarason's calls for theory-based work

They have helped us understand how support is linked to mental health. But all these investigators share an assumption—that what is most important about networks is the support functions they provide. Social support is one of the main ways social networks influence physical and mental health status: we do not dispute that. We do, however, argue that it is *not* the *only* critical pathway. Moreover, we believe that the exclusive study of more proximal pathways detracts from the need to focus on the social context and structural underpinning in which social support is provided. Furthermore, studying social support to the exclusion of other potential pathways does not help us understand the findings in which large and dense networks, or sometimes high levels of support, are associated with poorer health outcomes or less adaptive behaviors, (e.g., transmission of HIV, illicit drug use, alcohol consumption, and less prenatal care).

In order to have a comprehensive framework within which to explain these phenomena, we must move "upstream" and return to an orientation to network structure. Only then can we fully consider the multiple pathways by which social networks might profoundly influence health outcomes. It is also critical to maintain a view of social networks as lodged within those larger social and cultural contexts which shape the structure of networks.

In Figure 7–1, we present a conceptual model of how social networks impact health. We envision a cascading causal process beginning with the macrosocial to psychobiological processes that are dynamically linked together to form the processes by which social integration effects health. As suggested above, we start by embedding social networks in a larger social and cultural context in which upstream forces are seen to condition network structure. Serious consideration of the larger macrosocial context in which networks form and are sustained has been lacking in all but a small number of studies and is almost completely absent in studies of social network influences on health.

We then move downstream to understand the influences network structure and function have on social and interpersonal behavior. We argue that networks operate at the behavioral level through four primary pathways: *(1)* provision of social support, *(2)* social influence, *(3)* on social engagement and attachment, and *(4)* access to resources and material goods. These micropsychosocial and behavioral processes, we argue, then influence even more proximate pathways to health status. These include direct physiological stress responses; health-damaging behaviors such as tobacco consumption or high-risk sexual activity; health-promoting behavior such as appropriate health service utilization, medical adherence, and exercise; and finally, exposure to infectious disease agents such as HIV, other sexually transmitted diseases (STDs), or tuberculosis.

By embedding social networks in this larger chain of causation, we can integrate "upstream" macrosocial forces related to the political economy with social networks as mediating structures between the largest- and smallest-scale social forms. Thus, we can examine how labor markets, economic pressures, and organizational relations influence the structure of networks (Luxton 1980; Krause and Borwashi-Clark 1995; Bodemann 1988; Belle 1982). We can examine specifically how culture, rapid social change, industrialization, and urbanization affect the structure of networks. Perhaps the most critical findings to date in this area relevant to social epidemiology are whether "community" is dead or dying in postindustrial American society. In fact, this question has been central to many social network analysts. (See Wellman et al. 1988 for an excellent discussion of this question.)

The Assessment of Social Networks

Next we come to identifying critical domains of social networks. A social network might be defined as the web of social relationships that surround an individual and the characteristics of those ties (Fischer 1982; Mitchell 1969; Fischer et al. 1977; Laumann 1973). Burt has defined network models as describing "the structure of one or more networks of relations within a system of actors" (Burt 1982, p. 20). Thus, while we mainly have considered in this chapter egocentric networks (networks surrounding an individual), network analysis can easily examine networks of networks. Network characteristics (see Fig. 7–1) cover:

1. *Range* or *size* (number of network members)
2. *Density* (the extent to which the members are connected to each other)
3. *Boundedness* (the degree to which they are defined on the basis of traditional group structures such as king, work, neighborhood
4. *Homogeneity* (the extent to which individuals are similar to each other in a network)

Related to network structure, characteristics of individual ties include:

5. *Frequency of contact,* (number of face-to-face contacts and/or contacts by phone or mail)
6. *Multiplexity* (the number of types of transactions or support flowing through a set of ties)
7. *Duration* (the length of time an individual knows another)
8. *Reciprocity* (the extent to which exchanges or transactions are even or reciprocol)

Downstream Social and Behavioral Pathways

Social support

Moving downstream, we now come to a discussion of the mediating pathways by which networks might influence health status. Most obviously the structure of network ties influences health via the provision of many kinds of support. This framework immediately acknowledges that *not all* ties are supportive and that there is variation in the type, frequency, intensity, and extent of support provided. For example, some ties provide several types of support while other ties are specialized and provide only one type. Social support is typically divided into subtypes, which include emotional, instrumental, appraisal, and informational support (House 1981). Emotional support is related to the amount of "love and caring, sympathy and understanding and/or esteem or value available from others" (Thoits 1995). Emotional support is most often provided by a confidant or intimate other, although less intimate ties can provide such support under circumscribed conditions.

Instrumental support refers to help, aid, or assistance with tangible needs such as getting groceries, getting to appointments, phoning, cooking, cleaning, or paying bills. House (1981) refers to instrumental support as aid in kind, money, or labor. Appraisal support, often defined as the third type of support, relates to help in decision making, giving appropriate feedback, or help deciding which course of action to take. Informational support is related to the provision of advice or information in the service of particular needs. Emotional, appraisal, and informational support are often difficult to disaggregate and have various other definitions (e.g. self-esteem support).

We share the view of Kahn and Antonucci (1980), who view social support as transactional in nature, potentially involving both giving and receiving. Further, the process of giving and receiving support resources occurs within a normative framework of exchange in which behavior is guided by norms of interdependence, solidarity, and reciprocity (see George 1986). Support exchanges also take place within a life-course context and not simply in response to day-to-day contingencies. This helps explain patterns of continued support exchange in late life among persons who are disabled and unable to reciprocate. Moreover, support exchanges take place within the context of social network ties, which are long-standing and based on shared histories and not as isolated or atomized phenomenon. Measures of support frequently fail to assess such aspects of reciprocity and instead focus more attention on received support.

Apart from type of support, it is important to differentiate cognitive from behavioral aspects of support. That a person perceives support to be available upon need may or may not correspond with the actual provision of that support in circumstances in which such a request is made. Both the cognitions that surround one's sense of the availability and adequacy of potential support and the extent to which support is actually received appear to be different and equally important. Support that is received is an actual exchange related to a behavior. It is sometimes called enacted or experienced support (Dunkel-Schetter and Bennett 1990). A brisk debate persists over which is most important in what situations—behavioral or cognitive—in either case, it is clear that they tap different aspects of support and are only modestly correlated in most studies (Dunkel-Schetter and Bennett 1990).

Unlike emotional support, instrumental, appraisal, and informational support may influence health because these types of support improve access to resources and material goods. Classic examples would be Granovetter's study of the strength of "weak ties," in which ties that are personally less intimate but that bridge across networks provide for better access to jobs (1973). Another example is Howell's work (1969) on how women obtain abortions. Support conceived of in these ways provides economic

opportunity and access to health care and creates institutional liaisons.

Social influence

Networks may influence health via several other pathways. One pathway that is often ignored is based on *social influence*. Marsden asserts that the "proximity of two actors in social networks is associated with the occurrence of interpersonal influence between the actors" (1994, p. 3). As the term is used, influence need not be associated with face-to-face contact, nor does it require deliberate or conscious attempts to modify behavior (1994, p 4). Marsden refers to work by Erickson (1988) suggesting that under conditions of ambiguity "people obtain normative guidance by comparing their attitudes with those of a reference group of similar others. Attitudes are confirmed and reinforced when they are shared with the comparison group but altered when they are discrepant" (Marsden and Friedkin 1994, p. 5). Shared norms around health behaviors (e.g., alcohol and cigarette consumption, health care utilization, treatment adherence, and dietary patterns) might be powerful sources of social influence with direct consequences for the behaviors of network members. These processes of mutual influence might occur quite apart from the provision of social support taking place within the network concurrently. For instance, cigarette smoking by peers is among the best predictors of smoking for adolescents (Landrine et al. 1994). The social influence which extends from the network's values and norms constitutes an important and underappreciated pathway through which networks impact health.

Social engagement

A third and more-difficult-to-define pathway by which networks may influence health status is by promoting social participation and social engagement. Participation and engagement result from the enactment of potential ties in real-life activity. Getting together with friends, attending social functions, participating in occupational or social roles, group recreation, church attendance—these are all instances of social engagement. Thus, through opportunities for engagement, social networks define and reinforce meaningful social roles including parental, familial, occupational, and community roles, which in turn provide a sense of value, belonging, and attachment Those roles that provide each individual with a coherent and consistent sense of identity are only possible because of the network context, which provides the theater in which role performance takes place.

In addition, network participation provides opportunities for companionship and sociability. We, as well as others (Rook 1990), argue that these behaviors and attitudes are not the result of the provision of support per se but are the consequence of participation in a meaningful social context in and of itself. (See Rook 1990 for an excellent discussion of the difference between support and companionship.) We hypothesize that part of the reason measures of social integration or "connectedness" have been such powerful predictors of mortality for long periods of follow-up is that these ties give meaning to an individual's life by virtue of enabling him or her to participate in it fully, to be obligated (in fact, often to be the provider of support), and to feel attached to one's community. Despite the tendency of some researchers to classify "belonging" as another feature of support, this pathway is distinct from the level of support that is either received or even perceived, standing apart from cognitive and behavioral aspects of support. Such a pathway relates closely to the way in which social networks contribute to social cohesion. Through contact with friends and family and participation in voluntary activities, life acquires a sense of coherence, meaningfulness and interdependence.

Recent evidence from our longitudinal study of aging (Glass et al. in press; Bassuk et al. 1999) indicates that social engagement and participation is related to the maintenance of cognitive function in old age and to reductions in mortality independent of level of emotional or instrumental support.

Rook (1987) also reports that a measure of companionship was a more important antidote to minor life stresses than was social support. We suspect that this range of salutory benefits is associated directly and indirectly with increases in levels of activities related to social engagement itself. Thus, social engagement may activate physiologic systems which operate directly to enhance health as well as indirectly by contributing to a sense of coherence and identity which allows for a high level of well-being.

Person-to-person contact
Networks also influence disease by restricting or promoting exposure to infectious disease agents. In this regard the methodological links between epidemiology and networks are striking. What is perhaps most remarkable is that the same network characteristics that can be health-promoting can at the same time be health-damaging if they serve as vectors for the spread of infectious disease. Efforts to link mathematical modeling by applying network approaches to epidemiology are in their infancy and have started to appear over the last 10 years (Morris 1994; Morris et al. 1991; Laumann et al. 1989; Friedman 1995; Kloudahl 1985). In an insightful paper, Morris (1994) discusses how epidemiologists developed models of disease transmission by initially recognizing the biological characteristics of the disease agent. By the turn of the century, epidemiologists had recognized that the population dynamics of an epidemic are proportional to *(1)* the probability that one member of the contact is susceptible, *(2)* the probability that the other is infected, and *(3)* the number of effective contacts made between individuals per unit time (Morris 1994). By the 1920s, important contributions had been made which tied the outbreak of an epidemic to the density of susceptibles, and virtually all modern models of the spread of epidemics are centered on an understanding that the ratio of susceptibles to immunes is more critical to the spread and containment of epidemics than is the absolute number of susceptibles.

The contribution of social network analysis to the modeling of disease transmission is the understanding that in many, if not most cases, disease transmission is not spread randomly throughout a population. Social network analysis is well suited to the development of models in which exposure between individuals is not random but rather is based on geographic location, sociodemographic characteristics (age, race, gender), or other important characteristics of the individual (socioeconomic position, occupation, sexual orientation) (Laumann et al. 1989). Furthermore, because social network analysis focuses on characteristics of the network rather than on characteristics of the individual, it is ideally suited to the study of diffusion of transmissable diseases through populations via bridging ties between networks or uncovering characteristics of ego-centered networks that promote the spread of disease.

Perhaps the most successful example to date of the application of network analysis to the spread of infectious disease is work done on HIV transmission. Whether spread through sexual contact or intravenous drug use, HIV transmission results from selective rather than random mixing. It is clear that the potential for spread depended (and still depends) upon the "existence and size of a bridge population" (Morris et al. 1996). Thus, the early spread of AIDS in the United States from a predominantly gay male population to a heterosexual population depended on people who could bridge those populations.

Understanding the dynamics of disease spread predominantly by person-to-person contact requires an appreciation for the complex dynamics between individuals and their social networks. To date, few studies have capitalized on the rich methods developed by network analysts that might be directly applicable to the diffusion of socially patterned disease.

Access to material resources

Surprisingly little research has sought to examine differential access to material goods, resources, and services as a mechanism through which social networks might operate. This, in our view, is unfortunate given the work of sociologists showing that social networks operate by regulating an individual's access to life-opportunities by virtue of the extent to which networks overlap with other networks. Perhaps the most important among these studies is Granovetter's classic study of the power of "weak ties" that, on the one hand, lack intimacy, but on the other hand facilitate the diffusion of influence and information and provide opportunities for mobility (1973).

We speculate that participation in networks on the basis of shared work experiences (i.e., trade unions, professional organizations), health experiences (support groups for recovery from cancer, stroke, heart disease), or religious affiliation, for instance, provides access to resources and services which have a direct bearing on health outcomes. Quite apart from the support provided by these ties, even the instrumental support provided, membership in these groups may provide access to job opportunities, high-quality health care, and housing. While this pathway is closely allied with instrumental appraisal and financial support, we believe that further empirical work and increased understanding may show that it constitutes a linkage between networks and health not defined primarily by support.

We have identified five mechanisms by which the structure of social networks might influence disease patterns. Social support is the mechanism most commonly invoked, but social networks also influence health through additional behavioral mechanism, including (1) forces of social influence, (2) levels of social engagement and participation, (3) regulation of contact with infectious disease, and (4) access to material goods and resources. These mechanisms are not mutually exclusive. In fact, it is most likely that in many cases they operate simultaneously. The researcher starting an investigation in this area needs to develop clear hypotheses about which aspects of network structure and the mechanism(s) through which it may influence health a priori to maximize opportunities to understand the way in which social structures are linked to health.

Biological and Psychological Pathways Proximate to Health Status

Social networks operate through the above-described series of five behavioral mechanisms in shaping the health of individuals. In turn, these behavioral mechanisms affect other downstream factors via biologic and psychological pathways most proximate to the health outcome. Moving across our diagram (Fig. 7–1), we now turn our attention to these pathways. Three distinct pathways will be outlined, although again the reader is alerted to the distinct possibility, in fact, likelihood, that multiple pathways are involved simultaneously.

First, social networks via social influence or supportive functions influence health-promoting or health-damaging behaviors such as tobacco and alcohol consumption, physical activity, dietary patterns, sexual practices, and illicit drug use. Second, social networks via any number of pathways influence cognitive and emotional states such a self-esteem, social competence, self-efficacy, depression, and affect. Third, networks may have direct effects on health outcomes by influencing a series of physiologic pathways largely related to stress responses. (See Chapter 13, for a fuller discussion of these pathways.) We view pathways 1 and 2 as logical and valid; however, there is not a large literature to date on the links between networks and health behaviors or psychological attributes, so we will review them only briefly before turning to the third pathway. The reader is referred to two excellent recent reviews on the physiologic and behavioral processes linked to social networks and support (Uchino et al. 1996; Knox and Uvnas-Moberg 1998).

Health behaviors

Evidence suggests that, in general, social network size or "connectedness" is inverse-ly related to risk-related behaviors. Data from Alameda County (Fig. 7–2) show a steady gradient between increasing social disconnection and the cumulative prevalence of health-damaging behaviors such as tobacco and alcohol consumption, physical inactivity, and consequent obesity. Trieber and colleagues (1991) report that social support is related to physical exercise. Several studies have reported that social support is related to smoking cessation, especially among men (Hanson et al. 1990; Murray et al. 1995), but other studies have reported no associations (Mermelstein et al. 1986).

In general, behavioral pathways such as these do not appear to account for a large part of the relationship between social networks and morbidity or mortality. In most instances, relative risks are reduced about 20% when such behaviors are introduced into multivariate models (Berkman and Syme 1979; Kaplan et al. 1988; House et al. 1982; Seeman et al. 1993a). However, this may be due to the fact that we are most often measuring components of networks (size and support) that are less predictive of health behaviors. The addition of assessments of other mechanisms including social influence and social engagement may strengthen the explanatory power of our models.

Psychologic mechanisms

Self-efficacy, defined as the degree of confidence persons have in their ability to perform specific behaviors, has been shown to be associated with a variety of health and functional outcomes (Grembowski et al. 1993; AcAuley 1993; Mendes de Leon et al. 1996; Seeman et al. 1993b; Tinetti and Powell 1993). A considerable body of evidence undergirds the assertion that self-efficacy is one of the psychosocial pathways through which social support operates. For example, in a study of postpartum depression, the protective effect of social support was observed to occur primarily through its mediation of maternal feelings of self-efficacy (Cutrona and Troutman 1986). Other

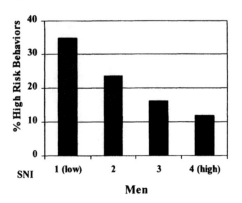

Figure 7–2. Distribution of health practices and risk factors such as cigarette smoking, alcohol consumption, physical inactivity, obesity and dietary patterns by level of social integration. Percent of men and woment who have several high risk behaviors (three of five) by level of social network index (Alameda County Study, n = 2229 men, n = 2496 women), ages 30–69 years.

studies have observed the indirect influence of social support through enhanced self-efficacy in coping with abortion (Major et al. 1990), smoking cessation (Gulliver et al. 1995), and depression (McFarlane et al. 1995). The association between social networks and health-promoting behavior such as exercise has also been shown to be mediated through self-efficacy Duncan and McAuley 1993).

Evidence suggests that ongoing network participation is essential for the maintenance of self-efficacy beliefs in late life. A study by McAvay et al. (1996) found that lower levels of social network contact were predictive of decline in the health and safety domains of self-efficacy, and the absence of instrumental support was also associated with decline in the productivity, health, and transportation domains. There is some evidence that the impact of self-efficacy and social support are reciprocal—meaning that while social support may bolster self-efficacy, it may also be the case that the self-efficacy is independently associated with higher levels of social support (Holahan and Holahan 1987). The complexity of these reciprocal dynamics have yet to be fully examined.

In addition to self-efficacy, social integration appears to operate through additional psychosocial pathways. For example, some evidence suggests that social support promotes functional and adaptive coping styles (Holahan and Moos 1987; Wolf et al. 1991). An influential study by Dunkel-Schetter et al. (1987) has shown, however, that these relationships are likely to be reciprocal. Their evidence suggests that in stressful situations, different coping styles elicit different responses from the social environment. Indeed, the tendency to ask for and make use of social support itself is one of many possible coping styles, and has numerous psychological antecedents and correlates (Dunkel-Schetter et al. 1992). In a review of patterns of attachment, Fonagy (1996) presents evidence that attachment relationships contribute to self-esteem and the perception that the individual is in control of his or her own destiny.

Social support may additionally operate through its influence on emotion, mood, and perceived well-being. Numerous studies have shown that social support is associated with symptoms of depression (Bowling and Browne 1991; Holahan et al. 1995, 1997; Lin and Dean 1984; Lomauro 1990; Matt and Dean 1993; Morris et al. 1991; George et al. 1989; Turner 1983; Oxman et al. 1992). This evidence is particularly important in light of the fact that social support, especially perceived emotional support, has been shown to buffer the deleterious influences of stressful life events on the risk of depression and depressive symptoms (Lin et al. 1986; Paykel 1994; Vilhjalmsson 1993). The evidence appears to be strong that those who are socially isolated are at increased risk of depression, especially in late life (Murphy 1982). The relationship in some cases is reciprocal, with support influencing depressive symptoms and vice versa (Oxman et al. 1992). In studies of psychological health, one consistent finding is that the perceived adequacy of social support, more so than the availability of support, appears to be most important (Henderson 1981).

Physiologic pathways
An examination of the pathways linking social networks to health outcomes yields a rich and complex lattice work of interlinking mechanisms—biological, psychological, and biophysiological—that cascades from the macro to the micro, from upstream to downstream, to generate potentially powerful influences on health and well-being across the lifecourse. One of the robust findings in the literature on networks and health is the broad impact network integration has on all-cause mortality. This may be related to the numerous pathways which more proximately impact disease onset or progression, but it is also possible that some more general phenomenon is at work. Our inability to address this question in a serious way has been the result in part of the lack of a larger theoretical model such as the one proposed here. By specifying a chain of interrelated pathways that range from the macro to the micro, we can expand the scope of our investigation and identify domains of influence that have previously remained unexplored. Below, we describe several promising areas where such expansion might profitably take place.

Accelerated aging and a lifecourse perspective. We speculate that social isolation, disintegration, and disconnectedness influence mortality and therefore longevity or life expectancy by influencing the rate of aging of the organism. In a review on aging from a social and biomedical perspective, Berkman (1988, p. 51) hypothesized that social isolation "was a chronically stressful condition to which the organism responded by aging faster. Isolation would then also be associated with age-related morbidity and functional decline. Thus, the cumulative conditions [that] tend to occur in very old age [would be] accelerated." Such "accelerated aging" hypotheses have also been applied to other social experiences, especially to racial differences in health in the United States (Jones 1995).

It is characteristic of changes related to aging that peak rises in response to stress or challenge are not as different between young and old as is the time it takes to return to prechallenge levels. Older animals take longer to return to a baseline state after challenge and therefore spend a greater amount of time "under the curve." This has implications for the cumulative wear and tear of life stressors in late life. Figure 7–3 illustrates this pattern in a hypothetical situation. For instance, Sapolsky et al. (1983) show that while older rats have slightly elevated levels of basal corticosterone, by far the most remarkable change with age is the impaired capacity of the older rats to adapt to and recover from stress. In a series of experiments, old and young rats exposed to cold or immobilization stress reacted initially in the same way, with dramatic increases in corticosterone, but after 90 minutes and even up to 150 minutes after exposure, the aged rats still maintained very high levels due to continued secretion, while the young rats had returned to basal levels.

Missing from our earlier conceptualization was a lifecourse perspective which has become much clearer with evidence accumulated since the 1988 review. Research on humans and animals (both primates and nonprimates) indicates that early experiences, especially social experiences between

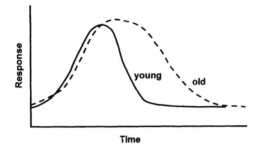

Figure 7–3. Hypothetical model of reactions to stress or challenge by age.

primary caregivers and infants, are powerful determinants of social, behavioral, and physiological development across the life span. In fact, many changes in function that are considered "normal aging" show variability related to early life experiences. It now appears that long-term neurobiological experiences which unfold in old age may have been shaped, in part, by experiences during early "critical" or "sensitive" experiences (Suomi 1997).

In a series of landmark studies, Meany and colleagues have shown that in rodents frequency of early handling and maternal separation contribute to stable differences throughout the life span in the hypothalamic–pituitary–adrenal (HPA) axis responses. These differences are especially marked in response to stressful stimuli (Francis et al. 1996; Meaney et al. 1985, 1988, 1996). The HPA axis response to stress is a classic adaptive mechanism in virtually all mammals. (See Chapter 13 for a detailed discussion.) Poor, inefficient, or exaggerated HPA axis response has been implicated in decreased sensitivity to insulin, risk of steroid-induced diabetes, hypertension, hyperlipidemia, arterial disease, impairment of growth and tissue repair, and immunosuppression (Francis et al. 1996). Briefly, these experiments show that rats handled during the postnatal period show faster adrenocortical recovery from stress than do nonhandled rats or those experiencing maternal separation. Furthermore, the aged rats that were not

handled showed age-related rises in basal glucorticoid levels that were not apparent among the aged handled rats (showing an "aging" effect). These findings suggest that the cumulative exposure to glucocorticoids over the life span was greater in the non-handled rats or those experiencing early maternal separation when compared to rats who were handled or spent extensive time with their mothers.

Most remarkable was that in old age there was marked hippocampal cell loss and cognitive impairment in the aged nonhandled rats. These results indicate that experiences involving maternal separation and withdrawal from handling—in general, a nurturant experience—influence the way rodents react to stress and appear to accelerate the aging of the organism. In addition, they point to the importance of a lifecourse perspective in which the influences of affiliation are developmental. We take these results to indicate the possibility that chronic social isolation throughout the lifecourse may produce persistent HPA axis response difference that induce faster aging. This hypothesis has yet to be fully addressed in humans.

In now-classic work Suomi and colleagues have studied rhesus monkeys to learn about development from infancy to adulthood. They conclude that early social relationships shape behavioral and physiologic functioning throughout the lifecourse in powerful ways (1997). Infant monkeys who were separated from their mothers and reared by peers were more likely to become "high reactors" and impulsive when compared to mother-reared controls. "High reactive monkeys are not only more likely to exhibit depressive-like behavioral responses to separation but also tend to show greater and longer HPA activation, more dramatic sympathetic arousal, more central noradrenergic turnover, and greater selective immunosuppresion" (Suomi 1991). While these monkeys have not been followed into old age, the pattern of the stress response is remarkably similar to that described by Meaney and his colleagues.

We know a lot about how early childhood attachment affects later psychological development in humans; however, not as much evidence is available with regard to physiologic concomitants or long-term health outcomes in terms of morbidity or mortality in late adulthood. Some of the strongest work in the area has been conducted by Gunnar and her colleagues at the University of Minnesota (Gunnar and Nelson 1994). With regard to physiologic reactivity, especially as assessed by salivary cortisol, they have reported that among young children who are behaviorally inhibited, secure attachment between parent and child prevents a heightened cortisol response to arousing and strange situations (Nachmias et al. 1996). In fact, only among children who are inhibited *and* insecurely attached are elevations in cortisol observed in response to exposure to a stressful situation. Gunnar reports that securely attached infants and toddlers (who have experienced "consistent, responsive, and sensitive" forms of relationships with their parents) tend to develop into socially competent children. Social competence predicts a pattern or hormonal stress activity in which cortisol levels are low in familiar situations but may be higher than average in new and uncertain situations. Gunnar cautions that not all elevated levels of hormonal stress response should be viewed as maladaptive since a healthy and realistic appreciation of new challenges may portend better adaptation as situations are mastered effectively (Gunnar et al. 1997).

The biological effects of adult social experiences: continuity and change. Early theories of aging assumed that plasticity was a characteristic of early phases of development and was virtually nonexistent by old age. In contrast, developmental neurobiologists, neuropsychologists, social scientists, and geriatricians now recognize that in most domains, change occurs through the lifecourse and is not restricted to early development. For instance, neuronal plasticity, especially following injury, has been the subject of a great deal of research, most of which suggests the aging brain is more plastic than we ever suspected (Moss and Albert 1988; Cotman 1985). Similarly, clinical trials of physical activity across adulthood show that interventions, even in very old age, have significant effects (Buchner et al. 1992; Emery and Gatz 1990; Wolinsky et al. 1995).

The impact of social attachments made in early years on health outcomes remains an intriguing and understudied area; however, the vast body of epidemiologic evidence produced to date indicates that it is adult social circumstances that are linked to poor health outcomes. Debates in which we pitch continuity (the effect of early development/environment) against discontinuity (the effect of recent events) are *not* likely to be fruitful since both have consequences for health outcomes. Furthermore, we know that large-scale social upheavals and transitions profoundly disrupt patterns of social organizations established in earlier life. Geographical relocation related to urbanization, housing policy, or employment opportunities; large-scale social change or depression such as seen in Russia and Eastern Europe; and job stress and corporate policies that are not "family" friendly represent environmental challenges that tear at the fabric of social networks, which in turn have deleterious consequences on health.

Chapter 13 of this volume discusses a range of biological mechanisms that link adult social experiences to poor health outcomes. In *this* chapter, we would like to emphasize only those that have been found to link aspects of social networks and support to health. The reader is referred to Chapter 13 for a fuller explanation of biological pathways.

Animals who are isolated have been shown to have more extensive athersclerosis than less isolated animals. This has been shown in both primates and nonprimates (Nerem et al. 1980). Shively and colleagues

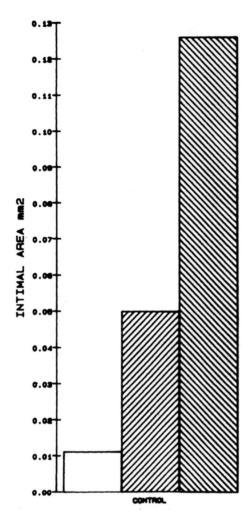

Figure 7–4. Mean coronary artery atherosclerosis extent as measured by intimal area in control-group females that were (1) dominant in social groups, (open bar), (2) subordinate in social groups (right hatched bar), and (3) housed in single cages. Shively, C.A., Clarkson, T.B., and Kaplan, J.R. (1989). Social deprivation and coronary artery atherosclerosis in female cynomologus monkey. *Atherosclerosis*, 77:69–76.

(1989) have reported that adult female cynomolgus monkeys housed alone compared to those housed in small groups had developed more atherosclerosis than other animals, yet there were no differences in lipid concentration. Figure 7–4 shows the mean intimal area effected in monkeys in

the social group who were dominant, subordinate, and isolated.

In recent studies, Shively and colleagues have continued their investigations to understand the mechanisms through which social isolation leads to cardiovascular disease. In recent studies, Watson (Watson et al. 1998) showed that chronic social isolation experienced by monkeys caged alone may influence atherosclerosis by altered autonomic activity. Adult monkeys housed alone had much higher heart rates under nonchallenge, average conditions than did monkeys housed in groups. These differences could not be explained by level of physical activity. The authors hypothesized that the lack of affiliative behavior may be a key component related to caging since upon reunion with other monkeys, rates of affiliative behavior increased compared to preseparation time.

With regard to cardiovascular reactivity in humans, several recent studies have identified remarkably strong relationships with support and reactivity assessed in terms of blood pressure response to stress or challenge. Among the clearest of these is an experiment conducted by Kamarck et al. (1991). In this experiment, they exposed all subjects to a challenge involving public speaking. They then randomly told half the group that social support was available by telling them before the "challenge" that someone was available for help if they needed it. They would be just outside the room. In fact, no support was actually provided; it was merely available if needed. People without support had higher systolic and diastolic pressure both *before* the actual challenge as well as during the challenge. Thus, support availability protects against increased blood pressure response associated with stressful situations.

This type of experiment has now been repeated, and several critical aspects of the design (the nature of the challenge, the type of support, the match between subject and supporter) have been varied. Some evidence suggests that support may moderate stress differentially for men and women (Kirschbaum et al. 1995). Although they are not completely consistent, the majority of these studies confirm the important role of support in moderating levels of reactivity, although the type of challenge and match between supporter and subject are important to outcomes (Uchino et al. 1996).

A few studies have reported variations in cortisol, epinephrine, or norepinephrine related to social isolation. Sapolsky et al. (1997) report that in their studies of baboons in the wild, the degree of affiliation was related to adrenocortical status. As found in most studies of humans, they note that it was not a single form of affiliation that was important but an aggregate measure of eight aspects of social connectedness. Sanchez et al. (1994) report that in rats isolated from contact, there are reduced corticosterone concentrations. In humans, work by our group from the MacArthur Foundation on Successful Aging (Seeman et al. 1994) indicates that among older men and women with relatively high functional status, social networks and support are related to basal levels of several neuroendocrine factors assayed from overnight urine samples. Studies by Knox and colleagues (1985) show measures of lack of attachment with intimate contacts as well as low number of contacts with acquaintances are associated with high resting-plasma adrenaline levels in young men. In this same study, the later measure of contact with acquaintances was related to heart rate variability. In a study of stress related to a nuclear power plant accident, Fleming (Fleming et al. 1982) showed that people with low social support had higher levels of urinary norepinephrine regardless of their level of stress. For further discussion of mechanisms related to cardiovascular disease, the reader is referred to a review by Knox and Uvnas-Moberg (1998).

Another pathway by which social relationships might influence health involves alteration in immune response. There is a growing body of knowledge in this area.

While immune function is a complex and multidimensional phenomenon and not detached from neurendocrine response, much progress has been made in the last decade or two in understanding how social ties influence immune function (see Cohen et al. 1997).

The largest body of evidence in this area links social support to changes in immune parameters. Early studies show the pervasive effects of bereavement or living with a severely ill spouse or child in terms of suppressed immune function, particularly cellular immunity. Work over the last few years by Kiecolt-Glaser and colleagues and others has found that less devastating aspects of relationships such as the quality of marital relationship or feelings of loneliness among medical students also compromise immunocompetence (Kiecolt-Glaser et al. 1984, 1987; Thomas et al. 1985; Glaser et al. 1985). The latter studies of medical students showed that those who were lonely had not only lower levels of natural-killer-cell activity but also significantly high Epstein-Barr virus (EBV) antibody titers. Thus, again we see provocative evidence that social isolation may regulate immune mechanisms involved in the regulation of latent infections. Finally, studies of affiliation in nonhuman primates further suggest that such intimate affiliative behaviors are associated with cellular immune response (Cohen et al. 1992).

ASSESSMENT OF SOCIAL INTEGRATION, SOCIAL NETWORKS, AND SOCIAL SUPPORT

The assessment of aspects of social relationships in epidemiologic studies often has not benefited enough from work in the social sciences. Our aim in this section is to introduce the reader to range of measures available with a brief commentary regarding their utility for a specific purpose. At the outset, it should be made explicit that we do not believe there is a single measure which is optimal or even appropriate for all purposes. The investigator must consider why he or she hypothesizes that social ties are important to the health outcome of interest and then select and potentially modify or tailor an instrument. For instance, evidence to date suggests that measures of social integration are related to mortality and perhaps to the development of atherosclerosis whereas emotional support is most highly related to survival in post-MI (myocardial infarction) patients. These findings and subsequent hypotheses for new studies necessitate the use of different measures. In a similar vein, studying HIV transmission or initiation of high-risk behaviors necessitates the use of still other types of instruments.

Following the logic of House and Kahn (1985), we have divided our discussion of measures into three sections: *(1)* those measures that primarily assess social ties or social integration, *(2)* measures that more formally assess aspects of social networks, and *(3)* measures assessing social support, both cognitively "perceived" and behaviorally

"received." Table 7–1 shows examples of these three domains along with references to the measures. The reader is referred to several lengthier reviews, especially in relation to social support. Several of these reviews include additional information on the psychometric properties of the scales (Orth-Gomér and Unden 1987; Heitzman and Kaplan 1988; House and Kahn 1985).

Measures of Social Ties and Integration

Several brief measures of social ties have been used in large prospective community-based studies. They consistently predict health outcomes, particularly mortality. These scales, consisting of between nine and 18 items, usually take between 2 and 5 minutes to administer. The instruments often tap the size of networks, frequency of contact, membership in voluntary and religious organizations and social participation. Perhaps the best conceptual framework in which to place these measures is that of social integration. From this perspective, the

Table 7.1. Ways of Assessing Social Relationships

Social Relations

Social Network Index	Berkman and Syme 1979
Social Relationships and Activity	House et al. 1982
Social Network Interaction Index	Orth-Gomér and Johnson 1987
Social Contacts and Resources	Donald and Ware 1982

Social Networks

Northern California Community Study	Fischer 1982
East York Social Network Study	Wellman and Leighton 1979
New Haven EPESE Network Assessment	Seeman and Berkman 1988
	Glass et al. 1997
A Convey Network Model	Antonucci 1986
Bonds of Pluralism	Laumann 1973

Social Support

Social Support Scale in OARS	Blazer et al. 1982
Interpersonal Support Evaluation List (ISEL)	Cohen and Hobermann 1983
Social Support Scale	Lin et al. 1979
Social Support Questionnaire (SSQ)	Sarason et al. 1983
Inventory of Socially Supportive Behaviors (ISSB)	Barrera et al. 1981
Interview Schedule for Social Interaction (ISSI)	Henderson et al. 1980
Perceived Social Support (PSS)	Procidano and Heller 1983
Perceived Social Support Scale (PSSS)	Blumenthal et al. 1987
Abbreviated ISSI	Unden and Orth-Gomér 1984
Medical Outcomes Study Social Support	Sherbourne and Stewart 1991

measures often assess domains of social network size and diversity and social engagement and participation. Because these measures are brief, they rarely include multiple items tapping a similar domain. Therefore, with the exception of the Orth-Gomér and Johnson instrument (1987), there are limited data on internal consistency from a psychometric standpoint. They do, however, have good test–retest reliability (Donald and Ware 1982), are modestly correlated with other psychosocial constructs in expected ways (Seeman and Berkman 1988; Berkman and Breslow 1983), and have solid construct validity in terms of consistency in predicting mortality.

The ease with which the instruments are administered, the degree to which they assess a broad range of levels of social integration from extreme isolation to high levels of integration, and their proven predictive validity are the major assets of this class of instruments. Their major disadvantages lie in not providing much insight into the mechanisms that might be health promoting (e.g., provision of emotional or instrumental support, social engagement, social influence) and in providing limited information on the depth and quality of social relationships. Since it is likely that the critical mechanisms vary among health outcomes, this can be a serious shortcoming of the measures.

Measures of Social Networks

Most classical measures of social networks have been developed without an eye toward how they might be used in studies of health outcomes. However, they provide the best measures of network structure and are often sensitively linked to aspects of social support and occasionally to patterns of social influence or person-to-person contact that enable transmission of infectious agents. Most instruments take between 20 minutes to an hour to complete and provide a rich understanding of the complex dynamics and morphology of networks. Classical examples are those developed by Fischer (1982), Wellman (Wellman and Leighton

1979), and Laumann (1973). If the aim of an investigator is to test hypotheses related to specific structural components of networks (i.e., homogeneity, multiplexity, density, reachability), these instruments are ideal and should be used more often in health-related research. In fact, before launching a study of networks, we recommend a review of several of these measures.

In the past decade, several network instruments have been adapted from these earlier assessments with modifications for use in epidemiology and health psychology. Antonucci's (1986) convoy measure makes excellent use of a bull's-eye mapping technique used in traditional network assessments. (See Boissevain for an early version, 1974.) Following the network assessment, the subject the provides information about individuals in the network regarding social support and sociodemographic characteristics. Similarly, measures from our group, based on the Yale Health and Aging Study, were adapted from question developed by Fischer in his California study (1982). The items tap critical dimensions of networks (size, homogenity, density, contact, proximity) and support (types, availability, adequacy, source) in an abbreviated fashion without asking to identify specific individuals (see Seeman and Berkman 1988 and Glass et al. 1997). These measures are not as lengthy to administer as the traditional network questionnaires but they are also not as rich in assessment of the full range of characteristics as are these traditional measures.

Measures of Social Support

Over the last 15 years, there has been a proliferation of social support measures. They often share a core set of orientations, particularly in the assessment of several types of support including emotional, instrumental or tangible, appraisal, and financial. Beyond that core, the measures are often different from one another in subtle yet important ways. Perhaps the most striking difference is in the orientation to the assessment of perceived support vs. received support. For instance, perceived support items are often oriented toward hypothetical conditions (if you need help, is there anyone you could count on for a small loan, help with a problem). Received support is often grounded in behavioral transactions occurring over a set period of time (in the last week, month, etc., did anyone talk to you about your feelings, lend you money). The investigator must choose between these orientations depending on the hypothesis and population being studied.

Social support instruments tend to have been better studied with regard to their psychometric status. Furthermore, since they commonly include multiple items tapping single domains, they have good internal validity. They usually include from 15 to 40 items and take between 10 and 20 minutes to administer. Their only weakness from the perspective of external validity is that they were often developed on a very small, often college-aged population. Their applicability to populations of heterogeneous middle-aged and older adults must be ascertained on a case-by-case basis. It should be noted that pure social support instruments such as those developed by Cohen (Cohen and Hoberman 1983), Procidano and Heller (1983), Barrera (Barrera et al. 1981), Sherbourne and Stewart (1991), Blumenthal et al. (1987), and Sarason et al. (1983) are excellent measures of support but do not measure network structure (and do not purport to do so). If the investigator is interested in a specific aspect of social support, these are excellent choices for use and ease of administration.

Early in the development of assessments of social interaction, Henderson (Henderson et al. 1980) developed an excellent measure encompassing a broad range of dimensions including social integration, social interactions, and attachment. This instrument has been used in a range of settings *primarily with regard to psychiatric status*. It has 52 items and takes about 30 minutes to complete. It has been modified by Unden and Orth-Gomér (1984) to take under 10 minutes and is very useful in covering a

range of dimensions not exclusively falling into any single domain.

Overview

Our aim in this section was to give the reader a brief overview of the spectrum of measures available to assess aspects of social networks and relationships. There are many instruments in this area now and our aim was not to be comprehensive but, on the contrary, to identify instruments we believe have a great deal of promise and utility to epidemiologists. We have not reviewed some promising new areas, especially those related to negative aspects of social relationships (see Rook 1984), nor have we reviewed more unstructured assessments which may be of great use in psychiatric or clinical studies. (See work by George et al. 1985; Fonagy et al. 1995.) These assessments have great value but may be difficult to incorporate in the broad-based structured interviews usually used by epidemiologists.

SOCIAL NETWORKS AND MORTALITY, MORBIDITY AND DISABILITY

Over the last 20 years a vast literature has accumulated that links social networks or social support and physical and mental health. A complete review of this literature is beyond the scope of this chapter and the reader is referred to several recent reviews covering a broad array of outcomes (Anderson et al. 1996; Berkman 1995; Bowling 1991; Ell 1996; Greenwood et al. 1996; Helgeson and Cohen 1996; Seeman 1996; Eriksen 1994). Our intention here is to review the evidence linking social networks and social support to selected outcomes, highlighting studies related to all-cause mortality, cardiovascular disease, stroke, and infectious diseases.

All-Cause Mortality

Over the last 20 years 13 large prospective cohort studies across a number of countries from the United States to Scandinavian countries to Japan have been conducted that show that people who are isolated or disconnected from others are at increased risk of dying prematurely. Each of these major studies is reviewed briefly below.

In the first of these studies—from Alameda County (Berkman and Syme 1979)—men and women who lacked ties to others (in this case, based on an index assessing contacts with friends and relatives, marital status, and church and group membership) were 1.9 to 3.1 times more likely to die in a 9-year follow-up period from 1965 to 1974 than those who had many more contacts.

The relative risks associated with social isolation were *not* centered in one cause of death; rather, those who lacked social ties were at increased risk of dying from ischemic heart disease (IHD), cerebrovascular and circulatory disease, cancer, and from other causes in a final category that included respiratory, gastrointestinal, and all other causes of death. Clearly, this social condition is not associated exclusively with increased risks from, say, coronary heart disease (CHD). The relationship between social isolation and mortality risk was independent of health behaviors such a smoking, alcohol consumption, physical activity, preventive health care, and a range of baseline comorbid conditions.

Another study—this one in Tecumseh, Michigan (House et al. 1982)—shows a similar strength of positive association for men, but not for women, between social connectedness/social participation and mortality risk over a 10–12-year period. An additional strength of this study was the ability to control for some biomedical predictors assessed from physical examination (e.g., cholesterol, blood pressure, and respiratory function). In the same year, Blazer (1982) reported similar results from an elderly sample of men and women in Durham County, North Carolina. He compared three measures of social support and attachment: *(1)* self-perceived impaired social support, including feelings of loneliness, *(2)* impaired social roles and attachments, and *(3)* low frequency of social interaction. The

relative risks for dying associated with these three measures was 3.4, 2.0, and 1.9, respectively.

In the last few years, results from several more studies have been reported—one from a study in the United States and three from Scandinavia. Using data from Evans County, Georgia, Schoenbach et al. (1986) used a measure of social contacts modified from the Alameda County Study and found risks to be significant in older white men and women even when controlling for biomedical and sociodemographic risk factors although some racial and gender differences were observed. In Sweden, the Goteborg study (Wellin et al. 1985) shows that in different cohorts of men born in 1913 and 1923, social isolation proved to be a risk factor for dying independent of age and biomedical risk factors. A report by Orth-Gomér and Johnson (1987) is the only study besides the Alameda County one to report significantly increased risks for women who have been socially isolated. Finally, in a study of 13,301 men and women in eastern Finland, Kaplan and associates (1988) have shown that an index of social connections almost identical to the Social Network Index used in Alameda County predicts mortality risk for men but not for women independent of standard cardiovascular risk factors.

Several recent studies of older men and women in the Alameda County study and the Established Populations for the Epidemiologic Study of the Elderly (EPESE) studies confirm the continued importance of these relationships into late life (Seeman et al. 1988, 1993a). Furthermore, two studies of large cohort of men and women in a large health maintenance organization (HMO) (Vogt et al. 1992) and 32,000 male health professionals (Kawachi et al. 1996) suggest that social networks are, in general, more strongly related to mortality than to the incidence or onset of disease.

Two very recent studies in Danish men (Pennix et al. 1997) and Japanese men and women (Sugisawa et al. 1994) further indicate that aspects of social isolation or social support are related to mortality. Virtually all of these studies find that people who are socially isolated or disconnected to others have between two and five times the risk of dying from all causes compared to those who maintain strong ties to friends, family, and community.

Cardiovascular Disease

There is conflicting albeit limited evidence that social networks or support is related to the onset of cardiovascular disease. One study of middle-aged Swedish men shows social integration to be related to the incidence of myocardial infarction (Orth-Gomér et al. 1993), but several other studies have reported no associations (Kawachi et al. 1996; Vogt et al. 1992).

In contrast, in the last 6 years, there have been a host of studies suggesting that social ties, especially intimate ties and emotional support provided by those ties, influence survival among people post-MI or with serious cardiovascular disease. In the first of these, Ruberman et al. (1984) explored 2320 male survivors of acute MI who were participants in the Beta-Blocker Heart Attack Trial. Patients who were socially isolated were more than twice as likely to die over a 3-year period than those who were less socially isolated. When this measure of social isolation was combined with a general measure of life stress, which included items related to occupational status, divorce, exposure to violent events, retirement, or financial difficulty, the risks associated with high-risk psychosocial status were even greater. Those in the high-risk psychosocial categories were four to five times as likely to die as those in the lowest risk categories. This psychosocial characteristic was associated with death from all causes and sudden deaths. It made large contributions to mortality risk in both the high-arrhythmia and low-arrhythmia groups. In this study (and most of the studies in which subjects are recruited post-event), the investigators were not able to determine the temporal association between the assessment of psychosocial resources

and the severity of disease. Nonetheless, it serves as a powerful model for future studies.

In a second Swedish study of 150 cardiac patients and patients with high-risk factor levels for CHD, the finding that lack of support predicts death was further confirmed (Orth-Gomér et al. 1988). Patients who were socially isolated had a 10-year mortality rate that was three times higher than did those who were socially active and integrated. Because these patients were examined extensively for prognostic factors at study entry, it was possible to disentangle effects of psychosocial and clinical characteristics.

In a third study, Williams et al. (1992), enrolled 1368 patients who were undergoing cardiac catheterization from 1974 through 1980 who had been found to have significant coronary artery disease. They examined survival time until cardiovascular death through 1989. In this study, men and women who were unmarried or without a confidant were over three times as likely to die within 5 years compared with those who had a close confidant or who were married (odds ratio [OR], 3.34; confidence interval [CI], 1.8–6.2). This association was independent of other clinical prognostic indicators and sociodemographic factors, including socioeconomic status.

Case et al. (1992) examined the association between marital status and recurrent major cardiac events among patients post-MI who were enrolled in the placebo arm of a clinical trial, the Multicenter Diliazem Post-Infarction Trial. These investigators reported that living alone was an independent risk factor with a hazard ratio of 1.54 (CI, 1.04–2.29) for recurrent major cardiac event, including both nonfatal infarctions or cardiac deaths.

In a fifth study, we explored the relationship between social networks and support and mortality among men and women hospitalized for MI between 1982 and 1988 who were participants in the population-based New Haven EPESE (Berkman et al. 1992). Over the study period, 100 mean and 94 women were hospitalized for an MI.

Thirty-four percent of women and 44% of men died in the 6-month period after MI.

Among both men and women, emotional support, measured prospectively, was related to both early in-hospital death and later death over a 1-year period. Among those admitted to the hospital, almost 38% of those who reported no source of emotional support died in the hospital compared with 11.5% of those with two or more sources of support. The patterns remained steady throughout the follow-up period. At 6 months, the major end point of the study, 52.8% of those with no source of support had died compared with 36.0% of those with one source and 23.1% of those with two or more sources of support. These figures did not change substantially at 1 year. As Figure 7–5 shows, the patterns were remarkably consistent for both men and women, younger and older people, and those with more or less severe cardiovascular disease, as assessed by a Killip classification system. In multivariate models that control for sociodemographic factors, psychosocial factors, including living arrangements, depressive symptoms, and clinical prognostic indicators, men and women who reported no emotional support had almost three times the mortality risk compared with subjects who reported at least one source of support (OR, 2.9; 95% CI, 1.2–6.9).

In a study of men and women undergoing coronary bypass surgery or aortic valve replacement, Oxman and colleagues (1995) found that membership in voluntary organizations, including religious organizations, and drawing strength and comfort from religious or spiritual faith were related to sur-

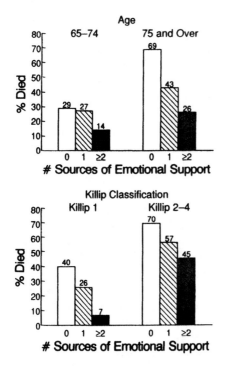

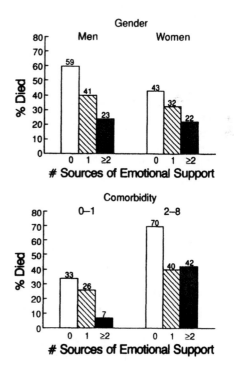

Figure 7–5. Percentage of patients with myocardial infarction who died within 6 months ranked by level of social support. Adjustments were made for age (top left), gender (top right), severity of myocardial infarction as defined by Killip class (bottom left), and comorbidity (bottom right). Adapted from Berkman, L.F., Leo-Summers, L., and Horowitz, R.I. (1992). Emotional support and survival after myocardial infarction. *Ann Internal Med*, 117:1003–9.

vival postsurgery. When these two dimensions were combined, people who endorsed neither of these items were over seven times as likely to die as those who belonged to such organizations and drew comfort from their faith. Though it is beyond the scope of the chapter to go into detail on the recent research on religiosity, this later study complements and balances the work on the importance of intimacy by illustrating that a sense of belonging to informal organizations that are rooted in common values and collective goals may also be an important influence on well-being and survival.

In a study of Mexican Americans and non-Hispanic whites in the Corpus Christi Heart Project (Farmer et al. 1996), social support was found to predict mortality for an average period of over 3 years; however, the relative risk was very strong in the Mexican-American men and women (3.38, CI 1.73–6.62).

These findings in post-MI populations, coupled with the strong data on long-term mortality and relatively weaker data on incidence, would suggest that social networks and support may have the greatest impact on determining not the onset of disease but rather prognosis and survival.

To date there are only a handful of studies related to other cardiovascular related diseases. A study of congestive heart failure (Krumholz et al. 1998) among older men and women in New Haven found emotional support to be related to survival for men but not women and found no association with risk for initial hospitalization (Chen et al., in press).

Stroke

As we noted with respect to cardiovascular disease, the evidence in favor of the view that social integration is associated with cerebrovascular disease is less compelling for incidence, and to some extent for mortality. However, the evidence that social networks and support are important in recovery from stroke is increasingly convincing.

Several studies have identified a trend toward higher risk of death from stroke among those who are socially isolated (Berkman and Breslow 1983; Kawachi et al. 1996), although these studies have lacked the strength to fully evaluate the associations. However, a number of additional studies have shown that social networks and support (particularly social isolation) are associated with case fatality in the poststroke period. For example, in a study by Vogt et al. (1992), social network measures were strong predictors of both cause-specific and all-cause mortality among persons who had incident cases of ischemic heart disease, cancer, and stroke. During 10 years of follow-up of a group of newly diagnosed stroke patients, clinical diagnosis of depression was associated with poor survival (Morris et al. 1993). In that study, patients who were both socially isolated and clinically depressed were at particular risk for poststroke fatality. To date, no studies have reported a link between social isolation and incidence of nonfatal stroke. In one study of 32,624 U.S. male health care workers, Kawachi found a trend in the association between risk of nonfatal stroke and social networks. However, it was not possible to conduct multivariate analyses due to inadequate statistical power (Kawachi et al. 1996). What seems clear is that the evidence in favor of a link between social ties and disease incidence has been shown only for certain infectious disease and, to a limited extent, for coronary heart disease. Efforts to identify an association in stroke have suffered from inadequate statistical power. In theory, the same mechanisms that are likely to be associated with protection against heart disease may operate in stroke, although they may be more difficult to detect when the number of events becomes small. Chief among them may be modulation of blood pressure (Strogatz et al. 1997) and stress-related vascular reactivity.

Numerous observational studies have reported that several aspects of social integration, particularly operating through emotional support, influence stroke recovery both in terms of physical functioning and psychological adjustment (Evans et al.

1987; Friedland and McColl 1987; Glass et al. 1993; McLeroy et al. 1984; Morris et al. 1991; Robertson and Suinn 1968). Several studies have found that social support predicts quality of life after stroke (Angeleri et al. 1993; Evans et al. 1994; King 1996; Hyman 1972). The absence of social support has been shown to be associated with a variety of negative responses to stroke including suicidal thoughts (Kishi et al. 1996) and poststroke depression (PSD) (Andersen et al. 1995). The availability of social support has also been shown to be an important predictor of hospital course, including length of stay and discharge disposition (Colantonio et al. 1993; Lehmann et al. 1975). In a cohort study of 152 stroke survivors, Brosseau and colleagues (1996) found that the presence of social support predicted both discharges to rehabilitation and discharge to nursing homes. The findings regarding the impact of social support on stroke recovery appear to be particularly robust in light of a recent review which discards those studies that failed to adhere to sound methodological principles (Kwakkel et al. 1996). In that study, social support was the only psychosocial factor to be retained.

In addition, several randomized clinical trials have shown that psychosocial interventions have led to improved adjustment in stroke patients (Evans et al. 1988) and longer survival in patients with other chronic illness (Oldenburg et al. 1985; Spiegel et al. 1989). Enhancement of available social supports has been an important element in these intervention approaches.

Infectious Disease

The centrality of social networks in the distribution of infectious disease is compactly described by Morris (1995) in a recent overview in which she argued that:

Infectious diseases spread by person-to-person contact may be strongly channeled by patterns of selective (or 'non-random') social mixing. The more intimate and extended the contact needed for disease transmission, the more impact selective mixing will have on the speed and direction of spread. Patterns of selective mixing at the population level are in turn the outcome of the heterogeneity in individual contact networks. (Morris 1995, p. 302)

The concern with social networks as a factor in the health status of populations is precisely the concern with the nature of these patterns of social mixing. As such, infectious diseases offer a strategic site to study several important pathways through which social network structure impacts health.

Studies of social networks and infectious disease have clumped in several discernable areas. In this selective review, we will highlight only two. First, we will briefly examine what is known about social network influences on the spread of HIV/AIDS as well as on risk factors for that spread. Second, we will examine important new evidence showing the influence of social support on susceptibility to infection by the common cold virus.

Social networks and HIV/AIDS
Research on the social networks of injection drug users illustrates the myth that social networks and support are inevitably health-promoting. (For an important recent review, see Neaigus et al. 1994.) Some evidence suggests that the overall density of risk-taking subnetworks is associated with higher levels of risk for the individual. Participation in risk networks socializes an individual to a health-compromising lifestyle and then reinforces that pattern through various channels of social influence. In a study of 293 inner city injecting drug users (IDUs), Latkin and colleagues (1995) found that network density and size of drug-using subnetwork were positively associated with frequency of drug use. That same study found that injectors whose personal networks contained a noninjecting spouse/lover/sex partner injected less frequently, suggesting that some kinds of ties may be protective against high risk exposure. These findings are corroborated by studies that show that supportive ties ameliorate the influence of high risk environments on drug

use (Newcomb and Bentler 1988; Zapka et al. 1993).

Numerous commentators have noted that one of the reasons that behavior change interventions appear to be ineffective among injection drug users is that the social networks of IDUs themselves are stark barriers to that effectiveness. This has led to calls for interventions that attempt to work *with* rather than *around* those networks (Friedman et al. 1992; Kelly et al. 1993). An innovative example is Kelly and collaborators (1991), who used key opinion leaders in high risk social settings to attempt to change norms around high-risk behaviors.

The study of the role of social support and infectious disease has also led to important evidence regarding potential biophysiological pathways through which social support may operate. For example, in one of the only studies of its type, Theorell and colleagues (1995) followed HIV-infected men in Sweden and tracked their decline in CD4 count over a 5-year period. This group found that men who reported lower "availability of attachments" at baseline declined more rapidly in CD4 levels, indicating the possibility that social support mediates primary immune system parameters.

Social scientists such as Roderick Wallace have noted that at the intersection of social networks and physical locations in space, sociogeographic matrices are formed through which and across which epidemics such as HIV travel (Wallace 1991). The structure of overlapping networks located in space acts as a system of conduits allowing for epidemic spread. At the micro level this phenomenon is visible in the rapid rates of saturation that occur within subnetworks of high-risk individuals. This phenomenon is also visible at a more macro level. For example, Hunt shows how patterns of HIV transmission vary within regions of Uganda according to patterns of migrant labor use, where these labor market patterns form the social network infrastructure which creates opportunities for the spread of the epidemic.

Social support and the common cold

That social contacts may confer a generalized host resistance against the development of infectious disease was suggested in early papers by, among others, Cassel (1976) and Selye (1956). More recently, a solid foundation of evidence has begun to show that social support appears to alter primary immune system parameters that regulate host resistance (Esterling et al. 1996; Glaser et al. 1992; Kiecolt-Glaser et al. 1994; Uchino et al. 1996).. In the most powerful evidence yet compiled, Cohen and colleagues (1997) conducted an experiment to test the hypothesis that the diversity of network ties is related to susceptibility to the common cold. In this experiment, after reporting the extent of participation in 12 types of social ties (e.g., spouse, parent, friend, workmate, member of social group), subjects were given nasal drops containing one of two rhinoviruses and monitored for the development of a common cold. Results indicated that those with more types of social ties were less susceptible to common colds, produced less mucus, fought infection more efficiently, and shed less virus even after controlling for prechallenge virus-specific antibody, virus type, age, sex, season, body mass index, education, and race. Susceptibility to colds decreased in a dose–response manner with increased diversity of the social network.

If indeed social integration and participation are associated with changes in immune system functioning, the implications are far-reaching. First, immune system functioning is directly linked to the development of infectious diseases, allergies, autoimmune diseases, and cancer (Cohen 1988). While the evidence is less compelling that lack of social support increases risk of cancer and autoimmune disease, the evidence compiled by Cohen and others has important implications for the likelihood of this effect. In addition, the discovery of the influence of social support on neuroendocrine function suggests that social support processes may contribute to the pathogenesis of cardiovascular disease due to the influence of immune system function on the health of the arterial system and on hemodynamic processes.

CONCLUSIONS

In this chapter, we have reframed discussions of the impact that different qualities or dimensions of social relationships have on health by placing them in the larger context of social networks. This is a very large undertaking, and when coupled with a search for a deeper understanding of how social networks influence health, it becomes even larger. It is incumbent upon the investigators wishing to work in this area to recast general ideas about networks and health into specific hypotheses which will be testable through the explicit identification and articulation of theories, pathways, and mechanisms through which social networks impact health. It is unlikely that any single measure or study design will be useful for all purposes, diseases, or behaviors. Rather, by articulating the "upstream" contextual influences of network structure and "downstream" pathways by which networks more directly and proximately influence health, investigators will make significant progress. Much of this work invoked earlier theories and often used measures that conceptually blurred domains of networks and functional aspects of such ties.

We have also brought together much of the literature on biological pathways linking social networks to a broad array of outcomes. In doing so, we hope to introduce the reader to the many potentially fruitful areas of research in this area. The literature on biological pathways is not as well developed as are other areas of social network research. We believe this is an excellent area in which to do research.

Finally, we believe that some of the most important questions in this field have to do with understanding the determinants of network structure and social support. Issues related to cultural, ethnic, and class-related variations in the structure and function of

networks will help us to develop critically needed interventions to improve health.

REFERENCES

Andersen, G., Vestergaard, K., Ingemann-Nielsen, M., and Lauritzen, L. (1995). Risk factors for post-stroke depression. *Acta Psychiatr Scand,* 92:193–8.

Anderson, D., Deshaies, G., and Jobin, J. (1996). Social support, social networks and coronary artery disease rehabilitation: a review. *Can J Cardiol,* 12:739–44.

Angeleri, F., Angeleri, V.A., Foschi, N., Giaquinto, S., and Nolfe, G. (1993). The influence of depression, social activity, and family stress on functional outcome after stroke. *Stroke,* 24:1478–83.

Antonnuci, T.C. (1986). Measure social support networks: hierarchical mapping techniques. *Generations,* X:10–12.

Antonucci, T., and Akiyama, H. (1987a). An examination of sex differences in social support among older men and women. *Sex Roles,* 17:737–49.

Antonucci, T., and Akiyama, H. (1987b). Social networks in adult life and a preliminary examination of the convoy model. *J Gerontol,* 42:519–27.

Antonucci, T.C., and Jackson, J.S. (1990). The role of reciprocity in social support. In Sarason, B.R., Sarason, I.G., and Pierce, G.R. (eds.), *Social support: an interactional view.* New York: John Wiley, pp. 173–98.

Barnes, J.A. (1954). Class and committees in a Norwegian island parish. *Hum Relations,* 7:39–58.

Barrera, M. Jr., Sandler, I.N., and Ramsey, T.B. (1981). Preliminary development of a scale of social support: studies on college students. *Am J Community Psychol,* 9:435–47.

Bassuk, S., Glass, T., and Berkman, L. (1999). Social disengagement and incident of cognitive decline in the community-dwelling elderly. *Ann Intern Med,* 131:165–73.

Belle, D.E. (1982). The impact of poverty on social networks and supports. *Marriage Family Rev,* 5:89–103.

Berkman, L.F. (1985). The relationship of social networks and social support to morbidity and mortality. In Cohen, S., and Syme, S.L. (eds.), *Social support and health.* Orlando, FL: Academic Press, pp. 241–62.

Berkman, L.F. (1986). Social networks, support and health: taking the next step forward. *Am J Epidemiol,* 123:559–62.

Berkman, L.F. (1988). The changing and heterogeneous nature of aging and longevity: a social and biomedical perspective. *Annu Rev Gerontol Geriatr,* 8:37–68.

Berkman, L.F. (1995). The role of social relations in health promotion. *Psychosom Med,* 57: 245–54.

Berkman, L.F., and Breslow, L. (1983). *Health and ways of living: the Alameda County Study.* New York: Oxford University Press.

Berkman, L.F., and Syme, S.L. (1979). Social networks, host resistance and mortality: a nine year follow-up study of Alameda County residents. *Am J Epidemiol,* 109:186–204.

Berkman, L.F., Leo-Summers, L., and Horwitz, R.I. (1992). Emotional support and survival following myocardial infarction: a prospective population-based study of the elderly. *Ann Intern Med,* 117:1003–9.

Bierstedt, R. (1966). *Emile Durkheim.* London: Weidenfeld and Nicolson.

Blazer, D.G. (1982). Social support and mortality in an elderly community population. *Am J Epidemiol,* 115:684–94.

Blumenthal, J.A., Burg, M.M., Barefoot J., William, R.B., Haney, T., and Zimmer, G. (1987). Social support, type A behavior and coronary artery disease. *Psychosom Med,* 49:331–40.

Bodemann, Y. M. (1988). Relations of product and class rule: the basis of patron/clientage. In Wellman B., and Berkowitz, S.D. (eds.), *Social structures: a network approach.* Cambridge, UK: Cambridge University Press, pp. 198–220.

Boissevain, J. (1974). *Friends of friends: networks, manipulators and coalitions.* New York: St. Martins Press.

Bott, E. (1957). *Family and social network.* London: Tavistock Press.

Bowlby, J. (1969). *Attachment and loss,* vol. 1: *Attachment.* London: Hogarth Press.

Bowlby, J. (1973). *Attachment and loss,* vol. 2: *Separation—anxiety and anger.* London: Hogarth Press.

Bowlby, J. (1980). *Attachment and loss,* vol. 3: *Loss—sadness and depression.* London: Hogarth Press.

Bowlby, J. (1988). *A secure base: clinical applications of attachment theory.* London: Routledge.

Bowling, A. (1991). Social support and social networks: their relationship to the successful and unsuccessful survival of elderly people in the community. An analysis of concepts and a review of the evidence. *Fam Pract,* 8: 68–83.

Bowling, A., and Browne, P.D. (1991). Social networks, health, and emotional well-being among the oldest old in London. *J Gerontol,* 46:S20–32.

Broadhead, W.E., Kaplan, B.H., James, S.A., Wagner, E.H., Schoenbach, V.J., Grimson, R., Heyden, S., Tibblin, G., and Gehlbach, S.H. (1983). The epidemiologic evidence for a relationship between social support and health. *Am J Epidemiol,* 117:521–37.

Brosseau, L., Potvin, L., Philippe, P., and Boulanger, Y.L. (1996). Post-stroke inpatient rehabilitation. II. Predicting discharge disposition. *Am J Phys Med Rehabil,* 75:431–6.

Buchner, D.M., Beresford, S.A., Larson, E.B., LaCroix, A.Z., and Wagner, E.H. (1992). Effects of physical activity on health status in older adults. II. Intervention studies. *Annu Rev Public Health,* 13:469–88.

Burt, R.S. (1982). *Toward a structural theory of action.* New York: Academic Press.

Case, R.B., Moss, A.J., Case, N., McDermott, M., and Eberly, S. (1992). Living alone after myocardial infarction. *JAMA,* 267–515.

Cassel, J. (1976). The contribution of the social environment to host resistance. *Am J Epidemiol,* 104:107–23.

Chen, Y.T., Vaccarino, V., Williams, C.S., Butler, J, Berkman, L.F., and Krumholz, H.M. (1999). Risk factors for heart failure in the elderly: a prospective community-based study. *AJM,* 106:605–12.

Cobb, S. (1976). Social support as a moderator of life stress. *Psychosom Med,* 38:300–14.

Cohen, S. (1988). Psychosocial models of the role of social support in the etiology of physical disease. *Health Psychol,* 7:269–97.

Cohen, S., and Hoberman, H.M. (1983). Positive events and social support as buffers of life change stress. *J Appl Soc Psychol,* 13:99–125.

Cohen, S., and Syme, S.L. (eds.). (1985). *Social support and health.* New York: Academic Press.

Cohen, S., Kaplan, J.R., Cunnick, J., Manuck, S.B., and Rabin, B.S. (1992). Chronic social stress, affiliation and cellular immune response in non-human primates. *Psychol Sci,* 4:301–10.

Cohen, S., Doyle, W.J., Skoner, D.P., Rabin, B.S., and Gwaltney, J.M. Jr. (1997). Social ties and susceptibility to the common cold. *JAMA,* 277:1940–4.

Colantonio, A., Kasl, S.V., Ostfeld, A.M., and Berkman, L.F. (1993). Psychosocial predictors of stroke outcomes in an elderly population. *J Gerontol,* 48:S261–8.

Cotman, C.W. (ed.). (1985). *Synaptic plasticity.* New York: Guilford Press.

Cutrona, C.E., and Troutman, B.R. (1986). Social support, infant temperament, and parenting self-efficacy: a mediational model of postpartum depression. *Child Dev,* 57:1507–18.

Dean, A., and Lin, N. (1977). The stress-buffering role of social support: problems and prospects for systematic investigation. *J Nerv Ment Dis*, 165:403–17.

Donald, C.A., and Ware, J.E. (1982). *The qualification of social contacts and resources*. Santa Monica, CA: Rand Corporation.

Duncan, T.E., and McAuley, E. (1993). Social support and efficacy cognitions in exercise adherence: a latent growth curve analysis. *J Behav Med*, 16:199–218.

Dunkel-Schetter, C., and Bennett, T.L. (1990). Differentiating the cognitive and behavioral aspects of social support. In Sarason, B.R., Sarason I.G., and Pierce G.R. (eds.), *Social support: an interactional view*. New York: John Wiley, pp. 267–96.

Dunkel-Schetter, C., Folkman, S., and Lazarus, R.S. (1987). Correlates of social support receipt. *J Pers Soc Psychol*, 53:71–80.

Dunkel-Schetter, C., Feinstein, L.G., Taylor, S.E., and Falke, R.L. (1992). Patterns of coping with cancer. *Health Psychol*, 11:79–87.

Durkheim, É. (1893). *The division of labor in society*. New York: Free Press.

Durkheim, E. (1895, 1982). *The rules of sociological method*, ed. Lukes, S. (tr. Halls, W.D., 1938). New York: Free Press.

Durkheim, É. (1897, 1951). *Suicide: a study in sociology*. Glencoe, IL: Free Press.

Ell, K. (1996). Social networks, social support and coping with serious illness: the family connection. *Soc Sci Med*, 42:173–83.

Emery, C.F., and Gatz, M. (1990). Psychological and cognitive effects of an exercise program for community-residing older adults. *Gerontologist*, 30:184–8.

Erickson, B.H. (1988). The relational basis of attitudes. In Wellman, B., and Berkowitz, S.D. (eds.), *Social structures: a network approach*. New York: Cambridge University Press, pp. 99–121.

Eriksen, W. (1994). The role of social support in the pathogenesis of coronary heart disease. A literature review. *Fam Pract*, 11:201–9.

Esterling, B.A., Kiecolt-Glaser, J.K., and Glaser, R. (1996). Psychosocial modulation of cytokine-induced natural killer cell activity in older adults. *Psychosom Med*, 58:264–72.

Evans, R.L., Bishop, D.S., Matlock, A.L., Stranahan, S., Halar, E.M., and Noonan, W.C. (1987). Prestroke family interaction as a predictor of stroke outcome. *Arch Phys Med Rehabil*, 68:508–12.

Evans, R.L., Matlock, A.L., Bishop, D.S., Stranahan, S., and Pederson, C. (1988). Family intervention after stroke: does counseling or education help? *Stroke*, 19:1243–9.

Evans, R.L., Connis, R.T., Bishop, D.S., Hendricks, R.D., and Haselkorn, J.K. (1994). Stroke: a family dilemma. *Disabil Rehabil*, 16:110–8.

Farmer, I., Meyer, P.S., Ramsey, D.J., Goff, D.C., Wear, M.L., Labarthe, D.R., and Nichaman, M.Z. (1996). Higher levels of social support predict greater survival following acute myocardial infarction: the Corpus Christi Heart Project. *Behav Med*, 22:59–66.

Fischer, C.S. (1982). *To dwell among friends: personal networks in town and city*. Chicago: University of Chicago Press.

Fischer, C.S., Jackson, R.M., Steuve, C.A., Gerson, K., Jones, L.M., and Baldassare, M. (1977). *Networks and places*. New York: Free Press.

Fleming, R., Baum, A., Gisriel, M.M., and Gatchel, R.J. (1982). Mediating influences of social support on stress at Three Mile Island. *J Hum Stress*, 8:14–22.

Fonagy, P. (1996). Patterns of attachment, interpersonal relationships and health. In Blane, D., Brunner, E., and Wilkinson, R. (eds.), *Health and social organization: towards health policy for the twenty-first century*, London: Routledge Press, pp. 125–51.

Fonagy, P., Steele, M., Steele, H., Leigh, T., Kennedy, R., Mattoon, G., and Target, M. (1995). Attachment, the reflective self, and borderline states: the predictive specificity of the Adult Attachment Interview and pathological emotional development. In Goldberg, S., Muir R., and Kerr, J. (eds.), *John Bowlby's attachment theory: historical, clinical and social significance*. New York: Analytic Press, pp. 233–78.

Francis, D., Diorio, J., LaPlante, P., Weaver, S., Seckl, J., and Meaney, M. (1996). The role of early environmental events in regulating neuroendocrine development. Moms, pups, stress and glucocorticoid receptors. *Ann N Y Acad Sci*, 794:136–52.

Friedland, J., and McColl, M.A. (1987). Social support and psychosocial dysfunction after stroke: buffering effects in a community sample. *Arch Phys Med Rehabil*, 68:475–80.

Friedman, S.R. (1995). Promising social network results and suggestions for a research agenda. *NIDA Res Monogr*, 151:196–215.

Friedman, S.R., Neaigus, A., Des Jarlais, D.C., Sotheran, J.L., Woods, J., Sufian, M., Stepherson, B., and Sterk, C. (1992). Social intervention against AIDS among injecting drug users. *Br J Addict*, 87:393–404.

George, C., Kaplan, N., and Main, M. (1985). The adult attachment interview. University of California at Berkeley (manuscript).

George, L.K. (1986). Caregiver burden: conflict between norms of reciprocity and solidarity. In Pillemar, K.A., and Wolf, R.D. (eds.), *Conflict and abuse in families of the elderly: theory, research and intervention*. Boston: Auburn House, pp. 67–92.

George, L.K., Blazer, D.G., Hughes, D.C., and Fowler, N. (1989). Social support and the outcome of major depression. *Br J Psychiatry,* 154:478–85.

Glaser, R., Kiecolt-Glaser, J.K., Speicher, C.E., and Holiday, J.E. (1985). Stress, loneliness and changes in herpes virus latency. *J Behav Med,* 8:249–60.

Glaser, R., Kiecolt-Glaser, J.K., Bonneau, R.H., Malarkey, W., Kennedy, S., and Hughes, J. (1992). Stress-induced modulation of the immune response to recombinant hepatitis B vaccine. *Psychosom Med,* 54:22–9.

Glass, T.A., Matchar, D.B., Belyea, M.J., and Feussner, J.R. (1993). Impact of social support on outcome in first stroke. *Stroke,* 24:64–70.

Glass, T.A., Mendes de Leon, C.F., Seeman, T.E., Berkman, L.F. (1997). Beyond single indicators of social networks: a LISREL analysis of social ties among the elderly. *Soc Sci Med,* 44:1503–18.

Glass, T.A., Mendes de Leon, C.F., Marottoli, R., and Berkman, L.F. (1999). Population based study of social and productive activities as predictors of survival among elderly Americans. *Br Med J* 319:478–483.

Granovetter, M. (1973). The strength of weak ties. *Am J Sociol,* 78:1360–80.

Granovetter, M. (1982). The strength of weak ties: a network theory revisited. In Marsden, P., and Lin, N. (eds.), *Social structure and network analysis.* Beverly Hills, CA: Sage, pp. 105–30.

Greenwood, D.C., Muir, K.R., Packham, C.J., and Madeley, R.J. (1996). Coronary heart disease: a review of the role of psychosocial stress and social support. *J Public Health Med,* 18:221–31.

Grembowski, D., Patrick, D., Diehr, P., Durham, M., Beresford, S., Kay, E., and Hecht, J. (1993). Self-efficacy and health behavior among older adults. *J Health Soc Behav,* 34:89–104.

Gulliver, S.B., Hughes, J.R., Solomon, L.J., and Dey, A.N. (1995). An investigation of self-efficacy, partner support and daily stresses as predictors of relapse to smoking in self-quitters. *Addiction,* 90:767–72.

Gunnar, M.R., and Nelson, C.A. (1994). Event-related potentials in year-old infants: relations with emotionality and cortisol. *Child Dev,* 65:80–94.

Gunnar, M.R., Tout K. deHaan, M., and Pierce, S. (1997). Temperament, social competence, and adreno cortical activity in preschoolers. *Dev Psychobiol,* 31:65–85.

Hall, A., and Wellman, B. (1985). Social networks and social support. In Cohen, S., and Syme, S.L. (eds.), *Social support and health.* Orlando: Academic Press, pp. 23–41.

Hanson, B.S, Isacsson, S.O., Janzon, L., and Lindell, S.E. (1990). Social support and quitting smoking for good: is there an association? Results from the population study "Men Born in 1914," Malino, Sweden. *Addict Behav,* 15:221–33.

Heitzmann, C.A., and Kaplan, R.M. (1988). Assessment of methods for measuring social support. *Health Psychol,* 7:75–109.

Helgeson, V.S., and Cohen, S. (1996). Social support and adjustment to cancer: reconciling descriptive, correlational, and intervention research. *Health Psychol,* 15:135–48.

Henderson, S. (1981). Social relationships, adversity and neurosis: an analysis of prospective observations. *Br J Psychiatry,* 138:391–8.

Henderson, S., Duncan-Jones, P., and Byrne, D. (1980). Measuring social relationships: the interview schedule for social interaction. *Psychol Med,* 10:723–34.

Holahan, C.J., and Moos, R.H. (1987). Personal and contextual determinants of coping strategies. *J Pers Soc Psychol,* 52:946–55.

Holahan, C.J., Moos, R.H., Holahan, C.K., and Brennan, P.L. (1995). Social support, coping, and depressive symptoms in a late-middle-aged sample of patients reporting cardiac illness. *Health Psychol,* 14:152–63.

Holahan, C.J., Moos, R.H., Holahan, C.K., and Brennan, P.L. (1997). Social context, coping strategies, and depressive symptoms: an expanded model with cardiac patients. *J Pers Soc Psychol,* 72:918–28.

Holahan, C.K., and Holahan, C.J. (1987). Self-efficacy, social support, and depression in aging: a longitudinal analysis. *J Gerontol,* 42:65–8.

Holmes, J. (1993). *John Bowlby and attachment theory.* London: Routledge.

House, J.S. (1981). *Work stress and social support.* Reading, MA: Addison-Wesley.

House, J.S., and Kahn, R. (1985). Measures and concepts of social support. In Cohen, S., and Syme, S.L.(eds.), *Social support and health.* Orlando: Academic Press, pp. 79–108.

House, J.S., Robbins, C., and Metzner, H.L. (1982). The association of social relationships and activities with mortality: prospective evidence from the Tecumseh community health study. *Am J Epidemiol,* 116:123–40.

House, J.S., Landis, K.R., and Umberson, D. (1988). Social relationships and health. *Science,* 241:540–5.

Howell, N.E. (1969). *The search for the abortionist.* Chicago: University of Chicago Press.

Hunt, C.W. (1989). Migrant labor and sexually

transmitted disease: AIDS in Africa. *J Health Soc Behav*, 30:353–73.

Hyman, M.D. (1972). Social isolation and performance in rehabilitation. *J Chronic Dis*, 25:85–97.

Jones, C.P. (1995). Systolic blood pressure and "race": are black folks aging faster? Paper presented at the American Public Health Association annual meeting in San Diego, California on October 30, 1995.

Kahn, R.L. (1979). Aging and social support. In Riley, M.W. (ed.), *Aging from birth to death: an interdisciplinary perspective*. Boulder, CO: Westview, pp. 72–92.

Kahn, R.L., and Antonucci, T.C. (1980). Convoys over the lifecourse: attachment, roles and social support. In Baltes, P.B., and Brim, O. (eds.), *Life span development and behavior*. New York: Academic Press, pp. 253–86.

Kamarck, T., Mannuck, S. B., and Jennings, J. (1991). Social support reduces cardiovascular reactivity to psychological challenge: a laboratory model. *Psychosom Med*, 52: 42–58.

Kaplan, G.A., Salonen, J.T., Cohen, R.D. Brand, R.J., Syme, S.L., and Puska, P. (1988). Social connections and mortality from all causes and from cardiovascular disease: prospective evidence from eastern Finland. *Am J Epidemiol*, 128:370–80.

Kawachi, I., Colditz, G.A., Ascherio, A., Rimm, E.B., Giovannucci, E., Stampfer, M.J., and Willett, W.C. (1996). A prospective study of social networks in relation to total mortality and cardiovascular disease in men in the USA. *J Epidemiol Community Health*, 50:245–51.

Kelly, J.A., St Lawrence, J.S., Diaz, Y.E., Stevenson, L.Y., Hauth, A.C., Brasfield, T.L., Kalichman, S.C., Smith, J.E., and Andrew, M.E. (1991). HIV risk behavior reduction following intervention with key opinion leaders of population: an experimental analysis. *Am J Public Health*, 81:168–71.

Kelly, J.A., Murphy, D.A., Sikkema, K.J., and Kalichman, S.C. (1993). Psychological interventions to prevent HIV infection are urgently needed. New priorities for behavioral research in the second decade of AIDS. *Am Psychol*, 48:1023–34.

Kiecolt-Glaser, J.K., Garner, W., Speicher, C.E., Penn, G.M., Holliday, J., and Glaser, R. (1984). Psychosocial modifiers of immunocompetence in medical students. *Psychosom Med*, 46:7–14.

Kiecolt-Glaser, J.K., Fisher, L.D., Ogrocki, P., Stout, J.C., and Speicher, C.E. (1987). Marital quality, marital disruption and immune function. *Psychosom Med*, 49:13–34.

Kiecolt-Glaser, J.K., Malarkey, W.B., Cacioppo, J.T., and Glaser, R. (1994). Stressful personal relationships: immune and endocrine function. In Glaser, R., and Kiecolt-Glaser, J.K., (eds.), *Handbook of human stress and immunity*. San Diego, CA: Academic Press, pp. 321–39.

King, R.B. (1996). Quality of life after stroke. *Stroke*, 27:1467–72.

Kirschbaum, C., Klauer, T., Filipp, S.H., and Hellhammer, D.H. (1995). Sex-specific effects of social support on cortisol and subjective responses to acute psychological stress. *Psychosom Med*, 57:23–31.

Kishi, Y., Kosier, J.T., and Robinson, R.G. (1996). Suicidal plans in patients with acute stroke. *J Nerv Ment Dis*, 184:274–80.

Kloudahl, A.S. (1985). Social networks and the spread of infectious diseases: the AIDS example. *Soc Sci Med*, 21:1203–16.

Knox, S.S., and Uvnas-Moberg, K. (1998) Social isolation and cardiovascular disease: an atherosclerotic pathway? *Psychoneuroendocrinology*. 23:877–90.

Knox, S., Theorell, T., Svensson, J., and Waller, D. (1985). The relation of social support and working environment to medical variables associated with elevated blood pressure in young males: a structural model. *Soc Sci Med*, 21:525–31.

Krause, N., and Borawshi-Clark, E. (1995). Social class differences in social support among older adults. *Gerontologist*, 35:498–508.

Krumholz, H.M., Butler, J., Miller, J., Vaccarino, V., Williams, C., Mendes de Leon, C.F., Seeman, T.E., Kasl, S.V., and Berkman, L.F. (1998). The prognostic importance of emotional support for elderly patients hospitalized with heart failure. *Circulation*, 97: 958–64.

Kwakkel, G., Wagenaar, R.C., Kollen, B.J., and Lankhorst, G.J. (1996). Predicting disability in stroke: a critical review of the literature. *Age Ageing*, 25:479–89.

LaCapra, D. (1972). *Emile Durkheim: sociologist and philosopher*. Ithaca, NY: Cornell University Press.

Landrine, H., Richardson, J.K., Klondoff, E.A., and Flay, B. (1994). Cultural diversity in the predictors of adolescent cigarette smoking: the relative influence of peers. *J Behav Med*, 17:331–6.

LaRocca, J.M., House, J.S., and French, J.R. Jr. (1980). Social support, occupational stress and health. *J Health Soc Behav*, 21:202–8.

Latkin, C., Mandell, W., Oziemkowska, M., Celentano, D., Vlahov, D., Ensminger, M., and Knowlton, A. (1995). Using social network analysis to study patterns of drug use among urban drug users at high risk for HIV/AIDS. *Drug Alcohol Depend*, 38:1–9.

Laumann, E.O. (1973). *Bonds of pluralism*. New York: John Wiley.

Laumann, E.O., Gagnon, J.H., Michaels, S., Michael, R.T., and Coleman, J.S. (1989). Monitoring the AIDS epidemic in the U.S.: a network approach. *Science*, 244:1186–9.

Lehmann, J.F., DeLateur, B.J., Fowler, R.S., Warren, C.G., Arnhold, R., Schertzer, G., Hurka, R., Whitmore, J.J., Massoch, A.J., and Chambers, K.H. (1975). Stroke rehabilitation: outcome and prediction. *Arch Phys Med Rehabil*, 56:383–9.

Lin, N., and Dean, A. (1984). Social support and depression: a panel study. *Soc Psychiatry*, 19:83–91.

Lin, N., Simeone, R., Ensel, W., and Kuo, W. (1979). Social support, stressful life events and illness: a model and an empirical test. *J Health Soc Behav*, 20:108–19.

Lin, N., Dean, A., and Ensel, W.M. (1981). Social support scales: a methodological note. *Schizophr Bull*, 7:73–89.

Lin, N., Woelfel, M.W., and Light, S.C. (1985). The buffering effect of social support subsequent to an important life event. *J Health Soc Behav*, 26:247–63.

Lin, N., Dean, A., and Ensel, W.M. (1986). *Social support, life events, and depression*. New York: Academic Press.

Link, B.G., and Phelan, J.(1995). Social conditions as fundamental causes of disease. *J Health Soc Behav*, Spec No:80–94.

Lomauro, T.A. (1990). Social support, health locus-of-control, and coping style and their relationship to depression among stroke victims. Doctoral Dissertation, St. John University US. *Dissertation Abstracts Int* 51:2628.

Luxton, M. (1980). *More than a labor of love*. Toronto: Women's Press.

Major, B., Cozzarelli, C., Sciacchitano, A.M., Cooper, M.L., Testa, M., and Mueller, P.M. (1990). Perceived social support, self-efficacy, and adjustment to abortion. *J Pers Soc Psychol*, 59:452–63.

Marsden, P.V., and Friedkin, N.E. (1994). Network studies of social influence. In Wasserman, S., and Galaskiewicz, J. (eds.), *Advances in social network analysis: research in the social and behavioral sciences*. Thousand Oaks, CA: Sage, pp. 3–25.

Matt, G.E., and Dean, A. (1993). Social support from friends and psychological distress among elderly persons: moderator effects of age. *J Health Soc Behav*, 34:197–200.

McAuley, E. (1993). Self-efficacy, physical activity, and aging. In Kelly, J.R., (ed.), *Activity and aging: staying involved in later life*. Newbury Park, CA: Sage, pp. 187–206.

McAvay, G.J., Seeman, T.E., and Rodin, J. (1996). A longitudinal study of change in domain-specific self-efficacy among older adults. *J Gerontol B Psychol Soc Sci*, 51: P243–53.

McFarlane, A.H., Bellissimo, A., and Norman, G.R. (1995). The role of family and peers in social self-efficacy: links to depression in adolescence. *Am J Orthopsychiatry*, 65:402–10.

McLeroy, K.R., DeVellis, R., DeVellis, B., Kaplan, B., and Toole, J. (1984). Social support and physical recovery in a stroke population. *J Soc Personal Relationships*, 1:395–413.

Meaney, M.J., Aitken, D.H., Bodnoff, S.R., Iny, L.J., and Sapolsky, R.M.(1985). The effects of postnatal handling on the development of the glucocorticoid receptor systems and stress recovery in the rat. *Prog Neuropsychopharmacol Biol Psychiatry*, 9:731–4.

Meaney, M.J., Aitken, D.H., VanBerkel, C., Bhatnagar, S., and Sapolsky, R.M. (1988). Effect of neonatal handling on age-related impairments associated with the hippocampus. *Science*, 239:766–8.

Meaney, M.J., Diorio, J., Francis, D., Widdowson, J., LaPlante, P., Caldji, C., Sharma, S., Seckl, J.R., and Plotsky, P.M. (1996). Early environmental regulation of forebrain glucocorticoid receptor gene expression: implications for adrenocortical responses to stress. *Developmental Neuroscience*, 18:49–72.

Mendes de Leon, C.F., Seeman, T.E., Baker, D.I., Richardson, E.D., and Tinetti, M.E. (1996). Self-efficacy, physical decline, and change in functioning in community-living elders: a prospective study. *J Gerontol B Psychol Sci Soc Sci*, 51:S183–90.

Mermelstein, R., Cohen, S., Lichtenstein, F., Beer, J.S., and Kamarck, T. (1986). Social support and smoking cessation maintenance. *J Consult Clin Psychol*, 54:447–53.

Mitchell, J.C. (1969). The concept and use of social networks. In Mitchell, J.C. (ed.), *Social networks in urban situations: analyses of personal relationships in Central African towns*. Manchester, England: Manchester University Press, pp. 1–50.

Morris, M. (1994). Epidemiology and social networks: modeling structured diffusion. In Wasserman, S., and Galaskiewicz, J. (eds.), *Advances in social network analysis: research in the social and behavioral sciences*. Thousand Oaks, CA: Sage, pp. 26–52.

Morris, M. (1995). Data driven network models for the spread of infectious disease. In Mollison, D. (ed.), *Epidemic models: their structure and relation to data*. Cambridge, UK: Cambridge University Press, pp. 302–22.

Morris, M., Podhisita, C., Wawer, M.J., and Handcock, M.S. (1996). Bridge populations in the spread of HIV/AIDS in Thailand. *AIDS*, 10:1265–71.

Morris, P.L., Robinson, R.G., Raphael, B., and Bishop, D. (1991). The relationship between the perception of social support and post-stroke depression in hospitalized patients. *Psychiatry*, 54:306–16.

Morris, P.L., Robinson, R.G., Andrzejewski, P., Samuels, J., and Price, T.R. (1993). Association of depression with 10-year poststroke mortality. *Am J Psychiatry*, 150:124–9.

Moss, M.B., and Albert, M.S. (1988). Future directions in the study of aging. In Albert, M.S., and Moss, M.B. (eds.), *Geriatric neuropsychology*. New York: Guilford Press, pp. 293–304.

Murphy, E. (1982). Social origins of depression in old age. *Br J Psychiatry*, 141:135–42.

Murray, R.P., Johnston, J.J., Dolce, J.J., Lee, W.W., and O'Hara, P. (1995). Social support for smoking cessation and abstinence: the Lung Health Study. The Lung Health Study Research Group. *Addict Behav*, 20:159–70.

Nachmias, M., Gunnar, M., Mangelsdorf, S., Parritz, R., and Buss, K. (1996). Behavioral inhibition and stress reactivity: the moderating role of attachment security. *Child Dev*, 67:508–22.

Neaigus, A., Friedman, S.R., Curtis, R., Des Jarlais, D.C., Furst, R.T., Jose, B., Mota, P., Stepherson, B., Sufian, M., Ward, T., and Wright, J.W. (1994). The relevance of drug injectors' social and risk networks for understanding and preventing HIV infection. *Soc Sci Med*, 38:67–78.

Nerem, R.M., Levesque, M.J., and Cornhill, J.F. (1980). Social environments as a factor in diet-induced atherosclerosis. *Science*, 208:1475–6.

Newcomb, M.D., and Bentler, P.M. (1988). Impact of adolescent drug use and social support on problems of young adults: a longitudinal study. *J Abnorm Psychol*, 97:64–75.

Oldenburg, B., Perkins, R.J., and Andrews, G. (1985). Controlled trial of psychological intervention in myocardial infarction. *J Consult Clin Psychol*, 53:852–9.

Orth-Gomér, K., and Johnson, J. (1987). Social network interaction and mortality: a six year follow-up of a random sample of the Swedish population. *J Chronic Dis*, 40:949–57.

Orth-Gomér, K., and Unden, A.L. (1987). The measurement of social support in populations surveys. *Soc Sci Med*, 24:83–94.

Orth-Gomér, K., Unden, A.L., and Edwards, M.E. (1988). Social isolation and mortality in ischemic heart disease. *Acta Med Scand*, 224:205–15.

Orth-Gomér, K., Rosengren, A, and Wilhelmsen, L. (1993). Lack of social support and incidence of coronary heart disease in middle-aged Swedish men. *Psychosom Med*, 55:37–43.

Oxman, T.E., Berkman, L.F., Kasl, S. Jr., Freeman, D.H., and Barrett, J. (1992). Social support and depressive symptoms in the elderly. *Am J Epidemiol*, 135:356–68.

Oxman, T.E., Freeman, D.H., Jr., and Manheimer, E.D. (1995). Lack of social participation or religious strength and comfort as risk factors for death after cardiac surgery in the elderly. *Psychosom Med*, 57:5–15.

Paykel, E.S. (1994). Life events, social support and depression. *Acta Psychiatr Scand*, Suppl 377:50–8.

Pennix, B.W., van Tilburg, T., Kriegsman, D.M., Deeg, D.J., Boeke, A.J., and van Eijk, J.T. (1997). Effects of social support and personal coping resources on mortality in older age: the Longitudinal Aging Study, Amsterdam. *Am J Epidemiol*, 146:510–9.

Procidano, M.E., and Heller, K. (1983). Measures of perceived social support from friends and family: three validation studies. *Am J Community Psychol*, 11:1–24.

Robertson, E.K., and Suinn, R.M. (1968). The determination of rate of progress of stroke patients through empathy measures of patient and family. *J Psychosom Res*, 12:189–91.

Rook, K.S., (1984). The negative side of social interaction. *J Pers Soc Psychol*, 46:1097–108.

Rook, K.S. (1987). Social support versus companionship: effects of life stress, loneliness and evaluations of others. *J Pers Soc Psychol*, 52:1132–47.

Rook, K.S. (1990). Social relationships as a source of companionship: implications for older adults' psychological well being. In Sarason, B.R., Sarason, T.G., and Pierce, G.R. (eds.), *Social support: an interactional view*. New York: John Wiley, pp. 221–50.

Ruberman, W., Weinblatt, E., Goldberg, J.D., and Chaudhary, B.S. (1984). Psychosocial influences on mortality after myocardial infarction. *N Eng J Med*, 311:552–9.

Sanchez, M.M., Aguado, F., Sanchez-Toscano, F., and Saphier D. (1994). Effects of prolonged social isolation on responses of neurons in the bed nucleus of the stria terminalis, preoptioc area, and hypothalamic paraventricular nucleus to stimulation of the medial amygdala. *Psychoneuroendocrinology*, 20:525–41.

Sapolsky, R.M., Krey, L.C., and McEwens, B.S. (1983). The adrenocortical stress-response in the aged male rat: impairment of recovery from stress. *Exp Gerontol*, 18:55–64.

Sapolsky, R.M., Alberts, S.C., and Altmann, J.

(1997). Hypercortisolism associated with social subordinance or social isolation among wild baboons. *Arch Gen Psychiatry*, 54: 1137–43.

Sarason, I.G., Levine, H.M., Bashem, R.B., and Sarason, B.R. (1983). Assessing social support: the social support questionnaire. *J Pers Soc Psychol*, 44:127–9.

Sarason, B.R., Sarason, I.G., and Pierce, G. (1990). *Social support: an interactional view*. New York: John Wiley.

Schaefer, C., Coyne, J., and Lazarus, R. (1981). The health-related functions of social support. *J Behav Med*, 4:381–406.

Schoenbach, V.J., Kaplan, B.G., Freedman, L., and Kleinbaum, D.G. (1986). Social ties and mortality in Evans County, Georgia. *Am J Epidemiol*, 123:577–91.

Seeman, T.E. (1996). Social ties and health: the benefits of social integration. *Ann Epidemiol*, 6:442–51.

Seeman, T.E., and Berkman, L.F. (1988). Structural characteristics of social networks and their relationship with social support in the elderly: who provides support. *Soc Sci Med*, 26:737–49.

Seeman, T.E., Kaplan, G., Knudsen, L. Cohen, R., and Guralnik, J. (1988). Social network ties and mortality among the elderly in the Alameda County study. *Am J Epidemiol*, 126:714–23.

Seeman, T.E., Berkman, L.F., Kohout, F., LaCroix, A., Glynn, R., and Blazer, D. (1993a). Intercommunity variations in the association between social ties and mortality in the elderly: a comparative analysis of three communities. *Ann Epidemiol*, 3:325–35.

Seeman, T.E., Rodin, J., and Albert, M.A. (1993b). Self-efficacy and functional ability: how beliefs relate to cognitive and physical performance. *J Aging Health*, 5:455–74.

Seeman, T.E., Berkman, L.F., Blazer, D., and Rowe, J.W. (1994). Social ties and support and neuroendocrine function: the MacArthur Studies of Successful Aging. *Ann Behav Med*, 16:95–106.

Selye, H. (1956). *The stress of life*. New York: McGraw-Hill.

Sherbourne, C.D., and Stewart, A.L. (1991). The MOS social support theory. *Soc Sci Med*, 32:705–14.

Shively, C.A., Clarkson, T.B., and Kaplan, J.R. (1989). Social deprivation and coronary artery atherosclerosis in female cynomolgus monkey. *Atherosclerosis*, 77:69–76.

Spiegel, D., Bloom, J.R., Kraemer, H.C., and Gottheil, E. (1989). Effect of psychosocial treatment on survival of patients with metastatic breast cancer. *Lancet*, 2:888–91.

Storr, A. (1991). *'John Bowlby,' Munks Roll*. London: Royal College of Physicians.

Strogatz, D.S., Croft, J.B., James, S.A., Keenan, N.L., Browning, S.R., Garrett, J.M., and Curtis, A.B. (1997). Social support, stress, and blood pressure in black adults. *Epidemiology*, 8:482–7.

Sugisawa, H., Liang, J., and Liu, X. (1994). Social networks, social support and mortality among older people in Japan. *J Gerontol*, 49:S3–13.

Suomi, S.J. (1991). Uptight and laid-back monkeys: individual differences in the response to social challenges. In Brauth, S.E., Hall, W. S., and Dooling, R.J. (eds.), *Plasticity of development*. Cambridge, MA: MIT Press.

Suomi, S.J. (1997). Early determinants of behaviour: evidence from primate studies. *Br Med Bull*, 53:170–84.

Theorell, T., Blomkvist, V., Jonsson, H., Schulman, S., Berntorp, E., and Stigendal, L. (1995). Social support and the development of immune function in human immunodeficiency virus infection. *Psychosom Med*, 57: 32–6.

Thoits, P.A. (1995). Stress, coping, and social support processes: where are we? what next? *J Health Soc Behav*, Spec No:53–79.

Thomas, P.D., Goodwin, J.M., and Goodwin, J.S. (1985). Effect of social support on stress-related changes in cholesterol levels, uric acid level and immune function in an elderly sample. *Am J Psychiatry*, 142:735–7.

Tinetti, M.E., and Powell, L. (1993). Fear of falling and low self-efficacy: a case of dependence in elderly persons. *J Gerontol*, 48 Spec No:35–8.

Trieber, F.A., Batanowski, T., Broden, D.S., Strong, W.B., Levy, M., and Knox, W. (1991). Social support for exercise: relationship to physical activity in young adults. *Prev Med*, 20:737–50.

Turner, J.H., Beeghley, L., and Powers, C.H. (1989). *The Emergence of Sociological Theory*. Chicago, IL: The Dorsey Press.

Turner, R.J. (1983). Direct, indirect and moderating effects of social support upon psychological distress and associated condition. In Kaplan, H. (ed.), *Psychosocial stress: trends in theory and research*. New York: Academic Press, pp. 105–55.

Uchino, B.N., Cacioppo, J.T., and Kiecolt-Glaser, J.K. (1996). The relationship between social support and physiological processes: a review with emphasis on underlying mechanisms and implications for health. *Psychol Bull*, 119:488–531.

Unden, A.L., and Orth-Gomér, K.(1984). Social support and health. (Report No. 2.) Development of a survey method to measure social support in population studies. (Stress Research Report. No. 178.) Stockholm: Karolinska Institute.

Vilhjalmsson, R. (1993). Life stress, social support and clinical depression: a reanalysis of the literature. *Soc Sci Med*, 37:331–42.

Vogt, T.M., Mullooly, J.P., Ernst, D., Pope, C.R., and Hollis, J.F. (1992). Social networks as predictors of ischemic heart disease, cancer, stroke and hypertension—incidence, survival and mortality. *J Clin Epidemiol*, 45:659–66.

Wallace, R. (1991). Traveling waves of HIV infection on a low dimensional "socio-geographic" network. *Soc Sci Med*, 32:847–52.

Watson, S., Shively, C.A., Kaplan, J.R., and Line, S.W. (1998). Effects of chronic social separation on cardiovascular risk factors in female cynomologus monkeys. *Atherosclerosis*, 137:259–66.

Welin, L., Tibblin, G., Svardsudd, K. Tibblin, B., Ander-Peciva, S., Larsson, B., and Wilhelmsen, L. (1985). Prospective study of social influences on mortality: the study of men born in 1913 and 1923. *Lancet*, 1:915–8.

Wellman, B. (1988). The community question reevaluated. In Smith, M.P. (ed.), *Power, community and the city*. New Brunswick, NJ: Transaction, pp. 81–107.

Wellman, B. (1993). An egocentric network tale: comment on Bien et al. *Soc Networks*, 15:423–36.

Wellman, B., and Leighton, B. (1979). Networks, neighborhoods and communities. *Urban Affairs Q*, 14:363–90.

Wellman, B., and Wortley, S. (1990). Different strokes from different folks: community ties and social support. *Am J Sociol*, 96:558–88.

Wellman, B., Carrington, P.J., and Hall, A. (1988). Networks as personal communities. In Wellman, B., and Berkowitz, S.D. (eds.), *Social structures: a network approach: structural analysis in the social sciences*. New York: Cambridge University Press, pp. 130–84.

Williams, R.B., Barefoot, J.C., Califf, R.M, Haney, T.L., Saunders, W.B., Pryor, D.B., Hlatky, M.A., Siegler, I.C., and Mark, D.B. (1992). Prognostic importance of social and economic resources among medially treated patients with angiographically documented coronary artery disease. *JAMA*, 267:520–4.

Wolf, T.M., Balson, P.M., Morse, E.V., Simon, P.M., Gaumer, R.H., Dralle, P.W., and Williams, M.H. (1991). Relationship of coping style to affective state and perceived social support in asymptomatic and symptomatic HIV-infected persons: implications for clinical management. *J Clin Psychiatry*, 52:171–3.

Wolinsky, F.D., Stump, T.E., and Clark, D.O. (1995). Antecedents and consequences of physical activity and exercise among older adults. *Gerontologist*, 35:451–62.

Zapka, J.G., Stoddard, A.M., and McCusker, J. (1993). Social network, support and influence: relationships with drug use and protective AIDS behavior. *AIDS Educ Prev*, 5:352–66.

8

Social Cohesion, Social Capital, and Health

ICHIRO KAWACHI AND LISA BERKMAN

THE SEARCH FOR SOCIAL FORCES ACTING ON HEALTH

An important task for the emerging field of social epidemiology is to identify the *collective* characteristics of communities and societies that determine population health status. Ever since Durkheim, social scientists have recognized that society is not simply the sum of individuals—that the factors which determine population well-being cannot be reduced to individual risk factors. In a passage from *The Rules of Sociological Method*, Durkheim contended: "The group thinks, feels and acts entirely differently from the way its members would if they were isolated. If therefore we begin by studying these members separately, we will understand nothing about what is taking place in the group" (1895, 1982, p. 129). Thus, if we wish to understand what keeps some societies healthy, yet others sick, we had better search among social facts for explanations. Durkheim put his own methods to test by investigating the underlying causes of one of

the most individualistic acts imaginable, suicide. He reasoned that if forces external to the individual played any role in their well-being, such influences would be evident even for a cause of death that was apparently entirely within the realm of individual volition. By a process of careful deduction and the elimination of competing hypotheses, Durkheim succeeded in demonstrating that the population rate of suicide is, in fact, related to collective features of society. Comparing suicide statistics in European countries across time and space, Durkheim concluded that the lowest rates of suicide occurred in societies with the highest degrees of social integration. Conversely, an excess of suicides occurred in societies undergoing various forms of dislocation and loosening of social bonds. Most importantly, whereas individuals at risk of committing suicide came and went, the *social suicide rate* in each society remained relatively constant—evidence of the power of social forces in shaping this social phenomenon. In a famous passage, Durkheim concluded that

The social suicide-rate can be explained only sociologically. At any given moment the moral constitution of society establishes the contingent of voluntary deaths. There is, therefore, for each people a collective force of a definite amount of energy, impelling men to self-destruction. The victim's act which at first seems to express only his personal temperament is really the supplement and prolongation of a social condition which they express externally. . . .

To explain his detachment from life the individual accuses his most immediately surrounding circumstances; life is sad to him because he is sad. Of course his sadness comes from him without in one sense, however not from one or another incident of his career *but rather from the group to which he belongs.* (1897, 1997, p. 299, emphasis added)

The search continues today for collective characteristics that shape individual and group outcomes. Social scientists have puzzled over the question of why some communities seem to prosper, possess effective political institutions, have law-abiding and healthy citizens, while other communities do not. Many societal characteristics have been identified which could account for variations in group-level outcomes (such as the degree of inequality in incomes, described in Chapter 4), but Durkheim's original focus on social integration, or social cohesion, remains as relevant as ever. The purpose of this chapter, then, is to outline the theoretical and empirical linkages between social cohesion (and its related concept, social capital) and health.

SOCIAL COHESION AND SOCIAL CAPITAL

Social cohesion refers to the extent of connectedness and solidarity among groups in society (a more formal attempt at definition will follow). According to Durkheim, a cohesive society is one that is marked by the abundance of "mutual moral support, which instead of throwing the individual on his own resources, leads him to share in the collective energy and supports his own when exhausted" (1897, 1997, p. 210). A cohesive society is also one that is richly endowed with stocks of *social capital.* Social capital is defined as those features of social structures—such as levels of interpersonal trust and norms of reciprocity and mutual aid—which act as resources for individuals and facilitate collective action (Coleman 1990; Putnam 1993a). Social capital thus forms a subset of the notion of social cohesion. Social cohesion refers to two broader, intertwined features of society, which may be described as: *(1) the absence of latent social conflict*—whether in the form of income/wealth inequality; racial/ethnic tensions; disparities in political participation; or other forms of polarization; and *(2) the presence of strong social bonds*—measured by levels of trust and norms of reciprocity (i.e., social capital); the abundance of associations that bridge social divisions ("civil society"); and the presence of institutions of conflict management (e.g., a responsive democracy, an independent judiciary, and so forth). Social cohesion and social capital are both collective, or ecological, dimensions of society, to be distinguished from the concepts of social networks and social support, which are characteristically measured at the level of the individual (see Chapter 7).

James Coleman was one of the first social scientists to attempt a formal definition of social capital (1988, 1990). According to Coleman, social capital consists of those features of social structures that facilitate the actions of members within them. Since this definition is explicitly functionalist ("the facilitation of actions"), it follows that social capital is not a single entity, but can take a variety of forms—just as the concept "chair" identifies certain physical objects by their function, despite differences in form, appearance, and construction (1988). Some examples of the forms of social capital described by Coleman (1988, 1990) include levels of trust within a social structure, "appropriable" social organizations, norms and sanctions, and information channels. Although seemingly disparate, some of these concepts are causally linked. For instance, the trustworthiness of the social environment is critical to the proper

Table 8–1. Definitions of Social Capital

Author	Definition
James Coleman, 1990	"Social capital is defined by its function. It is not a single entity, but a variety of different entities having two characteristics in common: They all consist of some aspect of social structure, and they facilitate certain actions of individuals who are within the structure. Like other forms of capital, social capital is productive, making possible the achievement of certain ends that would not be attainable in its absence." (p. 302) *Examples:* Level of trustworthiness, extent of obligations, norms and effective sanctions, appropriable social institutions, information channels
Pierre Bourdieu, 1986	"Social capital is the sum of resources, actual or virtual, that accrue to an individual or group by virtue of possessing a durable network of more or less institutionalized relationships of mutual acquaintance and recognition." (p. 119)
Glenn Loury, 1992	"[Social capital refers] to naturally occurring social relationships among persons which promote or assist the acquisition of skills and traits valued in the marketplace." (p. 100)
Robert Putnam, 1993a	"Social capital . . . refers to features of social organization, such as trust, norms, and networks, that can improve the efficiency of society by facilitating coordinated actions." (p. 167) *Indicators:* Levels of trust, perceived reciprocity, density of membership in civic associations.

functioning of obligations and expectations, which are themselves forms of social capital. If *A* does something for *B*, expecting *B* to reciprocate at some time in the future, this establishes an expectation in *A* and an obligation on the part of *B*; but the success of the transaction depends crucially on the level of trust between *A* and *B* (1988). As an example of an appropriable social organization, Coleman cites the case of a resident's association in an urban housing project which formed initially for the purpose of pressuring builders to fix various problems (leaks, crumbling sidewalks, etc.). After the problems were solved, the organization remained as available social capital to improve the quality of life for residents (1990). The point is that an organization, once brought into existence for one set of purposes, can also be appropriated for other uses, thus constituting a form of social capital.

Following Coleman's pioneering work, a number of other attempts to define social capital have been made, spanning the disciplines of economics (Loury 1992), sociology (Bourdieu and Wacquant 1992), and political science (Putnam 1993a,b) (Table 8–1). Although the definitions differ slightly, there is sufficient consensus to draw some important generalizations about the nature of social capital:

1. *It is social.* The distinctive feature of social capital is that it is external to the individual—i.e., it is not lodged within individuals (as is human capital) nor in the means of production (as is physical capital). Rather, social capital inheres in the structure of social relationships; in other words, it is an ecologic characteristic. A useful distinction can be drawn here between social capital and social networks. Social networks are a characteristic that can (and most often has been) be measured at the individual level, whereas social capital should be properly considered a feature of the collective (neighborhood, community, society) to which the individual belongs. It makes no sense to measure an individual's social capital. In theory, a well-connected individual

(one who has lots of friends and close relatives) could experience different life chances and health outcomes depending on whether he or she resides in an environment that is rich or poor in social capital.

2. *Social capital is a public good.* A corollary of the fact that social capital is a collective characteristic is that it is also a public good. The *sine qua non* of a public good is its aspect of nonexcludability in consumption. For example, the voluntary efforts of a parent liaison at a public school do not primarily benefit that parent, but rather the other children (and their parents) belonging to the same class. This is in contrast to other forms of capital. Physical capital is ordinarily a private good, and property rights make it possible for the person who invests in it to wholly capture the benefits it produces (Coleman 1988). Similarly, human capital also has features of a private good—i.e., the person who invests the time and resources in accumulating skills and knowledge reaps the benefits in the form of a higher-paying job or more satisfying or higher-status work. (Although an argument may also be made for human capital as a public good, i.e., citizens at large benefit in many ways from living in a society where every member has a generally high level of education).

The fact that the actors who generate a public good typically capture only a small part of its benefits tends to lead to the problem of underinvestment. In fact, social capital almost always arises as a *by-product* of social relationships, and not as the result of conscious investment on the part of members within a social structure. Incidentally, some scholars have objected to the use of the term social "capital," arguing that the language implies an economic basis for social exchange. In fact, our intent is exactly the opposite, i.e., to remind economists that not all forms of capital involve mercantile exchange. We agree with Bourdieu (1986) that

The structure and distribution of the different types and subtypes of capital at a given moment in time represents [*sic*] that immanent structure of the social world, i.e., the set of constraints, inscribed in the very reality of the world, which govern its functioning in a durable way, determining the chances of success for practices. *It is in fact impossible to account for the structure and functioning of the social world unless one reintroduces capital in all its forms and not solely in the one form recognized by economic theory.* Economic theory has allowed to be foisted upon it a definition of the economy of practices which is the historical invention of capitalism. (Bourdieu 1986, p. 242, *emphasis added*)

In other words, capital may be used to describe any stock of resources, be they tangible (as in the form of dollars) or not so tangible (as in the form of interpersonal trust and norms of reciprocity). Given the characteristics described above, what evidence can we adduce that social capital matters for the outcomes of societies, communities, and individuals?

RELATIONSHIPS OF SOCIAL CAPITAL TO COMMUNITY AND INDIVIDUAL OUTCOMES

The benefits of social capital have been examined in at least eight separate fields of inquiry: *(1)* families and youth behavior problems—for example, the prevention of delinquency and the promotion of successful child development (Parcel and Menaghan 1993; Hagan et al. 1995); *(2)* schooling and education (e.g., Coleman 1988); *(3)* community life—for example, norms of labor market attachment (Wacquant and Wilson 1989; Case and Katz 1991); *(4)* work and organizations—for example, occupational mobility and income attainment (Boxman et al. 1991; Fellmeth 1996); *(5)* democracy and governance (e.g., Putnam 1993a; Verba et al. 1995); *(6)* economic development (e.g., Fukuyama 1995); *(7)* criminology (e.g., Sampson et al. 1997); and *(8)* public health (Kawachi et al. 1997a, 1999a). For a review of research in these areas, see Woolcock (1998). In terms of relevance to public health, we will briefly review the contributions of three disciplines: criminology, political science, and epidemiology.

Social Capital and Crime

Nearly a half-century after Durkheim's treatise on suicide, two Chicago criminologists, Clifford Shaw and Henry McKay (1942), made a startling discovery: in their study of 21 U.S. cities, the same socioeconomically disadvantaged areas continued to exhibit high delinquency rates over a span of several decades despite changes in their racial and ethnic composition. Their discovery echoed Durkheim's earlier finding of the persistent effects of the social environment on certain social phenomena (suicide, crime), regardless of what populations experienced them. This observation led Shaw and MacKay to reject individualistic explanations of delinquency and focus instead on community processes which led to the apparent transgenerational transmission of criminal behavior.

What do suicides and crime have in common? In each instance, the investigators attributed the geographic variations in the occurrence of events to the strength (or absence) of social cohesion. Weak social controls and the disruption of local community organization were hypothesized to be the underlying factor producing increased rates of suicide (in the case of 19th-century Europe) and crime (in 20th-century America). Social disorganization has been defined as the "inability of a community structure to realize the common values of its residents and maintain effective social controls" (Sampson and Groves 1989). The social organizational approach views local communities and neighborhoods as complex systems of friendship, kinship, and acquaintanceship networks, as well as formal and informal associational ties rooted in family life and ongoing socialization processes (Sampson 1996). From the perspective of crime control, a major dimension of social disorganization is the ability of a community to supervise and control teenage peer groups, especially gangs. Thus Shaw and McKay (1942) argued that residents of cohesive communities were better able to control the youth behaviors that set the context for gang violence. Examples of such controls include the supervision of leisure-time youth activities, intervention in street-corner congregation, and challenging youth "who seem to be up to no good." Socially disorganized communities with extensive street-corner peer groups are also expected to have higher rates of adult violence, especially among younger adults who still have ties to youth gangs (Sampson 1996).

Recently, social disorganization theory has been explicitly linked to the concept of social capital. Sampson et al. (1997) surveyed 8782 residents of 343 Chicago neighborhoods in 1995 to ask about their perceptions of social cohesion and trust in the neighborhood. Respondents were asked how strongly they agreed (on a five point scale) that "People around here are willing to help their neighbors," "This is a close-knit neighborhood," "People in this neighborhood can be trusted," "People in this neighborhood generally don't get along with each other," and "People in this neighborhood do not share the same values" (the last two items were reverse-coded). The resulting scale was then combined with responses to questions about the level of informal social control (whether neighbors would intervene in situations where children were engaging in delinquent behavior) to produce a summary index of "collective efficacy." Collective efficacy turned out to be significantly ($P < 0.01$) related to organizational participation ($r = 0.45$) and neighborhood services ($r = 0.21$). In hierarchical statistical models adjusting for individual characteristics [age, socioeconomic status (SES), gender, ethnicity, marital status, home ownership, and years in neighborhood], the index of collective efficacy was significantly inversely associated with reports of neighborhood violence and violent victimization as well as homicide rates. For example, a 2 standard deviation (S.D.) elevation in neighborhood collective efficacy was associated with a 39.7% reduction in the expected homicide rate.

The link between social capital and violent crime/homicide has been further replicated at the state level (Kennedy et al. 1998; Kawachi et al., 1999b). In these ecological analyses, states with lower levels of trust (as gauged by responses to opinion surveys) exhibited higher rates of both violent crime and property crime, including homicide (r = 0.82), assault (0.61), and robbery (0.45), as well as burglary (0.54) (all correlation coefficients, $P < 0.05$) (Kawachi et al., 1999b).

Social Capital, "Civil Society," and the Functioning of Democracy

Independently of the discoveries made in criminology, social capital has emerged as a major focus of inquiry in political science. Ever since Tocqueville, American scholars have been fascinated by the role of civic associations in maintaining social cohesion. Having observed the Americans for 2 years during his visit in the 1830s, Tocqueville concluded that they were a "nation of joiners," and that "Americans of all ages, all conditions, and all dispositions constantly form associations" (1845, 1990, p. 114). Political scientists have theorized about the functions of civic associations, including their ability to bind together society and to minimize the disintegrative effects of conflict, as well as to provide individual members with a sense of personal identification and enhanced social status (Smith and Freedman 1972). The concept of "civil society" (or "civic culture") has been described by Ralf Dahrendorf in the following way:

The term "civil society" is more suggestive than precise. It suggests, for example, that people behave towards each other in a civilized manner; the suggestion is fully intended. It also suggests that its members enjoy the status of citizens, which again is intended. However, the core meaning of the concept is quite precise. Civil society describes the associations in which we conduct our lives, and that owe their existence to our needs and initiatives rather than to the state. (Dahrendorf 1995)

In other words, civil society is defined as that zone between the individual and the state which is occupied by a crisscrossing network of voluntary associations. The web of weak social ties created by voluntary associations acts as the social glue that holds society together. A variety of advantages have been claimed for civil society, such as keeping individuals from becoming isolated, protecting them from the state, meeting needs that cannot be filled by government, and encouraging more active engagement in the life of the community whilst preserving a degree of choice.

The recent surge of interest in civil society within political science can be traced to the publication in 1993 of a seminal work by the American political scientist Robert Putnam. His book *Making Democracy Work* (1993a) reports how Putnam sought to measure the strength of civil society—or more specifically, social capital—across the 20 regions of Italy. The purpose of his 20-year study was to attempt to explain the performance of local governments, which were introduced to Italy in 1970. Local government performance in each region of Italy was assessed by surveys, interviews, and a diverse set of policy indicators selected to gauge institutional responsiveness to constituents and their efficiency in conducting the public's business. Putnam's central finding was that the wide variations in the performance of regional governments was most closely related to the level of social capital in each region. In northern Italy, where citizens actively participate in civic associations—choral societies, soccer leagues, literary guilds, and the like—regional governments were "efficient in their internal operation, creative in their policy initiatives, and effective in implementing those initiatives" (Putnam 1993a, p. 81). By contrast, in southern Italy, where patterns of civic engagement were much weaker, local government tended to be corrupt and inefficient. Putnam explained his findings in terms of the way social capital enables citizens to cooperate with each other for mutual benefit and hence overcome the dilemmas of collective action. Citizens living in areas characterized by high levels of social capital were more likely to trust their fellow citizens and to value solidarity and equality.

By contrast, social relations in areas of low social capital were characterized by proverbs such as "Damned is he who trusts another," "Don't make loans, don't give gifts, don't do good, for it will turn out bad for you," and "When you see the house of your neighbor on fire, carry water to your own" (Putnam 1993a, p. 144).

The mechanisms by which social capital influences political participation and government performance have been detailed by Verba and colleagues (1995). According to their Civic Voluntarism Model, ordinary and routine activities that take place when citizens join voluntary associations may appear to have nothing to do with politics or public issues, but they can nonetheless develop organizational and communications skills that are relevant for politics and thus can facilitate political activity:

Organizing a series of meetings at which a new personnel policy is introduced, chairing a large charity benefit, or setting up a food pantry at a church are activities that are not in and of themselves political. Yet, they foster the development of skills that can be transferred to politics. (Verba et al. 1995, p. 18)

Moreover, participation in nonpolitical associations can act as the locus of attempts at political recruitment: Church and organization members make social contacts and thus become part of networks through which requests for participation in politics are mediated. Indeed, the *embeddedness* of political activity in the nonpolitical institutions of civil society has profound implications for the ability of communities to garner resources for themselves and to improve their level of well-being. An obvious example is the community which is able to organize and apply pressure to government to obtain resources—such as police and fire services and block grants—that in turn help to sustain neighborhood organization and crime control. Where political participation is depressed, the community correspondingly suffers. For example, Hill and Leighley used Census data to show a relationship between the voting turnout rate of the poor and the level of state spending on welfare programs (1992).

Again, ecological evidence bears out the connection between social capital and political participation. Putnam (1993a) and

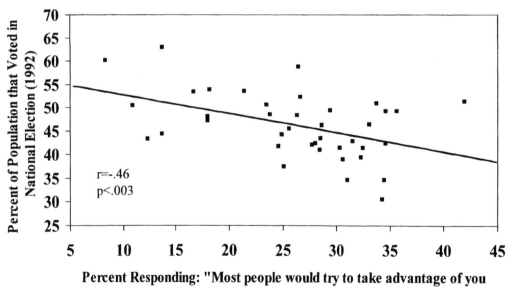

Figure 8–1. Relation between interpersonal trust and voter turnout in U.S. states (from Kawachi and Kennedy 1997).

Kawachi and Kennedy (1997) have noted the tight correlation between indicators of social capital and political activities such as voting. Within the United States, levels of civic trust and group membership are strongly correlated with geographic variations in voter turnout at elections (Fig. 8–1).

Although we have discussed the pathway running from social capital to human capital, the opposite is clearly possible: Educational attainment is one of the strongest individual predictors of group participation as well as trust (Brehm and Rahn 1997). The bidirectionality of the association suggests that there may be certain feedback and amplification effects of social capital on collective outcomes. In communities where stocks of social capital are being actively eroded, the associated underinvestment in human capital may lead to a further deterioration in civic activity. For instance, William Julius Wilson has suggested that racial segregation in urban residential neighborhoods, coupled with the progressive outmigration of successful working class families, resulted in the concentration of poverty, unemployment, crime, and ill-health in American inner-city ghettos (Wilson 1987; Wacquant and Wilson 1989). The flight of social capital in such areas—evidenced by the lack of norms of labor force attachment and other forms of "collective socialization"—threatens to keep residents in a perpetual state of disadvantage and despair.

Social Capital and Public Health

The latest area to which the notion of social capital has been applied is within the discipline of public health. Kawachi et al. (1997a) carried out an ecological analysis of social capital indicators across the United States in relation to state-level mortality rates. Indicators of social capital were the same ones used by Putnam (1993b; 1995): levels of interpersonal trust, norms of reciprocity, and density of associational membership (Table 8–1). Data were obtained from residents in 39 states from the General Social Surveys conducted by the National Opinions Research Center between 1986

and 1990. Among other questions, the survey asked about membership in a wide variety of voluntary associations—church groups, sports groups, hobby groups, fraternal organizations, labor unions, and so on. Per capita group membership in each state was strongly inversely correlated with age-adjusted all-cause mortality ($r = -0.49$, $P < 0.0001$). In regression analyses adjusted for household poverty rates, a one-unit increment in the average per capita group membership was associated with a lower age-adjusted overall mortality rate of 66.8 deaths per 100,000 population (95% confidence interval: 26.0 to 107.5). Density of civic associational membership was similarly a predictor of deaths from coronary heart disease, malignant neoplasms, and infant mortality. The General Social Surveys also asked questions related to levels of civic trust. Respondents in each state were asked which is true: "Most people can be trusted," or "You can't be too careful in dealing with people." The correlation of associational membership to civic trust was very high ($r = 0.65$). In turn, the level of distrust (the proportion of residents in each state agreeing that most people can't be trusted) was strikingly correlated with age-adjusted mortality rates ($r = 0.79$, $P < 0.0001$) (Fig. 8–2). In regression models, variations in the level of trust explained 58% of the variance in total mortality across states. Lower levels of social trust were associated with higher rates of most major causes of death, including coronary heart disease, malignant neoplasms, cerebrovascular disease, unintentional injury, and infant mortality. If these associations are causal, then an increase in level of trust by 1 S.D., or 10%, would be associated with about a 9% lower level of overall mortality.

Most recently, Kawachi et al. (1999a) carried out a multilevel study of the relationship between state-level social capital and individual self-rated health. Self-rated health ("Would you say your overall health is excellent, very good, good, fair, or poor?") was assessed among 167,259 individuals residing in 39 U.S. states, sampled

Age-Adjusted Mortality Rates by Social Capital (Social Trust)

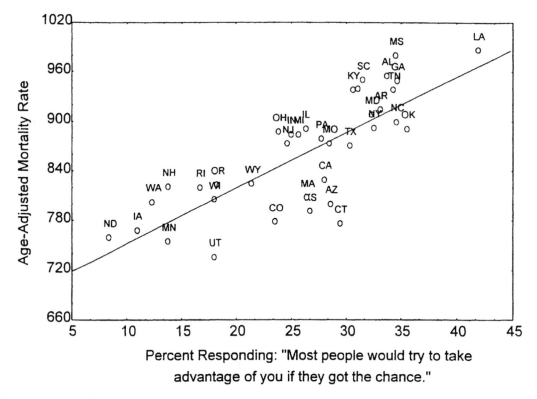

Figure 8–2. Relation between interpersonal trust and age-adjusted mortality rates in U.S. states (from Kawachi et al. 1997a).

by the Center for Disease Control's Behavioral Risk Factor Surveillance System (BRFSS). From this single item, a dichotomous outcome measure was created (1=fair or poor; 0=excellent, very good, or good). A recent review of 27 community studies concluded that even such a simple global assessment appears to have high predictive validity for mortality, independent of other medical, behavioral, or psychosocial risk factors (Idler and Benyamini 1997). For most studies, odds ratios for subsequent mortality ranged from 1.5 to 3.0 among individuals reporting poor health compared to excellent health. Self-rated health has also been demonstrated in longitudinal studies to predict the onset of disability (e.g., Idler and Kasl 1995).

Social capital indicators, aggregated to the state level, were obtained from the Na-

tional Opinion Research Center's General Social Surveys, described above (Kawachi et al. 1997a). Indicators of social capital included levels of interpersonal trust (percent of citizens responding "Most people can be trusted"), norms of reciprocity (percent of citizens responding "Most people are helpful"), and per capita membership in voluntary associations. Logistic regression was carried out with the SUDAAN procedure to estimate the odds ratios of fair/poor health (vs. excellent/good health). A strength of this particular study was the availability of information on individual-level confounds, including health insurance coverage, smoking status, overweight, as well as sociodemographic characteristics such as household income level, educational attainment, and whether the individual lived alone.

Table 8–2. Logistic regression results. Odds ratios and 95% confidence intervals (CI) of individuals reporting fair/poor health according to levels of social trust, adjusted for individual-level characteristics

Independent Variables	Odds ratio for fair/poor health	
	Model 1*	Model 2**
Low Trust***	1.68 (1.58–1.79)	1.41 (1.33–1.50)
Medium Trust	1.19 (1.13–1.26)	1.14 (1.08–1.21)
High Trust	1.00	1.00
Age (years)	1.04 (1.04–1.04)	
Age:		
25 years		0.74 (0.67–0.81)
<25–39		1.00
40–64		2.38 (2.26–2.50)
65+		4.80 (4.52–5.10)
Male	0.92 (0.88–0.95)	1.05 (1.01–1.09)
Race:		
Black	2.01 (1.91–2.11)	1.33 (1.27–1.40)
White	1.00	1.00
Other	1.84 (1.71–1.98)	1.43 (1.33–1.55)
Living alone		1.93 (1.34–2.80)
Income:		
<$10,000		5.95 (5.58–6.34)
$10,000–14,999		4.39 (4.00–4.60)
$15,000–19,999		3.01 (2.80–3.23)
$20,000–24,999		2.42 (2.25–2.60)
$25,000–34,999		1.88 (1.75–2.01)
$35,000+		1.00
Missing		2.97 (2.79–3.17)
Current smoker		1.51 (1.45–1.57)
Obese		1.70 (1.64–1.77)
Health Insurance Coverage		0.73 (0.70–0.78)
Recent Checkup		1.39 (1.32–1.46)

*Adjusted for age (as continuous variable), gender, and race.

**Adjusted for age (as categorical variable), gender, race, household income, living alone, current smoking status, obesity, health insurance coverage, and health checkup in last 2 years.

***Percent responding on the General Social Surveys that "Most people can't be trusted."

Low-trust states were AL, AR, LA, MS, TN, WV (mean % mistrust = 59.4%; range: 56.0%–61.6%).

Medium-trust states were AK, CA, CO, CT, FL, GA, IL, IN, IA, KY, MD, MA, MI, MO, NH, NJ, NY, NC, OH, OK, OR, PA, RI, SC, TX, UT, VA, WA (mean % mistrust = 42.9%; range: 33.4%–51.7%).

High-trust states were KS, MN, ND, WI, WY (mean % mistrust = 26.7; range: 21.2%–32.6%).

Source: reprinted from Kawachi et al., 1999a.

As expected, strong associations were found between individual risk factors (e.g., low income, low education, smoking, obesity, lack of access to health care) and poor self-rated health. However, even after adjusting for these proximal variables, individuals living in states with low social capital were at increased risk of poor self-rated health. For example, the odds ratio for fair/poor health associated with living in areas with the lowest levels of social trust was 1.41 (95% confidence interval: 1.33 to 1.50) compared to living in high-trust states (Table 8–2). In other words, these findings were consistent with an apparent contextual effect of state-level social capital on individual well-being, independent of the more proximal predictors of self-rated health.

MECHANISMS LINKING SOCIAL CAPITAL TO HEALTH

The mechanisms linking social capital to outcomes such as crime prevention and political participation have been articulated, and they appear plausible. But what about mechanisms linking social capital to health outcomes? It is useful here to distinguish between the *compositional* effects of social capital and its *contextual* effects (see Chapter 14 for a clear description of these effects).

On the one hand, an ecologic-level correlation between social capital and poor health can be explained by the fact that more socially isolated individuals reside in areas lacking in social capital (a compositional effect). Socially isolated individuals are more likely to be concentrated in communities that are depleted in social capital, because such places provide fewer opportunities for individuals to form local ties (Sampson 1988; Wacquant and Wilson 1989). There are well-established and biologically plausible links between social isolation (measured at the individual level) and poor health outcomes (e.g., Berkman and Syme 1979; Kawachi et al. 1996; see also Chapter 7 of this book). To date, no study

of social capital and health has simultaneously accounted for individual-level indicators of social isolation (e.g., not having contacts with friends or relatives, not attending church or belonging to groups). Hence, it is not possible to rule out a compositional effect of social capital on self-rated health.

A more challenging task is to identify the mechanisms by which social capital could exert a contextual effect on individual health. Social capital may affect health through different pathways depending on the geographic scale at which it is measured, e.g., neighborhoods vs. states. Considering effects at the neighborhood level, there are at least three plausible pathways by which social capital could affect individual health: *(1)* by influencing health-related behaviors; *(2)* by influencing access to services and amenities; and *(3)* by affecting psychosocial processes.

Health-Related Behaviors

First, social capital may influence the *health behaviors* of neighborhood residents by *(1)* promoting more rapid diffusion of health information (Rogers 1983) or increasing the likelihood that healthy norms of behavior are adopted (e.g., physical activity) and by *(2)* exerting social control over deviant health-related behavior. The theory of the diffusion of innovations suggests that innovative behaviors (e.g., use of preventive services) diffuse much more rapidly in communities that are cohesive and in which members know and trust each other (Rogers 1983). Alternatively, recent evidence from criminology (Sampson et al. 1997) suggests that the extent to which neighbors are willing to exert social control over deviant behavior (a characteristic that Sampson et al. termed collective efficacy) predicts their ability to prevent delinquency and crime. A similar process may also operate to prevent other forms of deviant behavior, such as adolescent smoking, drinking, and drug abuse. For instance, part of the reason why relatively little underage smoking occurs in Japan in spite of the ubiquitous presence of cigarette vending machines may be due to the close-knit nature of Japanese society and the extent to which neighbors, teachers, and strangers are willing to intervene when minors are caught breaking the law. (We shall turn later to the potentially coercive nature of societies characterized by high levels of social capital.)

Access to Services and Amenities

Access to local services and amenities is a second way in which neighborhood social capital may affect health. Again, evidence from criminology suggests that socially cohesive neighborhoods are more successful at uniting to ensure that budget cuts do not affect local services (Sampson et al. 1997). Residents of cohesive neighborhoods more readily band together to create the kinds of "appropriable" social organizations described earlier by Coleman (1990). The same kind of organizational processes could conceivably ensure access to services such as transportation, community health clinics, and recreational facilities that are directly relevant to health. Macintyre and colleagues (1993) have documented how poor and affluent neighborhoods differ systematically in terms of their access to such amenities and resources. Given such geographically based inequalities, the existence of local pressure groups to lobby for the provision of services could make all the difference.

Psychosocial Processes

Finally, neighborhood social capital could influence the health of individuals via psychosocial processes by providing affective support and acting as the source of self-esteem and mutual respect (Wilkinson 1996). Variations in the availability of psychosocial resources at the community level may help to explain the anomalous finding that socially isolated individuals residing in more cohesive communities—such as the East Boston community (Seeman et al. 1993), African Americans in rural Georgia (Schoenbach et al. 1986), and Japanese

Americans in Hawaii (Reed et al. 1983)—do not appear to suffer the same ill health consequences as those living in less cohesive communities.

Trusting social environments in turn tend to beget trustworthy citizens. The developmental processes by which the moral values of trust and reciprocity become instilled in children was described by Jane Jacobs in her classic work *The Death and Life of Great American Cities* (1961, 1992), which is where the earliest-known use of the term "social capital" occurs. Children growing up in a social-capital-rich neighborhood quickly learn that "people must take a modicum of public responsibility for each other even if they have no ties to each other." Moreover, "this is a lesson nobody learns by being told. It is learned from the experience of having *other people without ties or kinship or close friendship or formal responsibility to you* take a modicum of public responsibility for you" (p. 82, *emphasis* in the original). Jacobs went on to describe the benefits of neighborhood social capital for the preservation of sidewalk safety, the facilitation of child rearing, the enhancement of self-government, and the maintenance of the civility of public life in general.

Social Capital at the Level of the State

Turning finally to mechanisms linking social capital at the *state* level to individual health, it appears that the more cohesive states produce more egalitarian patterns of political participation that result in the passage of policies which ensure the security of all its members (Kawachi and Kennedy 1997; Kawachi et al. 1997b). Putnam (1993a) has demonstrated that social capital (measured by the same indicators used by Kawachi et al. 1997a) is indispensable to the responsiveness and smooth functioning of civic institutions. Low levels of interpersonal trust correlate strikingly with low levels of trust and confidence in public institutions (Brehm and Rahn 1997); low levels of political participation (as measured by voting and other forms of engagement in politics) (Kawachi and Kennedy 1997; Putnam 1993b; Verba et al. 1995); and ultimately, reduced efficacy of government institutions. United States data demonstrate that states with low levels of interpersonal trust are less likely to invest in human security and are likely to be less generous with their provisions for social safety nets. For example, mistrust was highly inversely correlated ($r = -0.76$) with the maximum welfare assistance as a percentage of per capita income in each state. Needless to say, less generous states are likely to provide less hospitable environments for vulnerable segments of the population.

REMAINING PROBLEMS WITH THE DEFINITION AND CONCEPT OF SOCIAL CAPITAL

We have attempted to provide a sense of the considerable progress that has been made in establishing the theoretical and empirical linkages between social capital and health. Several issues remain to be resolved, however.

Definitional and Measurement Issues

Both the definition and approaches to measurement of social capital are still evolving. Various commentators have highlighted ambiguities in the definition of the concept. For instance, the definitions listed in Table 8–1 seem to mix together indicators such as membership in civic associations with moral resources such as trust and reciprocity. As Woolcock has pointed out, "This leaves unresolved whether social capital is the infrastructure or the content of social relations, the 'medium,' as it were, or the 'message'" (1998, p. 156). In other words, the definition seemingly encompasses both the structure and function of social relations. If social capital in the form of trust is created as a by-product of participation in civic associations (which are themselves indicators of social capital), this leaves us with the problematic conceptual task of distinguishing between the *sources* of social capital and the *benefits* derived from them.

Measurement is a separate issue. Although there is virtually universal agreement that social capital is a collective characteristic and ought to be measured at the aggregate level, little or no work has been carried out to distinguish the concept from an array of existing neighborhood-level constructs in the field of community psychology (Lochner et al., in press). Constructs such as "psychological sense of community" (McMillan and Chavis 1986), "community competence" (Cottrell 1976; Eng and Parker 1994), and "neighboring" (Buckner 1988) all involve the assessment of neighborhood-level characteristics such as levels of trust, norms of reciprocity, and civic engagement. In short, further theoretical and empirical work is needed to sort out the issue of whether social capital represents an independent construct or is merely "old wine in new bottles" (Lochner et al. in press). (Regardless of the outcome of this debate, however, we note that the relevance of characterizing neighborhood social environment as a determinant of health remains undiminished.)

On a practical level, work remains to be carried out in selecting different indicators of social capital. Two types of approaches are possible: *(1)* using *aggregate* variables (i.e., aggregating individual responses to social surveys) and *(2)* using *integral* variables (i.e., direct social observation of neighborhoods). The latter approach has been scarcely tested. An observable indicator of reciprocity might be the number of instances in a city in which commuters block opposing traffic at busy intersections during rush hour compared to the number of instances when they do not. (We are indebted to Alvin Tarlov for this example.) An indicator of trust might be the proportion of gas stations in a community that require customers to pay up before letting them pump vs. those that do not. And so on.

Social Capital and Public Policy

Further ambiguity in the notion of social capital is evidenced by the fact that it has been used to justify contradictory policy prescriptions (Woolcock 1998). Conservatives regard state–society relations as zero-sum—i.e., "as the state waxes, other institutions wane" (George F. Will, quoted in Woolcock 1998). It has been argued that Big Government, through the paternalistic provision of a panoply of social services, tends to "crowd out" the activities of civic associations (McKnight 1995; Fukuyama 1995). By contrast, liberals tend to regard state–society relations as positive-sum—i.e., the state can nurture civil society. Skocpol (1996), for one, argues that many of the existing key civic associations in America came about as a result of deliberate government intervention and support. Thus, voluntary associations have historically operated in close symbiosis with the welfare state. Early in this century, the forerunner of the PTA (then the National Congress of Mothers) lobbied for historic breakthroughs in social policy, including mothers' pensions (which later became Aid to Families with Dependent Children) and the Sheppard–Towner program (which later became part of the Social Security Act). As Putnam (1993b) has noted: "Social capital is not a substitute for effective public policy but rather a prerequisite for it and, in part, a consequence of it" (p. 42).

Both liberals and conservatives alike have displayed a tendency to discuss social capital as an unqualified social good (Woolcock 1998). This is partly a consequence of the functionalist definition of the concept. (It "facilitates collective action for mutual benefit.") But, of course, it is quite possible to conceive of the downside of social capital, including its coercive aspects (caused by interlocking networks of obligations) as well as the inhibition of individual expression (created by the stifling atmosphere of public surveillance and meddlesome neighbors). And some forms of social capital (e.g., criminal gangs) may provide resources for its members but contribute little to (or be frankly disruptive of) social cohesion. The downside of social capital suggests that it is

a resource to be *optimized* rather than maximized (Woolcock 1998).

ACCESS TO SOCIAL CAPITAL

Although social capital has been earlier characterized as a public good whose benefits are available to all members within a social structure, this definition needs qualification. The extent of access to some forms of capital is undoubtedly unequal across income levels, gender, and race. Poor people, women, and African Americans may be excluded from access to social capital because of residential segregation, labor market segmentation, or other forms of discrimination both overt and covert. This suggests that an important task in research and policy is to identify those characteristics of civic associations that have the ability to *bridge* social divisions. Although new forms of civic association are being constantly generated (for example, in the form of suburban soccer leagues), their potential to serve the interests of society at large will remain limited so long as people's access to such forms of capital is restricted by other structuring processes such as residential segregation or segregation in the labor market or in schools.

An important agenda for research is therefore to identify the characteristics of civic associations that are more or less likely to serve the common interest. For instance, groups that are set up with other-regarding missions (e.g., charities) are more likely to serve the public interest than those characterized by self-regarding missions (e.g., hobby groups). Similarly, associations which involve face-to-face contact are more likely to foster trust and mutual aid than virtual communities (Internet discussion groups) or associations that require only the payment of membership dues (e.g., the American Medical Association [AMA]). (This is not to deny the real political clout wielded by tertiary associations such as the AMA, but whether they contribute to social cohesion is another matter.)

have schaly
erodes

HOW CAN WE INTERVENE TO BUILD SOCIAL CAPITAL?

Finally, how should we proceed to build social capital? There is an asymmetry to our state of knowledge of social capital; regrettably, we have a far better understanding of the forces that tend to destroy social capital but rather few notions of what kinds of interventions help to build it. One lesson is clear: social capital requires stability of social structure. Disruptions of social organization or of social relations can be highly destructive to social capital. As Jacobs emphasized, the basis of social cohesion must be "a continuity of people who have forged social networks. These networks are a city's irreplaceable social capital. Whenever the capital is lost, from whatever cause, the income from it disappears, never to return until and unless new capital is slowly and chancily accumulated" (1961, 1992, p. 138). Although we lack a complete understanding of how social capital is created, there is ample evidence of the destructive effects of residential instability and turnover. One of the unforeseen consequences of the urban renewal programs of the 1960s was the destruction of social capital following the breakup of cohesive inner-city neighborhoods.

Putnam (1995) has argued that social capital is generally on the decline in American society. According to time trend data obtained from the General Social Surveys, average group membership has dropped by a quarter in all social class groups over the last 25 years. The proportion of Americans agreeing that most people can be trusted fell by more than a third between 1960 (when 58% agreed) and 1993 (37%) (Putnam 1995). We have noted the general decline in social capital. The ways to rebuild civil society in America will depend less on calls to return to a romanticized Tocquevillian past than on identifying emerging forms of social capital and capitalizing on existing policy levers. Although beyond the scope of this chapter, it is possible to conceive of an array of top–down and bottom–up approaches to rebuild social capital. From a top–down perspective, state and federal government, as well as the private sector, could do much to directly subsidize local associations that foster social capital, such as neighborhood associations, cooperative childcare, and youth organizations. From a bottom–up perspective, existing institutions (such as faith communities, trade unions, and charitable foundations) could do much to encourage voluntarism and invest in the social infrastructure of distressed neighborhoods.

Many things determine the health status of communities and societies, but the power of social capital lies in its potential ability to explain an array of collective outcomes that directly or indirectly influence well-being. As Durkheim wrote more than a century ago:

A nation can be maintained only if, between the State and the individual, there is interspersed a whole series of secondary groups near enough to the individuals to attract them strongly in their sphere of action and drag them, in this way, into the general torrent of social life." (1893, 1997, p. 28)

REFERENCES

Berkman, L.F., and Syme, S.L. (1979). Social networks, host resistance and mortality: a nine-year follow-up study of Alameda County residents. *Am J Epidemiol*, 109:186–204.

Bourdieu, P. (1986). The forms of capital. In Richardson, J.G. (ed.), *The handbook of theory: research for the sociology of education.* New York: Greenwood Press, pp. 241–58.

Bourdieu, P., and Wacquant, L. (1992). *Invitation to reflexive sociology.* Chicago: Chicago University Press.

Boxman, E., De Graaf, P., and Flap, H. (1991). The impact of social and human capital on the income attainment of Dutch managers. *Soc Networks*, 13:51–73.

Brehm, J., and Rahn, W. (1997). Individual-level evidence for the causes and consequences of social capital. *Am J Polit Sci*, 41:999–1023.

Buckner, J.C. (1988). The development of an instrument to measure neighborhood social cohesion. *Am J Community Psychol*, 16:771–91.

Case, A.C., and Katz, L.F. (1991). *The company you keep: the effects of family and neighbor-*

hood on disadvantaged youths. (NBER Working Paper No. 3705.) Cambridge, MA: National Bureau of Economic Research.

Coleman, J.S. (1988). Social capital in the creation of human capital. *Am J Sociol,* 94 Suppl:S95–120.

Coleman, J.S. (1990). *Foundations of social theory.* Cambridge, MA: Harvard University Press.

Cottrell, L.S. Jr. (1976). The competent community. In Kaplan, B.H., Wilson, R.N., and Leighton, A.H. (eds.), *Further exploration in social psychiatry.* New York: Basic Books, pp. 195–209.

Dahrendorf, R. (1995). A precarious balance: economic opportunity, civil society, and political liberty. *The Responsive Community,* 5:13–39.

Durkheim, E. (1897, 1997). *Suicide: a study in sociology,* ed. Simpson, G. (tr. Spaulding, J.A., and Simpson, G., 1951). New York: Free Press.

Durkheim, E. (1893). *The division of labor in society* (tr. Simpson, G., 1933). Glencoe, IL: Free Press.

Durkheim, E. (1895, 1982). *The rules of sociological method,* ed. Lukes, S. (tr. Halls, W.D., 1938). New York: Free Press.

Eng, E., and Parker, E. (1994). Measuring community competence in the Mississippi Delta: the interface between program evaluation and empowerment. *Health Educ Q,* 21:199–220.

Fellmeth, A. (1996). Social capital in the United States and Taiwan: trust or rule of law. *Dev Policy Rev,* 14:151–71.

Fukuyama, F. (1995). *Trust: the social virtues and the creation of prosperity.* New York: Free Press.

Hagan, J., Merkens, H., and Boehnke, K. (1995). Delinquency and disdain: social capital and the control of right-wing extremism among east and west Berlin youth. *Am J Sociol,* 100:1028–52.

Hill, K.Q., and Leighley, J.E. (1992). The policy consequences of class bias in state electorates. *Am J Polit Sci,* 36:351–63.

Idler, E.L., and Kasl, S. (1995). Self-ratings of health: do they also predict change in functional ability? *J Gerontol B Pscyhol Sci Soc Sci,* 50:S344–53.

Idler, E.L., and Benyamini, Y. (1997). Self-rated health and mortality: a review of twenty-seven community studies. *J Health Social Behav,* 38:21–37.

Jacobs, J. (1961, 1992). *The death and life of great American cities.* New York: Vintage.

Kawachi, I., and Kennedy, B.P. (1997). Health and social cohesion: why care about income inequality? *BMJ,* 314:1037–40.

Kawachi, I., Colditz, G.A., Ascherio, A., Rimm, E.B., Giovannucci, E., Stampfer, M.J., and Willett, W.C. (1996). A prospective study of social networks in relation to total mortality and cardiovascular disease in men in the U.S. *J Epidemiol Community Health,* 50:245–51.

Kawachi, I., Kennedy, B.P., Lochner, K., and Prothrow-Stith, D. (1997a). Social capital, income inequality, and mortality. *Am J Public Health,* 87:1491–8.

Kawachi, I., Kennedy, B.P., and Lochner, K. (1997b). Long live community: social capital as public health. *Am Prospect,* November/December: 56–9.

Kawachi, I., Kennedy, B.P., and Glass, R. (1999a). Social capital and self-rated health: a contextual analysis. *Am J Public Health,* 89:1187–1193.

Kawachi, I., Kennedy, B.P., and Wilkinson, R.G. (1999b). Crime: social disorganization and relative deprivation. *Soc Sci Med.* 48:719–31.

Kennedy, B.P., Kawachi, I., Prothrow-Stith, D., Lochner, K., and Gupta, V. (1998). Social capital, income inequality, and firearm violent crime. *Soc Sci Med,* 47:7–17.

Lochner, K., Kawachi, I., and Kennedy, B.P. (1999). Social capital: a guide to its measurement. *Health and Place,* (in press).

Loury, G. (1992). The economics of discrimination: getting to the core of the problem. *Harvard J African Am Public Policy,* I:91–110.

Macintyre, S., MacIver, S., and Sooman, A. (1993). Area, class and health: should we be focusing on places or people? *J Soc Pol,* 22:213–34.

McKnight, J. (1995). *The careless society.* New York: Basic Books.

McMillan, D.W., and Chavis, D.M. (1986). Sense of community: a definition and theory. *J Community Psychol,* 14:6–23.

Parcel, T., and Menaghan, E. (1993). Family social capital and children's behavior problems. *Soc Psychol Q,* 56:120–35.

Putnam, R.D. (1993a). *Making democracy work: civic traditions in modern Italy.* Princeton, NJ: Princeton University Press.

Putnam, R.D. (1993b). The prosperous community: social capital and public life. *Am Prospect,* 13:35–42.

Putnam, R.D. (1995). Bowling alone: America's declining social capital. *J Democracy,* 6: 65–78.

Reed, D., McGee, D., Yano, K., and Feinleib, M. (1983). Social networks and coronary heart disease among Japanese men in Hawaii. *Am J Epidemiol,* 117:384–96.

Rogers, E. (1983). *Diffusion of innovations.* New York: Free Press.

Sampson, R.J. (1988). Local friendship ties and community attachment in mass society: a multilevel systemic model. *Am Sociol Rev*, 53:766–79.

Sampson, R.J. (1996). The community. In Wilson, J.Q., and Petersilia, J. (eds.), *Crime*. San Francisco: Institute for Contemporary Studies, pp. 193–216.

Sampson, R.J., and Groves, W.B. (1989). Community structure and crime: testing social-disorganization theory. *Am J Sociol*, 94:774–802.

Sampson, R.J., Raudenbush, S.W., and Earls, F. (1997). Neighborhoods and violent crime: a multilevel study of collective efficacy. *Science*, 277:918–24.

Schoenbach, V.J., Kaplan, B.H., Fredman, L., and Kleinbaum, D.G. (1986). Social ties and mortality in Evans County, Georgia. *Am J Epidemiol*, 123:577–91.

Seeman, T.E., Berkman, L.F., Kohout, F., LaCroix, A., Glynn, R., and Blazer, D. (1993). Intercommunity variations in the association between social ties and mortality in the elderly: a comparative analysis of three communities. *Ann Epidemiol*, 3:325–35.

Shaw, C., and McKay, H. (1942). *Juvenile delinquency and urban areas*. Chicago: University of Chicago Press.

Skocpol, T. (1996). Unravelling from above. *Am Prospect*, 25:20–5.

Smith, C., and Freedman, A. (1972). *Voluntary associations: perspectives on the literature*. Cambridge, MA: Harvard University Press.

Tocqueville, A., de (1835, 1990). *Democracy in America*, ed. Reeve, H., Bowen, F., and Bradley, P. (tr. Reeve, H., 1945). New York: Vintage.

Verba, S., Lehman Schlozman, K., and Brady, H.E. (1995). *Voice and equality: civic voluntarism in American politics*. Cambridge, MA: Harvard University Press.

Wacquant, L.J.D., and Wilson W.J. (1989). The cost of racial and class exclusion in the inner city. *Ann Am Acad Polit Soc Sci*, 501:8–25.

Wilkinson, R.G. (1996). *Unhealthy societies: the afflictions of inequality*. London: Routledge.

Wilson, W.J. (1987). *The truly disadvantaged*. Chicago: University of Chicago Press.

Woolcock, M. (1998). Social capital and economic development: toward a theoretical synthesis and policy framework. *Theory and Society*, 27:151–208.

9

Depression and Medical Illness

ROBERT M. CARNEY AND KENNETH E. FREEDLAND

DEFINITIONS OF DEPRESSION

Depression is an ambiguous term that can refer to an individual symptom (dysphoric mood), a syndrome, or any of several disorders. Dysphoric mood is a normal response to loss and other adverse circumstances. Thus, it is usually not regarded as clinically significant unless other depressive symptoms are also present. Syndromal depression is an unpleasant mood state involving multiple depressive symptoms. However, there is little agreement as to which symptoms comprise the syndrome, how many symptoms must be conjointly present to warrant the diagnosis, or how severe the symptoms must be for the individual to be considered "clinically depressed." This lack of consensus is reflected in the many different questionnaires and rating scales designed to assess syndromal depression.

The depressive disorders, in contrast, were defined by a psychiatric task force and delineated in the 4th edition of the American Psychiatric Association's *Diagnostic and Statistical Manual of Mental Disorders*

(DSM-IV) (American Psychiatric Association 1994). The task force based its definitions on studies of the epidemiology, course, outcome, and treatability of various forms of mood disturbance. Although the DSM-IV criteria have been somewhat controversial, they are widely utilized by researchers and clinicians in the United States and elsewhere. The criteria clearly specify the symptoms of each disorder and the diagnostic thresholds for the severity, number, duration, and functional impact of these symptoms. The DSM-IV also includes rules for determining whether to count physical symptoms such as fatigue in the diagnosis of psychiatric comorbidities in medically ill patients. The DSM-IV criteria are essentially a lingua franca for research on depression and other psychiatric disorders in medical populations.

Depression is one of the most common psychiatric problems in the United States (Blazer et al. 1994), yet it can be difficult to diagnose because there is no definitive laboratory test for it. The diagnosis is based primarily on the patient's self-reported

191

symptoms and on clinical observations. The DSM-IV provides a *descriptive* rather than an *etiological* nosology as it is based on the pattern, severity, and duration of symptoms rather than on inferences about the causes of the patient's distress or dysfunction. The descriptive approach is one of the keys to psychodiagnostic reliability since the causes of most psychiatric disorders are both poorly understood and controversial.

The most fundamental distinction in the differential diagnosis of depressive disorders is between the *bipolar* and *unipolar* disorders. Patients with bipolar disorders cycle between depressive and manic or hypomanic episodes, while those with unipolar depression never present with mania or hypomania. During manic or hypomanic episodes, the patient's mood is abnormally elevated or euphoric, and other features such as hyperactivity, press of speech, flight of ideas, grandiose ideation, inappropriate behavior, or decreased need for sleep may appear. The difference between mania and hypomania is one of degree: Manic episodes are serious psychiatric emergencies in which patients are often at great risk of harming themselves or others; hypomanic episodes are qualitatively similar to manic episodes but not severe enough to require hospitalization. The unipolar depressive disorders, the focus of this chapter, are considerably more prevalent than the bipolar depressive disorders.

Adjustment reaction with depressed mood is the mildest and most transient of the unipolar disorders. It typically occurs in the wake of an identifiable stressor, such as a divorce or a medical crisis, and persists no longer than 6 months after the stressor(s) that originally provoked it abates. Its symptoms consist of relatively mild emotional distress and limited social, occupational, or other functional impairment.

The symptoms of the other unipolar depressive disorders include *(1)* depressed mood; *(2)* markedly diminished interest or pleasure in almost all activities; *(3)* significant changes in appetite or weight; *(4)* in-

somnia (or, in some cases, hypersomnia); *(5)* psychomotor agitation or retardation; *(6)* fatigue; *(7)* feelings of worthlessness or excessive or inappropriate guilt; *(8)* diminished ability to think, concentrate, or make decisions; and *(9)* recurrent thoughts of death or suicide, which are often accompanied by a sense of hopelessness. *Minor depression* is the least severe of these disorders. A *minor depressive episode,* unlike an adjustment reaction, is not necessarily the consequence of an identifiable stressor. It may be present when between two and four symptoms (at least one of which must be depressed mood or loss of interest) continue for at least two weeks. Minor depression is listed in DSM-IV for research purposes only; it is not yet established as a clinical disorder (American Psychiatric Assocation 1994).

Dysthymia is a mild but chronic form of depression in which the symptoms persist for 2 years or longer. Unlike minor depression, diminished interest or pleasure in activities does *not* count toward the diagnosis, but hopelessness and low self-esteem do.

A *major depressive episode* may be present when five or more depressive symptoms (at least one of which must be depressed mood or loss of interest) are present almost daily for at least 2 weeks and cause clinically significant distress or functional impairment. Major depression is a debilitating psychiatric disorder that may persist for months or even years if left untreated. Whether treated or untreated, many patients relapse while recovering from major depressive episodes. Recurrences months or years after complete remission are also relatively common.

RELATIONSHIP BETWEEN DEPRESSION AND MEDICAL ILLNESS

Depression is common in patients with chronic medical conditions. Prevalence estimates vary depending upon the medical disorder, but they are nearly always higher than those observed in otherwise medically healthy individuals. In general medical practices, up to 40% of the patients have one or more depressive symptoms (Crum et al. 1994).

Some depressive episodes are reactions to the physical dysfunction or discomfort associated with medical illness, but many depressed patients have depressive episodes long before they develop any medical problems. Furthermore, depression may alter the course and outcome of a medical illness even if the depressive episode began as a reaction to the medical illness.

For example, patients who are depressed following a stroke (Feibel and Springer 1982), hip fracture (Shamash et al. 1992; Magaziner et al. 1990), or acute myocardial infarction (Stern et al. 1977) take longer to recover than do nondepressed patients with these conditions. Depression also contributes to the development and/or progression of a wide range of common medical conditions such as infertility (Lapane et al. 1995), temporomandibular joint pain (Vimpari et al. 1995), and pruritus (Gupta et al. 1994). Pruritus, or itching, is the most common symptom of dermatologic disease. It is associated with psoriasis and atopic dermatitis, among other common skin conditions. Gupta and colleagues (1994) found that depression was significantly related to pruritus in patients with atopic dermatitis, chronic idiopathic urticaria, and psoriasis. Although these conditions are not life-threatening, dermatosis patients rate pruritus second only to disfigurement as a source of distress, and severe pruritus is associated with an increased risk for suicide.

There are over 8 million cases of diabetes mellitus in the United States (Harris 1995). An estimated 15% (1.2 million) of these individuals have major depression, and nearly one-third have clinically significant depression (Gavard et al. 1993). Diabetes is a risk factor for neuropathy, kidney disease, peripheral vascular disease, and heart disease, and this risk is increased in patients whose diabetes is in poor control. Depression has been associated with poorer metabolic control both in cross-sectional (Jacobson et al. 1985) and prospective studies (Lustman et al. 1988). Not surprisingly, depression has also been shown to predict macrovascular complications and retinopathy (Kovacs et al. 1995).

Depression has also been associated with immunological dysfunction. Patients with major depression have been found to have blunted natural killer cell activity (Maes et al. 1994, 1995). This may increase the risk for many acute and chronic illnesses.

Depression may even have a causal role in the development of heart disease and cancer, two of the leading causes of death in the United States. There have been many epidemiologic investigations of the possible etiologic role of depression in various types of cancer. Unfortunately, these studies have provided mixed results.

One of the larger prospective studies using a standardized instrument to assess depression was conducted by Linkins and Comstock (1990), whose group administered the Center for Epidemiological Studies Depression Scale (CES-D) to 2264 participants from 1971 through 1974 in Washington County, Maryland. Those who were free of cancer 2 to 4 years later were followed over an additional 12-year period. Consistent with many of the previous studies, there was only a slight association between depressed mood and cancer incidence. However, the association was much stronger among cigarette smokers (relative risk = 4.5 for cancer in general, 2.9 for cancers not associated with smoking, and 18.5 for the types of cancer associated with cigarette smoking). Thus, depression may interact with smoking, and perhaps with other risk factors, to magnify the risk for cancer.

Knekt et al. (1996) studied over 7000 men and women who were free from cancer at baseline and reported similar findings. Using the General Health Questionnaire and the Present State Examination to assess psychiatric symptoms, the investigators found a strong interaction between depression and smoking. The relative risk of lung cancer given cigarette smoking was 3.38 in patients with minimal depression and 19.67 in patients with higher levels of depression. Comparable risk ratios remained after adjusting for other risk factors.

However, Friedman (1994) reported a follow-up of 923 patients with a depression diagnosis compared with over 140,000 patients without a depression diagnosis who received prescriptions from a pharmacy at the same time as did the depressed patients. Although there was a difference in the relative risk of cancer between the two groups, confounding demographic and medical factors may have accounted for the results of the unadjusted analysis. Thus, the prospective studies that have attempted to determine the relationship between depression and cancer risk have yielded mixed results.

In summary, comorbid depression has been found to have adverse effects on a variety of acute and chronic medical illnesses. Of all the medical illnesses studied to date, the relationship between depression and coronary heart disease (CHD) has received the most attention, primarily because CHD is one of the leading causes of morbidity, disability, and mortality among adults. Over 4,500,000 Americans have CHD, and at least 500,000 deaths are attributable to acute myocardial infarction (MI) annually (American Heart Assocation 1992). Because of its prevalence and its often-devastating consequences, heart disease remains one of the biggest challenges facing health care professionals today. The rest of this chapter deals with the current state of research on depression in CHD.

EPIDEMIOLOGY OF COMORBID DEPRESSION IN CORONARY HEART DISEASE

Depressive symptoms are very common in patients with CHD. Up to 65% of patients report depressive symptoms following acute myocardial infarction (American Heart Association 1992; Cassem and Hackett 1971; Cay et al. 1972; Croog and Levine 1982). Clinically significant depression is also com-mon. The estimated point prevalence of major and minor unipolar depressive episodes in post-MI patients is 45%, as defined by the Research Diagnostic Criteria (RDC), a predecessor of DSM-IV (Schleifer et al. 1989). Major depression alone is present in between 16% and 22% of these patients (Schleifer et al. 1989; Carney et al. 1990; Frasure-Smith et al. 1993; Forrester et al. 1992). This is considerably higher than the point prevalence of major depression in the community, which is estimated to be less than 5% (Robins and Regier 1991).

Although there have been relatively few follow-up studies of depression in the post-MI population, there is evidence that it tends to follow a chronic course during the first year after the MI (Schleifer et al. 1989; Stern et al. 1977; Travella et al. 1994), and that relapses are common in patients whose depression does not fully remit (Wells et al. 1992). For example, Stern et al. (1977) found that 22% of post-MI patients were depressed shortly after an acute MI and that 70% of these patients were still depressed 1 year later.

Many patients who are free of depression in the first few days and weeks following an acute MI go on to experience an episode of depression within a year. Lespérance et al. (1996) found that approximately one out of three patients develop major depression at some time during the 12 months following a myocardial infarction.

Depression is also quite common in patients who have not recently had a myocardial infarction or other significant cardiac event but who do have documented cardiac disease. The point prevalence of major depression is estimated to be between 17% and 23% in medically stable patients with coronary heart disease (Carney et al. 1987; Hance et al. 1995; Gonzalez et al. 1996) and about 17% of these patients have minor depression (Hance et al. 1995). Major depression also tends to be quite persistent unless treated in patients who have not had a recent cardiac event but who have stable coronary artery disease. Hance et al. (1995) found that half of the patients with major depression at the time of diagnostic cardiac catheterization either remained depressed or relapsed within 12 months. Approximately 50% of patients with CHD who have a current episode of major depression have had one or more prior episodes of major depression (Freedland et al. 1992a). For many of these patients, the first episode of depression predated the clinical onset of coronary disease by years or even decades. In the remaining 50% of the patients, the first episode of depression occurred sometime after the clinical onset of coronary disease.

In many cases, minor depression spontaneously remits without any intervention. In other cases, however, it is the harbinger of a more severe major depressive episode. In a study of patients with documented coronary disease but without a recent cardiac event, nearly 50% of the patients who initially presented with minor depression developed major depression within the next 12 months (Hance et al. 1995). Unfortunately, it is difficult to differentiate between patients who will remit without treatment and those who will deteriorate. Consequently, patients with minor depression should at least be monitored, if not treated, to reduce the risk of major depression.

There have been numerous studies of depression in patients undergoing coronary artery bypass graft (CABG) surgery, but none of them has evaluated the prevalence or effects of DSM-IV depressive disorders. Using a cutoff score of 16 or greater on the CES-D, point prevalence rates of "clinically significant" depression just prior to CABG range from 27% to 47% (McKhann et al. 1997; White et al. 1995; Langeluddecke et al. 1989). Within 6 months following CABG, CES-D depression estimates range from 26% to 61% (McKhann et al. 1997; White et al. 1995; Langeluddecke et al. 1989). Thus, depression may be even more common in CABG patients than in post-MI patients. Studies of DSM-IV depressive disorders in CABG patients are still needed, however.

In summary, depression is a common co-morbid condition in patients with CHD. Many patients who are found to be depressed after the clinical onset of CHD were already depressed prior to the clinical onset. Major depression, especially in post-MI patients, is not a transient adjustment reaction but rather a clinically significant psychiatric disorder that may persist for months or even years if left untreated.

Most studies of depression in CHD have been based on a series of patients recruited from coronary care units or cardiac catheterization laboratories. The majority of subjects have been white males. However, there is evidence that the risk of depression is twice as high among women with CHD as among men (Carney et al. 1990, 1987). There is also evidence that African-American CHD patients are as likely as Americans of European descent to be depressed. These conclusions are based on very limited samples, so further research is clearly needed on depression in female and ethnic minority CHD patients.

ADVERSE EFFECTS OF DEPRESSION

Psychosocial Morbidity

Most studies of psychosocial adjustment in post-MI patients have found that those who have moderate to severe depression during the first few weeks following the infarction are more likely than nondepressed controls to experience social adjustment problems over the first year of recovery. They are also slower to return to work and report more stress and emotional instability than do nondepressed patients (Cay et al. 1972; Mayou et al. 1978; Lloyd and Cawley 1983). Depression is also associated with poor psychosocial adjustment following coronary bypass surgery (Bryant and Mayou 1989).

In a study of the effects of chronic medical illness in a community sample, heart disease and gastrointestinal disorders were the two illnesses with the greatest negative impact on quality of life (Stewart et al. 1989). Individuals with comorbid depression reported worse psychosocial adjustment than nondepressed respondents across all chronic illnesses including heart disease (Wells et al. 1989b). Thus, depression further complicates the often difficult process of psychosocial adjustment to heart disease.

Medical Morbidity and Mortality

For more than 60 years, depression has been suspected of increasing the risk of cardiac events (Fuller 1935). Surprisingly, there have been very few studies of the relationship between depression and cardiac events, such as sudden cardiac death or myocardial infarction, until relatively recently. One of these, in a study of 3007 adults age 55 and over in the New Haven sample of the National Institute of Mental Health's multicenter Epidemiological Catchment Area (ECA) study, found that the 15-month mortality rate was four times higher in individuals with depressive disorders than in nondepressed subjects (Bruce and Leaf 1989). Sixty-three percent of the recorded deaths in the depressed sample were from heart disease or stroke. Similarly, a long-term study of cause-specific mortality showed that depressed subjects had more than twice the expected rate of cardiovascular mortality (Rabins et al. 1985).

Depression has a wide range of adverse effects on the course and outcome of coronary heart disease. For example, major depression at the time of the diagnosis of coronary artery disease doubles the risk that a major cardiac event will occur within the following 12 months (Carney et al. 1988a). Depression also increases the risks of reinfarction and mortality following MI (Stern et al. 1977; Ahern et al. 1990; Ladwig et al. 1991; Silverstone 1987; Denollet et al. 1995), and is associated with increased mortality rates in patients with ventricular arrhythmias (Kennedy et al. 1987).

As stated earlier, women with CHD may be twice as likely as men to be depressed (Carney et al. 1987, 1990). There is also evidence that women who are depressed or bereaved have an increased incidence of sudden cardiac death (Cottington et al. 1980; Talbott et al. 1977). We have speculated that depression may help to explain why

the mortality rate following MI is higher in women than in men (Carney et al. 1991), but further research is needed to confirm this.

In addition to increasing the risk of myocardial infarction and other major cardiac events, depression is associated with an increased rate of ventricular arrhythmias (Carney et al. 1993) and decreased heart rate variability (Carney et al. 1995c). Both of these are risk factors for sudden cardiac death.

Whether the effects of depression on cardiac event rates are independent of established risk factors is an issue of obvious importance in this line of research. It is quite conceivable, for example, that the CHD patients who become depressed tend to be the ones with the most severe heart disease and, consequently, the ones already most likely to die. However, in most of the studies cited above, efforts were made to control for various indices of disease severity as well as for other established cardiac risk factors. For example, in a study of cardiac events in the 12 months following diagnostic cardiac catheterization and angiography, Carney et al. (1988a) found that the rate of cardiac events was twice as high in depressed as in nondepressed patients. This effect was independent of severity of coronary artery disease, left ventricular dysfunction, smoking, and other cardiac risk factors. Similarly, Frasure-Smith et al. (1993) found depression to be associated with a more than fourfold increased risk for mortality during the first 6 months following acute MI, after adjusting for established risk factors including left ventricular dysfunction. Moreover, the prognostic significance of depression was equivalent to that of left ventricular dysfunction and of prior history of myocardial infarction, two well-known risk factors for mortality following acute MI.

Nevertheless, given the modest reliability of most techniques used to quantify the severity of coronary artery disease, it is possible, although unlikely, that there might still be an association between depression and disease severity. As more precise methods of quantifying coronary disease severity are developed, this question should be reconsidered.

SPECIFIC CHARACTERISTICS OF DEPRESSION ASSOCIATED WITH CARDIAC EVENTS

Although it is already clear that depressed post-MI patients are at increased risk of premature mortality and cardiac morbidity, research is still at an early stage on the question of whether these risks are limited to patients with particular depressive symptoms or depression subtypes or limited to cases of depression in which certain comorbid psychiatric disorders are present. For example, Lespérance et al. (1996) found that 40% of acute myocardial infarction (MI) patients with a prior history of major depression died in the year following the MI, compared to 10% of patients who were depressed for the first time. Thus, recurrent major depression may have different prognostic implications than would a single episode.

In a retrospective analysis, Schleifer et al. (1986) found that patients who met the diagnostic criteria for major depression even when the somatic symptoms of depression were disallowed were at greater risk for mortality than patients who met the criteria only if the somatic symptoms *were* allowed. Similarly, Lespérance et al. (1996) found that depression was even more predictive of mortality when sleep and appetite disturbances were eliminated from the diagnostic criteria. Nondepressed cardiac patients often report fatigue and sleep disturbance (Freedland et al. 1992b). Perhaps because the somatic symptoms are less specific to depression in cardiac patients, the cognitive and affective symptoms may be more predictive of mortality. Alternatively, the psychological symptoms may be central to the process underlying the relationship of depression to increased cardiac events.

Hopelessness, for example, has been found to predict fatal and nonfatal ischemic heart disease in a cohort of initially healthy American men and women (Anda et al. 1993) and mortality in a group of middle-aged Finnish men (Everson et al. 1996). In a study which compared depression, as measured by a self-report inventory of depressed mood, with hopelessness, hopelessness was the better predictor of myocardial infarction (Everson et al. 1996). However, other studies have shown that cardiac events are better predicted by depressive disorders than by depressed mood alone. It is possible that the presence of hopelessness may be a marker of severe depression and that its association with cardiac events may be related to its association with more severe depression. Another possibility is that hopelessness may reduce the patient's motivation to adhere to his or her medical treatment regimen. Poor adherence, in turn, may increase the risk for cardiac events, perhaps in addition to other effects of depression.

Some psychological symptoms that are commonly associated with depression are themselves risk factors for cardiac end points. For example, comorbid anxiety disorders are extremely common in depressed patients (American Psychiatric Association 1994). In recent studies, severe anxiety has been found to predict cardiac mortality (e.g., Kawachi et al. 1994).

Social isolation is another well-documented risk factor for cardiac morbidity and mortality (Berkman et al. 1992). Inadequate social support is a common complaint among depressed patients, one that has been confirmed by numerous studies in which social support has been systematically measured. Lack of social support can prolong depressive episodes (e.g., George et al. 1989), and depressive behavior can diminish whatever social support is available by alienating family and friends (Coyne et al. 1987; Keitner and Miller 1990). Unfortunately, most studies of social isolation and cardiac end points either have not measured depression at all or have done so inadequately. For example, Ruberman et al. (1984) used just three questions from a 20-item questionnaire to assess depression. They defined depression as a positive response to at least two of the three questions. Although the questions did cover several symptoms of depression (dysphoric mood, pessimism, and fatigue upon awakening), this scale is neither a specific nor even a particularly sensitive measure of clinical depression.

In a study which assessed both social support and depression with widely accepted, standardized instruments, Frasure-Smith et al. (1995) reported that only a diagnosis of major depression, a Beck Depression Inventory score (BDI) $\geq$ 10, a history of depression, and anxiety, as measured by the State-Trait Anxiety Inventory, were predictive of cardiac events in the year following an MI. Social support, as measured by the Blumenthal Social Support Scale, was not predictive of cardiac events in this study, but it did significantly correlate with the BDI.

Thus, it is unclear whether particular subtypes or symptoms of depression are more strongly related to cardiac end points. It is also unclear to what extent other psychosocial risk factors commonly associated with depression contribute to the effect of depression on mortality and medical morbidity. Future studies should measure these other risk factors carefully when depression is assessed.

The more severe forms of depression seem to be associated with a greater risk for cardiac events than are milder depressive disorders. For example, Barefoot et al. (1996) found that patients with documented coronary artery disease who had moderate to severe depression had an 84% greater risk for mortality than did nondepressed patients with coronary disease. In comparison, those with mild depression had a 57% greater risk. Pratt et al. (1996) conducted a follow-up of 1551 participants from the Baltimore site in the Epidemiological Catchment Area (ECA) study who were free of heart disease in 1981. The ECA study was an epidemiological survey of psychiatric disorders in the general population. Patients with a history of dysphoric mood had an odds ratio for MI of 2.07 (95% CI, 1.16–

3.71), whereas those with a history of major depression had an odds ratio of 4.54 (95% CI, 1.65 to 12.44). Thus, it appears that the risk imparted by depression exists along a continuum of severity, much like serum cholesterol or hypertension.

However, the severity of depression typically fluctuates over the course of a depressive episode, and residual symptoms are often present during interepisode phases. Since relatively mild depressive symptoms can evolve into major depression, CHD patients with relatively mild depression are "at risk of being at increased risk" for cardiac events.

In one of the better studies of depression as a predictor of morality following an MI, Frasure-Smith et al. (1993, 1995) found that major depression was the best predictor of cardiac-related mortality in the first 6 months, whereas a Beck Depression Inventory score of 10 or greater, indicating at least mild depression, was the better predictor at 18 months. However, in one of the few longitudinal studies of depression in CHD, Lespérance et al. (1996) interviewed the survivors in the Frasure-Smith et al. cohort 12 months following the index MI. They found that over 40% of the patients who were not depressed at index but who subsequently became depressed during the follow-up period had BDI scores of 10 or higher at index. This is consistent with the results of the Hance et al. (1995) study, which found that nearly half of the patients with minor depression at the time of diagnostic cardiac catheterization developed major depression in the following 12 months. Thus, many post-MI patients with depressed mood or other symptoms of depression will subsequently develop major depression. We do not yet know whether the patients with fewer or more depressive symptoms who do *not* go on to develop major depression are at any higher risk for mortality than are otherwise comparable nondepressed patients. This is a very important question and deserves attention.

Appels and his colleagues have described a condition which includes some of the symptoms of depression but which they call vital exhaustion. The symptoms of vital exhaustion include fatigue, feeling tired upon awakening, irritability, and demoralization. Although depressed mood is an associated feature, it is not a required symptom. In a series of studies, Appels and others have shown that vital exhaustion predicts cardiac events (Kop et al. 1994; Appels and Schouten 1991). However, it is not clear whether vital exhaustion predicts any events that are not also predicted by depression. It is possible, for example, that vital exhaustion may merely reflect cultural differences in the expression of depressive symptoms, as most of this research has been conducted in Europe.

Appels and his colleagues have provided evidence that vital exhaustion is not correlated with left ventricular ejection fraction, an index of cardiac pump function. However, since fatigue is a cardinal symptom of vital exhaustion, concerns about a possible confound between vital exhaustion and the severity of heart disease cannot be easily dismissed. In any case, no study yet completed has evaluated vital exhaustion and depression in the same population, using adequate assessments for both. The relationship between depression and vital exhaustion should be studied more carefully.

WHO BECOMES DEPRESSED?

A variety of medical, demographic, and psychiatric factors predict depression in CHD patients. Schleifer et al. (1991) found that patients who were free of depression shortly after an acute MI and who were subsequently placed on digitalis were more likely to become depressed within 3 to 4 months than were patients placed on other medications. In fact, no other medication, not even beta-blockers, predicted depression. The authors concluded that digitalis may have depressogenic central nervous system (CNS) side effects.

In samples recruited at the time of diagnostic cardiac catheterization, depressed patients are more likely to have a personal or family history of depression, to be fe-

male, and to be younger than nondepressed patients (Carney et al. 1987; Hance et al. 1995; Gonzalez et al. 1996). Ladwig et al. (1992) found that patients who were depressed following an MI reported experiencing fatigue and stressful life events just prior to the MI. Not surprisingly, similar predictors of depression have been found in psychiatric patient populations.

Similarly, Lespérance et al. (1996) found that post-MI patients who became depressed within 12 months after hospital discharge were more likely to have a history of depression, to have depressive symptoms during hospitalization, and to be under 65 years of age than patients who remained free of depression. However, a statistical model including these variables correctly identified only 15% of the patients who became depressed after hospital discharge. Thus, we are not yet able to predict depression in cardiac patients with the accuracy needed to guide prevention efforts. By identifying factors which increase vulnerability to depression, we may be able to recognize those at risk, develop strategies for preventing depression, and thereby prevent cardiac events in these patients. This is a high-priority area for research.

DEPRESSION, ATHEROSCLEROSIS, AND CARDIAC END POINTS

Depression clearly affects the risk of cardiac events in patients with established coronary disease, but does it also play a role in atherogenesis? Several prospective studies have shown that among community residents with no known history of coronary disease, those who are depressed are more likely to have an MI or to die of cardiac-related causes in the ensuing years than are otherwise comparable but nondepressed participants (Kawachi et al. 1994; Appels and Schouten 1991; Aromaa et al. 1994; Barefoot and Schrall 1996; Ford et al. 1998; Hippisley-Cox et al. 1998). However, it is unclear whether these findings truly show that depression is atherogenic. The results of these studies are also compatible with the possibility that depression increases the risk for cardiac events in patients who develop coronary artery disease for reasons unrelated to depression. Although this is a critical question, it will be difficult to conduct the studies needed to answer it until inexpensive and noninvasive methods of measuring coronary atherosclerosis are developed.

MECHANISMS

There are several different mechanisms that might explain how depression increases the risk for cardiac morbidity and mortality. These include *(1)* CHD severity, *(2)* side effects of antidepressant medications, *(3)* poor adherence to medical treatment regimens, *(4)* established cardiac risk factors, and *(5)* altered autonomic tone and neuroendocrine function. Efforts to determine which of these candidate mechanisms is responsible for the cardiotoxicity of depression have dominated much of our recent research.

Severity of Coronary Disease

One possibility is that the CHD patients who become depressed are the ones who have the most severe heart disease. Living with coronary disease may be depressing; if so, severe coronary disease is probably more depressing than is mild disease. If this is true, depressed patients have a worse medical outcome than nondepressed patients simply because they have more severe cardiac disease.

However, as discussed earlier, the effects of depression on cardiac events have been found in most studies to be independent of the severity of coronary artery disease, the size of the myocardial infarction (in post-MI patients), the degree of left ventricular dysfunction, and most other recognized indices of cardiac disease severity (Frasure-Smith et al. 1993; Stern et al. 1977; Carney et al. 1988a). In short, although this is an intuitively appealing explanation for the effects of depression in cardiac patients, there is very little evidence to support it. However-

er, as more sensitive measures of disease severity become available, this question should be revisited.

Side Effects of Antidepressant Medications

Many antidepressant medications, particularly tricyclic antidepressants and monoamine oxidase inhibitors (MAOIs), have cardiotoxic side effects (Sheline et al. 1997). In vulnerable cardiac patients, especially those with branch bundle block, the side effects of these medications could be fatal. However, it is very unlikely that antidepressants account for much of the increased mortality or morbidity associated with depression, for several reasons. First, the association between depression and cardiac mortality was reported long before any antidepressant medications had even been developed (Fuller 1935). Second, only in a minority of cases are cardiotoxic reactions to antidepressant medications fatal (Warrington et al. 1989; Pary et al. 1989). Third, many of the newer antidepressants (particularly the selective serotonin reuptake inhibitors) appear to be relatively free of cardiac side effects, and they have become the drugs of choice for depressed cardiac patients (Sheline et al. 1997). Finally, few depressed patients with coronary disease are recognized as being depressed either by their cardiologist or their primary care physician (Frasure-Smith et al. 1993; Carney et al. 1987; Freedland et al. 1992a). Consequently, relatively few cardiac patients ever receive antidepressant medications.

Adherence to Medical Treatment Regimens

Depression has been found to affect adherence to medical treatment regimens in patients with various chronic illnesses (Dunbar 1990; Richardson et al. 1987). More specifically, it has been found to predict poor adherence to exercise regimes in cardiac rehabilitation programs and to cardiac risk-factor modification programs (Guiry et al. 1987; Blumenthal et al. 1982).

We conducted a study to determine whether depression is associated with noncompliance with cardiac medication regimens in patients with CHD (Carney et al. 1995a). Using an electronic monitoring device to assess adherence to a prophylactic aspirin regimen during the first 3 weeks after coronary angiography, we found that depressed patients over age 65 adhered to the treatment regimen on significantly fewer days than did patients who were not depressed. Cognitively impaired patients were excluded from the study, and there were no differences between the groups in either the complexity of their medical treatment regimens or in the number or severity of comorbid medical conditions. Thus, depression was associated with a lower rate of adherence to a medication known to reduce the risk of MI. The extent to which reduced adherence to medical treatment regimens can account for the increased risk of mortality or morbidity remains an important area to study.

Association with Established Risk Factors

If well-established cardiac risk factors such as smoking, elevated serum cholesterol, and hypertension are more common in depressed than in nondepressed patients with coronary disease, the depressed patients might be at increased risk for cardiac events not because they are depressed, but because they smoke, have hypertension, or have hyperlipidemia. Increased serum cholesterol has not been found to have a consistent association with depression (Oxenkrug et al. 1983; Bajwa et al. 1992). However, the prevalence of hypertension has been found to be higher in depressed community residents (Wells et al. 1989a), depressed medical patients (Wells et al. 1991), and depressed psychiatric patients than in nondepressed controls (Pfohl et al. 1991). Depressed psychiatric patients are more likely to be cigarette smokers than nondepressed individuals (Glassman et al. 1990; Hughes et al. 1986). This has also been found in depressed patients with CHD (e.g., Carney et

al. 1987) compared to nondepressed controls.

Since cigarette smoking and hypertension may be more common in depressed than nondepressed patients, these established risk factors might explain why depressed CHD patients are at greater risk for cardiac events. However, depression has *not* been associated with these risk factors in some studies linking depression to cardiac events. In addition, depression has been shown to be an *independent* predictor of cardiac morbidity and mortality after controlling for these risk factors in several studies (Kawachi et al. 1994; Hippisley-Cox et al. 1998). Nevertheless, the role of hypertension and smoking in the increased risk for cardiac events associated with depression should be more carefully studied.

Altered Autonomic Tone and HPA Axis Dysunction

Dysregulation of the autonomic nervous system (ANS) and of the hypothalamic–pituitary–adrenal (HPA) axis is one of the most plausible explanations for the effects of depression on medical morbidity and mortality in CHD patients (Carney et al. 1995b). Dysregulation of the ANS and of the HPA axis has been found in medically well patients with major depressive disorder, as evidenced by elevated plasma and urinary catecholamines and their metabolites (Esler et al. 1982; Lake et al. 1982; Roy et al. 1988; Siever and Davis 1985; Veith et al. 1994; Wyatt et al. 1971), elevated plasma and urinary cortisol (Roy et al. 1988), elevated resting heart rate (Lake et al. 1982; Wyatt et al. 1971; Dawson et al. 1977; Lahmeyer and Bellier 1987), and decreased heart rate variability (Dallack and Roose 1990; Imaoka et al. 1985; Rechlin 1994).

Numerous studies have demonstrated that increased sympathetic and decreased parasympathetic nervous system activity predispose CHD patients to ventricular tachycardia, ventricular fibrillation, and sudden cardiac death (Kliks et al. 1975; Podrid et al. 1990; Schwartz et al. 1976;

Schwartz and Stone 1980; Schwartz and Vanoli 1981; Verrier et al. 1974). Increased sympathetic activity triggers myocardial ischemia in patients with coronary disease.

The physiological features of depression may have a variety of other adverse cardiovascular effects in CHD patients. For example, plasma catecholamines, when elevated, increase platelet aggregation, lower the myocardial ischemic threshold, and increase the risk of coronary thrombosis (Hjemdahl et al. 1991; Markovitz and Matthews 1991). Elevated metabolites of urinary and plasma thromboxane A_2, indicating increased platelet aggregation, play a critical role in myocardial infarction and are also found in patients with unstable angina (Grande et al. 1990). Furthermore, increased platelet aggregation may contribute to atherogenesis as a component of the response to endothelial injury. There is direct evidence for increased platelet activation in depressed patients who are medically well. For example, Musselman and colleagues (Musselman et al. 1996) found that depressed patients exhibit enhanced platelet activation and responsiveness compared to nondepressed subjects. Thus, altered autonomic tone in depressed patients with CHD may increase the incidence of transient myocardial ischemia and even myocardial infarction.

Because the relationship between altered cardiac autonomic tone and sudden cardiac death is so well documented, there has been intense interest in the development of inexpensive, noninvasive, and quantifiable measures of cardiac autonomic activity. Heart rate variability (HRV) analysis is one of the most promising technologies that is being developed to obtain such measures (Task Force 1996). Beat-to-beat variability in the heart's rhythm is determined primarily by ANS modulation of the intrinsic cardiac pacemakers. HRV is generally thought to reflect the balance between the sympathetic and parasympathetic regulatory control of the heartbeat such that low HRV suggests excessive cardiac sympathetic and/or inadequate cardiac parasympathetic tone. Furthermore, HRV is highly specific to cardiac autonomic tone, in contrast to plasma and urinary catecholamines and other measures of systemic autonomic activity.

Low HRV is an independent predictor of mortality in patients with a recent myocardial infarction (Kleiger et al. 1987), stable coronary artery disease (Rich et al. 1988), and congestive heart failure (Frey et al. 1993). Although HRV has not yet been studied in depressed post-MI patients, there is growing evidence that it is lower in depressed than in medically comparable nondepressed patients with stable coronary disease (Freedland et al. 1992b; Carney et al. 1988b; Stein et al., in press). In contrast, we did not find a difference between moderately depressed and nondepressed medically stable CHD patients in either resting norepinephrine or in norepinephrine response to orthostatic challenge (Carney et al. 1999).

If depression increases the risk of mortality in post-MI patients by disturbing the regulation of cardiac autonomic tone, it should confer an especially high risk upon patients who are already vulnerable to lethal arrhythmias and sudden cardiac death. Specifically, we would expect to find a disproportionately high cardiac mortality rate among post-MI patients who are not only depressed but who also have significant ventricular arrhythmias and/or significant ventricular dysfunction.

There is already some support for the hypothesis that the interaction between depression and these well-established post-MI risk factors is a stronger predictor of mortality than depression alone or these risk factors alone. Three of the studies that have documented a relationship between depression and increased mortality focused on patients with arrhythmias who were at high risk for sudden cardiac death (Ahern et al. 1990; Ladwig et al. 1991; Kennedy et al. 1987). Furthermore, in the Frasure-Smith et al. (1995) study, depressed post-MI patients who had 10 or more premature ventricular contractions (PVCs) per hour were at considerably higher risk for mortality than either depressed patients without PVCs or nondepressed patients with 10 or more PVCs per hour. Unfortunately, this was a post hoc analysis of a small number of end points. Further research is needed to test this hypothesis.

There is also some evidence that depression may be especially problematic in patients with left ventricular dysfunction. In a study of patients with congestive heart failure (CHF) (Freedland et al. 1998), many of whom developed CHF following an acute MI, survival appeared to be markedly reduced in patients with both major depression and low left ventricular ejection fraction (LVEF) compared to nondepressed patients with either low or normal LVEF and to depressed patients with normal LVEF. Additional research is needed to clarify the mechanism of this interaction between depression and left ventricular dysfunction.

In summary, altered cardiac autonomic tone is one of the most plausible explanations for the effect of depression on mortality in post-MI patients. If this is indeed the mechanism that underlies this relationship, then depression should be particularly onerous in patients who have poor ventricular function or who are predisposed to lethal arrhythmias. Furthermore, depressed patients with low HRV should be at greater risk for mortality than depressed patients with relatively high HRV. These hypotheses should be carefully tested.

INTERACTIONS AMONG MECHANISMS

Two well-controlled drug trials have shown that adherence is an independent predictor of outcome, even among patients who are administered a placebo (Coronary Drug Project Research Group 1980; Horwitz et al. 1990). In a letter to the editor following the publication of one of these studies, Kellet (1990) speculated that perhaps the patients who failed to adhere to the treatment regimen and who subsequently died may have been depressed. The depression may have responsible for the poor adherence and increased mortality. Although it is highly speculative, this possibility deserves consideration. In future clinical trials, researchers should assess depression in their participants to examine this question.

Anda et al. (1993) found that depressed affect and hopelessness were independent risk factors for CHD incidence and mortality among both smokers and nonsmokers. They therefore concluded that depression had an effect independent of smoking. However, they also found that smoking was a more significant risk factor for CHD in patients with depressed mood or feelings of hopelessness.

Anda et al.'s findings are consistent with those of Kaplan et al. (1992), who reported that the effect of smoking on the extent of carotid atherosclerosis in 1100 middle aged men was 3.4 times greater in depressed compared to nondepressed subjects. Kaplan and his colleagues also found that the effect of low-density lipoprotein (LDL) cholesterol level on atherosclerosis was increased almost twofold. Moreover, the effect for fibrinogen level was increased by nearly fourfold in depressed compared to nondepressed participants. Thus, although depression may be an independent risk factor for cardiac events, it also may potentiate the effects of other cardiac risk factors for reasons that are presently unclear. The relationship between depression and other risk factors, especially smoking, is clearly an intriguing one and defines an important area of study.

These studies are also similar to the ones reviewed earlier concerning depression, smoking, and cancer-related mortality (Linkins and Comstock 1990; Knekt et al. 1996). For example, although there was only a slight association between depressed mood and the incidence of cancer, among smokers the relative risk ranged from 2.9 for cancers not associated with smoking to 18.5 with cancers associated with cigarette smoking (Linkins and Comstock 1990). Thus, depression may interact with smoking, and perhaps with other risk factors, to increase the risk for both cancer and heart disease.

WILL TREATING DEPRESSION REDUCE CHD MORBIDITY AND MORTALITY?

Antidepressants

There are four major classes of antidepressant medications: tricyclic antidepressants (TCAs), monoamine oxidase inhibitors (MAOIs), heterocyclic antidepressants, and selective serotonin reuptake inhibitors (SSRIs). All four classes are effective against depression in psychiatric patients. However, the TCAs and MAOIs are known to affect cardiac conduction, contractility, rate, and rhythm, and may induce orthostatic hypotension (Warrington et al. 1989; Pary et al. 1989). These effects may be particularly troublesome in older patients and those with unstable angina, conduction disorders, heart failure, or other complications of coronary disease. Fortunately, some of the newer antidepressants, such as the SSRIs, are less cardiotoxic. Although the potential for drug–drug interactions must be taken into account, SSRIs are frequently prescribed for depressed CHD patients (Sheline et al. 1997).

Nevertheless, there have been very few randomized, controlled antidepressant efficacy studies in cardiac patients. It is possible that depression in these patients may be qualitatively different than psychiatric depression and that it may not respond to the same kinds of treatments. However, nearly all of the antidepressant trials conducted on depressed CHD patients have found that depression can be successfully treated in these patients (e.g., Veith et al. 1982; Roose et al. 1998).

For example, in a recent controlled clinical trial, paroxetine (an SSRI) was compared to nortriptyline (a TCA) in a group of 81 depressed patients with documented coronary disease (Roose et al. 1998). The drugs were equally effective in an intent-to-treat analysis a study which included results of all those initially enrolled, including drop outs (61% improved on paroxetine vs. 55% on nortriptyline), but there were significant differences between the groups in adverse cardiovascular effects. Only one (2%) of the 41 patients on paroxetine, compared to seven (18%) of the 40 patients on nortriptyline, had an adverse cardiac event.

Psychotherapy

Although numerous experts have recommended psychotherapy for depression and other psychiatric disorders in patients with CHD, especially following MI (e.g., Blumenthal and Emery 1988), there have not yet been any randomized, controlled trials. Several randomized treatment trials have shown that patients with CHD do benefit from psychotherapeutic interventions (Blumenthal and Emery 1988; Van Dixhoorn et al. 1990; Rahe et al. 1979; Oldenburg et al. 1985; Oldridge et al. 1991). However, most of these studies have evaluated the addition of a psychosocial intervention to usual care or to cardiac rehabilitation. The studies have tested a wide variety of psychotherapeutic and behavioral interventions, including traditional group psychotherapy, relaxation training, and even music therapy, and were intended to reduce distress, modify type A behavior, or promote psychosocial adjustment following a cardiac event. Unfortunately, none of these studies have specifically recruited depressed patients. Instead, most of the patients have been recruited from cardiac rehabilitation programs, coronary care units, or outpatient cardiac services without regard to whether they were experiencing significant depression or any other form psychological distress at the time. Although there is little doubt that some depressed patients were enrolled in at least some of these studies, it is difficult to determine how beneficial these interventions were for the depressed patients.

Overall, the patients in these studies generally become somewhat less depressed and anxious as a result of treatment. However, most of the randomized trials have failed to show a significantly greater reduction in depression in the intervention than in the control groups (e.g., Rahe et al. 1979). Unfortunately, most of these studies have employed psychotherapeutic interventions that are not considered optimal treatments for depression. Studies of depressed CHD patients which evaluate the efficacy of recognized psychotherapeutic interventions for depression are clearly needed.

In a quantitative review of 16 randomized, controlled trials, Linden et al. (1996) found that CHD patients who received a psychotherapeutic intervention had lower 2-year morbidity (odds ratio 1.84) and mortality (1.70) rates compared to patients who were not treated with psychotherapy. Unfortunately, many of the studies included in the meta-analysis had serious methodological limitations. For example, the two largest trials—which, respectively, accounted for 77% and 37% of the treated subjects included in the meta-analyses of mortality and morbidity outcomes—have been criticized for flawed randomization procedures (Linden et al. 1996; Powell 1989).

Three large randomized studies have been published since the Linden et al. meta-analysis. The first was an attempt by Frasure-Smith et al. (1997) to replicate their successful stress management study, this time using more appropriate randomization procedures. Not only did the authors fail to find a lower rate of mortality in the intervention compared to the control group—they actually found *higher* cardiac and all-cause mortality rates among the older women in the intervention group. The patients were selected for "nonspecific distress" rather than for depression. However, many (if not most) of the participants undoubtedly were depressed. Nevertheless, the intervention had little effect on depression.

The second study was a multicenter controlled treatment trial conducted in Wales. Jones and West (1996) randomized 1168 patients with a recent MI to a psychological treatment group and 1160 patients to a usual care control group. Like the Frasure-Smith et al. study, there were no significant differences between the treated and control patients in self-reported depression. Furthermore, no difference in 12-month mortality was found between the treated and control patients.

Finally, Blumenthal and his colleagues (1997) randomly assigned 107 patients with documented coronary disease who developed myocardial ischemia during a laboratory-based mental stress test either to exercise training or to a stress management group. Patients who lived at a considerable distance from the medical center were selected as a usual-care comparison group. Although there were differences in cardiac events between the usual-care comparison group and the stress management groups, there were no significant differences between the stress management and exercise groups at the end of the treatment. Unfortunately, because a geographic criterion rather than random assignment was used to form the usual-care comparison group, it cannot be concluded with confidence that the treatment was responsible for the outcome. It is possible that the usual-care patients may not have received the same quality of medical care as the patients who lived nearer to the medical center.

Two randomized clinical trials in progress are investigating the effects of depression treatment on medical morbidity and mortality in post-MI patients. The Sertaline and Depression Heart Attack Randomized Trial (SADHART) is investigating the effects of the SSRI antidepressant sertaline. Enhancing Recovery In Coronary Heart Disease (ENRICHD) is using cognitive behavior therapy to treat both depression and inadequate social support. The details of these trials are not yet available to the public, and, unfortunately, no results are expected from either trial for several more years. Furthermore, these trials are not designed to compare the effects of medication and psychotherapy, or of other antidepressants and other forms of psychotherapy, on psychosocial and medical outcomes. Clearly, much work remains to be done in this area.

CONCLUSIONS AND RECOMMENDATIONS FOR FURTHER RESEARCH

Major and minor depression and dysthymia are common disorders in patients with chronic medical illness, including coronary heart disease. Major depression is associated with increased risks for further cardiac morbidity and mortality, increased functional impairment, and poor quality of life. We still know very little about who is at risk for developing depression; which features of depression are most strongly associated with myocardial infarction, sudden cardiac death, or other cardiac events; how depression increases the risk for cardiac events; and what effects depression treatments have on psychosocial and medical outcomes. Although recent developments in the treatment of coronary heart disease have improved survival and functioning in CHD patients, heart disease remains the most common cause of death and physical disability among older adults in the United States. Thus, the search for answers to these questions will remain a high priority for the next decade.

One of the biggest mistakes new investigators make in undertaking research in this area is to initiate studies without the requisite multidisciplinary collaboration. Studies of depression and medical illness are, of necessity, multidisciplinary. The complexities of measuring medical and psychological variables cannot be exaggerated. A team with expertise in psychiatry or psychology, epidemiology, and medicine is essential for high-quality research in this area. Many researchers have unfortunately learned this the hard way.

One of the limitations of most of the studies linking depression or any psychosocial risk factor to increased mortality or medical morbidity is small sample size. With small samples, it is often difficult to control adequately for confounding variables, and all else being equal, the results of smaller studies are less convincing than those of larger ones. This concern and the relative ease of working from existing datasets have led some newer investigators to examine data from previous studies which were intended for other purposes. Unfortunately, many of these parent studies did an inadequate job of assessing either depression (Ruberman et al. 1984) or cardiac events (Appels and Schouten 1991) because investigating the relationship between depression and cardiac events was not one of the purposes.

Other studies have failed to adequately assess depression, because it was not the primary psychological risk factor under study. Future studies must employ state-of-the-art measures of *all* variables of interest, psychological as well as medical. For very little additional cost, depression can be assessed well enough to inspire confidence in the findings, even if the relationship between depression and cardiac end points is not the primary focus of the study.

The National Heart, Lung, and Blood Institute (NHLBI) frequently sponsors large, multicenter studies that enroll thousands of patients to evaluate new medical risk factors or to assess new diagnostic procedures and treatments. Without compromising the primary goals of these studies, it should be possible to add psychosocial assessments to the medical measures already being obtained. The addition of psychosocial assessments would enable us to address questions of considerable interest in a cost-effective way.

ACKNOWLEDGMENTS

Preparation of this chapter was supported in part by grant No. 1U0-1HL58946 from the National Heart, Blood and Lung Institute, Bethesda, Maryland, Robert M. Carney, Ph.D., principal investigator.

REFERENCES

Ahern, D.K., Gorkin, L., Anderson, J.L., Tierney, C., Ewart, C., Capone, R.J., Schron, E., Kornfeld, D., Herd, J.A., Richardson, D.W., and Follick, M.J. (1990). Biobehavioral variables and mortality or cardiac arrest in the Cardiac Arrhythmia Pilot Study (CAPS). *Am J Cardiol*, 66:59–62.

American Heart Association. (1992). *1992 Heart and stroke facts.* (Pub. No. 55-0386.) Dallas: American Heart Association.

American Psychiatric Association. (1994). *Diagnostic and statistical manual of mental disorders* (4th ed., rev.). Washington, DC: American Psychiatric Association.

Anda, R., Williamson, D., Jones, D., Macera, C., Eaker, E., Glassman, A., and Marks, J. (1993). Depressed affect, hopelessness, and the risk of ischemic heart disease in a cohort of U.S. adults. *Epidemiology*, 4:285–94.

Appels, A., and Schouten, E. (1991). Waking up exhausted as risk indicator of myocardial infarction. *Am J Cardiol*, 68:395–8.

Aromaa, A., Raitasalo, R., Reunanen, A., Impivaara, O., Heliovaara, M., Knekt, P.K., Lehtinen, V., Joukamaa, M., and Maatela, J. (1994). Depression and cardiovascular diseases. *Acta Psychiatr Scand*, Suppl 377: 77–82.

Bajwa, W.K., Asnis, G.M., Sanderson, W.C., Irfan, A., and van Praag, H.M. (1992). High cholesterol levels in patients with panic disorder. *Am J Psychiatry*, 149:376–8.

Barefoot, J.C., and Schrall, M. (1996). Symptoms of depression, acute myocardial infarction, and total mortality in a community sample. *Circulation*, 93:1976–80.

Barefoot, J.C., Helms, M.J., Mark, D.B., Blumenthal, J.A., Califf, R.M., Haney, T.L., O'Connor, C.M., Siegler, I.C., and Williams, R.B. (1996). Depression and long-term mortality risk in patients with coronary artery disease. *Am J Cardiol*, 78:613–7.

Berkman, L.F., Leo-Summers, L., and Horwitz, R.I. (1992). Emotional support and survival after myocardial infarction: a prospective, population-based study of the elderly. *Ann Int Med*,117:1003–9.

Blazer, D.T.G., Keller, R.C., McGonagle, K.A., and Swartz, M.S. (1994). The prevalence and distribution of major depression in a national community sample: the national comorbidity survey. *Am J Psychiatry*, 151:979–86.

Blumenthal, J.A., and Emery, C.F. (1988). Rehabilitation of patients following myocardial infarction. *J Consult Clin Psychol*, 56:374–81.

Blumenthal, J.A., Williams, R.S., Wallace, A.G., Williams, R.B., and Needles, T.L. (1982). Physiological and psychological variables predict compliance to prescribed exercise therapy in patients recovering from myocardial infarction. *Psychosom Med*, 44:519–27.

Blumenthal, J.A., Jiang, W., Babyak, M.A., Krantz, D.S., Frid, D.J., Coleman, R.E.,

Waugh, R., Hanson, M., Appelbaum, M., O'Connor, C., and Morris, J.J. (1997). Stress management and exercise training in cardiac patients with myocardial ischemia. *Arch Intern Med*, 157:2213–23.

Bruce, M.L., and Leaf, P.J. (1989). Psychiatric disorders and 15-month mortality in a community sample of older adults. *Am J Public Health*, 79:727–30.

Bryant, B., and Mayou, R. (1989). Prediction of outcome after coronary artery surgery. *J Psychosom Res*, 33:419–27.

Carney, R.M., Rich, M.W., teVelde, A., Freedland, K.E., Saini, J., Simeone, C., and Clark, K. (1987). Major depressive disorders in coronary artery disease. *Am J Cardiol*, 60:1273–5.

Carney, R.M., Rich, M.W., Freedland, K.E., teVelde, A., Saini, J., Simeone, C., and Clark, K. (1988a). Major depressive disorder predicts cardiac events in patients with coronary artery disease. *Psychosom Med*, 50:627–33.

Carney, R.M., Rich, M.W., teVelde, A., Saini, J., Clark, K., and Freedland, K.E. (1988b). The relationship between heart rate, heart rate variability and depression in patients with coronary artery disease. *J Psychosom Res*, 32:159–64.

Carney, R.M., Freedland, K.E., and Jaffe, A.S. (1990). Insomnia and depression prior to myocardial infarction. *Psychosom Med* 52:603–9.

Carney, R.M., Freedland, K.E., Lustman, P.J., and Jaffe, A.S. (1991). Relation of depression and mortality after myocardial infarction in women. *Circulation*, 84:1876–7.

Carney, R.M., Freedland, K.E., Rich, M.W., Smith, L.J. and Jaffe, A.S. (1993). Ventricular tachycardia and psychiatric depression in patients with coronary artery disease. *Am J Med*, 95:23–8.

Carney, R.M., Freedland, K.E., Eisen, S., Rich, M.W., and Jaffe, A.S. (1995a). Major depression and medication adherence in elderly patients with coronary artery disease. *Health Psychol*, 14:88–90.

Carney, R.M., Freedland, K.E., Rich M.W., and Jaffe, A.S. (1995b). Depression as a risk factor for cardiac events in established coronary heart disease: a review of possible mechanisms. *Ann Behav Med*,17:142–9.

Carney, R.M., Saunders, R.D., Freedland, K.E., Stein, P., Rich, M.W., and Jaffe, A.S. (1995c). Depression is associated with reduced heart rate variability in patients with coronary heart disease. *Am J Cardiol*, 76:562–4.

Carney, R.M., Freedland, K.E., Veith, R.C., Cryer, P.E., Skala, J.A., Lynch, T., and Jaffe, A.S. (1999). Major, depression, heart rate, and plasma norepinephrine in patients with coronary heart disease. *Biol Psychiatry,* 45:458–63.

Cassem, H., and Hackett, T.P. (1971). Psychiatric consultation in a coronary care unit. *Ann Intern Med,* 75:9–14.

Cay, E.L., Vetter, N., Philip, A.E., and Dugard, P. (1972). Psychological status during recovery from an acute heart attack. *J Psychosom Res,* 16:425–35.

Coronary Drug Project Research Group. (1980). Influence of adherence to treatment and response of cholesterol on mortality. *N Engl J Med,* 303:1038–41.

Cottington, E.M., Matthews, K.A., Talbott, E., and Kuller, L.H. (1980). Environmental events preceding sudden death in women. *Psychosom Med,* 42:567–75.

Coyne, J.C., Kessler, R.C., Tal, M., Turnbull, J., Wortman, C.B., and Greden, J.F. (1987). Living with a depressed person. *J Consult Clin Psychol,* 55:347–52.

Croog, S.H., and Levine, S. (1982). *Life after heart attack.* New York: Human Sciences Press.

Crum, R.M., Cooper-Patrick, L., and Ford, D.E. (1994). Depressive symptoms among general medical patients: prevalence and one-year outcome. *Psychosom Med,* 56:109–17.

Dallack, G.W., and Roose, S.P. (1990). Perspectives on the relationship between cardiovascular disease and affective disorder. *J Clin Psychiatry,* 51 Suppl:4–9.

Dawson, M.E., Schell, A.M., and Catania, J.J. (1977). Autonomic correlates of depression and clinical improvement following electroconvulsive shock therapy. *Psychophysiol,* 14:569–78.

Denollet, J., Sys, S.U., and Brutsaert, D.L. (1995). Personality and mortality after myocardial infarction. *Psychosom Med,* 57:582–91.

Dunbar, J. (1990). Predictors of patient adherence: patient characteristics. In Shumaker, S. A., Schron, E. B., and Ockene, J. K. (eds.), *The handbook of health behavior change.* New York: Springer, pp. 348–60.

Esler, M., Turbott, J., Schwarz, R., Leonard, P., Bobik, A., Skews, H., and Jackman, G. (1982). The peripheral kinetics of norepinephrine in depressive illness. *Arch Gen Psychiatry,* 39:285–300.

Everson, S.A., Goldberg, D.E., Kaplan, G.A., Cohen, R.D., Pukkala, E., Tuomilehto, J., and Salonen, J.T. (1996). Hopelessness and risk for mortality an incidence of myocardial infarction and cancer. *Psychosom Med,* 58:113–21.

Feibel, J.H., and Springer, C.J. (1982). Depression and failure to resume social activities after stroke. *Arch Phys Med Rehabil,* 63:276–78.

Ford, D.E., Mead, L.A, Change, P.P., Cooper-Patrick, L., Wang, N.Y., and Klag, M.J. (1998). Depression is a risk factor for coronary artery disease in men. *Arch Intern Med,* 158:1422–6.

Forrester, A.W., Lipsey, J.R., Teitelbaum, M.L., DePaulo, J.R., Andrzejewski, P.L., and Robinson, R.G. (1992). Depression following myocardial infarction. *Int J Psychiatry, Med,* 22:33–46.

Frasure-Smith, N., Lesperance, F., Talajic, M. (1993). Depression following myocardial infarction: impact on 6 month survival. *JAMA,* 270:1819–25.

Frasure-Smith, N., Lesperance, F., and Talajic, M. (1995). Depression and 18-month prognosis after myocardial infarction. *Circulation,* 91:999–1005.

Frasure-Smith, N., Lesperance, F., Prince, R., Verrier, P., Garber, R.A., Juneau, M., Wolfson, C., and Bourassa, M.G. (1997). Randomized trial of home based psychosocial nursing intervention for patients recovering from myocardial infarction. *Lancet,* 350:473–9.

Freedland, K.E., Carney, R.M., Lustman, P.J., Rich, M.W., and Jaffe, A.S. (1992a). Major depression in coronary artery disease patients with versus without a prior history of depression. *Psychosom Med,* 54:416–21.

Freedland, K.E., Lustman, P.J., Carney, R.M., and Hong, B.A. (1992b). Underdiagnosis of depression in patients with coronary artery disease: the role of nonspecific symptoms. *Int J Psychiatry Med,* 22:221–9.

Freedland, K.E., Carney, R.M., Davila-Roman, V.G., Rich, M.W., Skala, J.A., and Jaffe, A.S. (1998). Major depression and survival in congestive heart failure. *Psychosom Med,* 60:118.

Frey, B., Binder, T., and Teufelsbauer, H. (1993). Heart rate variability and patient outcome in advanced heart failure. *J Am Coll Cardiol,* 21:286A.

Friedman, G.D. (1994). Psychiatrically-diagnosed depression and subsequent cancer. *Cancer Epidemiol Biomarkers Prev,* 3:3–11.

Fuller, R.G. (1935). What happens to mental patients after discharge from hospital? *Psychiatry Q,* 9:95–104.

Gavard, J.A, Lustman, P.J, and Clouse, R.E. (1993). Prevalence of depression in adults with diabetes. An epidemiological evaluation. *Diabet Care,* 16:1167.

George, L.K., Blazer, D.G., Hughes, D.C., and Fowler, N. (1989). Social support and the outcome of major depression. *Br J Psychiatry* 154:478–85.

Glassman, A.H., Helzer, J.E., Covey, L.S., Cottler, L.B., Stetner, F., Tipp, J.E., and Johnson,

J. (1990). Smoking, smoking cessation, and major depression. *JAMA*, 264:1546–9.

Gonzalez, M.B., Snyderman, T.B., Colket, J.T, Arias, R.M., Jiang, J.W., O'Connor, C.M., and Krishnan, K.R. (1996). Depression in patients with coronary artery disease. *Depression*, 4:57–62.

Grande, P., Grauholt, A., and Madsen, J. (1990). Unstable angina pectoris: platelet behavior and prognosis in progressive angina. *Circulation*, 81:16.

Guiry, E., Conroy, R.M., Hickey, N., and Mulcahy, R. (1987). Psychological response to an acute coronary event and its effect on subsequent rehabilitation and lifestyle change. *Clin Cardiol*, 10:256–60.

Gupta, M.A., Gupta, A.K., Schork, N.J., and Ellis, C.N. (1994). Depression modulates pruritus perception: a study of pruritus in psoriasis, atopic dermatitis, and chronic idiopathic urticaria. *Psychosom Med*, 56:36–40.

Hance, M., Carney, R.M., Freedland, K.E., and Skala, J. (1995). Depression in patients with coronary heart disease: a twelve month follow-up. *Gen Hosp Psychiatry*, 18:61–5.

Harris, M.I. (1995). Classification, diagnostic criteria, and screening for diabetes. In Harris, M.I., Cowie, C.C., Stern, M.P., et al. (eds.), *Diabetes in America* (2nd ed.). (NIH Pub. No. 95-1468.) Bethesda, MA.: National Institutes of Health, pp. 15–35.

Hippisley-Cox, J., Fielding, K., and Pringle, M. (1998). Depression as a risk factor for ischaemic heart disease in men: population based case-control study. *BMJ*, 316:1714–9.

Hjemdahl, P., Larrson, T., and Wallen, N.H. (1991). Effects of stress and B-blockade on platelet function. *Circulation*, 84:44–61.

Horwitz, R.I., Viscoli, C.M., and Berkman, L. (1990). Treatment adherence and risk of death after a myocardial infarction. *Lancet*, 336:542–5.

Hughes, J.R., Hatsukami, D.K., Mitchell, J.E., and Dahlgren, C.A. (1986). Prevalence of smoking among psychiatric outpatients. *Am J Psychiatry*, 57:43–9.

Imaoka, K., Inoue, H., Inoue, Y., Hazama, H., Tanaka, T., and Yamane, N. (1985). R-R intervals of ECG in depression. *Folia Psychiatrica Neurol Jpn*, 39:485–8.

Jacobson, A.M., Rand, L.I., and Hauser, S.T. (1985). Psychologic stress and glycemic control. A comparison of patients with and without proliferative diabetic retinopathy. *Psychosom Med*, 47:372–81.

Jones, D.A., and West, R.R. (1996). Psychological rehabilitation after myocardial infarction: multicentre randomised controlled trial. *BMJ*, 313:1517–21.

Kaplan, G.A., Cohen, R.D., Wilson, T.W.,

Kauhanen, J., Salonen, J.T., and Salonen, R. (1992). Depression amplifies the association between carotid atherosclerosis and age, hypertension, low density liproteins, and platelet aggregability. Paper presented at the 32nd Annual Conference on Cardiovascular Disease Epidemiology, American Heart Association, March 19–21, 1992.

Kawachi, I., Sparrow, D., Vokanas, P.S., and Weiss, S.T. (1994). Symptoms of anxiety and risk of coronary heart disease the normative aging study. *Circulation*, 90:2225–9.

Keitner, G.I., and Miller, I.W. (1990). Family functioning and major depression: an overview. *Am J Psychiatry*, 147:1128–37.

Kellet, J.M. (1990). Compliance and clinical trials in heart disease (letter). *Lancet*, 336:1003.

Kennedy, G.J., Hofer, M.A., Cohen, D., Shindledecker, M.A, and Fisher, J.D. (1987). Significance of depression and cognitive impairment in patients undergoing programmed stimulation of cardiac arrythmias. *Psychosom Med*, 49:410–21.

Kleiger, R.E., Miller, J.P., Bigger, J.T., and Moss, A.J. (1987). Decreased heart rate variability and its association with mortality after myocardial infarction. *Am J Cardiol*, 113:256–62.

Kliks, B.R., Burgess, M.J., and Abildskov, J.A. (1975). Influence of sympathetic tone on ventricular fibrillation threshold during experimental coronary occlusion. *Am J Cardiol*, 36:45–9.

Knekt, P., Raitasalo, R., Heliovaara, M., Lehtinen, V., Pukkala, E., Teppo, L., Maatela, J., and Aromaa, A. (1996). Elevated lung cancer risk among persons with depressed mood. *Am J Epidemiol*, 144:1096–103.

Kop, W.J., Appels, A.P., Mendes de Leon, C.F., deSwart, H.B., and Bar, F.W. (1994). Vital exhaustion predicts new cardiac events after successful coronary angioplasty. *Psychosom Med*, 56:281–7.

Kovacs, M., Mukerji, P., Drash, A., and Iyengar, S. (1995). Biomedical and psychiatric risk factors for retinopathy among children with IDDM. *Diabetes Care*, 18:1592–9.

Ladwig, K.H., Kieser, M., Konig, J., Breithardt, G., and Borggrefe, M. (1991). Affective disorders and survival after acute myocardial infarction. *Eur Heart J*, 12:959–64.

Ladwig, K.H., Lehmacher, W., Roth, R., Breithardt, G., Budde, T.H., and Borggrefe, M. (1992). Factors which provoke post-infarction depression: results from the post-infarction late potential study (PILP). *J Psychosom Med*, 36:723–9.

Lahmeyer, H.W., and Bellier, S.N. (1987). Cardiac regulation and depression. *Psychiatr Res*, 21:1–6.

Lake, C.R., Pickar, D., Ziegler, M.G., Lipper, S., Slater, S., and Murphy, D.L. (1982). High plasma NE levels in patients with major affective disorder. *Am J Psychiatry,* 139: 1315–8.

Langeluddecke, P., Fulcher, G., Baird, D., Hughes, C., and Tennant, C. (1989). A prospective evaluation of the psychosocial effects of coronary artery bypass surgery. *J Psychosom Res,* 33:37–45.

Lapane, K.L., Zierler, S., Lasater, T.M., Stein, M., Barbour, M.M., and Hume, A.L. (1995). Is a history of depressive symptoms associated with an increased risk of infertility in women? *Psychosom Med,* 57:509–13.

Lespérance, F., Frasure-Smith, N., and Taljic, M. (1996). Major depression before and after myocardial infarction: its nature and consequences. *Psychosom Med,* 58:99–110.

Linden, W., Stossel, C., and Maurice, J. (1996). Psychosocial interventions for patients with coronary artery disease: a meta analysis. *Arch Intern Med,* 156:745–52.

Linkins, R.W., and Comstock, G.W. (1990). Depressed mood and development of cancer. *Am J Epidemiol,* 132:962–72.

Lloyd, G.G., and Cawley, R.H. (1983). Distress or illness? a study of psychosocial symptoms after myocardial infarction. *Br J Psychiatry,* 142:120–5.

Lustman, P.J., Griffity, L.S., and Clouse, R.E. (1988). Depression in adults with diabetes: results of a 5-year follow-up study. *Diabetes Care,* 11:605–12.

Maes, M., Meltzer, H.Y., Stevens, W., Calabrese, J., and Cosyns P. (1994). Natural killer cell activity in major depression: relation to circulating natural killer cells, cellular indices of the immune response, and depressive phenomenology. *Prog Neuropsychopharmacol Biol Psychiatry,* 18:717–30.

Maes, M., Bosmans, E., and Meltzer, H.Y. (1995). Immunoendocrine aspects of major depression. Relationships between plasma interleukin-1 and soluble interleukin-2 receptor, prolactin and cortisol. *Eur Arch Psychiatry Clin Neurosci,* 245:172–8.

Magaziner, J., Simonsick, E.M., Kashner, T.M., Hebel, J.R., and Kenzora, J.E. (1990). Predictors of functional recovery one year following hospital discharge for hip fracture: a prospective study. *J Gerontol,* 45:M101–7.

Markovitz, J.H., and Matthews, K.A. (1991). Platelets and coronary heart disease: potential psychophysiologic mechanisms. *Psychosom Med,* 53:643–68.

Mayou, R., Foster, A., and Williamson, B. (1978). Psychosocial adjustment in patients one year after myocardial infarction. *J Psychosom Res,* 22:447–53.

McKhann, G.M., Borowicz, L.M., Goldsborough, M.A., Enger, C., and Seines, O.E. (1997). Depression and cognitive decline after coronary artery bypass grafting. *Lancet,* 349:282–4.

Musselman, D.L., Tomer, A., Manatunga, A.K., Knight, B.T., Porter, M.R., Kasey, S., Marzec, U., Harker, L.A., and Nemeroff, C.B. (1996). Exaggerated platelet reactivity in major depression. *Am J Psychiatry,* 153:1212–7.

Oldenburg, B., Perkins, R.J., and Andrews, G. (1985). Controlled trial of psychological intervention in myocardial infarction. *J Consult Clin Psychol* 53:852–9.

Oldridge, N.B., Guyat, G., Jones, N., Crowe, J., Singer, J., Feeny, D., McKelvie, R., Runions, J., Streiner, D., and Torrance, G. (1991). Effects on quality of life with comprehensive rehabilitation after acute myocardial infarction. *Am J Cardiol,* 67:1084–9.

Oxenkrug, G.F., Branconnier, R.J., Harto-Truax, N., and Cole, J.O. (1983). Is serum cholesterol a biological marker for major depressive disorder? *Am J Psychiatry,* 40:920–1.

Pary, R.P., Tobias, C.R., and Lippmann, S. (1989). Antidepressants and the cardiac patient: selecting an appropriate medication. *Postgraduate Med,* 85:267–9.

Pfohl, B., Rederer, M., Coryell, W., and Stangl, D. (1991). Association between post dexamethasone cortisol level and blood pressure in depressed inpatients. *J Nerv Ment Dis,* 179:44–7.

Podrid, P.J., Fuchs, T., and Candinas, R. (1990). Role of the sympathetic nervous system in the genesis of ventricular arrhythmia. *Circulation,* 82 Suppl 1:103–10.

Powell, L.H. (1989). Unanswered questions in the Ischemic Heart Disease Life Stress Monitoring Program (editorial). *Psychosom Med,* 51:479–84.

Pratt, L.A., Ford, D.E., Crum, R.M., Armenian, H.K., Gallo, J.J., and Eaton, W.W. (1996). Depression, psychotropic medication, and risk of myocardial infarction: prospective data from the Baltimore ECA follow-up. *Circulation,* 94:3123–9.

Rabins, P.V., Harvis, K., and Koven, S. (1985). High fatality rates of late-life depression associated with cardiovascular disease. *J Affect Disord,* 9:165–7.

Rahe, R.H., Ward, H.W., and Hayes, V. (1979). Brief group therapy in myocardial infarction rehabilitation: three to four year follow-up of a controlled trial. *Psychsom Med,* 41: 229–42.

Rechlin, T. (1994). Are affective disorders associated with alterations of heart rate variability? *J Affect Disord,* 32:271–5.

Rich, M.W., Saini, J.S., Kleiger, R.E., Carney,

R.M., teVelde, A., and Freedland, K.E. (1988). Correlation of heart rate variability with clinical and angiographic variables and late mortality after coronary angiography. *Am J Cardiol*, 62:714–17.

Richardson, J.L., Marks, G., Johnson, C.A., Graham, J.W., Chan, K.K., Selser, J.N., Kishbaugh, C., Barranday, Y., and Levine, A.M. (1987). Path model of multidimensional compliance with cancer therapy. *Health Psychol*, 6:183–207.

Robins, L.N., and Regier, D.A. (1991). *Psychiatric disorders in America*. New York: Free Press.

Roose, S.P., Laghrissi-Thode, F., Kennedy, J.S., Nelson, J.C., Bigger, J.T., Pollock, B.G., Gaffney, A., Narayan, M., Finkel, M.S., McCafferty, J., and Gergel, I. (1998). Comparison of paroxetine and nortriptyline in depressed patients with ischemic heart disease. *JAMA*, 279:287–91.

Roy, A., Pickar, D., De Jong, J., Karoum, F., and Linnoila, M. (1988). NE and its metabolites in cerebrospinal fluid, plasma, and urine. *Arch Gen Psychiatry*, 45:849–57.

Ruberman, W., Weinblatt, E., Goldberg, J.D., and Chaudhary, B.S. (1984). Psychosocial influences on mortality after myocardial infarction. *N Eng J Med*, 311:552–9.

Schleifer, S.J., Macari, M.M., Slater, W., Kahn, M., Zucker, H., and Gorlin, R. (1986). Predictors of outcome after myocardial infarction: role of depression. *Circulation*, 74, Supp, II-10.

Schleifer, S.J., Macari-Hinson, M.M., Coyle, D.A., Slater, W.R., Kahn, M., Gorlin, R., and Zucker, H.D. (1989). The nature and course of depression following myocardial infarction. *Arch Int Med*, 149:1785–9.

Schleifer, S.J., Slater, W.R., Macari-Hinson, M.M., Coyle, D.A., Kahn, M., Zucker, H.D., and Gorlin, R. (1991). Digitalis and β-blocking agents: effects on depression following myocardial infarction. *Am Heart J*, 121:1397–1402.

Schwartz, P.J., and Stone, H.L. (1980). Left stellectomy in the prevention of ventricular fibrillation caused by acute myocardial ischemia in conscious dogs with anterior myocardial infarction. *Circulation*, 62:1256–65.

Schwartz, P.J., and Vanoli, E. (1981). Cardiac arrhythmias elicited by interaction between acute myocardial ischemia and sympathetic hyperactivity: a new experimental model for the study of antiarrhythmic drugs. *J Cardiovasc Pharmacol*, 3:1251–9.

Schwartz, P.J., Snebold, N.G., and Brown, A.M. (1976). Effects of unilateral cardiac sympathetic denervation on the ventricular fibrillation threshold. *Am J Cardiol*, 37:1034–40.

Shamash, K., O'Connell, K., Lowy, M., and Katona, C.L.E. (1992). Psychiatric morbidity and outcome in elderly patients undergoing emergency hip surgery: a one-year follow-up study. *Int J Geriatr Psych*, 7:505–9.

Sheline, Y., Freedland, K.E., and Carney, R.M. (1997).How safe are serotonin reuptake inhibitors for depression in patients with coronary heart disease? *Am J Med*, 102:54–9.

Siever, L., and Davis, K. (1985). Overview: toward a dysregulation hypothesis of depression. *Am J Psychiatry*, 142:1017–31.

Silverstone, P.H. (1987). Depression and outcome in acute myocardial infarction. *Br Med J*, 294:219–20.

Stein, P.E., Carney, R.M., Freedland, K.E., Skala, J.A., Kleiger, R.E., Rottman, J.N, and Jaffe, A.S. (submitted). Severe depression is associated with markedly reduced heart rate variability in patients with stable coronary heart disease.

Stern, M.J., Pascale, L., and Ackerman, A. (1977). Life adjustment post myocardial infarction: determining predictive variables *Arch Intern Med*,137:1680–5.

Stewart, A.L., Greenfield, S., Hays, R.D., Wells, K., Rogers, W.H., Berry, S.D, McGlynn, E.A., and Ware, J.E. (1989). Functional status and well-being of patients with chronic conditions: results from the Medical Outcomes Study. *JAMA*, 262:907–13.

Talbott, E., Kuller, L.H., Detre, K., and Perper, J. (1977). Biologic and psychosocial risk factors for sudden death from coronary disease in white women. *Am J Cardiol*, 39:858–64.

Task Force of the European Society of Cardiology and the North American Society for Pacing and Electrophysiology. (1996). Heart rate variability: standards of measurement, physiological interpretation an clinical use. *Circulation*, 93:1043–65.

Travella, J.I., Forrester, A.W., Schultz, S.K., and Robinson, R.G. (1994). Depression following myocardial infarction: a one year longitudinal study. *Int J Psychiatry Med*, 24 Suppl 4:357–69.

Van Dixhoorn, J., Duivenvoorden, H.J., Pool, J., and Verhage, F. (1990). Psychic effects of physical training and relaxation therapy after myocardial infarction. *J Psychsom Res*, 34:327–37.

Veith, R.C., Raskind, M.A., Caldwell, J.H., Barnes, R.F., Gumbrecht, G. and Ritchie, J.L. (1982). Cardiovascular effects of tricyclic antidepressants in depressed patients with chronic heart disease. *N Engl J Med*, 306:954–9.

Veith, R.C., Lewis, N., Linares, O.A., Barnes, R.F., Raskind, M.A., Villacres, E.C., Murburg, M.M., Ashleigh, E.A., Castillo, S., Peskind, E.R., Pascualy, M., and Halter, J.B. (1994). Sympathetic nervous system activity in major depression. *Arch Gen Psychiatry,* 51:411–22.

Verrier, R.L., Thompson, P.L., and Lown, B. (1974). Ventricular vulnerabiliity during sympathetic stimulation: role of heart rate and blood pressure. *Cardiovasc Res,* 8:602.

Vimpari, S.S., Knuuttila, M.L.E., Sakki, T.K., and Kivela, S.L. (1995). Depressive symptoms associated with symptoms of the temporomandibular joint pain and dysfunction syndrome. *Psychosom Med,* 57:439–44.

Warrington, S.J., Padgham, C., and Lader, M. (1989). The cardiovascular effects of antidepressants. *Psychol Med Monograph,* Suppl 16:1–40.

Wells, K.B., Golding, J.M., and Burnam, M.A. (1989a). Affective, substance use, and anxiety disorders in persons with arthritis, diabetes, heart disease, high blood pressure, or chronic lung conditions. *Gen Hosp Psychiatry,* 11:320–27.

Wells, K.B., Stewart, A., Hays, R., Burnam, M.A., Rogers, W., Daniels, M., Berry, S., Greenfield, S., and Ware, J. (1989b). The functioning and well-being of depressed patients. Results from the Medical Outcomes Study. *JAMA,* 262:914–9.

Wells, K.B., Rogers, W., Burnam, A., Greenfield, S., and Ware, J.E. (1991). How the medical comorbidity of depressed patients differs across health care setttings. Results from the Medical Outcomes Study. *Am J Psychiatry,* 148:1688–96.

Wells, K.B., Burnam, M.A., Rogers, W., Hays, R., and Camp, P. (1992). The course of depression in adult outpatients. Results from the Medical Outcomes Study. *Arch Gen Psychiatry,* 149:788–94.

White, W., Smith, L.R., Croughwell, N., Schell, R., Newman, M., and Reves, J.G. (1995). Depression in male and female patients undergoing cardiac surgery. *Br J Psychol Soc,* 34:119–28.

Wyatt, R.J., Portnoy, B., Kupfer, D.J., Snyder, F., and Engelman, K. (1971). Resting plasma catecholamine concentrations in patients with depression and anxiety. *Arch Gen Psychiatry,* 24:65–70.

10

Affective States and Health

LAURA D. KUBZANSKY AND ICHIRO KAWACHI

> Let no one persuade you to cure his headache until he has first given you
> his soul to be cured, for this is the great error of our day in the treatment
> of the human body, that physicians separate the soul from the body.
>
> Socrates, from *Charmides* (in Plato 1927)

EMOTIONS AND THE SOCIAL CONTEXT

Growing evidence suggests that the social environment, including conditions experienced in the family, neighborhood, and workplace, can influence health (Taylor et al. 1997). The question remains, How can social conditions that are external to the individual get inside the body to influence health? One pathway is through emotions and the physiological, cognitive, and behavioral responses they evoke. Emotions mediate an individual's response to events in the external world, especially when the event is particularly meaningful to him or her; they have been linked to both upstream social factors such as position in the socioeconomic hierarchy (Kemper 1993; Anderson and Armstead 1995; Williams et al. 1996) and individual health outcomes downstream (Kamarck and Jennings 1991; Cohen et al. 1993; Leventhal and Patrick-Miller 1993; Kawachi et al. 1995; Taylor et al. 1997; Kubzansky et al. 1998). As a re-

sult, emotions provide a critical window through which to examine the translation of social conditions into individual health status. Moreover, the social context plays an important role in determining which emotions are likely to be experienced, how they are expressed, and what their consequences will be. Kemper (1993) has suggested that many emotions are responses to power and status differentials embedded within social situations. As a result, even emotions that feel highly personal and unique to the individual may be conditioned by external social factors and are likely to be socially patterned.[1] For example, previous research has found that black men and women and those who come from lower socioeconomic status (SES) groups generally report higher levels of negative emotions like depression than do other individuals (Warheit et al. 1973; Mirowsky and Ross 1980; Thoits 1982; Turner and Noh 1983; Kessler and Neighbors 1986; Ulbrich et al. 1989). Thus, the study of emotions may help to explain both how social conditions "get under the skin" to affect health and how health status is systematically patterned according to the social context.

EMOTIONS AND HEALTH: A BRIEF HISTORY

Links between emotion and health have been described for over 2000 years. For example, the Talmud mentions the potentially destructive effects of anger on one's physical and spiritual well-being (described in Siegman 1994b). Similarly, Rabbi Joshua ben Hananya, a first- and second-century (C.E.) scholar, maintained that hostility and hatred of others are among the factors that shorten the life span (*Tractate Avot* 2:15, cited in Siegman 1994b). In ancient times, Hippocrates considered the four bodily humors (blood, black bile, yellow bile, and phlegm) to be the basis of personality, and these elements were subsequently believed to relate also to the causes of disease (Allport 1961). The prevailing humor in a person was thought to produce that person's temperament (involving predispositions toward particular emotions), while the excess of a humor led to disease. For example, an excess of black bile produced a tendency to be melancholy, eventually leading to depression and finally physical illness. Though medical diagnosis no longer relies on the theory of humors, in many ways the basic typology has survived: We talk about the hopeless, depressed "melancholic"; the angry hostile "choleric"; the apathetic, alexithymic "phlegmatic"; and the ruddy, optimistic "sanguine" (Friedman and Booth-Kewley 1987). In 1628 William Harvey, one of the pioneers in cardiovascular physiology, wrote: "A mental disturbance provoking pain, excessive joy, hope or anxiety extends to the heart, where it affects its temper, and rate, impairing general nutrition and vigor" (1628/1928, Harvey 1928, p. 106). More recently, psychoanalytic theory has suggested that psychological conflicts could trigger or contribute to disease processes, whereby somatic symptoms represent symbolic expressions of underlying repressed psychological conflicts. Thus, conflicts about expressing anger were postulated to lead to heart disease, conflicts about dependency needs to ulcers, and repressed depression to dermatological disorders (Alexander et al. 1968). Unfortunately, empirical tests of these psychoanalytically inspired hypotheses produced inconsistent results at best, and research on emotion and health fell out of favor (Siegman 1994b).

With advances in research methodology, investigators in recent decades have identified a number of mechanisms by which emotions might influence health, including the activation of the hypothalamic–pituitary–adrenocortical (HPA) axis and the sympathetic–adrenal–medullary (SAM) system. Researchers have begun again to focus on emotion, building a strongly suggestive case for a causal relationship between emotion and health. While there is clearly a reciprocal relationship between health and emotion (e.g., ill-health may lead to negative emotions), the focus of this chapter is on the role of emotions in the etiology of disease (and health) rather than viewing them as a consequence of disease or as part of the process of disease management.

DIFFERENTIATING BETWEEN STRESS AND EMOTION

Stress has often been proposed as one way social conditions may get inside the body. External circumstances or events are hypothesized to cause psychological and/or physical stress which in turn may cause physiological changes related to disease processes. Most stress theories assume that stress is detrimental to health because the experience of stress triggers physiological changes.[2] The physiological basis of stress was first proposed by Hans Selye, who suggested that physical and psychosocial stressors both elicit the same pattern of physiological responding (Selye 1950). Selye described a General Adaptation Syndrome that consists of three stages: *(1) alarm,* in which initial reactions necessary to meet the demands of the stressor are mobilized (fight-or-flight reaction), *(2) resistance,* in which the full adaptation to the stressor occurs with improvement or disappearance of physiological symptoms (return to homeostasis), and *(3) exhaustion,* when the stressor is sufficiently severe and prolonged that somatic defenses become overtaxed and depleted.

One problem with the general stress theory is that all stressors are presumed to have the same physiologic effects. For example, prolonged exposure to a loud noise is considered functionally similar to experiencing the death of one's spouse. The theory also focuses primarily on the physiological set of reactions elicited by noxious stimuli (external stressors) and does not address the psychological or emotional side of the stress reaction. Moreover, the theory cannot account for individual differences in reactions to stressors.

In response to some of the inadequacies of the general stress theory, investigators put forth a psychological theory of stress, which attempts to explain when an individual will experience stress and links psychological processes to the physiological processes described by Selye (Lazarus 1990). Stress is experienced when individuals perceive that external demands exceed their ability to cope. The interpretation of an event as stressful triggers a series of physiological changes. Tests of the stress hypothesis have examined the health effects of the accumulation of major life events (e.g., moving house, birth of a baby) as well as daily hassles (everyday manifestations of chronic and lower-intensity stressors such as concern about paying bills) (Dohrenwend and Dohrenwend 1974; Brown and Harris 1978; DeLongis et al. 1982; Williams et al. 1992).

However, some puzzles in studies of stress and health have not been adequately addressed by the research. For example, psychological theories of stress cannot fully explain why some individuals undergo many stressful events with few health consequences while others with seemingly trivial problems experience poor health outcomes.

Defining stress is difficult. What does it mean to experience stress? Are there different kinds of stress, such as "good" stress (e.g., planning a wedding) vs. "bad" stress (e.g., death of a spouse)? Investigators have tried to define stress objectively by adding up the number of potentially stressful events or daily hassles people experience. What one individual considers stressful, however, another may not. Thus, simply summing numbers of "stressful" events may not tell us much about an individual's life experience, particularly because not all individuals are stressed in the same situation. Many studies conceptualize stress as relatively unidimensional and assume the effects of a stressor are similar for everyone. But to know if someone is "stressed," we need to know the individual's interpretation of the potentially stressful event and its meaning for his or her life. Here, the study of emotions may provide some clues. While there is some overlap between stress and emotion and their relationships to health, there are important distinctions between them. In this chapter, environmental events are considered stressors and emotions are considered responses to stressors (Cohen et al. 1995b). A negative emotional response typically occurs if demands are perceived to exceed one's ability to cope (Lazarus 1991b; Cohen et al. 1995b). Clearly, potentially stressful events can be associated with a variety of different emotions. For example, losing one's job may provoke anger in some individuals and depression in others. Thus, emotions can be considered products of stress as well as mediators of its effects (Spielberger and Sarason 1978), thereby providing a more nuanced way of understanding an individual's interaction with the environment.

EMOTION THEORY: AN OVERVIEW

Emotions may be conceptualized as having cognitive, neurobiological, and behavioral components (Scherer 1982; Frijda 1986; Barlow 1988; Leventhal and Patrick-Miller 1993). Emotion theorists have suggested that specific emotions are biologically based, arise as a product of the interaction between the person and the environment, and mediate between continually changing situations and the individual's behavior (Arnold 1960; Lazarus 1968; Scherer 1982; Frijda 1986; Ellsworth 1991). As such, emotions are a process that motivates individuals to respond to their environment and that allows an adaptive flexibility of response that is not available to organisms which rely on instinct (Scherer 1982; Ellsworth and Smith 1988). Thus, emotions are considered to be functionally appropriate processes which may have dysfunctional consequences when the system is taxed beyond the limits of its capability (Frijda 1993).

Expressed emotions serve to communicate the person's emotional state and likely behavior to others in the social environment (Scherer 1982; Frijda 1986). The state of subjective feeling serves as a compelling signal that a person is faced with a particular type of challenge and motivates the person to respond to this challenge (Frijda 1986). For example, fear motivates a person to escape danger, sadness motivates a person to disengage from loss, and so on (Lazarus 1991b). Each emotion depends on an individual's construal and evaluation of the environment; events are appraised in terms of their importance and the demands they place on the individual, as well as the person's options and prospects for coping (Lazarus 1991a). More specifically, individuals appraise events in terms of whether they are potentially harmful (e.g., associated with threat or loss) or beneficial (e.g., associated with actual or potential gain) (Scherer 1982; Roseman 1984; Smith and Ellsworth 1985; Frijda 1986; Lazarus 1991a; Smith and Lazarus 1993). In addition, emotions are associated with urges to act in particular ways called *action tendencies,* which enable the individual to cope with environmental demands (Frijda 1986; Fredrickson 1998). In turn, specific action tendencies are associated with patterns of physiological activity that support subsequent adaptive behavior (Plutchik 1980;

Scherer 1982; Frijda 1986; Lazarus 1991a; Levenson 1994). It has been theorized that specific patterns of physiological responses are associated with each emotion (Lazarus 1991a; Leventhal and Patrick-Miller 1993; Levenson 1994b). For example, the behavioral and physiological consequences of feeling anger vs. feeling sadness may be very different. However, empirical evidence for this is not conclusive. Each emotion, moreover, is not tied in a one-to-one correspondence with specific objective stimuli or specific behaviors. While particular urges to act may be associated with specific emotions, people do not invariably act out these urges when experiencing particular emotions. Antecedents and consequences of emotions vary widely as a function of the demands, resources, and constraints in the environment; the imminence, duration, and uncertainty of events; and individuals' motives and beliefs about themselves and the world (Lazarus 1991a). Despite this heterogeneity, the cognitive, neurobiological, and behavioral components of emotions vary systematically and can be identified with a sufficient understanding of the emotion process (Smith and Pope 1992).

Regulating emotions includes modifying the expression, behavior, or physiological sequelae associated with an emotion, as well as manipulating opportunities for experiencing any given emotion (Gross and Levenson 1993). Various theories have postulated that effective emotion regulation is also critically related to health outcomes. Research on the inhibition of emotion (i.e., suppression, repression) suggests that the process of inhibiting thoughts and feelings entails physiological work. This effort is considered to be a cumulative stressor that increases susceptibility to a variety of illnesses over time (Weinberger et al. 1979; Pennebaker and Beall 1986; Temoshok 1987; Pennebaker and Susman 1988; Shedler et al. 1993).

Most emotions may be seen either as transitory *states* brought on by specific situations, or as *traits,* i.e., stable and general dispositions to experience particular emotions (Spielberger and Sarason 1978; Barlow 1988; Lazarus 1994; Miller et al. 1996).[3] Individuals high in trait anger, for example, experience the transitory state of anger more frequently and intensely than individuals low in trait anger (Spielberger et al. 1985). Thus, certain personality types are hypothesized to be vulnerable to disease in part because these individuals are predisposed to experience particular emotions. For example, hostility is considered a personality trait which predisposes individuals to experience more episodes of anger, suspicion, and cynicism than other individuals. In addition, some researchers have hypothesized that hostile individuals may create hostile environments by virtue of their cynical, mistrusting, and aggressive behavior, thereby creating more opportunities to experience anger (Smith and Frohm 1985).

APPROACHES FOR INVESTIGATING THE RELATIONSHIP BETWEEN EMOTION AND HEALTH

Emotions are hypothesized to influence health directly because they evoke physiological processes (e.g., activation of the hypothalamic–pituitary–adrenocortical axis and the sympathetic-adrenal-medullary system), and indirectly because they influence health and other behaviors (Fig. 10–1). Elevations in serum norepinephrine levels associated with negative emotions may increase blood lipids, free fatty acids, blood pressure, and heart rate, as well as constriction of peripheral blood vessels and the suppression of cellular immune function. Negative emotions such as anxiety and depression may also lead to altered autonomic regulation of the heart (specifically, reduced heart rate variability), which may in turn explain their association with fatal coronary heart disease (CHD) (Lown and Verrier 1976; Kleiger et al. 1987; Fei et al. 1994; Kawachi et al. 1995). Other direct emotion–disease pathways may be through effects on the immune system. The activation of the HPA axis and the sympathetic nervous system results in elevated serum

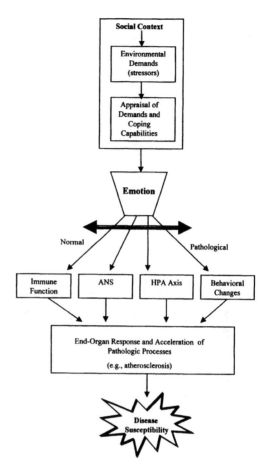

Figure 10–1. A model of the stress–emotion–health process.

levels of cortisol and catecholamines (Baum and Grunberg 1995). Since immune cells have receptors for these hormones (Rabin et al. 1989; Ader et al. 1991), cortisol, epinephrine, and norepinephrine are directly implicated in the regulation of immune function (O'Leary 1990). Over time, recurring activation of these systems may set disease-related physiological processes in motion.

Negative emotions may also indirectly affect health through associations with behavioral and other risk factors such as smoking, excessive alcohol consumption, greater body mass, lower physical activity, and higher levels of blood lipids and blood pressure (Carney et al. 1987; Leiker and

Hailey 1988; Smith 1992; Siegler 1994; Hayward 1995; Kawachi et al. 1996; Miller et al. 1996; Kubzansky et al. 1998). Everson and colleagues (1997a) found that behavioral risk factors (smoking, alcohol consumption, physical activity, body mass index) appeared to mediate the relationship between hostility (conceptually related to anger) and cardiovascular morbidity and mortality. Similarly, Hayward (1995) recently reviewed the literature on the relationship between negative emotion (clinical levels) and cardiovascular risk factors and found consistent evidence for an association of anxiety and depression with a number of these factors (see also Kasl et al. 1968; Everson et al. 1997a). Thus, emotions may trigger cognitive, behavioral, or social processes, which in turn affect health. A more elaborate discussion of indirect and direct pathways can be found in Chapter 13.

Figure 10–1 presents a heuristic model designed to illustrate the stress–emotion–health process. For the purposes of parsimony we have presented a unidirectional model; however, the exclusion of alternative paths is not intended to reject hypotheses about their existence.

Much of the literature on emotion and health relates to the mechanisms connecting emotion to physiology and pathology, but an important task for social epidemiologists is to put emotions in a social context. There is evidence that the experience of emotions is systematically patterned by social structures (for related work, see Lynch et al. 1997; Taylor et al., 1997). Investigators are beginning to examine simultaneously the upstream determinants and downstream effects of health. For example, one recent study tried to delineate the pathway from the social context → emotions → physiological substrates. Kubzansky and colleagues (in press) examined the relationships between socioeconomic position (as measured by educational attainment), anger (and hostility), and a cluster of risk factors associated with CHD in an ongoing study of community-dwelling men. Results indicated

that lower levels of educational attainment and greater hostility were both associated with the risk factor cluster. Results of path analyses further suggested that the effects of socioeconomic position on cardiovascular functioning may be mediated by anger.

Research on the direct health consequences of emotion states has typically focused on the immediate physiological responses associated with emotion experiences, in contrast to research on emotion traits, which tends to examine the long term health effects of recurring emotion experiences. Short-term effects of acute emotion states are generally examined in the laboratory to identify physiological parameters hypothesized to be related to disease processes. However, while it is generally assumed that the short-term effects of emotions are related to their long-term health consequences, research demonstrating such linkages remains sparse (Davison and Petrie 1997). For example, research on cardiovascular reactivity has tended to measure the individual's propensity to react to acute stress or negative emotions with increased heart rate and blood pressure (e.g., Matthews et al. 1986; Houston 1994; Everson et al. 1997a). While some work has suggested that short-term cardiovascular reactivity is associated with poor health outcomes in the long run, the evidence is far from conclusive (Manuck and Krantz 1986; Manuck et al. 1988; Houston 1994). Other laboratory and experimental research has examined the acute effects of emotion on parameters such as platelet aggregation, coronary vascular tone, various aspects of autonomic functioning, and a number of immune effects (see O'Leary 1990, for reviews; Kamarck and Jennings 1991). In order to examine the effects of acute emotions on major disease outcomes like myocardial infarction, different study designs are needed, e.g., the case-crossover design, in which exposure to a transient risk factor (such as an episode of anger) is contrasted with exposure during a "control" period within the same individual (e.g., at the same time the previous day) (Mittleman et al. 1995). This type of research is relatively new but has offered promising results.

By contrast, more traditional case-control (cross-sectional) and longitudinal study designs have been used to examine the relationship between chronic emotions and health. Although emotions are usually measured at a single point in time, the measurement approaches used in these studies are designed to identify the chronic nature of the emotion experience.[4] Because causality between emotion and health goes in both directions and effects accumulate over a long period of time, prospective studies are best suited for investigating the risk of disease associated with chronic emotion states. The most convincing design is to measure emotions among initially disease-free individuals, thereby preserving the temporal order of the linkage between emotion and disease onset. Given the lack of feasibility to conduct true experiments in which people can be assigned to experience one emotion or another, prospective cohort studies present the strongest evidence for the hypothesis that emotions influence health.

Much of the research on emotion and health has been carried out the context of coronary heart disease (CHD). Coronary heart disease is the leading cause of death in many countries (Myerburg and Castellanos 1992), and the traditional risk factors (e.g., smoking, hypertension, hypercholesterolemia, obesity, physical activity, diabetes, and hormonal factors) explain only about 40% of the occurrence of CHD (Marmot and Winkelstein 1975; Syme 1993). The emphasis on CHD in research is therefore not surprising. Evidence for associations between emotions and other health outcomes is much more sparse. As a result, in the sections to follow, the emotion–CHD relationship is emphasized largely because the bulk of the evidence has been collected in this area. In describing research on emotions and health outcomes other than CHD, we highlight what has been done and give some consideration to potential barriers to

Table 10–1. Unresolved issues in the study of emotion and health

- Role of emotions in the onset vs. clinical course of disease
- Clinical vs. subclinical levels of emotion
- Expressed vs. nonexpressed emotions
- Negative vs. positive emotions
- Acute vs. chronic levels of emotions (state vs. trait)

research. We subsequently discuss some unresolved questions (Table 10–1), measurement issues, and directions for future research on emotion and health.

THE EPIDEMIOLOGICAL EVIDENCE ON EMOTION AND CHD

In the 1950s, two cardiologists, Friedman and Rosenman, proposed a new risk factor for CHD called the type A behavioral (TAB) pattern (Friedman and Rosenman 1959). As formulated by Friedman (Friedman 1969), TAB is an action–emotion complex that requires an environmental challenge to serve as the trigger for expression. The overt manifestations of the behavior include a free-floating but well-rationalized hostility, hyperaggressiveness, and a sense of time urgency. Several large-scale epidemiological studies conducted during the 1960s and 1970s appeared to corroborate the Type A hypothesis, culminating in a National Institutes of Health panel that concluded in 1981 that TAB was an independent risk factor for CHD (Review Panel on Coronary-Prone Behavior and Coronary Heart Disease 1981). However, enthusiasm for the TAB concept started to wane in the mid-1980s following the publication of a series of cohort studies that failed to find a relationship with CHD (see Matthews 1988; Allan and Scheidt 1996, for excellent reviews). The conflicting evidence on TAB and CHD may be partly due to the fact that the self-rated TAB questionnaires used in negative studies did not inquire about the full range of behaviors associated with the action–emotion complex (Kawachi et al.

1998). The videotaped structured interview is regarded as the most sensitive approach to diagnosing the TAB pattern, but it has obvious limitations in the context of large-scale longitudinal studies. Although a meta-analysis of 18 controlled trials concluded that psychological treatment for TAB resulted in a 50% reduction in recurrent coronary events (Nunes et al. 1987), the focus of research on psychological predictors of CHD has gradually shifted away from TAB toward examining the relationships between specific negative emotions and CHD (Friedman 1969; Dembroski et al. 1978; Krantz and Durel 1983).

Given the similarities between certain emotional states, Booth-Kewley and Friedman (1987) suggested that a number of negative emotions may be risk factors for CHD, and recent research has begun to corroborate this hypothesis. Links between CHD incidence and specific emotions like anxiety, anger, and depression have emerged. (See Chapter 9 of this volume for a discussion of depression and CHD; also Goldstein and Niaura 1992; Kawachi et al. 1994a, 1996; Kubzansky et al. 1997, 1998). Emotion suppression, i.e., the suppression of visible manifestations of emotions like anger and anxiety, has also been found to be a risk factor for CHD (Haynes et al. 1980; Denollet et al. 1996).

Anger and CHD

Chronic anger and hostility have long been suspected in the etiology of CHD (Smith and Frohm 1985; Siegman 1994b). Recent laboratory and epidemiological studies, both cross-sectional and prospective, have suggested that high levels of anger increase the risk of CHD. Anger and hostility are strongly associated with one another and have been implicated as "toxic" components in the relationship between the Type A behavior pattern and CHD (Matthews et al. 1977; Haynes and Feinleib 1980; Williams et al. 1980; Barefoot et al. 1983, 1991; Shekelle et al. 1983; Matthews 1985; Smith and Frohm 1985; Dembroski et al. 1989; Miller et al. 1996). In this research

hostility has been considered as a long-standing attitudinal disposition, as opposed to anger, which is considered an emotion and a component of the broader hostility complex (Buss 1961; Zillman 1979; Matthews 1985; Spielberger et al. 1985). Anger has been defined as an unpleasant emotion arising in response to events that are perceived as unjust, and accompanied by physiological arousal and the activation of action tendencies or impulses toward aggression. Most research in this area has focused primarily on hostility rather than on anger per se. (For a broad overview of this work, see Helmers et al. 1994.) Although anger has been frequently implied as an important component of the hostility–CHD relationship, prospective studies that focus explicitly on anger as a risk factor for CHD are still few in number.

In a comprehensive meta-analytic review, Miller et al. (1996) found support for the hypothesis that chronic anger and hostility are independent risk factors for the development of CHD and premature mortality. Kawachi and colleagues (1996) examined the association between anger and CHD in a 7-year follow-up study of 1305 men in the Normative Aging Study. Compared with men reporting the lowest levels of anger, the relative risk (RR) for men with the highest levels of anger was 2.66 (95% confidence interval [CI]: 1.26 to 5.61) for incident coronary events (including nonfatal myocardial infarction [MI], fatal CHD, and angina pectoris). A dose–response relation was found between level of anger and overall CHD risk, even after relative risks were adjusted for other major cardiovascular risk factors. A 3-year follow-up study of 3750 Finnish men aged 40 to 59 also found that high levels of self-rated irritability and easily aroused anger were associated with increased CHD mortality, although the excess risk was confined to men with preexisting heart disease (Koskenvuo et al. 1988).

Anxiety and CHD

Because the word "anxiety" represents both a lay construct and a scientific term, confusion has frequently arisen about the precise meaning of the term (Barlow 1988). Anxiety has been defined as a future-oriented negative affective state resulting from perceptions of threat, characterized by a perceived inability to predict, control, or obtain desired results in upcoming situations (Barlow 1988).

A recent review of the literature concluded that there is strongly suggestive evidence for anxiety as a risk factor for CHD (see Kubzansky et al. 1998). The Northwick Park Heart Study, which followed 1457 initially healthy men for a period of 10 years, reported a striking association between self-reported symptoms of phobic anxiety and fatal CHD (Haines et al. 1987). Compared with men with the lowest level of anxiety, those with the highest levels had a relative risk of fatal CHD of 3.77 (95% CI: 1.64 to 8.64) (Haines et al. 1987). This association persisted after controlling for several cardiovascular risk factors. Kawachi et al. (1994a) similarly examined the association between phobic anxiety and CHD in the Health Professionals Follow-Up Study, an ongoing cohort of 33,999 male health professionals free of diagnosed CHD at baseline. The multivariate relative risk of fatal CHD among the most anxious men was 2.45 (95% CI: 1.00 to 5.96) compared with the least anxious men. An additional prospective study of self-reported anxiety symptoms in relation to risk of CHD was conducted within the Normative Aging Study (Kawachi et al. 1994b). Compared with men reporting no anxiety symptoms, men reporting at least two had elevated risks of fatal CHD, particularly sudden cardiac death (multivariate odds ratio [OR] = 4.46; 95% CI: 0.92 to 21.6; the estimates of risk in this study were imprecise due to the small number of events). In the Framingham Heart Study, a 20-year follow-up of 749 initially healthy women found that anxiety symptoms were significantly associated with MI and coronary death among homemakers, but not among employed women (Eaker et al. 1992). The relative risks of CHD (adjusted for other cardiovas-

cular risk factors) in homemakers who reported any tension or symptoms of anxiety compared with those who reported none were 6.2 (95% CI: 1.7 to 23.2) for tension and 7.8 (95% CI: 1.9 to 32.3) for anxiety symptoms (Eaker et al. 1992). Most recently, in a 20-year follow-up of 1759 initially healthy men in the Normative Aging Study, Kubzansky et al. (1997) examined the relationship between CHD and worry, an important cognitive component of anxiety (Barlow 1988; Borkovec et al. 1983). Five domains of worry were considered including social conditions, health, finances, self-definition, and aging. Compared with men reporting the lowest levels of worry about social conditions, those reporting the highest levels had a multivariate adjusted RR of 2.41 (95% CI: 1.40 to 4.13) for nonfatal MI, with a dose–response relationship between level of worry and overall CHD risk. Some associations were also evident between the health and financial worries subscales and CHD (Kubzansky et al. 1997). Other studies, using both diagnostic and questionnaire scales to assess clinical and subclinical anxiety, have also linked anxiety disorders and symptoms to CHD (Talbott et al. 1981; Coryell et al. 1982, 1986; Weissman et al. 1990).

Depression and CHD

Depression is generally considered a mixture of several emotions, such as sadness, loneliness, hopelessness, guilt, and shame, and is often associated with some kind of loss (Lazarus 1991b; Shaver and Brennan 1991). For an extensive discussion of depression (and related emotions) and its relationship to medical illness, readers are referred to Chapter 9 in this volume. Here we briefly highlight only the most relevant research on the role of depression in CHD incidence.

Some prospective studies have found a modest association between depression and risk of incident heart disease (Anda et al. 1993; Barefoot and Schroll 1996; Pratt et al. 1996; Ford et al. 1998; Sesso et al. 1998). Anda and colleagues (1993) examined prospectively the relationship between depressed affect and ischemic heart disease (IHD) incidence in 2832 healthy adults in the National Health Examination Follow-up Study. Depressed affect was associated with a significantly increased risk of fatal (RR = 1.5; 95% CI: 1.0 to 2.3) as well as nonfatal (RR = 1.6; 95% CI: 1.1 to 2.4) IHD. Another prospective study of 409 men and 321 women in Denmark found an association between depression and CHD (Barefoot and Schroll 1996). Increased depression scores over time were significantly associated with excess risk of total MI over a 27-year follow-up period (RR = 1.71; 95% CI: 1.19 to 2.44) among both men and women. In a further 40 year follow-up of 1190 male medical students, men who reported clinical depression were at significantly greater risk for subsequent CHD (RR = 2.12; 95% CI: 1.24 to 3.63) (Ford et al. 1998). Most recently, in a 7-year follow-up of 1305 men within the Normative Aging Study, Sesso and colleagues (1998) found an association between depression and incident CHD, including dose–response relationships, using three depression scales. Compared with men reporting the lowest level of depression, those in the highest level had multivariate-adjusted RRs of incident CHD ranging from 1.46 (95% CI: 0.83 to 2.57) to 2.07 (95% CI: 1.13 to 3.81) depending on which measure of depression was used.

However, not all studies have found an association between depression and increased risk of CHD. For example, using their own depression index, Vogt and colleagues (1994) followed 2573 men and women in a northwest HMO over the course of 15 years. The highest tertile of depressive symptoms was not associated with an increased risk of IHD compared with the lowest depression tertile (relative hazard = 0.94; 95% CI: 0.70 to 1.28). In a 5-year follow-up study of 4367 men and women aged 60 or older with hypertension, Wassertheil-Smoller et al. (1996) similarly failed to find increased risk of myocardial infarction among depressed individuals. Despite the mixed findings, further research seems warranted given the number of plausible biologic mechanisms by which depression may increase risk of incident CHD, (described more fully in Chapter 9).

Suppressed Emotion and CHD

Researchers have hypothesized that not only are high levels of expressed anger or anxiety toxic, but so also is the suppression (or inhibition) of these emotions. The association between emotion suppression and CHD has been examined in a number of studies. In the Framingham study, the single item "inability to discuss angry feelings" predicted subsequent CHD risk (Haynes et al. 1980). In a 10-year prospective epidemiologic study of approximately 1400 people in Yugoslavia, Grossarth-Maticek and colleagues (1985a,b) found that suppression of emotions was the best single predictor of CHD. Those who scored high on a scale measuring suppression and denial of emotion were at ten times greater risk for CHD than those who scored lower. A recent follow-up study of patients with established CHD examined the association between the so-called type D personality and mortality (Denollet et al. 1996). Type D personality was defined by anxiety suppression—individuals who scored high on an anxiety trait scale and who also reported a high degree of social inhibition. Controlling for biomedical predictors of mortality, risk of cardiac death was increased fourfold for individuals with type D personality compared to those who did exhibit the type D personality (OR = 4.1; 95% CI: 1.9 to 8.8) (Denollet et al. 1996).

Acute Emotions and CHD

A separate set of mechanisms by which emotion may lead to cardiovascular disease involves acute or "triggering" effects. (See Kamarck and Jennings 1991, for a related review.) For example, acute anxiety states may lead to hyperventilation, which then may trigger coronary vasospasm (Rasmussen et al. 1986). It has also been hypothesized that acute hemodynamic stress caused by transient, intense emotional states may cause rupture of atherosclerotic plaques on the vessel wall of coronary arteries, which may then initiate acute coronary events including sudden cardiac death (Falk 1983; Davies and Thomas 1984; Gorlin et al. 1986). An increasing number of studies have begun to test the triggering hypothesis (e.g., Weiss and Engel 1971; Reich et al. 1981; Falk 1983; Tofler et al. 1990; Gelernt and Hochman 1992). The recent development of the case-crossover study design has enabled investigators to examine directly the triggering effects of acute emotions. In the Determinants of Myocardial Infarction Onset Study, a case-crossover study involving 1623 patients, episodes of anger were found to be potent triggers of acute MI (Mittleman et al. 1995). The relative risk of MI in the 2 hours after an episode of anger was 2.3 (95% CI: 1.7 to 3.2). The study also found that the relative risk for MI associated with an episode of anxiety occurring 0–2 hours before the onset of MI was 1.6 (95% CI: 1.1 to 2.2) (Mittleman et al. 1995).

Platelet aggregation associated with increased psychological stress may also lead to thrombosis and ischemia (Kamarck and Jennings 1991). Kamarck and Jennings (1991) review a number of studies that examined the relationship between environmental stressors and platelet aggregation (Gordon et al. 1973; Fleischman et al. 1976; Haft and Arkel 1976; Mest et al. 1982; Levine et al. 1985). Most of these studies found an increase in platelet aggregation associated with stressful tasks. We mention these studies because, although emotions were not directly measured, the tasks used to simulate environmental stress (public speaking, exam stress, medical diagnostic procedures) have frequently been associated with negative emotions (Spielberger and Sarason 1978; Neiss 1988; Leventhal and Patrick-Miller 1993). In fact, several recent studies have found a relationship between hostility and trait anger and platelet activation (Markovitz et al. 1996; Wenneberg et al. 1997; Markovitz 1998). Increased circu-lating levels of adrenaline appear to be the mechanism underlying the relationship between acute psychological stress and increased platelet aggregation.

Emotion and the Atherosclerotic Process

Emotion and hypertension

Numerous studies have examined the relationship of anxiety and anger to raised blood pressure. With few exceptions (Dunner 1985; Charney and Heninger 1986), studies in psychiatric settings largely support the notion that individuals with anxiety disorders have a higher incidence of hypertension (Noyes et al. 1978; Katon 1986; Wells et al. 1989; Hayward 1995). A number of investigators have also reported that trait anxiety is a predictor of a subsequent rise in blood pressure (Jenkins et al. 1983; Markovitz et al. 1991; Pernini et al. 1991). For example, in a study of 468 middle-aged normotensive women, those with more anxiety symptoms had greater increases in systolic blood pressure over the course of 3-year follow-up (Markovitz et al. 1991). Additional recent evidence also suggests that elevated anxiety levels among middle-aged men and women are predictive of the incidence of hypertension (Markovitz et al. 1993; Jonas et al. 1997).

Many of the studies examining anger as a risk factor for hypertension are retrospective or cross-sectional in design, rendering the results somewhat inconclusive (Niaura and Goldstein 1992). Generally, research on anger and hypertension in minority communities has found a consistent relationship between high levels of anger and increased rates of hypertension (see Kumanyika and Adams-Campbell 1991). In other populations, however, evidence for this association has been mixed (Siegler 1994; Jorgensen et al. 1996).

The effects of anxiety or anger on blood pressure may be even greater than research to date has suggested. Anxious and angry individuals who suppress or repress their emotions are not identified as being anxious or angry by the usual measures (Shedler et al. 1993). Research designed explicitly to identify those who inhibit their emotion, has often found that inhibited emotion is associated with increased risk for hypertension (e.g., Harburg et al. 1979; Gentry 1985; Julius et al. 1985; Manuck et al. 1985; Rosenman 1985; Sommers-Flanagan and Greenberg 1989; Warrenburg et al. 1989; King et al. 1990).

Emotion and atherosclerotic progression
Coronary heart disease is the end result of underlying atherosclerotic processes (Goldberg 1992), and a number of investigators have hypothesized that negative emotions may contribute directly to the progression of atherosclerosis (Matsumoto et al. 1993; Julkunen et al. 1994; Agewall et al. 1996). Angiographic studies have examined the relationship between anxiety and anger (and their suppression) and the severity of atherosclerosis in patients with established coronary disease. Some though not all, studies have found associations between severity of disease and anxiety (Zyzanski et al. 1976; Blumenthal et al. 1979; Tennant and Langeluddecke 1985; Tennant et al. 1987), anger and hostility (Williams et al. 1980; Tennant and Langeluddecke 1985; Tennant et al. 1987), depression (Zyzanski et al. 1976), and suppressed anger (Dembroski et al. 1985).

A growing number of studies have begun to examine relationships between emotions and atherosclerosis using B-mode carotid sonography (a noninvasive method for measuring atherosclerosis). In a cross-sectional analysis, Matsumoto and colleagues (1993) found that self-reported anger was strongly positively correlated with severity of carotid atherosclerosis in a sample of 34 patients, and the association remained significant in multivariate analyses controlling for a range of cardiovascular risk factors. In a sample of 119 middle-aged men followed for 2 years, Julkunen et al. (1994) found an association between hostility and suppression of anger as the carotid atherosclerosis progressed. A twofold acceleration in ultrasonographically assessed progression of atherosclerosis was found for individuals with high levels of

anger suppression and hostility compared with those reporting lower levels. Matthews and colleagues (1998) found similar results in a sample of 200 postmenopausal women, although baseline levels of atherosclerosis were not assessed. High levels of anger suppression at baseline significantly predicted high levels of atherosclerosis 10 years later, while high hostility was associated with increased atherosclerosis over 1.5 year follow-up, when standard cardiovascular risk factors were controlled. Another recent study found discontent to be predictive of the progression of atherosclerosis over 3-year follow-up, using ultrasonographic measures of atherosclerosis (Agewall et al. 1996).

EMOTION AND CANCER

Despite the long-held beliefs about a link between emotion and cancer, empirical support for the role of emotion in the development of cancer has remained sparse. Based on work with cancer patients, Temoshok (1987) proposed a model of the cancer-prone individual (type C personality) as one who is stoic, has difficulty in expressing emotions, and has an attitude of resignation or helplessness/hopelessness. However, examination of psychological factors in cancer *incidence* has proved difficult on several grounds. Cancer comprises a heterogeneous group of diseases of multiple etiologies that vary in their tissue of origin, cell type, biological behavior, anatomic site, and degree of differentiation (Anderson et al. 1994). Depending on the cancer site, some tumors may be more susceptible to psychological factors than others (Anderson, Kiecolt-Glaser et al. 1994). Cancers, in contrast to CHD, typically involve longer induction times between exposure and disease onset, so longer follow-up times are required. Much of the evidence for a link between emotion and cancer rests on cross-sectional or retrospective studies (see Fox et al. 1988; Gross 1989), from which it is difficult to convincingly demonstrate that the effects of the emotion preceded the development of the disease. The few prospective studies that exist present a mixed picture of a link between emotion and cancer risk. For example, in a 17-year follow-up study of 2020 middle-aged employed men, higher levels of depression were associated with a twofold increase in the odds of cancer death (Shekelle et al. 1981). This increase in risk persisted after adjustment for smoking, alcohol consumption, occupational status, and family history of cancer. No single site appeared to be more strongly associated with depression. However, another prospective study of depression and cancer in a representative U.S. sample found no such association (Kaplan and Reynolds 1988). This study followed participants for 17 years and tested whether the link between depression and cancer might only exist in particular subgroups of the population or depend on demographic differences between the cohorts under study. After examining these possibilities, the authors found no support for an association between depression and cancer. In another prospective study, investigators examined whether Yugoslav men and women who suppressed their emotions were significantly more likely to die from cancer during the follow-up period (Grossarth-Maticek et al. 1985a). This study presented evidence for a strong association between emotion inhibition and cancer mortality, and these findings were replicated in another study by the same researchers in Heidelberg, Germany (Grossarth-Maticek and Eyesenck 1990). Findings in these two studies also suggested an interaction between smoking and depression, such that depressed individuals who smoked were at greatly increased risk of dying from cancer.

Studies of cancer mortality are unable to distinguish between the effects of emotion on cancer *incidence* vs. *survival* following the diagnosis of cancer. The mechanisms linking emotion to cancer survival may be very different from those linking emotion to cancer incidence. For instance, survival following cancer diagnosis may reflect psychosocial adjustment, adherence to treatment, and the availability of social support,

all of which are plausibly related to the patient's emotional state. (In fact, there is a great deal of research on and evidence for the role of emotion in the progression of and adjustment to cancer. See for example, Greer and Morris 1975; Pettingale 1985; Anderson et al. 1994.) By contrast, the link between emotion and cancer incidence (if one exists) may be mediated through health behavior differences (e.g., smoking) (Fox et al. 1988) or through effects on immune functioning (Pennebaker and Susman 1988; O'Leary 1990; Herbert and Cohen 1993a). There is some skepticism however, about any link between emotion and cancer incidence, because of the lack of convincing prospective evidence (Anderson et al. 1994; Davison and Petrie 1997).

EMOTION AND THE COMMON COLD

Psychological distress and stressors appear to be reliably associated with immune function downregulation, although fewer studies have examined the effects of specific emotions (Kiecolt-Glaser and Glaser 1988; O'Leary 1990; Herbert and Cohen 1993b). Negative emotions are thought to alter susceptibility to infectious diseases like the common cold through their effects (both direct and indirect) on immune function (Cohen 1996). Some work has examined the relationship between depression and immunity (see O'Leary 1990, for review; Herbert and Cohen 1993a). In a meta-analysis, Herbert and Cohen (1993a) found strong evidence for a "dose–response" relation between depression (clinical depression and depressed mood) and immune function, measured by a variety of parameters, including lymphocyte function, natural killer cell activity, and circulating white blood cells. Participants in these studies were identified in terms of their depressed status, and immunological assays were conducted. The health implications of such measures of immune functioning among healthy individuals are not known, however (Herbert and Cohen 1993a). In an effort to address this issue, some investigators have used a viral challenge methodology in a controlled laboratory setting to examine more directly the association between stress, emotion, and the common cold (Cohen et al. 1991, 1993; Cohen 1996). In these studies, emotion and stress are sometimes, but not always, considered separately. Given that only a proportion of people exposed to an infectious agent will develop clinical disease, investigators have examined whether individuals with higher levels of negative emotion were more likely to catch a cold. In one study healthy subjects were exposed to a common cold virus, quarantined, and monitored for the development of biologically verified clinical illness (Cohen et al. 1993). Prior to exposure, levels of negative emotions were measured. Even after controlling for health behaviors, age, gender, and educational attainment, individuals with higher levels of negative emotions were more likely to develop clinical illness (Cohen et al. 1993). Among other studies examining susceptibility to a cold, most but not all have replicated these findings. (For null findings see Smith et al. 1992; Cohen et al. 1995a.) However, because of the methodological and logistical complexities in conducting such studies, research in this area is not extensive.

EMOTION AND OTHER HEALTH OUTCOMES

Studies examining the role of emotion in the etiology of other health outcomes are surprisingly sparse. One meta-analysis considered the effects of anxiety, depression, and anger on several illnesses that have traditionally been considered psychosomatic, including asthma, peptic ulcer, rheumatoid arthritis, and headache (Friedman and Booth-Kewley 1987). Based on their review, the authors concluded there was suggestive evidence for a number of emotion–disease associations, including *(1)* anxiety and asthma, ulcer, arthritis and headache, *(2)* depression and asthma, ulcer (weak), arthritis, and headache, *(3)* anger and asthma, and

arthritis (weak). However, most of the published studies were cross-sectional, with small sample sizes, and could not distinguish whether the emotion was cause or effect of the diseases. For some diseases, such as asthma, there is good evidence that emotions can trigger an attack or exacerbate existing symptoms. But evidence implicating emotion in the onset of asthma is lacking. In general, while research has been published on emotion and illnesses ranging from asthma, tension and migraine headaches, genital herpes, AIDS, rheumatoid arthritis, and multiple sclerosis, most of this work has examined the effect of emotion on disease progression or adjustment to diagnosis (see, for example, O'Leary 1990; Lehrer et al. 1993).

UNRESOLVED ISSUES IN EMOTION– HEALTH RESEARCH

There are numerous unresolved issues which leave our current understanding of the emotion–health relationship incomplete (see Table 10–1), and a consideration of theoretically based emotion research may enrich our understanding and help to address gaps in our knowledge. The role of emotions in the onset vs. the clinical course of many diseases (even including CHD) is not clearly understood. For example, there is good evidence that depression adversely affects the prognosis of many diseases once they are established, but its role in disease onset is less clear. The level of emotion at which disease occurs has not yet been determined (e.g., clinical vs. subclinical levels of anxiety or depression). Similarly, the differential effects of acute vs. chronic emotions and the different pathways by which they may influence health outcomes have not been fully explored. Investigators have not considered the full spectrum of emotions; most of the research has focused on health effects of negative emotions. Finally, the different effects of expressed vs. suppressed or repressed emotions on health outcomes are not fully understood. The following sections highlight a few of these issues.

Pathological vs. Normal Experiences of Emotion

The experience of most emotions occurs along a continuum, ranging from normal to clinical/pathological levels. There is a range within which emotion levels are considered to be normal; but when they occur in inappropriate contexts and at high intensities, they may be identified as pathological (Frijda 1994). Anxiety and depression are commonly experienced emotions that can also underlie clinical disorders. For example, an anxiety disorder is considered to be present when the experience of anxiety is *(1)* recurrent and persistent; *(2)* of an intensity far above what is considered reasonable, given the objective danger or threat; *(3)* paralyzing so that individuals feel helpless and unable to cope; and *(4)* the cause of impaired psychological or physiological functioning (Lader and Marks 1973; Ohman 1993). Psychological research has suggested that pathological anxiety (clinically diagnosed conditions like panic disorder or generalized anxiety disorder) and normal anxiety reactions are essentially similar in their cognitive, neurobiological, and behavioral components (Clark and Watson 1994; Frijda 1994). Thus, according to Barlow (1988) and others (e.g., Spielberger and Sarason 1978; Ohman 1993), anxiety can refer to both the normal and pathological spectrum of symptomatology. Much of the epidemiologic research on anxiety and CHD to date has focused on subclinical (in the range of normal) manifestations of anxiety (Barlow 1988; Frijda 1994). Hence, the link between anxiety and increased risk of CHD has implications for a broad group of individuals. Anxiety is used here as an exemplar; similar relationships are hypothesized between pathological and normal experiences of other emotions.

Emotion Interrelationships

Considerable overlap occurs in the cognitive, neurobiological, and behavioral components of emotions. For example, appraisals of threat may be common to both anxiety and anger, while anxiety and elation may both be accompanied by cardiovascular arousal. How do these similarities affect the ability of researchers to detect specific health effects of specific emotions? Specificity of emotion/disease associations may be especially difficult to establish because emotions rarely occur in isolation (Lazarus 1991a; Robinson et al. 1991). For example, anxiety and depression often occur together, but few studies that have examined the association of anxiety with CHD have simultaneously accounted for the overlap between anxiety and depression in either self-report rating scales or diagnoses of clinical disorders (Breier et al. 1984; Barlow 1988; Clark 1989). Clear evidence that "pure" anxiety (as independent of depression) plays a role in CHD has yet to be demonstrated.

A greater understanding of the relationship between emotion and health may be gained by understanding the patterns of situational evaluations that are associated with specific emotion experiences. Research on emotion has suggested that when evaluating the harm or benefit of a situation, individuals make a number of more specific appraisals in terms of how much control one has, who is responsible for the situation, and so on (Lazarus 1968; Scherer 1982; Smith and Ellsworth 1985; Frijda 1986). Reliable associations between unique patterns of situational appraisals and specific emotions have been identified (e.g., see Scherer 1982; Roseman 1984; Smith and Ellsworth 1985; Smith and Lazarus 1993), and certain appraisals may particularly critical in defining emotion effects (Roseman 1984). For example, a sense of control has been identified as a key appraisal for a number of emotions (Smith and Ellsworth 1985), and has also been related to health and mortality (Rodin 1986; Barlow 1988; Reich and Zautra 1990). Based on the similarity of emotions across these dimensions, more similar health outcomes might be expected.

Some work has succeeded in identifying specific physiological patterns associated with particular emotions (Ekman et al. 1983; Levenson et al. 1990; Levenson 1992;

Cacioppo et al. 1993), although the reliability of these differences has been debated (Schwartz and Weinberger 1980; LeDoux 1994). Investigations to date have looked at only a limited array of physiological parameters, and technological and methodological advances in our ability to measure physiological changes may yield more conclusive evidence in the future (Baum et al. 1992). Levenson (1994b) suggests that whether autonomic response differs reliably across emotions depends on whether the emotions reliably call forth different patterns of behavior and whether these behavior patterns require different configurations of autonomic support. Even among emotions which seem to call forth similar physiological responses such as anxiety and excitement, there may be subtle differences. For example, in the presence of a stressor, negative and positive emotions are associated with appraisals of threat and challenge, respectively (Smith and Ellsworth 1987; Tomaka et al. 1993). Laboratory studies have further suggested that individuals who feel challenged by a stressful task exhibit greater cardiac reactivity and decreased vascular resistance, whereas those who feel threatened exhibit relatively less cardiac reactivity (measured by heart rate, cardiac contractility, cardiac output) and higher vascular resistance (Tomaka et al. 1993). Thus, the mobilization of physiological resources may depend in part on whether individuals perceive a situation to be threatening or challenging.

Efforts at differentiating between specific emotions may also focus on multiple aspects of emotion. Work that has attempted to distinguish between anxiety and depression, for example, has suggested that anxiety is associated with active efforts to cope with difficult situations (and with physiological responses mobilized to support these efforts), whereas depression is more likely to be characterized by behavioral retardation and with a related *lack* of mobilization of physiological resources (Barlow 1988; Clark and Watson 1991). Similarly, while anger and anxiety are related in that they share similar behavioral and physiological

components (Eriksen 1966; Barlow 1988; Ellsworth 1991), the action tendencies and coping strategies may differ sharply between the two emotions. Anger may be associated with an impulse to aggress while anxiety may be associated with the desire to withdraw from social situations. These different forms of coping may have very different health implications.

Expression, Inhibition, Denial, Ambivalence

Regardless of the nature of an emotion, three general types of emotion experience have been conceptualized: *(1)* failure to attend to emotions—repression, *(2)* conscious inhibition of the expression of emotion when one is emotionally aroused—suppression, *(3)* willingness to express or disclose an emotion—expression (Pennebaker and Beall 1986; Gross and Levenson 1993; Davison and Petrie 1997). Both repression and suppression have been linked, albeit inconsistently, with adverse health outcomes (Weinberger et al. 1979; Gentry 1985; Grossarth-Maticek et al. 1985b; Davison and Petrie 1997). The notion that "bottling up" one's emotions is harmful to health can be traced to the "hydraulic" model of emotion which posits that when expressive signs of emotion are inhibited, they are discharged through other channels (i.e., physiological) (Cannon 1927; Marshall 1972). Similarly, other investigators have suggested that the act of inhibiting the outward expression of emotion entails physiological work, which over time may place cumulative stress on an individual (Pennebaker and Beall 1986). These types of theories suggest that people who chronically inhibit (or suppress) their emotions may be more prone to disease than those who are emotionally expressive (Alexander 1939; Freud 1961; Pennebaker and Beall 1986; Shedler et al. 1993). Similar reasoning is applied to those who repress or deny their emotion experiences, where repression is considered to involve a more unconscious level of emotional inhibition (Davison and Petrie 1997).

If repression and inhibition are associated with increased vulnerability to illness, then it stands to reason that being emotionally expressive may confer some health benefits. The ability to disclose one's feelings is hypothesized to be particularly important in the face of traumatic events (Pennebaker and Beall 1986). By talking about or confronting a traumatic event individuals may be better able to organize, assimilate, or give meaning to the trauma (Pennebaker and Beall 1986). Some empirical support for this hypothesis has been obtained, where writing or talking about emotional topics have been found to have beneficial influences on immune function, short-term changes in autonomic activity, significant decreases in physician visits, and long-term improvements in mood and indicators of well-being. (For a summary of this literature, see Pennebaker 1997.)

Not all forms of emotional expression are healthy, however. For example, Siegman (1994a) distinguishes between the experience, expression, and repression of anger and argues that expressing anger has toxic cardiovascular consequences while repressing anger has toxic effects on the immune system. The appropriate emotion regulation or control then rests on avoiding the extremes of inhibition and expression (Siegman, 1994a, see also Blotcky et al. 1983, for similar formulations; King and Emmons 1991). Methodologically, it is difficult to distinguish between the forms of emotion nonexpression. Lack of expression may be due to repression, suppression, or simply the failure to experience an emotion (Davison and Petrie 1997). Although some measures have been developed which try to differentiate between these constructs, more conceptual clarity is needed to distinguish between the theoretical possibilities and their effects (e.g., see Barefoot and Lipkus 1994; Davison and Petrie 1997, for further discussion; Gross and John 1998).

Emotion and Health: Positive vs. Negative Emotions

The literature on the relationship between emotion and health has focused primarily on negative emotions as predictors of health outcomes. Research tends to be problem driven and while negative emotions pose a wide array of problems for individuals and for society, this focus has come at the expense of the neglect of positive affect. Thus, despite the folk wisdom which has extolled the benefits of positive emotion (e.g., laughter and humor, see Cousins 1979), research on positive emotions in health has lagged behind that on negative emotions (Fredrickson 1998). Some empirical work suggests that positive emotions may be associated with lowered susceptibility to disease (Bovard 1985; Cohen and Rodriguez 1995; Myers and Diener 1995; Seeman and McEwen 1996). A sense of optimism (related to the emotions of hope and happiness) has been linked to enhanced well-being (Scheier and Carver 1987; Reker 1997). For example, one study examined the association between optimism and recovery from coronary bypass surgery in 54 patients not suffering from any major psychiatric difficulties (Scheier and Carver 1987). On the day preceding surgery, patients filled out questionnaires that assessed their levels of optimism. Rates of recovery from the surgery were considerably faster among individuals who were more optimistic, controlling for patients' physical health status prior to the operation.

Exactly how positive emotions promote health is not well understood. Fredrickson (1998) has proposed a "broaden and build" model that posits that positive emotions build an individual's resources in multiple domains. With positive emotion experiences, individuals may develop physical skills that build strength, cognitive skills that enhance coping, and social–affective skills that aid in building and strengthening relationships. Such resources are in turn hypothesized to promote health and well-being. Positive emotions may also function as an antidote to the lingering effects (both cognitive and physiological) of negative emotions (Fredrickson 1998). Whereas negative emotions narrow an individual's thinking and behavior, positive emotions may help to undo the psychological and physiological effects of negative emotion, thereby loosening its hold on the individual's mind and body (Fredrickson and Levenson 1998). Experimental tests of this hypothesis have examined differences in speed of recovery from emotion-related cardiovascular arousal where recovery is defined as the degree to which one's physiological responses return to pre-arousal levels. In one study, investigators examined the dissipation of fear-related cardiovascular arousal (Fredrickson and Levenson 1998). After a fear induction, investigators induced one of three states: contentment, sadness, or a neutral state. Cardiovascular arousal dissipated more quickly when feelings of contentment were induced than when sadness or a neutral state was induced. The authors suggested that by neutralizing lingering autonomic arousal sparked by negative emotions, positive emotions may then interrupt or cut short the damaging impact of reactivity on the cardiovascular system. Other work has also suggested that positive emotion may be associated with better immune function (Stone et al. 1987, 1994).

Finally, positive emotions may have a more indirect influence on health by promoting social interactions (Malatesta 1989; Rime et al. 1992; Frijda 1994; Fredrickson 1998). For example, the expression of emotions such as joy, laughter, and sympathy involves the company of others and shows an inclination to associate (Malatesta 1989). Happy people have been found to be more loving, forgiving, trusting, energetic, decisive, creative, helpful, and sociable. These are prosocial behaviors and actions that promote and strengthen social bonds, which in turn may enhance health (Myers and Diener 1995). Readers are referred to Chapter 7 on the relation between social integration and health.

Measurement Issues

Most epidemiological studies on emotion and health have relied on self-reports of emotion, using a specific emotions approach. This approach theorizes that there are many different types of emotions, each with different characteristics and specific response patterns (Tomkins 1963; Izard 1977). Measures that result in scales with labels like "happiness," "sadness," and "anxiety" have been derived using this approach. Measures in this tradition generally include adjective checklists or lists of statements that respondents endorse in terms of the extent to which each statement applies to them.[5] A number of reliable and well-validated scales of emotions exist for measuring anger, anxiety, and depression (see for example, Robinson et al. 1991; Barefoot and Lipkus 1994; Stone 1995), and fewer for positive emotions.

Self-report assessments have a number of problems, however. Study subjects must be willing to disclose what may feel like private information. Some subjects may want to present themselves in the best light possible and therefore fail to respond accurately to the questions (a phenomenon called social desirability). Or individuals may lack insight into themselves and may fail to give an accurate report of the emotions they experience. Other investigators have argued that self-report data are problematic because they cannot distinguish between genuine mental well-being (i.e., low anxiety) and the façade of health created by psychological defenses (Shedler et al. 1993). A further issue in measurement is what to include in the domain of emotion. Many scales ask about somatic symptoms (e.g., racing heart), since emotions in general seem highly correlated with physical symptom reports (Leventhal and Patrick-Miller 1993). Given this strong association, using emotion scales that include symptom assessments to predict certain types of health outcomes (e.g., general symptomatology) may be somewhat misleading. Scales should be carefully screened on whether their content is appropriate for the study being undertaken. Measures other than self-report are possible. These include peer reports such as asking spouses to provide emotion ratings for study subjects, and observer ratings, in which trained interviewers observe and rate subjects on their emotions.

More generally, whatever type of emotion measure is used, it is not always evident how to define someone as "not exposed" to emotions like anxiety or anger or happiness, since almost everybody generally experiences some level of each emotion. Even the definitions of emotionally based psychiatric disorders are somewhat loose. For example, in his review of the anxiety disorders, Barlow (1988) suggests that the diagnosis and differentiation of the various anxiety disorders are not yet well understood (although for treatment purposes the diagnostic criteria draw important distinctions). Clearly identifying the aspects of emotion that have pathophysiological consequences will involve careful consideration of the instruments used to measure each emotion, as different measures may be appropriate depending on the hypothesis being investigated. Moreover, in choosing a measure, the psychometric properties of each instrument (e.g., reliability and validity) should be carefully evaluated. (See Stone 1995, for more detailed discussion of these issues.) Consideration of the measurement of emotion should also take into account possible variation across gender, race/ethnicity, and age. While it is not within the scope of this chapter to review the large literature addressing these issues, investigators should be aware of them when choosing appropriate measures. Ultimately, the choice of method used to measure emotion will be based largely on the theoretical and practical needs of each study.

CONCLUSIONS

Growing evidence supports the role of negative emotions in pathogenesis and disease prognosis, in particular, for coronary heart disease. In this chapter, we have attempted to leaven the findings from recent epidemiological studies with theoretical insights provided by mainstream psychological research on emotions. We have highlighted key issues for further interdisciplinary research, where greater conceptual clarity promises to yield greater understanding of the mechanisms by which the experience of

emotions—both positive and negative—leads to differential health outcomes. Although the bulk of empirical research to date has concentrated on the relation of negative emotions to coronary disease, the field is poised for a much broader expansion in the scope of inquiry. Researchers have begun to turn their attention to the role of positive emotions, as well as to the influence of emotions on the maintenance of good health—for example, the extension of vigorous and productive aging in later years.

Continued research on emotions is critical to the advancement of social epidemiology for at least three reasons: first, because the social patterning of emotions offers researchers an important clue about how variations in the external social environment produce differences in individual health status; second, because emotions represent a crucial link in the chain of causation that runs from stressors to biological responses within individuals (the so-called sociobiological translation); and last but not least, because research on emotions provides a basis for the development of psychosocial interventions which aim to break the link between social conditions and illness outcomes. Recently, several studies have begun to test the hypothesis that emotions may mediate the relationship between social conditions and individual health (Lynch et al. 1996; Ickovics et al. 1997; Kubzansky et al. in press). Further work of this nature will firmly set the emotion and health relationship into the broader social context, lay the groundwork for modes of intervention, and provide new directions for future research.

NOTES

1. However, not all individuals in the same environment are affected by the environment in the same way. While emotions may be socially patterned, they are not determined solely by social conditions but rather by the interaction between the individual and his or her environment (Lazarus 1991a; Taylor et al. 1997).

2. In some theories once individuals considers themselves to be stressed, the physiological and biological changes are considered to be largely similar regardless of the nature of the stressor. Bi-

ological changes that occur during the stress process may then place individuals at increased risk for disease.

3. Emotions are considered separate psychological entities from moods or attitudes. Emotions are generally considered to have an object, so they are "about" something, whereas moods have been defined as being more diffuse, lower in intensity, and of longer duration than emotions (Frijda 1993). Emotions are one component of attitudes, which have been defined as learned predispositions to respond in a consistent manner with respect to a given object (Fishbein and Ajzen 1975; Breckler 1993).

4. The ongoing interaction between emotion and health may be particularly difficult to capture in research investigations that measure emotion at a single point in time. As a result, reports of the relationship between emotion and health may be underestimates.

5. In contrast, a dimensional emotion approach builds on the notion that there are a small number of dimensions which describe all emotions (i.e., pleasantness, activation), and specific emotions are derived from combinations of these basic dimensions. (See Stone 1995, for greater discussion of dimensional measures.) Research on emotion and health, however, benefits from the specific emotion approach, because dimensional approaches miss much of the richness of affective life and do not convey differences in how different emotions are experienced in physiological and behavioral domains (Lazarus 1991a).

REFERENCES

Ader, R., Felten, D.L., and Cohen, N. (eds.). (1991). *Psychoneuroimmunology*. San Diego, CA: Academic Press.

Agewall, S., Wikstrand, J., Dahlof, C., and Fagerberg, B. (1996). Negative feelings (discontent) predict progress of intima-media thickness of the common carotid artery in treated hypertensive men at high cardiovascular risk. *Am J Hypertens*, 9:545–50.

Alexander, F.G., French, T.M., and Pollack, G.H. (1968). *Psychosomatic specificity: experimental study and results*. Chicago: The University of Chicago Press.

Alexander, R. (1939). Psychological aspects of medicine. *Psychosom Med*, 1:7–18.

Allan, R., and Scheidt, S. (1996). Stress, anger, and psychosocial factors for coronary heart disease. In Manson, J.E., Ridker, P.M., Gaziano, J.M., and Hennekens, C.H. (eds.), *Prevention of myocardial infarction*. New York: Oxford University Press, pp. 274–307.

Allport, G.W. (1961). *Pattern and growth in personality*. New York: Holt, Rinehart, & Winston.

Anda, R., Williamson, D., Jones, D., Macea, C., Eaker, E., Glassman, A., and Marks, J. (1993). Depressed affect, hopelessness, and the risk of ischemic heart disease in a cohort of U.S. adults. *Epidemiology*, 4:285–94.

Anderson, B.L., Kiecolt-Glaser, J.K., and Glaser, R. (1994). A biobehavioral model of cancer stress and disease course. *Am Psychol*, 49(5):389–404.

Anderson, N.B., and Armstead, C.A. (1995). Toward understanding the association of socioeconomic status and health: a new challenge for the biopsychosocial approach. *Psychosom Med*, 57:213–25.

Arnold, M.B. (1960). *Emotion and personality*. New York: Columbia University Press.

Barefoot, J.C., and Lipkus, I.M. (1994). The assessment of anger and hostility. In Siegman, A.W., and Smith, T.W. (eds.), *Anger, hostility and the heart*. Hillsdale, NJ: Lawrence Erlbaum, pp. 43–66.

Barefoot, J.C., and Schroll, M. (1996). Symptoms of depression, acute myocardial infarction, and total mortality in a community sample. *Circulation*, (93):1976–80.

Barefoot, J.C., Dahlstrom, W.G., and Williams, R.B. Jr. (1983). Hostility, CHD incidence, and total mortality: a 25-year follow-up study of 255 physicians. *Psychosom Med*, 45(1):59–63.

Barefoot, J.C., Peterson, B.L., Dahlstrom, W.G., Siegler, I.C., Anderson, N.B., and Williams, R.B. Jr. (1991). Hostility patterns and health implications: correlates of Cook-Medley Hostility Scale scores in a national survey. *Health Psychol*, 10(1):18–24.

Barlow, D.H. (1988). *Anxiety and its disorders*. New York: The Guilford Press.

Baum, A., and Grunberg, N. (1995). Measurement of stress hormones. In Cohen, S., Kessler, R.C., and Gordon, L.U. (eds.), *Measuring stress: a guide for health and social scientists*. New York: Oxford University Press, pp. 175–93.

Baum, A., Grunberg, N.E., and Singer, J.E. (1992). Biochemical measurements in the study of emotion. *Psychol Sci*, 3(1):56–60.

Blotcky, A.D., Carscaddon, D.M., and Grandmaison, S.L. (1983). Self-disclosure and physical health: in support of curvilinearity. *Psychol Reports*, 53:903–6.

Blumenthal, J.A., Thompson, L.W., Williams, R.B., and Kong, Y. (1979). Anxiety-proneness and coronary heart disease. *J Psychosom Res*, 23:17–21.

Booth-Kewley, S., and Friedman, H.S. (1987).

Psychological predictors of heart disease: a quantitative review. *Psychol Bull,* 101:343–62.

Borkovec, T.D., Robinson, E., Pruzinsky, T., Dupree, J. (1983). Preliminary explanation of worry: some characteristics and processes. *Behav Res Ther,* 21:9–16.

Bovard, E.W. (1985). Brain mechanisms in effects of social support on viability. In Williams, R.M. (ed.), *Perspectives on behavioral medicine.* Orlando, FL: Academic Press, pp. 103–29.

Breckler, S.J. (1993). Emotion and attitude change. In Lewis, M., and Haviland, J.M. (eds.), *Handbook of emotions.* New York: The Guilford Press, pp. 461–74.

Breier, A., Charney, D.S., and Heninger, G.R. (1984). Major depression in patients with agoraphobia and panic disorder. *Arch Gen Psychiatry,* 41:1129–35.

Brown, G.W., and Harris, T. (1978). *Social origins of depression.* London: Tavistock.

Buss, A.H. (1961). *The psychology of aggression.* New York: Wiley.

Cacioppo, J.T., Klein, D.J., Berntson, G.G., and Hatfield, E. (1993). The psychophysiology of emotion. In Lewis, M., and Haviland, J.M., (eds.), *Handbook of emotion.* New York: Guilford Press, pp. 119–42.

Cannon, W.B. (1927). The James-Lange theory of emotion: a critical examination and alternative theory. *Am J Psychol,* 39:106–24.

Carney, R.M., Rich, M.W., te Velde, A., Saini, J., Clark, K., and Jaffe, A.S. (1987). Major depressive disorder in coronary artery disease. *Am J Cardiol,* 60(16):1273–5.

Charney, D.S. and Heninger, G.R. (1986). Abnormal regulation of noradrenergic function in panic disorders: effects of clonidine in healthy subjects and patients with agoraphobia and panic disorder. *Arch Gen Psychiatry,* 43:1042–54.

Clark, L.A. (1989). The anxiety and depressive disorders: descriptive psychopathology and differential diagnosis. In Kendall, P.C., and Watson, D. (eds.), *Anxiety and depression: distinctive and overlapping features.* New York: Academic Press, pp. 83–129.

Clark, L.A., and Watson, D. (1991). Tripartite model of anxiety and depression: psychometric considerations and taxonomic implications. *J Abnorm Psychol,* 100:316–36.

Clark, L.A., and Watson, D. (1994). Distinguishing functional from dysfunctional affective responses. In Ekman, P., and Davidson, R.J. (eds.). *The nature of emotion.* New York: Oxford University Press, pp. 131–7.

Cohen, S. (1996). Psychological stress, immunity, and upper respiratory infections. *Curr Directions Psychol Sci,* 5(3):86–90.

Cohen, S., and Rodriguez, M.S. (1995). Pathways linking affective disturbances and physical disorders. *Health Psychol,* 14:374–80.

Cohen, S., Tyrrell, D.A.J., and Smith, A.P. (1991). Psychological stress in humans and susceptibility to the common cold. *N Engl J Med,* 325:606–12.

Cohen, S., Tyrrell, D.A.J., and Smith, A.P. (1993). Negative life events, perceived stress, negative affect, and susceptibility to the common cold. *J Person Soc Psychol,* 64:131–40.

Cohen, S., Doyle, W.J., Skoner, D.P., Fireman, P., Gwaltney, J.M., and Newsom, J.T. (1995a). State and trait negative affect as predictors of objective and subjective symptoms of respiratory viral infections. *J Person Soc Psychol,* 68(1):159–69.

Cohen, S., Kessler, R.C., and Gordon, L.U. (1995b). Strategies for measuring stress in studies of psychiatric and physical disorders. In Cohen, S., Kessler, R.C., and Gordon, L.U. (eds.), *Measuring stress: a guide for health and social scientists.* New York: Oxford University Press. pp. 3–26.

Coryell, W., Noyes, R., and Clancy, J. (1982). Excess mortality in panic disorder. *Arch Gen Psychiatry,* 39:701–3.

Coryell, W., Noyes, R., and House, J.D. (1986). Mortality among outpatients with anxiety disorders. *Am J Psychiatry,* 143:508–10.

Cousins, N. (1979). *The anatomy of an illness, as perceived by the patient.* New York: Norton.

Davies, M.J., and Thomas, A. (1984). Thrombosis and acute coronary-artery lesions in sudden cardiac ischemic death. *N Engl J Med,* 310:1137–40.

Davison, K., and Petrie, K. (1997). Emotional expression and health. In Baum, A., Newman, S., Weinman, J., West, R., and McManus, C. (eds.), *Cambridge handbook of psychology, health, and medicine.* Cambridge: Cambridge University Press, pp. 103–6.

DeLongis, A., Coyne, J.C., Dakof, G., Folkman, S., and Lazarus, R.S. (1982). Relationship of daily hassles, uplifts, and major life events to health status. *Health Psychol,* 1:119–36.

Dembroski, T.M., Weiss, S.M., Shields, J.L., Haynes, S., and Feinleib, M. (eds.). (1978). *Coronary-prone behavior.* New York: Springer-Verlag.

Dembroski, T.M., MacDougall, J.M., Williams, R.B., Haney, T.L., and Blumenthal, J.A. (1985). Components of type A, hostility, and anger-in: relationship to angiographic findings. *Psychosom Med,* 47(3):219–33.

Dembroski, T.M., MacDougall, J.M., Costa,

P.T.J., and Grandits, G.A. (1989). Components of hostility as predictors of sudden death and myocardial infarction in the Multiple Risk Factor Intervention Trial. *Psychosom Med*, 51:514–22.

Denollet, J., Sys, S.U., Stroobant, N., Rombouts, H., Gillebert, T.C., and Brutsaert, D.L. (1996). Personality as an independent predictor of long-term mortality in patients with coronary heart disease (see comments). *Lancet*, 347(8999):417–21.

Dohrenwend, B.S., and Dohrenwend, B.P. (1974). *Stressful life events: their nature and effects*. New York: Wiley.

Dunner, D. (1985). Anxiety and panic: relationship to depression and cardiac disorders. *Psychosomatics*, 26 Suppl 11:18–22.

Eaker, E.D., Pinsky, J., and Castelli, W.P. (1992). Myocardial infarction and coronary death among women: psychosocial predictors from a 20-year follow-up of women in the Framingham Study. *Am J Epidemiol*, 135(8): 854–64.

Ekman, P., Levenson, R.W., and Friesen, W.V. (1983). Autonomic nervous system activity distinguishes among emotions. *Science*, 221: 1208–10.

Ellsworth, P.C. (1991). Some implications of cognitive appraisal theories of emotion. In Strongman, K.T. (ed.), *International Review of Studies of Emotion*. New York: John Wiley, pp. 143–61.

Ellsworth, P.C., and Smith, C.A. (1988). From appraisal to emotion: differences among unpleasant feelings. *Motivation Emotion*, 12(3):271–302.

Eriksen, C.W. (1966). Cognitive responses to internally cued anxiety. In Spielberger, C.D. (ed.), *Anxiety and behavior*. New York: Academic Press, pp. 327–60.

Everson, S.A., Kauhanen, J., Kaplan, G.A., Goldberg, D.E., Julkunen, J., Tuomilehto, J., and Salonen, J.T. (1997a). Hostility and increased risk of mortality and acute myocardial infarction: the mediating role of behavioral risk factors. *Am J Epidemiol*, 146:142–52.

Everson, S.A., Lynch, J.W., Chesney, M.A., Kaplan, G.A., Goldberg, D.E., Shade, S.B., Cohen, R.D., Salonen, R., and Salonen, J.T. (1997b). Interaction of workplace demands and cardiovascular reactivity in progression of carotid atherosclerosis: population based study. *Br Med J*, 314:553–8.

Falk, E. (1983). Plaque rupture with severe preexisting stenosis precipitating coronary thrombosis: characteristics of coronary atherosclerotic plaques underlying fatal occlusive thrombi. *Br Heart J*, 50:127–34.

Fei, L., Anderson, M.H., Katritsis, D., Sneddon,

J., Statters, D.J., Malik, M., and Camm, A.J. (1994). Decreased heart rate variability in survivors of sudden cardiac death not associated with coronary artery disease. *Br Heart J*, 71:16–21.

Fishbein, M., and Ajzen, I. (1975). *Belief, attitude, intention, and behavior: an introduction to theory and research*. Reading, MA: Addison-Wesley.

Fleischman, A.I., Bierenbaum, M.L., and Stier, A. (1976). Effect of stress due to anticipated minor surgery upon in vivo platelet aggregation in humans. *J Hum Stress*, 2:33–7.

Ford, D.E., Mead, L.A., Chang, P.P., Cooper-Patrick, L., Wang, N.-Y., and Klag, M.J. (1998). Depression is a risk factor for coronary artery disease in men. *Arch Int Med*, 158:1422–6.

Fox, B.H., Temoshok, L., and Dreher, H. (1988). Mind-body and behavior in cancer incidence. *Advances*, 5(4):41–56.

Fredrickson, B.L. (1998). What good are positive emotions? *Rev Gen Psychol*, 2:300–19.

Fredrickson, B.L., and Levenson, R.W. (1998). Positive emotions speed recovery from the cardiovascular sequelae of negative emotions. *Cognition Emotion*, 12:191–220.

Freud, S. (1961). *Civilization and its discontents*. New York: Norton.

Friedman, H.S., and Booth-Kewley, S. (1987). The "disease-prone personality": a meta-analytic view of the construct. *Am Psychol*, 42(6):539–55.

Friedman, M. (1969). *Pathogenesis of coronary artery disease*. New York: McGraw-Hill.

Friedman, M., and Rosenman, R.H. (1959). Association of specific overt behavior pattern with blood and cardiovascular findings. *J Am Med Assoc*, 169:1286–96.

Frijda, N.H. (1986). *The emotions*. Cambridge: Cambridge University Press.

Frijda, N.H. (1993). Moods, emotions episodes, and emotions. In Lewis, M., and Haviland, J.M. (eds.), *Handbook of emotions*. New York: The Guilford Press, pp. 381–405.

Frijda, N.H. (1994). Emotions are functional, most of the time. In Ekman, P., and Davidson, R.J. (eds.), *The nature of emotion*. New York: Oxford University Press, pp. 112–22.

Gelernt, M.D., and Hochman, J.S. (1992). Acute myocardial infarction triggered by emotional stress. *Am J Cardiol*, 69:1512–3.

Gentry, W.D. (1985). Relationship of anger-coping styles and blood pressure among Black Americans. In Chesney, M.A., and Rosenman, R.H. (eds.), *Anger and hostility in cardiovascular and behavioral disorders*. New York: McGraw-Hill International Book Company, pp. 139–48.

Goldberg, R.J. (1992). Coronary heart disease:

epidemiology and risk factors. In Ockene, I.S., and Ockene, J.K. (eds.), *Prevention of coronary heart disease.* Boston: Little, Brown, pp. 3–41.

Goldstein, M.G., and Niaura, R. (1992). Psychological factors affecting physical condition: cardiovascular disease literature review. *Psychosomatics,* 33:134–5.

Gordon, J.L., Bowyer, D.E., Evans, C.W., and Mitchinson, M.J. (1973). Human platelet reactivity during stressful diagnostic procedures. *J Clin Pathol,* 26:958–62.

Gorlin, R., Fuster, V., and Ambrose, J.A. (1986). Anatomic-physiologic links between acute coronary syndromes. *Circulation,* 74:6–9.

Greer, S., and Morris, T. (1975). Psycholgocial attributes of women who develop breast cancer: a controlled study. *J Psychosom Res,* 19:147–53.

Gross, J. (1989). Emotional expression in cancer onset and progression. *Soc Sci Med,* 28(12):1239–48.

Gross, J.J., and John, O.P. (1998). Mapping the domain of expressivity: multimethod evidence for a hierarchical model. *J Person Soc Psychol,* 74(1):170–91.

Gross, J.J., and Levenson, R.W. (1993). Emotional suppression: physiology, self-report, and expressive behavior. *J Person Soc Psychol,* 64(6):970–86.

Grossarth-Maticek, R., and Eyesenck, H.J. (1990). Personality, stress and disease. *Psychol Rep,* 66:355–73.

Grossarth-Maticek, R., Bastiaans, J., and Kanazir, D.T. (1985a). Psychosocial factors as strong predictors of mortality from cancer, ischemic heart disease, and stroke: the Yugoslav prospective study. *J Psychosom Res,* 29:167–76.

Grossarth-Maticek, R., Kanazir, D.T., Schmit, P., and Vetter, H. (1985b). Psychosocial and organic variables as predictors of lung cancer, cardiac infarct and apoplexy: some differential predictors. *Personality Individual Differences,* 6:313–21.

Haft, J.I., and Arkel, Y.S. (1976). Effect of emotional stress on platelet aggregation in humans. *Chest,* 70:501–5.

Haines, A.P., Imeson, J.D., and Meade, T.W. (1987). Phobic anxiety and ischaemic heart disease. *Br Med J Clin Res Ed,* 295(6593): 297–9.

Harburg, E., Blakelock, E.H., and Roeper, P.J. (1979). Resentful and reflective coping with arbitrary authority and blood pressure: Detroit. *Psychosom Med,* 41:189–202.

Harvey, W. (1928). *Exercitatio anetomica de motu cordis et sanguinis [An anatomical exercise conerning the movement of heart and blood].* London: Baillieve, Tindall, & Cox.

Haynes, S.G., and Feinleib, M. (1980). Women, work, and coronary heart disease: prospective findings from the Framingham heart study. *Am J Public Health,* 70:133–41.

Haynes, S.G., Feinleib, M., and Kannel, W.B. (1980). The relationship of psychosocial factors to coronary heart disease in the Framingham study. III. Eight-year incidence of coronary heart disease. *Am J Epidemiol,* 111(1):37–58.

Hayward, C. (1995). Psychiatric illness and cardiovascular disease risk. *Epidemiol Rev,* 17:129–38.

Helmers, K.F., Posluszny, D.M., and Krantz, D.S. (1994). Associations of hostility and coronary artery disease: a review of studies. In Siegman, A.W., and Smith, T.W. (eds.), *Anger, hostility, and the heart.* Hillsdale, NJ: Lawrence Erlbaum.

Herbert, T.B., and Cohen, S. (1993a). Depression and immunity: a meta-analytic review. *Psychol Bull,* 113(3):472–86.

Herbert, T.B., and Cohen, S. (1993b). Stress and immunity in humans: a meta-analytic review. *Psychosom Med,* 55:364–79.

Houston, B.K. (1994). Anger, hostility, and psychophysiological reactivity. In Siegman, A.W., and Smith, T.W. (eds.), *Anger, hostility, and the heart.* Hillsdale, NJ: Lawrence Erlbaum.

Ickovics, J.R., Viscoli, C.M., and Horwitz, R.I. (1997). Functional recovery after myocardial infarction in men: the independent effects of social class. *Ann Internal Med,* 127:518–25.

Izard, C. (1977). *Human emotions.* New York: Plenum.

Jenkins, C.D., Sooervell, P.D., and Hames, C.G. (1983). Does blood pressure rise with age? . . . or with stress? *J Hum Stress,* 9:4–12.

Jonas, B.S., Franks, P., and Ingram, D.D. (1997). Are symptoms of anxiety and depression risk factors for hypertension? Longitudinal evidence from the National Health and Nutrition Examination Survey I Epidemiologic Follow-Up Study. *Arch Family Med,* 6:43–9.

Jorgensen, R.S., Johnson, B.T., Kolodziei, M.E., and Schreer, G.E. (1996). Elevated blood pressure and personality: a meta-analytic review. *Psychol Bull,* 120(2):293–320.

Julius, S., Schneider, R., and Egan, B. (1985). Suppressed anger in hypertension: facts and problems. In Chesney, M.A., and Rosenman, R.H. (eds.), *Anger and hostility in cardiovascular and behavioral disorders.* New York: McGraw-Hill, pp. 127–38.

Julkunen, J., Salonen, R., Kaplan, G.A., Chesney, M.A., and Salonen, J.T. (1994). Hostility and the progression of carotid atherosclerosis. *Psychosom Med,* 56:519–25.

Kamarck, T., and Jennings, J.R. (1991). Biobehavioral factors in sudden cardiac death. *Psychol Bull*, 109:42–75.

Kaplan, G.A., and Reynolds, P. (1988). Depression and cancer mortality and morbidity: prospective evidence from the Alameda County Study. *J Behav Med*, 11(1):1–13.

Kasl, S.V., Cobb, S., and Brooks, G.W. (1968). Changes in serum uric acid and cholesterol levels in men undergoing job loss. *J Am Med Assoc*, 206:1500–7.

Katon, W. (1986). Panic disorder: epidemiology, diagnosis, and treatment in primary care. *J Clin Psychiatry*, 10 Suppl:21–7.

Kawachi, I., Colditz, G.A., Ascherio, A., Rimm, E.B., Giovannucci, E., Stampfer, M.J., and Willett, W.C. (1994a). Prospective study of phobic anxiety and risk of coronary heart disease in men. *Circulation*, 89(5):1992–7.

Kawachi, I., Sparrow, D., Vokonas, P.S., and Weiss, S.T. (1994b). Symptoms of anxiety and risk of coronary heart disease. The Normative Aging Study. *Circulation*, 90(5): 2225–9.

Kawachi, I., Sparrow, D., Vokonas, P.S., and Weiss, S.T. (1995). Decreased heart rate variability in men with phobic anxiety (data from the Normative Aging Study). *Am J Cardiol*, 75(14):882–5.

Kawachi, I., Sparrow, D., Spiro, A., Vokonas, P., and Weiss, S.T. (1996). A prospective study of anger and coronary heart disease. The Normative Aging Study. *Circulation*, 94(9): 2090–5.

Kawachi, I., Sparrow, D., Kubzansky, L.D., Spiro, A.I., Vokonas, P.S., and Weiss, S.T. (1998). Prospective study of a self-report Type A scale and risk of coronary heart disease. Test of the MMPI-2 Type A scale. *Circulation*, 98:405–12.

Kemper, T.D. (1993). Sociological models in the explanation of emotions. In Lewis, M., and Haviland, J.M. (eds.), *Handbook of emotions*. New York: The Guilford Press, pp. 41–52.

Kessler, R.C., and Neighbors, H.W. (1986). A new perspective on the relationships among race, social class, and psychological distress. *J Health Soc Behav*, 27:107–15.

Kiecolt-Glaser, J.K., and Glaser, R. (1988). Psychological influences on immunity: implications for AIDS. *Am Psychol*, 43:892–8.

King, A.C., Barr Taylor, C., Albright, C.A., and Haskell, W.L. (1990). The relationship between repressive and defensive coping styles and blood pressure responses in healthy, middle-aged men and women. *J Psychosom Res*, 34(4):461–71.

King, L.A., and Emmons, R.A. (1991). Psychological, physical, and interpersonal correlates of emotional expressiveness, conflict, and control. *Eur J Person*, 5:131–50.

Kleiger, R.E., Miller, J.P., Bigger, J.T. Jr. and Moss, A.J. (1987). Decreased heart rate variability and its association with increased mortality after acute myocardial infarction. *Am J Cardiol*, 59(4):256–62.

Koskenvuo, M., Kaprio, J., Rose, R.J., Kesaniemi, A., Sarna, S., Heikkila, K., and Langinvainio, H. (1988). Hostility as a risk factor for mortality and ischemic heart disease in men. *Psychosom Med*, 50(4):330–40.

Krantz, D.S., and Durel, L.A. (1983). Psychobiological substrates of the Type A behavior pattern. *Health Psychol*, 2:393–411.

Kubzansky, L.D., Kawachi, I., Spiro, A. 3rd, Weiss, S.T., Vokonas, P.S., and Sparrow, D. (1997). Is worrying bad for your heart? A prospective study of worry and coronary heart disease in the Normative Aging Study. *Circulation*, 95(4):818–24.

Kubzansky, L.D., Kawachi, I., and Sparrow, D. (in press). Stress and adaptation: psychosocial predictors of allostatic load in the Normative Aging Study. *Ann Behav Med*.

Kubzansky, L.D., Kawachi, I., Weiss, S., and Sparrow, D. (1998). Anxiety and coronary heart disease: a synthesis of epidemiological, psychological, and experimental evidence. *Ann Behav Med*, 20:47–58.

Kumanyika, S., and Adams-Campbell, L.L. (1991). Obesity, diet and psychosocial fators contributing to cardiovascular disease in Blacks. *Cardiovasc Clin*, 21:47–73.

Lader, M., and Marks, I. (1973). *Clinical anxiety*. London: Heinemann.

Lazarus, R. (1994). The stable and the unstable in emotion. In Ekman, P., and Davidson, R.J. (eds.), *The nature of emotion*. New York: Oxford University Press, pp. 70–85.

Lazarus, R.L. (ed.). (1968). *Emotions and adaptation: conceptual and empirical relations*. Nebraska Symposium on Motivation, 1968. Lincoln, NE, U.S.A., University of Nebraska Press.

Lazarus, R.S. (1990). Target article: theory-based stress measurement. *Psychol Inquiry*, 1(1):3–13.

Lazarus, R.S. (1991a). *Emotion and adaptation*. New York: Oxford University Press.

Lazarus, R.S. (1991b). Progress on a cognitive-motivational-relational theory of emotion. *Am Psychol*, 46(8):819–34.

LeDoux, J.E. (1994). Emotion-specific physiological activity: don't forget about CNS physiology. In Ekman, P., and Davidson, R.J. (eds.), *The nature of emotions*. New York: Oxford University Press, pp. 248–52.

Lehrer, P.M., Isenberg, S., and Hochron, S.M. (1993). Asthma and emotion: a review. *J Asthma*, 30(1):5–21.

Leiker, M., and Hailey, B.J. (1988). A link between hostility and disease: poor health habits? *Behav Med,* 3:129–33.

Levenson, R.W. (1992). Autonomic nervous system differences among emotions. *Psychol Sci,* 3:23–7.

Levenson, R.W. (1994a). Human emotions: a functional view. In Ekman, P., and Davidson, R.J. (eds.), *The nature of emotion: fundamental questions.* New York: Oxford University Press, pp. 123–6.

Levenson, R.W. (1994b). The search for autonomic specificity. In Ekman, P., and Davidson, R.J. (eds.), *The nature of emotion.* New York: Oxford University Press, pp. 252–8.

Levenson, R.W., Ekman, P., and Friesen, W.V. (1990). Voluntary facial action generates emotion-specific autonomic nervous system activity. *Psychophysiology,* 27:363–84.

Leventhal, H., and Patrick-Miller, L. (1993). Emotion and illness: the mind is in the body. In Lewis, M., and Haviland, J.M. (eds.), *Handbook of emotions.* New York: The Guilford Press, pp. 365–80.

Levine, S.P., Towell, B.L., Suarez, A.M., Knieriem, L.K., Harris, M.M., and George, J.N. (1985). Platelet activation and secretion associated with emotional stress. *Circulation,* 71:1129–34.

Lown, B., and Verrier, R.L. (1976). Neural activity and ventricular fibrillation. *N Engl J Med,* 294(21):1165–70.

Lynch, J.W., Kaplan, G.A., and Salonen, J.T. (1997). Why do poor people behave poorly? Variation in adult health behaviours and psychosocial characteristics by stages of the socioeconomic life course. *Soc Sci Med,* 44(6):809–19.

Lynch, J.W., Kaplan, G.A., Cohen, R.D., Tuomilehto, J., and Salonen, J.T. (1996). Do cardiovascular risk factors explain the relation between socioeconomic status, risk of all-cause mortality, cardiovsacular mortality, and acute myocardial infarction? *Am J Epidemiol,* 144:934–42.

Malatesta, C.Z. (1989). Differential emotions model for the study of health and illness processes in aging. In Carsten, L.L., and Neale, J.M. (eds.), *Mechanisms of psychological influence on physical health.* New York: Plenum Press, pp. 105–28.

Manuck, S.B., and Krantz, D.S. (1986). Psychophysiologic reactivity in coronary heart disease and essential hypertension. In Matthews, K.A., Weiss, S.B., Detre, T., Dembroski, T.M., Falkner, B., and Manuck, S.B. (eds.), *Handbook of stress, reactivity, and cardiovascular disease.* New York: John Wiley, pp. 11–34.

Manuck, S.B., Morrison, R.I., Bellack, A.S., and Polefrone, J.M. (1985). Behaviour factors in

hypertension: cardiovascular responsivity, anger, and social competence. In Chesney, M.A., and Rosenman, R.H. (eds.), *Anger and hostility in cardiovascular and behavioral disorders.* New York: McGraw-Hill, pp. 149–72.

Manuck, S.B., Kaplan, J.R., Adams, M.R., and Clarkson, T.B. (1988). Studies of psychosocial influences on coronary artery atherosclerosis in cynomolgus monkeys. *Health Psychol,* 7(114):113–24.

Markovitz, J.H. (1998). Hostility is associated with increased platelet activity in coronary heart disease. *Psychosom Med,* 60:586–91.

Markovitz, J.H., Matthews, K.A., Wing, R.R., Kuller, L.H., and Meilahn, E.N. (1991). Psychological, biological and health behavior predictors of blood pressure changes in middle-aged women. *J Hypertension,* 9(5):399–406.

Markovitz, J.H., Matthews, K.A., Kannel, W.B., Cobb, J.L., and D'Agostino, R.B. (1993). Psychological predictors of hypertension in the Framingham Study. Is there tension in hypertension? (see comments). *J Am Med Assoc,* 270(20):2439–43.

Markovitz, J.H., Matthews, K.A., Kiss, J., and Smitherman, T. (1996). Effects of hostility on platelet reactivity to psychological stress in coronary heart disease patients and healthy controls. *Psychosom Med,* 58:143–9.

Marmot, M., and Winkelstein, W. Jr. (1975). Epidemiologic observations on intervention trials for prevention of coronary heart disease. *Am J Epidemiol,* 101(3):177–81.

Marshall, J.R. (1972). The expression of feelings. *Arch Gen Psychiatry,* 27:786–90.

Matsumoto, Y., Uyama, O., Shimizu, S., Michishita, H., Mori, R., Owada, T., and Sugita, M. (1993). Do anger and aggression affect carotid atherosclerosis? *Stroke,* 24:983–6.

Matthews, K.A. (1985). Assessment of Type A behavior, anger, and hostility in epidemiological studies of cardiovascular disease. In Ostfeld, A.M., and Eaker, E.D. (eds.), *Measuring psychosocial variables in epidemiologic studies of cardiovascular disease.* Washington, DC: U.S. Department of Health and Human Services, National Institutes of Health. NIH Publication No. 85-2270, pp. 153–84.

Matthews, K.A. (1988). Coronary heart disease and Type A behaviors: update on and alternative to the Booth-Kewley and Friedman (1987) quantitative review. *Psychol Bull,* 104:373–80.

Matthews, K.A., Glass, D.C., Rosenman, R.H., and Bortner, R.W. (1977). Competitive drive, Pattern A, and coronary heart disease: a further analysis of some data from the Western Collaborative Group Study. *J Chronic Dis,* 30:489–98.

Matthews, K.M., Manuck, S.B., and Saab, P.G. (1986). Cardiovascular responses of adolescents during a naturally occurring stressor and their behavioral and psychophysiological predictors. *Psychophysiology,* 23(2): 198–209.

Matthews, K.A., Owens, J.F., Kuller, L.H., Sutton-Tyrrell, K., and Jansen-McWilliams, L. (1998). Are hostility and anxiety associated with carotid atherosclerosis in healthy postmenopausal women? *Psychosom Med,* 60(5): 633–8.

Mest, H.J., Zehl, U., Sziegoleit, W., Taube, C., and Forster, W. (1982). Influence of mental stress on plasma level of prostaglandins, thromboxane B, and on circulating platelet aggregates in man. *Prostaglandins Leukot Med,* 8:553–63.

Miller, T.Q., Smith, T.W., Turner, C.W., Guijarro, M.L., and Hallet, A.J. (1996). A meta-analytic review of research on hostility and physical health. *Psychol Bull,* 119(2): 322–48.

Mirowsky, J.I., and Ross, C.E. (1980). Minority status, ethnic culture, and distress: a comparison of Blacks, Whites, Mexicans, and Mexican-Americans. *Am J Sociol,* 86(3):479–95.

Mittleman, M.A., Maclure, M., Sherwood, J.B., Mulry, R.P., Tofler, G.H., Jacobs, S.C., Friedman, R., Benson, H., and Muller, J.E. (1995). Triggering of acute myocardial infarction onset by episodes of anger. Determinants of Myocardial Infarction Onset Study Investigators (see comments). *Circulation,* 92(7):1720–5.

Myerburg, R., and Castellanos, A. (1992). Cardiac arrest and sudden cardiac death. In Braunwald, E. (ed.), *Heart disease: a textbook of cardiovascular medicine.* Philadelphia: W.B. Saunders, pp. 756–89.

Myers, D.G., and Diener, E. (1995). Who is happy? *Psychol Sci,* 6(1):10–9.

Neiss, R. (1988). Reconceptualizing arousal: psychobiological states in motor performance. *Psychol Bull,* 103(3):345–66.

Niaura, R., and Goldstein, M.G. (1992). Psychological factors affecting physical condition: cardiovascular disease literature review. *Psychosomatics,* 33(2):146–55.

Noyes, R., Clancy, J., Hoenk, P.R., and Slymen, D.R. (1978). Anxiety neurosis and physical illness. *Comprehensive Psychiatry,* 19:407–13.

Nunes, E.V., Frank, K.A., and Kornfield, D.S. (1987). Psychologic treatment for Type A behavior pattern and for coronary heart disease: a meta-analysis of the literature. *Psychosom Med,* 48:159–73.

Ohman, A. (1993). Fear and anxiety as emotional phenomena: clinical phenomenology, evolutionary perspectives, and information-processing mechanisms. In Lewis, M., and Haviland, J.M. (eds.), *Handbook of emotions.* New York: The Guilford Press, pp. 511–36.

O'Leary, A. (1990). Stress, emotion, and human immune function. *Psychol Bull,* 108:363–82.

Pennebaker, J.W. (1997). Writing about emotional experiences as a therapeutic process. *Psychol Sci,* 8(3):162–66.

Pennebaker, J., and Beall, S.K. (1986). Confronting a traumatic event: toward an understanding of inhibition and disease. *J Abnorm Psychol,* 95:274–81.

Pennebaker, J., and Susman, J. (1988). Disclosure of traumas and psychosomatic processes. *Soc Sci Med,* 26:327–32.

Pennebaker, J., Kiecolt-Glaser, J., and Glaser, R. (1988). Disclosure of trauma and immune function: health implications for psychotherapy. *J Consult Clin Psychol,* 56:239–45.

Pernini, C., Muller, F.B., and Buhler, F.R. (1991). Suppressed aggression accelerates early development of essential hypertension. *J Hypertens,* 9:499–503.

Pettingale, K.W. (1985). Towards a psychobiological model of cancer: biological considerations. *Soc Sci Med,* 20(8):779–87.

Plato (1927). *(Dialogues. English & Greek) Charmides; Alcibiades I and II; Hipparchus; The lovers; Theages; Minos; Epinomis/ Plato.* Cambridge, MA: Harvard University Press.

Plutchik, R. (1980). *Emotion: a psychoevolutionary synthesis.* New York: Harper & Row.

Pratt, L.A., Ford, D.E., Crum, R.M., Armenian, H.K., Gallo, J.J., and Eaton, W.W. (1996). Depression, psychotropic medication, and risk of myocardial infarction: prospective data from the Baltimore ECA follow-up. *Circulation,* 94:3123–9.

Rabin, B.S., Cohen, S., Ganguli, R., Lysle, D.R., and Cunnick, J.E. (1989). Bidirectional interaction between the central nervous system and the immune system. *Crit Rev Immunol,* 9:279–312.

Rasmussen, K., Ravnsbaek, J., Funch-Jenson, P., and Bagger, J.P. (1986). Oesophageal spasm in patients with coronary artery spasm. *Lancet,* 1(8474):174–6.

Reich, J.W., and Zautra, A.J. (1990). Dispositional control beliefs and the consequences of a control-enhancing intervention. *J Gerontol,* 45(2):46.

Reich, P., DeSilva, R.A., Lown, B., and Murawski, B.J. (1981). Acute psychological disturbance preceding life-threatening ventricular arrhythmias. *J Am Med Assoc,* 246: 233–5.

Reker, G.T. (1997). Personal meaning, optimism, and choice: existential predictors of depression in community and institutional elderly. *Gerontologist*, 37(6):709–16.

Review Panel on Coronary-Prone Behavior and Coronary Heart Disease. (1981). Coronary-prone behavior and coronary heart disease: a critical review. *Circulation*, 63:1169–215.

Rime, B., Philippot, P., Boca, S., and Mesquita, B. (1992). Long-lasting cognitive and social consequences of emotion: social sharing and rumination. In Stroebe, W., and Hewstone, M. (eds.), *European review of social psychology*. New York: John Wiley, p. 3.

Robinson, J.P., Shaver, P.R., and Wrightsman, L.S. (eds.). (1991). *Measures of personality and social psychological attitudes*. Measures of social psychological attitudes. New York: Academic Press.

Rodin, J. (1986). Aging and health: effects of the sense of control. *Science*, 233:1271–6.

Roseman, I. (1984). Cognitive determinants of emotions: a structural theory. In Shaver, P. (ed.), *Emotions, relationships and health*. Beverly Hills: Sage, 5:11–36.

Rosenman, R.H. (1985). Health consequences of anger and implications for treatment. In Chesney, M.A., and Rosenman, R.H. (eds.), *Anger and hostility in cardiovascular and behavioral disorders*. New York: McGraw-Hill, pp. 103–26.

Scheier, M.F., and Carver, C.S. (1987). Dispositional optimism and physical well-being: the influence of generalized outcome expectancies on health. *J Person*, 55(2):169–210.

Scherer, K.R. (1982). Emotion as a process: function, origin and regulation. *Soc Sci Inform*, 21(4–5):555–70.

Schwartz, G.E., and Weinberger, D.A. (1980). Patterns of emotional responses to affective situations: relations among happiness, sadness, anger, fear, depression, and anxiety. *Motivation Emotion*, 4:175–91.

Seeman, T.E., and McEwen, B.S. (1996). Impact of social environment characteristics on neuroendocrine regulation. *Psychosom Med*, 58:459–71.

Selye, H. (1950). *The physiology and pathology of exposure to stress*. Montreal: Acta.

Sesso, H.D., Kawachi, I., Vokonas, P.S., and Sparrow, D. (1998). Depression and the risk of coronary heart disease in the Normative Aging Study. *Am J Cardiol*, 82:851–56.

Shaver, P.R., and Brennan, K.A. (1991). Measures of depression and loneliness. In Robinson, J.P., Shaver, P.R., and Wrightsman, L.S. (eds.) *Measures of personality and social psychological attitudes*. New York: Academic Press, pp. 195–290.

Shedler, J., Mayman, M., and Manis, M. (1993). The illusion of mental health. *Am Psychol*, 48(11):1117–31.

Shekelle, R.B., Raynor, W.J.J., Ostfeld, A.M., Garron, D.C., Bieliauskas, L.A., Liu, S.C., Maliza, C., and Paul, O. (1981). Psychological depression and 17-year risk of death from cancer. *Psychosom Med*, 43(2):117–25.

Shekelle, R.B., Gale, M., Ostfeld, A.M., and Paul, O. (1983). Hostility, risk of coronary heart disease, and mortality. *Psychosom Med*, 45:109–14.

Siegler, I.C. (1994). Hostility and risk: demographic and lifestyle variables. In Siegman, A.W., and Smith, T.W. (eds.), *Anger, hostility, and the heart*. Hillsdale, NJ: Lawrence Erlbaum, pp. 199–214.

Siegman, A.W. (1994a). Cardiovascular consequences of expressing and repressing anger. In Siegman, A.W., and Smith, T.W. (eds.), *Anger, hostility and the heart*. Hillsdale, NJ: Lawrence Erlbaum, pp. 173–98.

Siegman, A.W. (1994b). From Type A to hostility to anger: reflections on the history of coronary-prone behavior. In Siegman, W., and Smith, T.W. (eds.), *Anger, hostility and the heart*. Hillsdale, NJ: Erlbaum, pp. 1–21.

Smith, A., Tyrrell, D.A., Barrow, G.I., Higgins, P.G., Bull, S., Trickett, S., and Wilkins, A.J. (1992). Mood and experimentally-induced respiratory virus infections and illnesses. *Psychol Health*, 6(3):205–12.

Smith, C.A., and Ellsworth, P.C. (1985). Patterns of cognitive appraisal in emotion. *J Person Soc Psychol*, 48(4):813–38.

Smith, C.A., and Ellsworth, P.C. (1987). Patterns of appraisal and emotion in taking an exam. *J Person Soc Psychol*, 52(3):1–14.

Smith, C.A., and Lazarus, R.S. (1993). Appraisal components, core relational themes, and the emotions. *Cognition Emotion*, 7(3/4):233–69.

Smith, C.A., and Pope, L.K. (1992). Appraisal and emotion: the interactional contributions of dispositional and situational factors. In Clark, M.S. (ed.), *Emotion and Social Behavior*. Newbury Park, CA: Sage, 14: pp. 32–62.

Smith, T.W. (1992). Hostility and health: current status of a psychosomatic hypothesis. *Health Psychol*, 11:139–50.

Smith, T.W., and Frohm, K.D. (1985). What's so unhealthy about hostility? Construct validity and psychosocial correlates of the Cook and Medley Ho scale. *Health Psychol*, 4(6):503–20.

Sommers-Flanagan, J., and Greenberg, R.P. (1989). Psychosocial variables and hypertension: a new look at an old controversy. *J Nerv Mental Dis*, 177(1):15–24.

Spielberger, C.D., and Sarason, J.G. (1978).

Stress and anxiety. Washington, DC: Hemisphere.

Spielberger, C.D., Johnson, E.H., Russell, S.F., Crane, R.J., Jacobs, G.A., and Worden, T.J. (1985). The experience and expression of anger: construction and validation of an anger expression scale. In Chesney, M.A., and Rosenman, R.H. (eds.), *Anger and hostility in cardiovascular and behavioral disorders.* Washington, DC: Hemisphere, pp. 5–30.

Stone, A.A. (1995). Measurement of affective response. In Cohen, S., Kessler, R.C., and Gordon, L.U. (eds.), *Measuring stress.* New York: Oxford University Press, pp. 148–71.

Stone, A.A., Cox, D.S., Valdimarsdottir, H., and Jansdorf, L. (1987). Evidence that secretory IgA antibody is associated with daily mood. *J Person Soc Psychol,* 52:988–93.

Stone, A.A., Neale, J.M., Cox, D.S., and Napoli, A. (1994). Daily events are associated with a secretory immune response to an oral antigen in men. *Health Psychol,* 13:440–18.

Syme, S.L. (1993). *The social environment and health.* The 11th Honda Foundation Discoveries Symposium: prosperity and Well-Being, Toronto, Canada.

Talbott, E., Kuller, L.H., Perper, J., and Murphy, P.A. (1981). Sudden unexpected death in women: biologic and psychosocial origins. *Am J Epidemiol,* 114:671–82.

Taylor, S.E., Repetti, R.L., and Seeman, T. (1997). Health psychology: what is an unhealthy environment and how does it get under the skin? *Ann Rev Psychol,* 48:411–47.

Temoshok, L. (1987). Personality, coping style, emotion, and cancer: toward and integrative model. *Cancer Surv,* 6:545–67.

Tennant, C.C., and Langeluddecke, P.M. (1985). Psychological correlates of coronary heart disease. *Psychol Med,* 15:581–8.

Tennant, C.C., Langeluddecke, P.M., Fulcher, G., and Wilby, J. (1987). Anger and other psychological factors in coronary atherosclerosis. *Psychol Med,* 17:425–31.

Thoits, P.A. (1982). Life stress, social support, and psychological vulnerability: epidemiological considerations. *J Commun Psychol,* 10:341–62.

Tofler, G.H., Stone, P.H., Maclure, M., Edelman, E., Davis, V.G., Robertson, T., Antman, E.H., and Muller, J.E. (1990). Analysis of possible triggers of acute myocardial infarction (the MILIS Study). *Am J Cardiol,* 66:22–7.

Tomaka, J., Blascovich, J., Kelsey, R.M., and Leitten, C.L. (1993). Subjective, physiological, and behavioral effects of threat and challenge appraisal. *J Person Soc Psychol,* 65(2):248–60.

Tomkins, S. (1963). *Affect, imagery, and con-sciousness,* vol. 11: *the negative affects.* New York: Springer.

Turner, R.J., and Noh, S. (1983). Class and psychological vulnerability among women: the significance of social support and personal control. *J Health Soc Behav,* 24:2–15.

Ulbrich, P.M., Warheit, G.J., and Zimmerman, R.S. (1989). Race, socioeconomic status, and psychological distress: an examination of differential vulnerability. *J Health Soc Behav,* 30:131–46.

Vogt, T., Pope, C., Mullooly, J., and Hollis, J. (1994). Mental health status as a predictor of morbidity and mortality: a 15 year follow-up of members of a health maintenance organization. *Am J Public Health,* 84:227–31.

Warheit, G.J., Holzer, C.E.I., and Schwab, J.J. (1973). An analysis of social class and racial differences in depressive symptomatology: a community study. *J Health Soc Behav,* 14:291–99.

Warrenburg, S., Levine, J., Schwartz, G.E., Fontana, A.F., Kemp, R.D., Delaney, R., and Mattson, R. (1989). Defensive coping and blood pressure reactivity in medical patients. *J Behav Med,* 12(5):407–24.

Wassertheil-Smoller, S., Applegate, W.B., Berge, K., Chang, C.J., Davis, B.R., Grimm, R.J., Kostis, J., Pressel, S., and Schron, E. (1996). Change in depression as a precursor of cardiovascular events. SHEP Cooperative Research Group (Systolic hypertension in the elderly). *Arch Intern Med,* 156:553–61.

Weinberger, D., Schwartz, G., and Davidson, R. (1979). Low anxious, high-anxious, and repressive coping styles: psychometric patterns and behavioral and physiological responses to stress. *J Abnorm Psychol,* 88:369–80.

Weiss, T., and Engel, B.T. (1971). Operant conditioning of heart rate in patients with premature ventricular contractions. *Psychosom Med,* 33:301–21.

Weissman, M.M., Markowitz, J.S., Ouellette, R., Greenwald, S., and Kahn, J.P. (1990). Panic disorder and cardiovascular/cerebrovascular problems: results from a community survey. *Am J Psychiatry,* 147:1504–8.

Wells, K.B., Golding, J.M., and Burnam, M.A. (1989). Affective, substances use, and anxiety disorders in persons with arthritis, diabetes, heart disease, high blood pressure, or chronic lung conditions. *Gen Hosp Psychiatry,* 11:320–7.

Wenneberg, S.R., Schneider, R.H., Walton, K.G., MacLean, C.R., Levitsky, D.K., Mandarino, J.V., Waziri, R., and Wallace, R.K. (1997). Anger expression correlates with platelet aggregation. *Behav Med,* 22(4):174–7.

Williams, S.J., and Bendelow, G. (1996). Emotions, health and illness: the 'missing link' in sociology? In James, V., and Gabe, J. (eds.), *Health and the sociology of emotions*. Cambridge, MA: Blackwell, pp. 25–54.

Williams, R.B., Haney, T.L., Lee, K.L., Kong, Y.H., Blumenthal, J.A., and Whalen, R.E. (1980). Type A behavior, hostility, and coronary atherosclerosis. *Psychosom Med,* 42:539–49.

Williams, R., Zyzanski, S.J., and Wright, A.L. (1992). Life events and daily hassles and uplifts as predictors of hospitalization and outpatient visitation. *Soc Sci Med,* 34:763–8.

Zillman, D. (1979). *Hostility and aggression.* Hillsdale, NJ: Lawrence Erlbaum.

Zyzanski, S.J., Jenkins, D., Ryan, T.J., Flessas, A., and Everist (1976). Psychological correlates of coronary angiographic findings. *Arch Intern Med,* 136:1234–7.

11

Health Behaviors in a Social Context

KAREN M. EMMONS

The impact of health behaviors on chronic disease morbidity and mortality is well known. The recent Harvard Report on Cancer Prevention concluded that two-thirds of all cancer deaths can be linked to modifiable behaviors, such as smoking, diet and obesity, and lack of exercise (Colditz et al. 1996). An extension of this analysis concluded that, by utilizing currently available intervention and early detection strategies, it should be possible to reduce cancer mortality in the United States by approximately 60% (Willett et al. 1996). Strong relationships also exist between health behaviors and risk for cardiovascular disease (American Heart Association 1996). Current recommendations call for substantial changes in the lifestyles of the American population in order to reduce the incidence of chronic disease (U.S. Department of Health and Human Services [DHHS] 1990; 1996a,b; Greenwald et al. 1995; U.S. Preventive Services Task Force 1996). For example, the latest health promotion guidelines include accumulation of at least 30 minutes of moderate physical activity on most days of the week, consumption of 30% or less of calories from fat, consumption of 20–30 g of fiber per day, and consumption of five or more servings of fruits and vegetables per day. In addition, the Healthy People 2000 goals include reduction of smoking prevalence in the United States to 15% or less and an increase in the use of sunscreen and other sun protection strategies to 60% of the population.

The purpose of this chapter is to review selectively data on risk factor change and to examine some of the factors that may explain the relatively low rate of long-term change produced by most health promotion interventions. Social contextual factors (e.g. educational attainment, socioeconomic status, role responsibilities, living circumstances, personal and community material resources) play a critical role in adoption and maintenance of preventive health behaviors; the impact of these factors on intervention outcomes will be explored. In particular, the need to integrate individual and population-based approaches will be emphasized, and examples and recommendations for integrated intervention approaches will be discussed. It will be argued that innovations in behavior change treatment must also draw upon insights from social epidemiology and integrate population-based strategies for dealing with social factors together with those developed for individual-level change. Some researchers have argued that health promotion interventions have failed and thus should not continue to be the focus of substantial research efforts; the premise of this chapter is that a great deal has been learned and that the potential exists to produce more effective intervention outcomes if what we already know is incorporated appropriately into health promotion intervention efforts, particularly at the population level.

RISK FACTOR PREVALENCE

Although there have been significant changes in health behaviors of the United States population over the last 25 years, the prevalence of many such behaviors is still far from recommended levels. In 1992, the most recent year that physical activity levels were measured in relation to the Healthy People 2000 Goals, only 24% of Americans were reaching recommended levels of activity; this represents just a 2% increase in prevalence of physical activity from 1985 (U.S. DHHS 1996a). Sedentary behavior is pervasive. Over 29% of adults in the United States report that they get little or no regular physical activity (U.S. DHHS 1996a). Despite the strong scientific evidence supporting the role of fruit and vegetable intake as a protective factor against cancer, only 20%–30% of Americans consume the recommended five or more servings per day (Subar et al. 1992, 1995; Serdula et al. 1995; Krebs-Smith et al. 1995). Further, recent data suggests that nearly 26% of the U.S. population continue to smoke (Centers for Disease Control [CDC] 1996). Although smoking prevalence has steadily declined among adults in the United States, the smoking rate among adolescents has remained relatively constant, fluctuating between 27.5% and 22.9% from 1987 through 1994, with rates increasing in recent years.

DISPROPORTIONATE RISK BY INCOME AND RACE/ETHNICITY— POCKETS OF RISK AND RISK FACTOR PREVALENCE

Chronic disease morbidity and mortality is disproportionately high among lower socioeconomic groups and some ethnic groups. For example, cancer incidence among white males in 1989 was 157.2 per 100,000, compared to 230.6 in black males; and 110.7 per 100,000 among white females, compared to 130.9 among black females (ACS, 1997). Cancer morbidity is also consistently associated with socioeconomic status (SES), regardless of how SES is measured (Tomatis 1992). Many risk factors for chronic disease are also more prevalent among lower-SES groups, and some important health behavior patterns vary by race and ethnicity (Emmons et al. 1994b; Osler 1993). For example, in relation to total food expenditures in 1990–1991, blacks devoted a greater proportion of their food expenditures to meats, poultry, fish, and eggs (37%) compared to Hispanics (29%) and whites (26%) (Interagency Board for Nutrition Monitoring and Related Research 1993). Hispanics had the greatest proportion of food expenditures for fruits and vegetables, relative to other ethnic groups. In a nationally representative sample of the U.S. population surveyed in 1989–1991, those with household incomes less than $10,000 consumed a mean of 3.6 servings of fruits and vegetables per day, compared with 4.8 servings among those with incomes greater than $50,000 (Krebs-Smith et al. 1995). Adjusting for caloric intake, only 16.3% of those in the low-income group met the Healthy People 2000 goal for fruit and vegetable consumption, compared to 28.9% of the higher-income group. Similarly, low-income households experienced less reduction in red meat consumption between 1978 to 1988 (Interagency Board 1993). Regarding physical activity, racial/ethnic minority populations are less active than white Americans, with the largest differences found among women (Caspersen et al. 1986; Caspersen and Merritt 1992; DiPietro and Caspersen 1991). Patterns of physical activity are also directly related to educational level and income (Caspersen et al. 1986; Siegal et al. 1993; CDC 1990; Folsom et al. 1985). Educational status is the strongest predictor of smoking status (Pierce et al. 1989; Novotny et al. 1988); in addition, African Americans are more likely to smoke than whites and Hispanics, while Hispanics have the lowest smoking prevalence. White smokers, however, have the highest cigarette consumption rate of smokers in any racial group (CDC 1996b,c).

HEALTH BEHAVIOR CHANGE INTERVENTIONS

In the last two decades, there has been a large volume of health behavior intervention research targeting chronic disease risk factors. These interventions have primarily focused on individuals, although a more recent generation of research has utilized community intervention trials and studies that target change among both organizations and individuals.

Individually Targeted Interventions

Reviews of behavior change interventions suggest that more intensive programs and those targeted at high-risk populations have the strongest outcome effects (Sorensen et al., 1998; Bowen et al. 1994; Bowen and Tinker 1995). These intervention strategies are typically studied in a reactive model, where participants who are ready to change are more likely to approach a specialty clinic or respond to advertisements for study programs. An examination of trends in smoking cessation outcomes, for example, revealed that the average 6- and 12-month abstinence rates are roughly 30%–35% (Shiffman 1993). The development of behavioral intervention strategies for smoking

cessation in the 1960s and 1970s represented a true innovation in treatment (Bernstein 1969). However, as noted by Shiffman, with the exception of nicotine replacement therapy there have since been few real innovations in smoking treatment (1993). Further, the most effective smoking cessation approaches have utilized intensive clinic-based models; a major drawback of these reactive intervention approaches is that the population impact is quite limited, because only a relatively small proportion of the target population participates in clinic-based programs (Abrams et al. 1997; Lichtenstein et al. 1996). The importance of intervention strategies that maximize intervention intensity, while increasing both the reach and impact of intervention efforts, has been recognized (Sorensen et al., in press; Abrams et al. 1996).

A number of more recent studies have utilized population-based approaches to delivery of smoking cessation and other types of health behavior interventions (Lichtenstein and Glasgow 1997; Lichtenstein et al. 1996). One strategy that has received increasing attention has been the use of tailored interventions that utilize technologic strategies to deliver intervention messages designed especially for a particular individual based on relevant and important personal information (Rimer and Glassman 1997). These are often proactive interventions that deliver tailored materials to a defined population (e.g., HMO members), regardless of whether or not the individuals are seeking to change. Two strategies that have received considerable research attention are tailored print communications (Rimer et al. 1994; King et al. 1994; Velicer et al. 1993) and tailored telephone counseling (Curry et al. 1995). Tailored interventions are typically algorithm-based and utilize computer-based "expert systems" programs that match a large library of messages to patient information needs, combining specific statements and graphics into a personalized intervention. Some tailored interventions have been found to increase short-term behavior change rates (Rimer and Glassman 1997; King et al. 1994; Davis et al., in press; Curry et al. 1995). The impact of tailored interventions, particularly telephone-based interventions, on long-term behavior change is less clear (Lichtenstein et al. 1996).

Tailored interventions have tremendous advantages over more intensive clinical interventions because they can accomplish the same kind of patient-matching of intervention strategies but can be delivered on a population level. However, these types of interventions do have limits for the types of populations to which they may be applicable to. For example, tailored interventions typically rely on completion of extensive questionnaire batteries either by telephone or in person (Velicer et al. 1993). Chronic disease risk factors are concentrated in lower-income populations that are less likely to be accessible by telephone (Resnicow et al. 1996) and more likely to have low literacy skills (Williams et al. 1995; Kirsch et al. 1993). Another problem with tailored interventions is that they rarely consider social contextual factors that may be critical for health behavior change to occur among socioeconomically and politically disadvantaged groups. The transition from clinical to population-based approaches may be limited if intervention innovations continue to ignore issues related to the social environment in which target populations live, and which can profoundly impact on health behaviors. Tailored intervention strategies could be an effective means of targeting the pockets of heightened prevalence in which disease risk is clustered (Feinleib 1996; Fisher 1995); however, unless such interventions are perceived as relevant to the issues faced on a daily basis by the target population, the likelihood of achieving either short-term or sustained intervention impact is greatly diminished. Addressing these social factors in the context of tailored interventions may require the use of alternative intervention delivery strategies, such as using peer health advisors to deliver interventions in workplace (Dacey Allen et al., submitted), or home-based settings (Emmons 1994a). This issue is discussed in further detail in the sections that follow.

Community-Based Interventions

Community-based health promotion interventions that utilize the organization as the unit of analysis have been conducted in the context of large community trials, in workplaces, in schools, and in health care settings. This population-based intervention approach is considered by many to be superior to those targeting only high-risk or highly motivated individuals (Rose 1992; McKinlay 1993). Community-based population-level approaches do have a much greater potential for impacting behavior among a larger number of people, although these interventions are typically much less intensive than individually targeted interventions, and therefore the intervention effects for the individual tend to be much smaller. Some of the community-based studies conducted to date have found no intervention effects across all studied risk factors (see Glasgow et al. 1995), and others have found effects only on some of the targeted behaviors (see Sorensen et al. 1996; 1998, for a full discussion of the effects of community-based trials). Overall, community interventions have yielded many significant effects; however, the magnitude of those effects has been small at the individual level.

Limits of Behavior Change Interventions

Several reasons have been put forth to explain why the risk-factor reduction interventions studied to date have had limited effects. First, there are strong *secular trends* in the United States related to most behavioral risk factors (Sorensen et al. 1998). In the presence of strong secular trends, it may be very difficult for most health behavior interventions to demonstrate strong effects because enormous effect sizes would be required to outperform the secular trends. The history of smoking in the United States provides an interesting case study of this issue. For example, in the past 30 years, smoking prevalence in the United States has dropped from 52% to 25.5% (CDC 1996a). Intervention trials have observed large smoking cessation rates in the control groups (e.g., Sorensen et al. 1996; Terborg and Glasgow, in press). There have also been concomitant changes in social norms related to smoking that have led to much greater restrictions in smoking in both public and private settings. The tobacco industry had been seemingly impervious to legal action and threats of regulation (Kluger 1996). However, the scientific, legal, political, and advocacy events of the last decade have for the first time in its history placed the tobacco industry in the position of having to negotiate with legal, public health, and governmental representatives regarding the regulation of nicotine, advertisement of smoking, and development of extensive strategies for prevention of tobacco use among youth.

These unprecedented changes related to cigarette smoking and its regulation are still unfolding, but it is clear that the social environment related to smoking has been dramatically changed in the United States. The impact of these societal norms on smoking outperforms any intervention outcomes found to date at the population level, and it is likely that these strong secular trends will continue. However, one question that arises is, To what extent will these societal changes affect smoking prevalence among less educated, underserved populations. There is an inverse relationship between social class and smoking prevalence (Winkleby et al. 1990; Pierce et al. 1989, Novotny et al. 1988); smoking prevalence is more than three times higher among those with only 11 years of education, compared to college graduates (38.2% vs. 12.3%, respectively) (CDC 1996b). Similar inverse relationships have also been observed between education and other behavioral risk factors (Patterson and Block 1988; Interagency Board 1995; Emmons et al. 1994). Historically, both community- and clinic-based efforts to reduce behavioral risk factors have not been effective with lower socioeconomic status groups, although a few notable exceptions

are reviewed in the next section. Although an extensive social epidemiological literature addresses the relationship between social factors and health outcomes, little attention has been paid in the context of intervention research to social contextual factors that influence health behaviors. This is discussed in greater detail below.

A concern that has been raised by public health advocates regarding health behavior change interventions is the strong focus on the individual level and *the limited focus on environmental or organizational variables*. Although studies conducted in organizational settings have the advantage of being able to affect the organizational environment and policies, relatively few studies have capitalized on this opportunity or have reported outcomes of environmental interventions. Notable exceptions are population-based studies that utilize the organization (e.g., work site or school) as the unit of intervention and randomization. For example, the COMMIT study, a community intervention trial targeting smoking cessation, focused on work sites, among other community organizations, as a key intervention channel. The intervention was aimed at increasing the prevalence of worksite tobacco control policies, increasing access to smoking cessation resources, and increasing worksite participation in other community cessation efforts. Work sites in the intervention communities reported offering more smoking cessation resources for employees compared to those in the control communities (Glasgow et al. 1996); there were no differences observed in the prevalence of worksite smoking policies.

The Working Well Trial also utilized the work site as the unit of randomization and intervention (Heimendinger et al. 1995; Abrams et al. 1994; Sorensen et al. 1996), and it provided outcome data related to environmental outcomes. The Working Well intervention led to significant increases in the availability of fruit and vegetables and more access to nutrition information at work; no intervention effects were observed for smoking policies (Biener et al., submitted). Interestingly, these environmental changes tracked well with the employee behavior changes, in which significant improvements were observed for the dietary outcomes but not for smoking (Sorensen et al. 1996). Other studies have found that increased smoking policy restrictions can lead to reduced cigarette consumption rates and to increased smoking cessation (Biener et al. 1989; Sorensen et al. 1989).

The recently completed CATCH study is another excellent example of a multiple-level intervention strategy that simultaneously targeted change at the individual, environmental, and community levels. The CATCH study targeted smoking, nutrition, and physical activity in 96 schools in four states. The baseline cohort was 5106 third graders, who were followed through fifth grade. The intervention focused on children's health behaviors, as well as on changing the availability of fruit, vegetables, low-fat foods, and opportunities for physical activity. Social norms and policies related to smoking were also targeted. Significant changes were found in nutrient content of school lunches, children's nutrient intakes, and levels of moderate-to-vigorous physical activity engaged in during physical education classes. Other school-based physical activity studies that targeted the organizational level found a significant improvement in children's ability to perform on a fitness test (Kelder et al. 1993).

The results of these studies suggest that environmental and organizational interventions are a key component of behavior change efforts and should be systematically integrated with individually oriented interventions whenever possible. The importance of targeting multiple levels of intervention has been highlighted in the social ecological model, which posits that effective and lasting health behavior change at the individual level requires interventions that target the individual; the individual's environment, social relationships, and communities; and governmental policies (Stokols 1996; McLeroy et al. 1988). Efforts to determine how to maximize change at the en-

vironmental level will be an important part of the next generation of studies targeting individual health behavior change.

Social Context

Health promotion interventions have traditionally limited their focus to the target health behavior and have been relatively inattentive to social contextual factors that are related to health behaviors in general. In the area of smoking, for example, there has been a heavy emphasis on nicotine dependence and the physiologic and pharmacological mechanisms that are associated with smoking initiation and maintenance (Pomerleau et al. 1993; Fagerstrom 1978; Carmelli et al. 1992; Perkin et al. 1989; Pomerleau and Pomerleau 1984; Shiffman 1989, 1991). Relatively little emphasis has been placed on the sociocultural factors that are associated with smoking. Although one should not overlook the contributions of work in nicotine pharmacology to the development of smoking cessation treatment strategies, development of effective intervention strategies should not be limited to a focus on individual physiological and psychological factors. As the other chapters in this volume aptly illustrate in detail (see Chapters 3, 4, 7 and 8), a number of social factors have been found to be related to health behaviors as well as chronic disease morbidity and mortality. A large quantity of research has documented the impact of social conditions, such as class, race, education, and gender, on health (Marmot and Davey Smith 1997; Adler et al. 1994; Marmot et al. 1978, 1996; Wilkinson 1992; Kennedy et al. 1996; Krieger et al. 1993). For example, controlling for behavioral status, an independent relationship has been found between social class and low birth weight (Roberts 1997; O'Campo et al. 1997). Social pathways such as social integration, social structure, residential characteristics, access to healthcare resources, and the division of labor chart the impact of these social factors on health outcomes (Amick et al.1995; McKinlay 1995; Kaplan 1995; Anderson and Armstead 1995; Wallack and Wallerstein 1987; Robertson and Minkler 1994).

It is not surprising that health behaviors as well as health outcomes are strongly related to social conditions. As recently noted by Sorensen et al. (1998) and Kaplan (1995), distal social structural forces clearly shape people's day-to-day experiences in ways that are typically not considered by health promotion interventions (Amick et al.1995). Even when individuals are interested in changing their health habits, it may be difficult to control the target health behaviors. For example, middle class neighborhoods have proportionally more pharmacies, restaurants, banks, and specialty stores, while low-income areas have more fast food restaurants, check cashing stores, liquor stores, and laundromats. The population density per food market is much greater in poor neighborhoods compared to middle- and upper-class neighborhoods; the typical cost of food is approximately 15%–20% higher in poor neighborhoods, while the quality of food available is poorer (Troutt 1993). As a result of access and transportation issues, the barriers to making healthier food choices in poor communities may be insurmountable. As Levine eloquently noted:

> Communities may provide safe, convenient jogging trails or confront residents with potholes, air pollution, and dangerous automobile traffic. People are encouraged to avoid cigarettes, to live "clean" lives, and to avoid accidents, but they are exposed to extreme dangers in the workplaces, on the highways, and in the communities where they live. (1981, p. 271)

Hillary Graham has conducted an excellent analysis of the impact of the social context on smoking among women in England (1994). Graham concluded that different dynamics drive the smoking habits of low-income women compared to middle- and upper-income women. She identified four categories of influence, including (1) everyday responsibilities (e.g., child care, caring for other family members) and patterns of paid work; (2) materials circumstances

(e.g., housing situation, partner's employment, income and benefit status, access to transportation and telephone); (3) social support and social networks (e.g., relationships with partner, family, and friendship networks; feelings of belonging); and (4) personal and health resources (e.g., physical and psychosocial health, health beliefs, health behaviors, alternative coping strategies). Following an extensive qualitative study and analysis, she concluded that low-income women use smoking as a means of coping with their economic pressures and the resulting demands placed on them to care for others. Smoking was not associated with minority group membership; smoking was primarily a factor for low-income white women. Having to care for more, while simultaneously living on less, provided the context in which relatively few women attempted or succeeded at smoking cessation. Compared to women who had never smoked or who had successfully quit smoking, the continuing smokers tended to be caring for others in circumstances that constrained rather than supported lifestyle change. Graham concluded that the overall pattern of difficulties and disadvantage faced by low-income women who smoke suggests that their adaptive capacity may already be taxed to the limit. Further, the results suggest that a focus on health-related risks of smoking may not on its own be effective with this group but rather that the crucial connection with smoking lay in the women's material and social circumstances. As a result, Graham concluded that the issue of how working class women live is a major and urgent issue for health promotion policy and practice. Interventions that help to reduce the burden of heavy caring responsibilities and improve women's material circumstances may be a step toward lifting the barriers that prevent low income women from quitting smoking. A qualitative study conducted in Chicago public housing developments supports these conclusions, in that the participants emphasized that smoking cessation would be more relevant to them if it was part of broader so-

Table 11–1. The social context of smoking among low-income populations

"Effects" of smoking	Characteristics of social environment
Reduces stress	High stress
Relatively low cost	Few economic resources
Provides social connection	Social norms support smoking
Causes disease/death in long run	Causes disease/death in short *and* long run

cial support efforts geared to improve their lives (Lacey et al. 1993).

Graham's analysis is compelling, and illustrates that, in the socioeconomic environments where smoking is concentrated, this behavior can be very adaptive in terms of helping individuals meet the immediate demands of their life circumstances. Table 11–1 compares the physiological and psychological effects of smoking to the stressors of poverty. From a short-term cost–benefit perspective, smoking may in fact be an adaptive behavior in impoverished circumstances, which further highlights the importance of addressing the social context in intervention design and delivery. Another study that evaluated the impact of stressors associated with having inadequate economic resources found that experience of daily hassles or stressors was related to smoking status among an urban, relatively low-income African-American sample (Romano et al. 1991). Cigarette consumption rate was also associated with experience of hassles. These findings further illustrate the possible functional value of smoking under conditions of economic and environmental stress.

McKinlay argues that many of the current approaches to health promotion decontextualize the ways in which at-risk behaviors are generated and sustained (1993). He further argues that social system contributions, including governmental policies, organizational priorities, and behaviors and practices of health care professionals represent intervention strategies that have considerable potential for yielding lasting health benefits. Existing data demonstrate that much of health promotion research has been conducted in a social vacuum, with lit-

tle attention to the influence of sociopolitical and regulatory factors (Altman 1995; Wallack and Winkleby 1986). It is becoming increasingly clear that effective health promotion interventions can no longer ignore social contextual factors. However, I would argue that in our efforts to address the broader social context we should not totally abandon efforts to intervene at the individual level. As Altman (1995) states, the key point in prevention research is to identify the web of causation and to intervene on as many levels as possible in the web. The most effective intervention strategies are likely to incorporate both the individual whose health behavior is in question and the larger community and governmental forces that influence the life of that individual. Further, studies that integrate individual interventions with larger systems intervention strategies may result in methodological innovations that will further our understanding of how best to conceptualize, intervene upon, and assess health behavior change efforts.

It is the premise of this volume, and of this chapter in particular, that efforts to intervene upon health behaviors without considering the social context in which they occur will be limited in their effectiveness, particularly with lower-income populations that have achieved less benefit from the behavior-specific risk-factor interventions that have been conducted to date. Fortunately, more attention has recently been paid to social contextual factors, and there is a growing literature that provides guidance on these types of interventions. The remainder of this chapter is devoted to a review of *(1)* theoretical issues related to the health behavior change interventions targeting the social context; *(2)* the social ecological model, which provides a framework for interventions targeting the social context; and *(3)* a selected discussion of published and ongoing studies utilizing innovative strategies to address the social context of health behavior change.

THEORETICAL ISSUES IN HEALTH BEHAVIOR CHANGE RESEARCH

Theoretical models of health behavior have received substantial research attention over the past two to three decades (Glanz et al. 1997; Abrams et al. 1997). Careful attention to theoretical constructs is considered to be an essential component of efforts to develop more effective intervention strategies (Baranowski et al., in press; Sorensen et al., in press). Specification of a theoretical model is essential in order to clarify the ways in which the "black box" of an intervention is expected to work (Koepsell et al. 1992). Although the level of specificity of theoretical models has increased, a large number of intervention studies have not been based on any theoretical underpinnings nor used well-articulated theoretical constructs to guide the intervention development, implementation, or evaluation.

Further, few studies have clearly articulated key hypothesized mediating variables, and fewer still have measured and evaluated the impact of mediating mechanisms (Baranowski et al., in press; Hansen and McNeal 1996). Those studies that have longitudinally assessed mediating variables often show that interventions have not substantially effected change in those hypothesized mechanisms (e.g., Baranowski et al., in press). The ability of interventions to yield change in mediating variables will determine to some extent the ability of the intervention to impact on the target outcome behaviors (Baranowski et al., in press). For example, the recent CATCH trial did demonstrate a substantial impact on mediating mechanisms, as well as on behavioral outcomes. However, knowledge of how to affect mediating variables is in its early stages of development. Baranowski et al. (in press) call for

a priority to be placed on research that increases our understanding of the relationships between theoretical variables and outcomes, and of the impact of community-based interventions on these mediating variables. This move is necessary if we are to take our intervention effects to the next level of effectiveness. Recent qualitative work examining social and cultural factors influencing health behavior across the life span emphasizes the importance of a "lifecourse" or developmental perspective in theory development, because the influencing factors are likely to vary with different phases of life (Backett and Davison 1995).

Another critical problem is that the majority of theoretical models addressing health behavior change have been developed and evaluated on middle-income and homogenous populations (Folsom et al. 1985). Relatively little attention has been paid to how mainstream theoretical constructs translate to low-income, diverse populations. Considerable research is needed in order to maximize the effectiveness of health behavior change interventions. Current theoretical models are further limited by their focus on the individual level, with little consideration of community-, organizational-, or systems-level factors that impact on the individual. Although some heuristic frameworks and models suggest strategies for targeting multiple levels of change (Gritz and Bastani 1993; Curry and Emmons 1994), they do not typically elucidate the specific mechanisms by which change should occur. Development of theoretical models that integrate individual-level factors with community and social context factors are needed to provide the basis for the next generation of research in this area. The social ecological model, which addresses multiple levels of influence on behavior, provides a mechanism for broadening theoretical developments.

SOCIAL ECOLOGICAL MODEL

The social ecological model offers a framework for addressing theoretical perspectives targeting multiple levels of influence on behavior. An ecological framework recognizes that behavior is affected by multiple levels of influence, including intrapersonal factors, interpersonal processes, institutional factors, community factors, and public policy. As Breslow recently wrote,

The aim must be to establish a health-promoting environment in the social space in which persons make health-significant decisions. The struggle is for the relevant space that various forces, some unconcerned with health and some actually detrimental to it, have thus far too largely preempted. Social ecology for health means deliberately occupying more of that social space and using it in the interest of health. (1996, p. 255)

Examples of interventions targeting each of the levels in the social ecological model are provided in Table 11–2. In a recent review of this approach, Stokols articulated several operating guidelines for adaptations of this model to health behavior change interventions. Examples of the application of these principles are provided in Table 11–3.

At each of the five levels of the social ecological model, individual theoretical perspectives can be integrated. On the *intrapersonal* level, where individual behavior change is the primary goal, applications of the social ecological model might integrate principles from the health beliefs model, social learning theory, the theory of reasoned action, the transtheoretical model, and behavioral choice theory (Becker 1979; Becker and Rosenstock 1984; Leventhal 1970; Leventhal and Hirschman 1982; Leventhal et al. 1983; Azjen and Fishbein 1980; Bandura 1986; Prochaska and DiClemente 1983). Common among these theories is the supposition that behavior change is a function of attitudes, perceived norms, and perception of one's ability to initiate change. The risk assessment literature also contributes to the theoretical perspectives at the individual level; this literature suggests that efforts to educate people about risks must go beyond generalized risk information (e.g., high-fat diets are bad for you) and focus on personalization of risk across multiple dimensions (Slovic 1987) (e.g., demonstration of specific ways in which the

Table 11–2. Social Ecological Model: Intervention Design

Intrapersonal Level

⇒ Motivational interventions
⇒ Skills building opportunities
⇒ Tailored intervention materials

Interpersonal Level

⇒ Interventions targeting social norms and social networks

Organizational/Environmental Level

⇒ Interventions in health care system
⇒ Interventions in workplaces
⇒ Interventions in schools

Community Level

⇒ Networking with community resources
⇒ Social service advocacy
⇒ Structural/environmental interventions in communities

Policy Level

⇒ Local, state, and federal laws
⇒ Intervention with federal regulatory agencies

individual is being impacted). The Precaution Adoption Model articulates several stages through which individuals make choices about continuing their risk behaviors or deciding to adopt healthier alternatives (e.g., precautions) (Weinstein 1988).

At the *interpersonal* level, substantial literatures document the impact of social support and social networks on health status and behaviors (Gore 1981, 1985; House 1981; Jacobson 1986; Berkman and Syme 1979). Families, for example, can provide a range of support for health behavior change, including information, appraisal, emotional, and instrumental support (Israel and Schurman 1990). Social norms within one's social network may structure and influence health behaviors and one's motivation and ability to change those behaviors (Sorensen et al. 1986; Macario et al., in press). In particular, health behaviors tend to cluster in families, further demonstrating the importance of including a focus on the family in behavior change interventions (Sallis et al. 1988a,b; Baranowksi, in press). To date, relatively little is known about fam-

Table 11–3. The Application of the Social Ecological Model to Health Behavior Interventions

Operating guidelines	Application in Health Behavior Interventions
Encompass multiple settings and life domains	• Provide methods/strategies to involve participants' families, friends, community • Design interventions that span multiple settings and have enduring positive effects on well-being • Integrate biomedical, behavioral, regulatory, and environmental interventions
Reinforce health-promoting social norms through existing social networks	• Provide cues for healthy behaviors throughout target community • Involve health care providers; engage family members and significant others; provide follow-up counseling • Connect participants with community organizations that support the individual's target goals
Target changes in the organization and environment in support of participant health	• Utilize input from advisory boards of constituents/representatives of target population to develop appropriate intervention methods and materials • Identify behavioral and organizational "leverage points" for health promotion • Train key community gate-keepers to deliver cancer prevention messages (e.g., health care providers, teachers, community leaders, preachers, camp counselors) • Provide key community leaders with materials and resources for extending their intervention efforts • In target organizational settings, review policies that can impact on norms for health behaviors (e.g., choice of foods for vending machines, smoking policies, youth access to cigarettes), and make recommendations • Utilize "other-directed," passive policy intervention strategies
Tailor programs to the setting through community participation and ownership	• Develop Community Advisory Boards, comprised of key leaders and representatives of target population • Collaborate with Community Advisory Board to develop appropriate resources and networks of community organizations that can support participants' behavior change goals • Develop interventions that enhance the fit between people and their surroundings
Empower individuals to make behavior change	• Provide motivational strategies to empower participants to make changes • Provide opportunities for making small steps toward target changes • Impact on social norms related to targeted changes
Utilize multiple delivery points for intervention messages	• Deliver interventions through multiple channels, and embed interventions into ongoing community programs and activities

ily influences on health behaviors, and there are further limits on what is known about how these influences operate at different developmental stages (Baranowski, in press). The best strategies for incorporating social networks in general and family in particular into health behavior change interventions deserve substantial research attention.

At the *institutional* level, the organization is the intervention target. Recent work to deliver smoking interventions in the context of the health care setting provide a good example of organizational-level interventions (Kottke et al. 1988). Efforts to formalize cancer prevention interventions as part of the standard of care have been found to be an effective way to affect both physician and patient behavior (Dietrich et al. 1992). Office systems interventions, guided by the literature on the diffusion of innovations and organizational change (Murray 1986; Rogers 1983), have been utilized and found to increase physician involvement in advice-giving, counseling, and screening (Kottke et al. 1988). In addition, policies and practices in physician offices that promote health can affect social norms within the practice and the community (e.g., smoking bans, provision of information and materials about cancer prevention, etc.).

As Tarlov (1996) recently noted, the interaction of people with the social and physical environment is a predominant determinant of health. Therefore, an emphasis on community and regulatory factors that influence health are critical. At the *community and policy levels*, conceptual models are influenced by literatures in the areas of community organization, social capital, program planning, the concept of reciprocal determinism from the social cognitive theory, and the socioecological framework. Models of community organization focusing on locality planning, social planning, and social action (Rothman and Tropman 1987), collaborative empowerment (Himmelman 1992), culturally relevant practice (e.g., Gutierrez and Lewis 1995; Rivera and Erlich 1995; Braithwaite et al. 1994), and coalition building (Goodman et al. 1993, 1996; Kaye and Wolff 1995) have also been used.

Using a social ecological framework, efforts which focus on multiple levels to structure intervention delivery can "infuse" the intervention across multiple levels of influence via multiple delivery points and extend it into participants' social networks (Gardner 1991). There are several recent examples that suggest that this is an important concept to build into behavior change interventions (Gardner 1991; Fiore 1996). The concept of infusion fits well into a social ecological model, which does not focus solely on the persons who are making health choices but rather engages the social processes and agencies that profoundly influence those choices (Breslow 1996). By doing so, interventions can maximize the infusion of the health promotion messages into the individual's social environment while simultaneously impacting on larger social and governmental factors that influence individual health behaviors.

INTERVENTION STUDIES TARGETING THE SOCIAL CONTEXT OF HEALTH BEHAVIORS

There is an increasing recognition of the role that social factors play in health behavior change; a number of studies have recently been completed or are currently underway that address these issues. The remainder of this chapter is devoted to a selected review of several examples of studies targeting social contextual factors in an effort to illustrate the importance and feasibility of such approaches. This review is not intended to be inclusive but rather to highlight several innovative interventions that target challenging populations and/or novel intervention delivery systems. Studies are included that examine church-based interventions, smoking interventions for pregnant women, access and policy interventions for health-related resources, and tobacco control.

Church-Based Interventions

With increasing disparities in chronic disease morbidity and mortality among black and white Americans (Lundberg 1991; Thomas et al. 1994; McBeath 1991; NRC 1989), public health researchers have begun to investigate alternative strategies for delivering health interventions to black communities. The black church has historically been a major focus of the spiritual, social, and political life of black Americans (Thomas et al. 1994). Further, social networks and social support provide the foundation for church activities and fellowship. Therefore, the church is a very important setting in which social factors associated with health behaviors can be addressed. Of particular importance, the church has a long history of addressing unmet health and human service needs of the black community (Thomas et al. 1994; Wiist and Flack 1990; Eng et al. 1994; Levin 1984; Dacey Allen, in review), and therefore health behavior interventions are likely to fit well within the church's priorities. Several recent studies, including those described below, suggest that church-based interventions are an important strategy for contextualizing health behavior interventions (Thomas et al. 1994; Depue et al. 1990; Davis et al. 1994; Voorhees et al. 1996; Wiist and Flack 1990; Eng et al. 1985; Levin 1984).

The Black Church Family Project was a

multiyear national study of community outreach programs sponsored by a large sample of black churches (Thomas et al. 1994). Over 40% of the churches surveyed operated three or more community outreach activities; 67% operated at least one of these types of activities. Over 50% of activities were focused on adult and family support programs, targeting provision of basic human services (e.g., food, shelter, child care) and preventive care and counseling (e.g., AIDS risk reduction counseling, drug abuse prevention, domestic violence). Thirty percent of activities were oriented to children and youth (e.g., AIDS education, drug abuse prevention, pregnancy prevention, and mental health), 9% were targeted to community development, and 9% were for the elderly (e.g., home health care, food delivery, medical care). Strong evidence for collaborative relationships between churches and secular service agencies was documented. Multivariate examination of church organizational characteristics suggested that churches that were larger and had more educated clergy were more likely to conduct community outreach programs.

The church was also utilized as the intervention channel in two recent studies targeting breast and cervical cancer screening. Davis et al. (1994) reported the results of an uncontrolled study in which 24 black and Hispanic churches participated in a screening intervention implemented by lay health leaders. The church participation rate was 96%. Seventy-eight percent of the churches organized support structures for participants who attended the intervention (e.g., child care, lunch/snacks, transportation). Ninety percent of the women who completed the baseline survey and were targeted for recruitment presented for screening. Fifty-two percent of the churches continued the cancer prevention campaign in the two years following the program period. In a second study, Dacey Allen and colleagues conducted a process evaluation of a church-based peer health advisor (PHA) intervention for breast cancer education (Dacey Allen et al., in review). Within each of the two participating churches, three women members were trained to serve as PHAs; these women delivered breast health education via small group education sessions and outreach activities. In-depth interviews with the PHAs indicated that substantial time is needed to acclimate to the role of PHA before conducting program activities, that not all PHAs were comfortable with all educational formats (e.g., small group vs. one-to-one outreach), that more involvement of and support from church leaders was desired, and that there was a strong commitment among the PHAs to continue outreach and education efforts after study completion. High rates of participation in the intervention and evaluation were found.

Perhaps the most rigorous studies of church-based interventions to date have been conducted by Becker and her colleagues. A randomized controlled design was used to evaluate the Heart, Body, and Soul Program, a church-based smoking cessation intervention targeted African Americans (Voorhees et al. 1996). This study was conducted in East Baltimore in 21 contiguous census tracts in which 88% of the population is African American, 46% of the population's income is less than poverty level, and 65% report being regular churchgoers. A convenience sample of 23 churches was selected, based on the church being known to pastors on the Steering Committee and the church being active in social and health issues; 96% of the invited churches participated. Twenty-two churches were randomly assigned to either an intensive culturally specific intervention or to a minimal self-help intervention. The intensive intervention included "environmental" interventions (e.g., pastoral sermons on smoking, testimony during church services, training of volunteers as lay smoking cessation counselors) and individually oriented interventions (individual and group support supplemented with spiritual audiotapes containing gospel music, a day-by-day scripturally guided stop-smoking booklet, and health fairs targeting cardiovascular risk and personalized health feedback). The self-help intervention included health fairs, personalized feedback, and an American Lung Association smoking cessation pamphlet designed for African Americans; the self-help intervention was disseminated through strategies selected by each of the churches in the self-help condition. There were no significant differences in smoking cessation rate between the intensive (27% self-reported quit rate; 19.6% validated quit rate) and self-help intervention (21.5% self-reported quit rate; 15% validated quit rate) conditions in terms of smoking cessation rate, although power for detecting these outcomes may have been limited. However, both conditions yielded higher cessation rates than those found among churchgoers in a community reference sample (2.9% self-reported quit rate). There was more positive movement in motivation to quit smoking among the intensive intervention group, and less regression or lack of movement in motivation, compared to the self-help group. Baptists in the intensive intervention condition were three times more likely to make progress than all other denominations; the authors suggest that the strong social norms and sanctions against substance use in Baptist religious organizations (Ahmed et al. 1994) may have placed the intervention more directly in the social context of the religion and thus have been more effective in this group.

The LIGHT Way (Living in God's Healthy Temple) Project, a church-based intervention targeting nutrition and physical activity, is an ongoing study being conducted by Becker and her colleagues. Twenty-six churches have been randomly assigned to receive an intensive environmental intervention (including sermons, testimony, spiritual guidance support books, gospel aerobics ["Movin' with the Spirit"] and support groups), or a control group. This multiple risk factor intervention will provide additional information about how spirituality and organized religion can be used to contextualize health behavior interventions.

The series of studies described above demonstrates that the church is a viable setting for conducting health interventions. In particular, interventions that place health in the context of religion and emphasize the church's religious values have been particularly effective. Utilization of peer health advisors and church volunteers for intervention design and delivery is particularly promising, because these strategies not only help to contextualize the intervention messages but also increase the likelihood of program institutionalization within both the church culture and its ministry.

Smoking During Pregnancy

Smoking during pregnancy is another challenging public health problem that has recently been addressed using interventions that target the social context. Quitting smoking before or during pregnancy is one of the most effective strategies for reducing the public health issue of low birth weight and other preventable causes of infant morbidity and mortality. However, traditional efforts to affect this problem have had a less than optimal impact on long-term cessation rates, and smoking cessation during pregnancy remains an elusive public health goal. Most approaches to smoking cessation have paid little attention to the role of smoking in a broader life context. Low-income and undereducated women are more likely to smoke during pregnancy but may not view smoking as a priority in light of other pressing life issues. Interventions that place smoking cessation in the context of other life issues may be more effective at reaching pregnant smokers, as illustrated by the three ongoing studies outlined below.

The Healthy Baby Second-Hand Smoke Study,[1] funded by Robert Wood Johnson Foundation's Smoke-Free Families Initiative, is an ongoing collaborative research effort between the Dana-Farber Cancer Institute (K. Emmons, principal investigator), Boston's Public Health Commission, and the Healthy Baby Program. The Healthy Baby Program (HBP) is a community-based home visitation and outreach program based in Boston's Public Health Commission that provides medical and social ser-

Table 11–4. Healthy Baby Second-Hand Smoke Study: Intervention Design

---

Intrapersonal Level

• *Motivational intervention delivered by Healthy Baby home visitation nurse, including:*
⇒ Use of motivational interviewing strategies
⇒ Feedback about levels of nicotine in participant's household
⇒ Goal-setting with feedback regarding impact of changes on household nicotine levels
⇒ Tailored follow-up counseling and intervention materials

• *Skills building opportunities*

Interpersonal Level

• *Incorporation of strategies for handling smoking among members of participant's social network*

Organizational/Environmental Level

• *Intervention placed in health care system*

Community Level

• *Networking with community resources*
• *Social service advocacy*

---

vices to high-risk pregnant women. The HBP nurses and public health advocates follow women throughout their pregnancy and up to 1 year after delivery, focusing on both medical and social needs. As part of the second-hand smoke study, HBP's nurses have been trained to provide a motivational smoking intervention as part of their usual home visitation practices. The smoking intervention includes measurement of and feedback about both the woman's health status and household nicotine concentrations, as well as linkages to the health care system. By incorporating a smoking intervention into a program that deals with the larger social context of pregnant women's lives, it is hypothesized that the intervention may be more effective in increasing smoking cessation during pregnancy, in affecting motivation for cessation, and in reducing household levels of environmental tobacco smoke. The intervention design, which draws heavily on a social ecological framework, is outlined in Table 11–4. Intervention outcomes are assessed during pregnancy and 1-month postpartum. This study represents another example of an effort to integrate individual- and systems-level interventions for health behavior change.

Another study which is currently under-

way recognizes the important role that both health care providers and a pregnant smoker's partner can play in a woman's willingness to quit smoking and her success at staying quit. This focus is particularly important, because partner's smoking status and support regarding smoking cessation during pregnancy are important predictors of both short- and long-term cessation. McBride and colleagues are utilizing a three-group design to compare *(1)* usual care, which consists of provider advice to quit and written self-help guide *(2)* enhanced self-help, which consists of provider advice, a written self-help guide, a late pregnancy relapse prevention gift kit, and six counseling calls from a health counselor; and *(3)* partner-assisted enhanced self-help, which consists of the enhanced self-help condition plus *(1)* couples counseling regarding supporting the woman in the quitting process, *(2)* a support skills booklet, *(3)* a follow-up counseling call, *(4)* five tailored newsletters concerning support skills, communication and smoking, *(5)* cessation materials, and *(6)* free nicotine replacement for partners who smoke. This study will provide important information about how to contextualize smoking interventions in the context of the woman's relationships with her partner.

An excellent example of an intervention that incorporates all levels within the health care system as part of an intervention to reduce smoking during pregnancy is the ongoing Provider-Delivered Smoking Intervention Project (PDSIP), which is being conducted by Ockene and colleagues. Most smoking interventions in the health care setting have targeted one type of provider (e.g., primary care physicians, obstetric providers), and there is typically little carryover of cessation counseling across different types of providers (e.g., obstetricians to pediatricians). In the PDSIP, Ockene and her colleagues are targeting three channels for intervention delivery: (1) WIC (Women, Infants, and Children) nutritionists who see women both during pregnancy and postpartum, (2) obstetricians and their staff who provide prenatal care, and (3) pediatricians and their staff who provide care to the infants. This study will evaluate outcomes related to the woman's smoking and awareness of the risks of smoking/benefits of stopping, providers' delivery of smoking cessation interventions, and association of psychosocial and social network characteristics with outcomes. This is an important example of a systems approach that is likely to increase the delivery of consistent messages and provision of assistance to women who are seen in public health clinics.

Access and Policy Interventions

Social contextual interventions have also targeted both sides of the access issue: (1) increasing access to health care and health promotion resources among underserved populations and (2) decreasing access to opportunities to develop behavioral risk factors among at-risk populations. The Massachusetts Farmers' Market Coupon Program for low-income elders (Webber et al. 1995) is an excellent example of an intervention designed to increase access to health promotion resources. Concerned about health outcomes for older adults, the Massachusetts Department of Public Health teamed up with the state's Department of Food and Agriculture, which is committed to encour-

aging the local production and consumption of agricultural commodities. The farmers' market coupons, which are distributed through Elderly Nutrition Projects throughout the state, are redeemable for fruit, vegetables, and other edible farm products at the state's 70 farmers' markets. In 1992, almost $86,000 in coupons were distributed by 23 agencies to 17,200 older adults; 73% of the coupons were redeemed. Thirty-eight percent of respondents in a survey of coupon recipients indicated that they continued to shop at the farmers' markets after spending their coupons; 32% of the seniors reported buying significantly more fruit and vegetables since receiving the coupons. The coupon program has also brought significant benefits to the state's farmers; coupons distributed through this program brought an additional $62,000 to farmers' markets in addition to the money seniors spent at the markets after the coupons had been spent. Farmer participation in the program grew by over 130% between 1987 and 1992. This is an excellent example of a social contextual, systems-level intervention that targets both individual behavior and organizational- and policy-level change, building on an interagency collaboration that addresses separate and overlapping goals of each agency.

A different perspective on access comes from the work targeting reduction of youth access to tobacco products. One very innovative intervention, Tobacco Policy Options for Prevention (TPOP), has recently been conducted by Forester and colleagues (Forester et al., in review). The TPOP intervention tested the hypothesis that the generation, adoption, and implementation of local youth tobacco-access policies can influence youth smoking. A community organizing strategy was used to implement a media advocacy campaign as well as to change ordinances, merchant policies and practices, and law enforcement practices regarding youth access to tobacco. By the end of the 3-year intervention period, each of the seven intervention communities had passed an ordinance restricting youth access, compared to only three of the control communities; the changes enacted in the control communities were also considerably weaker than those in intervention communities. Compared to the control communities, significantly greater decreases were found in the intervention communities in terms of tobacco availability, ability of underage youth to purchase cigarettes, and adolescent smoking prevalence. Perhaps most importantly, the intervention resulted in sharp decreases in adolescents' _perceived_ accessibility of tobacco through commercial sources, which the authors posit may have been an important mechanism by which the reductions in smoking prevalence were accomplished.

Social contextual interventions can also be targeted at the policy level. For example, tobacco use is a particular problem among Native American tribes in the northwestern United States: Their rates of tobacco use are more than 50% higher than those of the region's general population (Lichtenstein et al. 1995). Lichtenstein, Glasgow, and colleagues have conducted ongoing work related to tobacco control policies within Native American tribes. In one study (1995), 39 tribes were randomized into early and late intervention conditions. The intervention consisted of a policy consultation process delivered by two Indian staff members of the area Indian Health Board, regional workshops for tribal representatives, and visits to each of the tribes. The primary intervention goal was establishment of a tobacco policy resolution by tribal councils. Seventy-four percent of the tribes participated in at least one regional meeting. Participating tribes had a median of two in-person policy consultations and six telephone consultations. The early intervention tribes showed significantly higher implementation rates of more restrictive tobacco policies compared to the later-intervention tribes. There was also a significant increase in the number of articles on tobacco control that appeared in tribal newsletters. By placing the issue of tobacco control within the context of issues that are relevant to the leadership of the tribe, the intervention was successful in increasing the prevalence of tobacco control policies.

These three examples of community-based access and policy interventions highlight the powerful role that policy change and community organizing can have on purchase and consumption of both health-promoting and health-harming products. Both the Farmers' Market Coupon Program and the TPOP study were collaborations with the private sector that were formed in order to advance the economic and health goals of the community. Such strategies further embed the intervention messages into the community's value system and impact on social norms for health behaviors.

Although there has been considerable attention to policy in the area of tobacco control, policy innovations related to other health behaviors have been relatively unexplored. King et al. argue that passive approaches to promoting physical activity (e.g., restricting downtown centers for foot or bicycle traffic, placing parking lots at a distance from buildings, and making stairways more convenient and safe), for example, have important potential for achieving widespread increases in physical activity at the population level (King et al. 1995). Substantial work conducted in Australia in the area of skin cancer prevention emphasizes the importance of structural strategies (e.g., erecting canopies or shaded areas, planting shade trees) for reducing sun exposure. Breslow (1996) emphasizes the importance of utilizing macrosocial environments, represented by social agencies, national organizations, and federal regulatory agencies, as partners for health promotion. He cites the example of the U.S. Department of Agriculture and how its policies have historically favored excessive production of fatty foods, which were purchased and distributed in school lunch programs. Stemming partly from the substantial lobbying conducted by public health representatives, there have been recent changes in the requirements for the National School Lunch and Breakfast Programs. The changes require that, in order to receive federal subsidies, these programs must comply with the 1995 Dietary Guidelines for Americans and meet specified recommended dietary allowances. These changes in federal policies have a direct and strong impact on the health of U.S. children, similar to the potential impact of the tobacco settlement that is currently being negotiated between the federal government and the tobacco industry. Development and evaluation of macrolevel policy and environmental interventions for promotion of health behaviors are critical for improving health behavior outcomes.

CONCLUSIONS

Recent reviews of the status of health promotion interventions highlight the urgent need for treatment advances that target new insights through innovative study designs, careful qualitative and process evaluations, and partnerships with the community rather than incremental improvements of existing approaches (Shiffman 1993; Fisher et al. 1993). The purpose of this chapter has been to argue that innovations in behavior change treatment must also draw upon insights from social epidemiology and integrate strategies for dealing with social factors with those developed for individual-level change. Historically, there has been a divergence between epidemiologists, who focus on documenting the relationship between social conditions and health outcomes, and social scientists, who develop health-related interventions that are often devoid of social contextual factors. Although the need for interventions that address the social context may be less apparent in the predominantly white, middle-income populations in which many intervention models have been developed and tested, they are critical in interventions that target lower-income and ethnically diverse populations. Further, failure to include a social contextual focus in interventions for middle-income populations may, in part, explain the modest treatment effects found in many individually based intervention programs.

A recent article by Chamberlain (1997) highlights the relative inattention that health psychology has given to social contextual factors in general, and to the role of socioeconomic status on health outcomes in particular. Chamberlain conducted a qualitative study examining the impact of socioeconomic differences on conceptualization and meaning of health. Based on a detailed analysis of in-depth interviews about the meaning of health, four different views of health were identified. Low-income individuals were most likely to endorse either a *solitary view,* in which only physical aspects of health (e.g., having energy, lack of symptoms) were used to identify the nature of health, or a *dualistic view,* in which both physical and mental/emotional components of health were included but were regarded as separate and independent functions. In contrast, upper-income individuals were more likely to endorse either a *complementary view,* where physical and mental elements were integrated and considered interacting, or a *multiple view,* in which physical, mental, social, and spiritual health were regarded as in balance, as interdependent and interconnected. This work is very important in that it argues further that theoretical formulations of health behaviors must begin to take socioeconomic status into account and that without doing so interventions are likely to be targeting factors that may be irrelevant for the target groups. Factors such as social class can no longer be considered simple demographic variables (Chamberlain 1997), and many of our traditional theoretical models of health behavior will continue to have limited explanatory value if we do not begin to investigate theoretical processes by which social factors can influence health.

The work of Rose (1992) provides a particularly good illustration of the paradox of health promotion and prevention efforts. Individually based interventions may be more effective for the individual participants, but they have limited population coverage. In contrast, population-based efforts target a large percentage of the population but typically have lower levels of effectiveness compared to individually based intervention approaches. However, small changes at the population level can lead to large effects on disease risk. In evaluating health promotion interventions, the level of intervention impact must be judged as a function of the intervention's efficacy in terms of producing individual change, as well as its reach, or the penetration within the population (Abrams et al. 1996).

Although considerable resources have been spent focusing on the individual level, there have been relatively few efforts at incorporating social contextual factors into these intervention strategies. It is clear that the social context of health behavior cannot be ignored. Intervention research must begin to address the role of social factors in health behaviors, to expand our theoretical models to incorporate social factors, and to develop innovative intervention designs that will help to elucidate the most effective strategies for intervening within this context. Intervention research that represents a collaboration with existing community groups, social service agencies, and health care providers and which utilizes existing social networks and relationships to creatively design interventions that address social contextual factors is critical if we are to make a significant impact on health risk factors in the United States. However, as recently noted by Syme (1997) and Altman (1995), efforts to develop the next generation of prevention interventions must focus on building relationships with communities and developing interventions that derive from the communities' assessments of their needs, rather than the experts' assumptions about what is needed. Health behavior research also needs to stretch beyond the individual and interpersonal levels and begin to explore ways to work together with communities to systemically integrate social, governmental, and policy-level factors into behavior change interventions. At the same time, individually based intervention strategies should not be abandoned; rather, these approaches should be fully integrated into efforts to intervene at other levels. Elucidation and evaluation of mediating mechanisms related to social contextual interventions are also essential if we are to develop more effective intervention strategies.

NOTES

1. The Healthy Baby Second-Hand Smoke Study scientific team is comprised of the following individuals: Karen M. Emmons, PI, Glorian Sorensen, co-PI, S. Katherine Hammond, co-PI, Neal Klar, biostatistician, Kaydee Schmidt, co-investigator, Jackie Nolan and Gillian Barclay, project directors. The Healthy Baby Program Advisory Team is comprised of the following individuals: Kaydee Schmidt, director of Public Health Nursing, Marjorie Perkins, Healthy Baby program director, and Maggie Bonet, Sherry White, Patricia Whitworth, and the public health nurses who implemented the program.

ACKNOWLEDGMENTS

The author would like to thank Glorian Sorensen, Mary Kay Hunt, Douglas Johnston, Jackie Nolan, and Elizabeth Gonzalez Roberts for their contributions to the conceptualization of this manuscript and ongoing contributions to the author's research.

This work was supported by grants from the Robert Wood Johnson Foundation, Liberty Mutual Insurance group, NYNEX, Aetna, the Boston Foundation, and NIH grants 1RO1CA73242 and 1RO1HL50017.

REFERENCES

Abrams, D.B., Boutwell, W.B., Grizzle, J., Heimendinger, J. Sorensen, G., and Varnes, J. (1994). Cancer control at the workplace: the working well trial. *Prev Med,* 23:15–27.

Abrams, D.B., Orleans, C.T., Niaura, R., Goldstein, M., Prochaska, J., and Velicer W. (1996). Integrating individual and public health perspectives for treatment of tobacco dependence under managed health care: a combined stepped-care and matching model. *Ann Behav Med,.* 18:290–304.

Abrams, D., Emmons, K., and Linnan, L. (1997). Health behavior and health education: the past, present, and future. In Glanz, K., Lewis, F.M., and Rimer, B.K. (eds.), *Health behavior and health education: theory, research and practice* (2nd ed.). San Francisco: Jossey-Bass, pp. 453–78.

Adler, N.E., Boyce, T., Chesney, M.A., Cohen, S., Folkman, S., Khan, R.L., and Syme, S.L. (1994). Socioeconomic status and health: the challenge of the gradient. *Am Psychol,* 49:15–24.

Ahmed, F., Brown, D.R., Gary, L.E., and Saadatmand, F. (1994). Religious predictors of cigarette smoking: findings for African-American women of childbearing age. *J Behav Med,* 20:34–43.

Altman, D.G. (1995). Strategies for community health intervention: promises, paradoxes, pitfalls. *Psychosom Med,* 57:226–33.

American Heart Association. (1996). *1997 Heart and stroke statistical update.* Washington, DC: American Heart Association.

Amick, B.C., Levine, S., Tarlov, A., and Walsh, D. (1995). *Community and health.* Society and health. In Patrick, D.L., and Wickizer, T.M. (eds.), Oxford: Oxford University Press, pp. 46–92.

Anderson, N., and Armstead, C. (1995). Toward understanding the association of socioeconomic status and health: a new challenge for the biopsychosocial approach. *Psychosom Med,* 57:213–25.

Azjen, I., and Fishbein, M. (1980). *Understanding attitudes and predicting social behavior.* Englewood Cliffs, NJ: Prentice Hall.

Backett, K.C., and Davison, C. (1995). Lifecourse and lifestyle: the social and cultural location of health behaviors. *Soc Sci Med,* 40:629–38.

Bandura, A. (1986). *Social foundations of thought and action: a social cognitive theory.* Englewood Cliffs, NJ: Prentice Hall.

Baranowski, T., Lin, L.S., Wetter, D.W., Resnico, W.K., and Davis Hearn, M.D. (in press). Theory as mediating variables. *Am Psychologist,* 51:42–51.

Becker, M.H. (1979).Understanding patient compliance: the contribution of attitudes and other psychosocial factors. In Cohen, S.J. (ed.), *New directions in patient compliance.* Lexington, MA: Lexington Books: Health, c1979.

Becker, M.H., and Rosenstock, I.M. (1984). Compliance with medical advice. In Steptoe, A., and Mathews, A. (eds.), *Health care and human behavior.* London: Academic Press.

Berkman, L.D., and Syme, S.L. (1979). Social networks, host resistance and mortality: a nine year follow-up of Alameda County residents. *Am J Epidemiol,* 109:186–204.

Bernstein, D.A. (1969). Modification of smoking behavior: an evaluative review. *Psychol Bull,* 71:418–40.

Biener, L., Abrams, D., Emmons, K.M., and Pollick, H.J. (1989). A comparative evaluation of a restrictive smoking policy in a general hospital. *Am J Pub Health,* 79:192–5.

Bowen, D., and Tinker, L. (1995). Controversies in changing dietary behavior. In Bronner, F.

(ed.), *Nutrition and health: topics and controversies.* Boca Raton, FL: CRC Press.

Bowen, D., Henderson, M., Iverson, D., Burrows, E., and Henry, K. (1994). Reducing dietary fat: understanding the success of the women's health trial. *Cancer Prev Int,* 1: 21–30.

Braithwaite, R.L., Bianchi, C., and Taylor, S.E. (1994). Ethnographic approach to community organization and health empowerment. *Health Educ Q,* 21:407–16.

Breslow, L. (1996). Social ecological strategies for promoting healthy lifestyles. *Am J Health Promot,* 10:253–7.

Carmelli, D., Swan, G.E., Robinette, D., and Fabsitz, R.R. (1992). Genetic influence on smoking: a study of male twins. *N Engl J Med,* 327:829–33.

Caspersen, C.J., and Merritt, R.K. (1992). Trends in physical activity patterns among older adults: the Behavioral Risk Factor Surveillance System, 1986–1990. *Med Sci Sports Exerc,* 1992:24 (Suppl):S26.

Caspersen, C.J., Christenson, G.M., and Pollard, R.A. (1986). The status of the 1990 Physical Fitness Objectives: evidence from NHIS 85. *Public Health Rep,* 101:587–92.

Centers for Disease Control and Prevention (CDC). (1990). Coronary heart disease attributable to sedentary lifestyle: selected states, 1988. *JAMA,* 264:1390–2.

Centers for Disease Control and Prevention. (1996). Cigarette smoking among adults: United States, 1994. *Mor Mortal Wkly Rep,* 45:588–90.

Chamberlain, K. (1997). Socio-economic health differentials: from structure to experience. *J Health Psychol,* 2:399–411.

Colditz, G.A., DeJong, D., Hunter, D.J., Trichopoulos, D., and Willett, W.C. (eds.). (1996). Harvard report on cancer prevention, vol. 1: causes of human cancer. *Cancer Causes Control,* 7 Suppl 1.

Curry, S., and Emmons, K. (1994). Theoretical models for predicting and improving compliance with breast cancer screening. *Ann Behav Med,* 16:302–16.

Curry, S., McBride, C.M., Grothaus, L.C., Louis, D., and Wagner, E.H. (1995). A randomized trial of self-help materials personalized feedback and telephone counseling with nonvolunteer smokers. *J Consult Clin Psychol,* 63:1005–14.

Dacey Allen, J., Sorensen, G., Peterson, K., Stoddard, A.M., and Colditz, G. (submitted). Reach Out for Health: a church-based pilot breast cancer education program.

Davis, D.T., Bustamante, A., Brown, C.P., Wolde-Tsadik, G., Savage, E.W., Cheng, X., and Howland, L. (1994). The urban church

and cancer control: a source of social influence in minority communities. *Public Health
Rep*, 109:500–6.

DePue, J.D., Wells, B.L., Lasater, T.M., and Carleton, R.A. (1990). Volunteers as providers of
Heart Health Programs in churches: a report
on implementation. *Am J Health Prom*,
4:361–6.

Dietrich, A.J., O'Connor, G.T., Keller, A., Carney, P.A., Levy, D., Whaley, F.S. (1992). Cancer: improving early detection and prevention. A community practice randomized trial.
BMJ, 304:687–91.

DiPietro, L., and Caspersen, C.J. (1991). National estimates of physical activity among
white and black Americans. *Med Sci Sports
Exerc*, 23 (Suppl):S105.

Emmons, K.M., Hammond, S.K., and Farrell, N.
(1994a). A motivational intervention to reduce children's smoking exposure to environmental tobacco smoke. Paper Presented
at the Annual Meeting of the Society of Behavioral Medicine, Boston, March 26–28,
1994.

Emmons, K.M., Marcus, B.H., Linnan, L.,
Rossi, J.S., and Abrams, D. B. (1994b).
Mechanisms in multiple risk factor interven-
tions: smoking, physical activity, and dietary
fat intake among manufacturing workers.
Prev Med, 23:481–9.

Eng, E., Hatch, J., and Callan, A. (1994). Institutionalizing social support through the
church and into the community. *Health Educ
Q*, 12:81–92.

Fagerstrom, K.O. (1978). Measuring degree of
physical dependence to tobacco with reference to individualization of treatment. *Addic
Behav*, 3:235–41.

Feinleib, M. (1996). New directions for community intervention studies (editorial). *Am J
Pub Health*, 86:1696–7.

Fiore, M.C. (1996). *Smoking cessation: clinical
practice guideline: 18.* (DHHS Pub. No.
(PHS) AHCPR 96-0692.) Washington, DC:
U.S. Department of Health and Human Services.

Fisher, E. (1995). The results of the COMMIT
Trial (editorial). *Am J Public Health*,
85:159–60.

Fisher, E., Lichtenstein, E., Haire-Joshu, D.,
Morgan, G.D., and Rehberg, H.R. (1993).
Methods, success, and failures of smoking
cessation programs. *Annu Rev Med*, 44:481–
513.

Folsom, A.R., Casperson, C.J., Taylor, H.L, Jacobs, D.R. Jr., Luepker, R.V., Gomez-Marin,
O., Gillum, R.F., and Blackburn, H. (1985).
Leisure time physical activity and its relationship to coronary risk factors in a population-based sample. The Minnesota Heart
Survey. *Am J Epidemiol*, 121:570–9.

Forster, J., Murray, D.M., Wolfson, M., Blaine,
T.M., Wagenaar, A.C., and Hennrikus, D.J.
(1998). The effects of community policies to
reduce youth access to tobacco. *Am J Publi
Health*, 88:1193–8.

Gardner, H. (1991). *The unschooled mind*. New
York: Basic Books.

Glanz, K., Lewis, F.M., and Rimer, B.K. (1997).
*Health behavior and health education: theo-
ry, research, and practice* (2nd ed.). San Francisco: Jossey-Bass.

Glasgow, R.E., Terborg, J.R., Hollis, J.F., Sever-
son, H.H., and Boles, S.M. (1995). Take
heart: results from the initial phase of a worksite wellness program. *Am J Public Health*,
85:209–16.

Glasgow, R.E., Sorensen, G., Giffen, C., Shipley,
R., Corbett, K., and Lynn, W. (1996). Promoting worksite smoking control policies
and actions: the community intervention trial for smoking cessation (COMMIT) experience. *Prev Med*, 25:186–94.

Goodman, R., Burdine, J., Meehan, E., and
McLeroy, K. (1993). Coalitions. *Health Educ
Res*, 8:313–4.

Goodman, R., Wasserman, A., Chinman, M.J.,
Imm, P.S., and Morrisey, E. (1996). An ecological assessment of community coalitions:
approaches to measuring community-based
interventions for prevention and health promotion. *Am J Community Psychol*, 24:
33–61.

Gore, S. (1981). Stress-buffering functions of social supports: an appraisal and clarification
of research models. In Dohrenwend, B.S.,
and Dohrenwend, B.P. (eds.), *Stressful life
events and their context*. New York: Neale
Watson Academic.

Gore, S. (1985). Social support and styles of coping with stress. In Cohen, S., and Syme, S.L.
(eds.), *Social support and health*, Orlando,
FL: Academic Press.

Graham, H. (1994). *When life's a drag*. London:
Her Majesty's Stationery Office.

Greenwald, P., Kramer, B.S., and Weed, D.L.
(eds.). (1995). *Cancer prevention and control*. New York: Marcel Dekker.

Gritz, E.R., and Bastani, R. (1993). Cancer prevention—behavior changes: the short and
the long of it. *Prev Med*, 22:676–88.

Gutierrez, L., and Lewis, E. (1995). Community
organizing with women of color: a feminist
approach. *J Community Pract*, 1:23–43.

Hansen, W.B., and McNeal, R.B. Jr. (1996). The
law of maximum expected potential effect:
constraints placed on program effectiveness
of mediator relationships. *Health Educ Res
Theory Pract*, 11:501–7.

Heimendinger, J., Feng, Z., Emmons, K., Stoddard, A., Kinne, S., Biener, L., and Sorensen,
G. (1995). The working well trial: baseline

dietary and smoking behaviors of employees and related worksite characteristics. *Prev Med*, 24:180–93.

Himmelman, A.T. (1992). Communities working collaboratively for a change. Himmelman Consulting Group, Minneapolis, MN.

House, J.S. (1981). *Work, stress and social support*. Reading, MA: Addison Wesley.

Interagency Board for Nutrition Monitoring and Related Research. (1993). *Nutrition monitoring in the United States. Chartbook I: Selected findings from the National Nutrition Monitoring and Related Research Program.* Hyattsville, MD: Public Health Service.

Interagency Board for Nutrition Monitoring and Related Research. (1995). *Third report on nutrition monitoring in the United States.* Washington, DC.

Israel, B.A., and Schurman, S.J. (1990). Social support, control, and the stress process. In Glanz, K., Lewis, F.M, and Rimer, K. (eds.), *Health behavior and education*. San Francisco: Jossey-Bass.

Jacobson, D.E. (1986). Types and timing of social support. *J Health Soc Behav*, 27:250–64.

Kaplan, G. (1995). Where do shared pathways lead? some reflections on a research agenda. *Psychosom Med*, 57:208–12.

Kaye, G., and Wolff, T. (eds.). (1995). *From the ground up: a workbook on coalition building and community development*. Amherst, MA: Area Health Education Center/Community Partners.

Kelder, S.H., Perry, C.L., and Klepp, K.I. (1993). Community-wide youth exercise promotion: long-term outcomes of the Minnesota heart health program and the class of 1989 study. *J School Health*, 63:218–23.

Kennedy, B.P., Kawashi, I., and Prothrow-Stith, D. (1996). Income distribution and mortality: cross-sectional ecologic study of the Robin Hood index in the United States. *BMJ*, 312:1004–7.

King, A.C., Jeffery, R.W., Fridinger, F., Dusenbury, L., Provence, S., Hedlund, S.A., and Spangler, K. (1995). Environmental and policy approaches to cardiovascular disease prevention through physical activity: issues and opportunities. *Health Educ Q*, 22:499–511.

King, E., Rimer, B., Seay, J., Balshem, A., and Enstrom, P. (1994). Promoting mammography use through progressive interventions: is it effective? *Am J Public Health*, 84:104–6.

Kirsch, I.S., Jungeblut, A., Jenkins, L., and Kolstad, A. (1993). *Adult literacy in America: a first look at the results of the National Adult Literacy Survey*. Washington, DC: National Center for Education Statistics Educational Testing Service.

Kluger, R. (1996). *Ashes to ashes*. New York: Knopf, pp. 639–42.

Koepsell, T.D., Wagner, E.H., Cheadle, A.C., Patrick, D.L., and Martin, D.C. et al. (1992). Selected methodological issues in evaluating community-based health promotion and disease prevention programs. *Annu Rev Public Health*, 31:31–57.

Kottke, T.E., Battista, R.N., DeFriese, G.H., and Brekke, M.L. (1988) Attributes of successful smoking cessation interventions in medical practice. A meta-analysis of 39 controlled trials. *JAMA*, 259:2883–9.

Krebs-Smith, S.M., Cook, A., Subar, A.F., Cleveland, L., and Friday, J. (1995). U.S. adults fruit and vegetable intakes, 1989 to 1991: a revised baseline for the Healthy People 2000 objective. *Am J Public Health*, 85:1623–9.

Krieger, N., Rowley, D., Hermann, A.A., Avery, B., and Phillips, M.T. (1993). Racism, sexism, and social class: implications for studies of health, disease, and well-being. *Am J Prev Med*, 9 Suppl 6:82–122.

Lacey, L.P., Manfredi, C., Balch, G., Warnecke, R.B., Allen, K., and Edwards, C. (1993) Social support in smoking cessation among black women in Chicago public housing. *Public Health Rep*, 109:387–94.

Leventhal, H. (1970). Finding and theories in the study of fear communication. In Berkowitz, L. (ed.), *Advances in experimental social psychology*. New York: Academic Press.

Leventhal, H., and Hirschman, R.S. (1982). Social psychology and prevention. In Sanders, G., and Suls, J. (eds.), *Social psychology of health and illness*. Hillsdale, NJ: Lawrence Erlbaum, pp. 183–226.

Leventhal, H., Safer, M.A., and Panagis, D.M. (1983). The impact of communications on the self-regulation of health beliefs, decisions, and behavior. *Health Educ Q*, 10:3–29.

Levin, J. (1984). The role of the black church in community medicine. *JAMA*, 76:477–83.

Levine, S. (1981). Preventive health behavior. In Lamont-Havers, R. and Cahill, G. Jr. (eds.), *The social context of medical research*. Cambridge, MA: Ballinger.

Lichtenstein, E., and Glasgow, R. (1997). A pragmatic framework for smoking cessation: implications for clinical and public health programs. *Psych Addict Behav*, 11:142–51.

Lichtenstein, E., Glasgow, R., Lopez, K., Hall, R., McRae, S.G., Bruce Meyers, G. (1995). Promoting tobacco control policies in Northwest Indian Tribes. *Am J Public Health*, 85:991–4.

Lichtenstein, E., Glasgow, R., Lando, H., Ossip-Klein, D., and Boles, S. (1996). Telephone counseling for smoking cessation: rationales and meta-analytic review of evidence. *Health Educ Re Theory Pract*, 11:243–57.

Lundberg, G. (1991). National health care reform: an aura of inevitability is upon us (editorial). *JAMA*, 265:2566–7.

Macario, E., Emmons, K., Hunt, M.K., Sorensen, G., and Rudd, R. (1998). Factors influencing nutrition education for patients with low literacy. *J Am Diet Assoc*, 98: 559–64.

Marmot, M.G., and Davey Smith, G. (1997). Socio-economic differentials in health: the contribution of the Whitehall Studies. *J Health Psych*, 2:283–96.

Marmot, M.G., Adelstein, A.M., Robinson, N., and Rose, G. (1978). The changing social class distribution of heart disease. *BMJ*, 2:1109–12.

Marmot, M.G., Bobak, M., and Davey Smith, G. (1995). Explanations for social inequalities and health. In Amick, B.C. Levine, S., Tarlov, A., and Walsh, D.C. (eds.), *Society and health*. London: Oxford University Press, pp. 172–210.

McBeath, W.H. (1991). Health for all: a public health vision (editorial). *Am J Public Health*, 81:1560–5.

McKinlay, J.B. (1993). The promotion of health through planned sociopolitical change: challenges for research and policy. *Soc Sci Med*, 36:109–17.

McKinlay, J. (1995). The new public health approach to improving physical activity and autonomy in older populations. In Heikkinon, E. (ed.), *Preparation for aging*. New York: Plenum Press.

McLeroy, K.R., Bibeau, D., Steckler, A., and Glanz, K. (1988). An ecological perspective on health promotion programs. *Health Educ Q*, 15:351–77.

Morris, P.M., Neuhauser, L., and Campbell, C. (1992). Food security in rural America: a study of the availability and costs of food. *J Nutr Educ*, 24 (Suppl):52–8.

Murray, D.M. (1986). Dissemination of community health promotion programs: the Fargo-Moonhead Heart Health Program. *J School Health*, 56:375–81.

National Research Council. (1989). A common destiny: blacks and American society. Washington, DC: National Academy of Sciences.

Novotny, T.E., Warner, K.E., Kendrik, J.S., and Remington, P.L. (1988). Smoking by blacks and whites: socioeconomic and demographic differences. *Am J Psychiatry*, 78:1187–9.

O'Campo, P., Xue, X., Wang, M.C., and Caughy, M. (1997). Neighborhood risk factors for low birthweight in Baltimore: a multilevel analysis. *Am J Pub Health*, 87:1113–8.

Osler, M. (1993). Social class and health behaviour in Danish adults: a longitudinal study. *Public Health*, 107:251–60.

Patterson, B., and Block, G. (1988). Food choic-

es and the cancer guidelines. *Am J Public Health*, 78:282–6.

Perkin, K.A., Epstein, L.H., Stiller, R.L., Marks, B.L., and Jacob, R.G. (1989). Chronic and acute tolerance to the heart rate effects of nicotine. *Psychopharmacology*, 97:529–34.

Pierce, J.P., Fiore, M.C., Novotny, T.E., Hatziandreu, E.J., and Davis, R.M. (1989). Trends in cigarette smoking in the United States: educational differences are increasing. *JAMA*, 26:56–60.

Pomerleau, O.F., and Pomerleau, C.S. (1984). Neuroregulators and the reinforcement of smoking: towards a biobehavioral explanation. *Neurosci Biobehav Rev*, 8:503–13.

Pomerleau, O.F., Collins, A.C., Shiffman, S., and Pomerleau, C.S. (1993). Why some people smoke and others do not: new perspectives. *J Consult Clin Psychol*, 61:723–31.

Prochaska, J.D., and DiClemente, C.C. (1983). Stages and processes of self-change of smoking: toward an integration model. *J Consult Clin Psychol*, 51:390–5.

Resnicow, K., Futterman, R., Weston, R.E., Royce, J., Parms, C., Freeman, H.P., and Orlandi, M.A. (1996). Smoking prevalence in Harlem, NY. *Am J Health Promot*, 10: 343–6.

Rimer, B., and Glassman, B. (1997). Tailored communications for cancer prevention in managed care settings. *Outlook*, 4–5.

Rimer, B., Orleans, C.T., Fleisher, L., Cristinzio, S., Resch, N., Telepchak, J., and Keintz, M. (1994). Does tailoring matter? the impact of a tailored guide on ratings and short-term smoking related outcomes for older smokers. *Health Educ Res Theory Pract*, 9:69–84.

Rivera, F., and Erlich, J. (1995). An option assessment framework for organizing in emerging minority communities. In Tropman, J., Erlich, J., and Rothman J. (eds.), *Tactics and techniques of community intervention* (3rd ed.). Itasca, IL: Peacock.

Roberts, E.M. (1997). Neighborhood social environments and the distribution of low birthweight in Chicago. *Am J Public Health*, 87:597–603.

Robertson, A., and Minkler, M. (1994). New health promotion movement: a critical examination. *Health Educ Q*, 21:295–312.

Rogers, E.M. (1983). *Diffusion of innovations* (3rd ed.). New York: Free Press.

Romano, P.S., Bloom, J., and Syme, L. (1991). Smoking, social support, and hassles in an urban African-American community. *Am J Public Health*, 81:1415–22.

Rose, G. (1992). *The strategy of preventive medicine*. New York: Oxford University Press.

Rothman, L., and Tropman, J.E. (1987). Models of community organization and macro practice: their mixing and phasing. In Cox, F.M., Erlich, J.L., Rothman, J., and Tropman, J.E. (eds.), *Strategies of community organization* (4th ed.). Itasca, IL: Peacock.

Sallis, J.F., and Nader, P.R. Family determinants of health behaviors. (1988a). In Gochman, D.S. (ed.), *Health behavior: emerging research perspectives*. New York: Plenum, pp. 107–124.

Sallis, J.F., Patterson, T.L., Buono, M.J., Atkins, C. J., and Nader, P.R. (1988b). Aggregation of physical activity habits in Mexican-American and Anglo families. *J Behav Med*, 11:31–41.

American Cancer Society Surveillance Research, 1997. Cancer Facts and Figures—1997. Atlanta, GA.

Serdula, M.K., Coates, R.J., Byer, T., Mokdad, A., and Subar, A. (1995). Fruit and vegetable intake among adults in 16 states: results of a brief telephone survey. *Am J Public Health*, 85:236–9.

Shiffman, S. (1989). Tobacco "chippers": individual differences in tobacco dependence. *Psychopharmacology*, 97:539–47.

Shiffman, S. (1991). Refining models of dependence: variations across persons and situations. *Br J Addict*, 86:611–5.

Shiffman, S. (1993). Smoking cessation treatment: any progress? *J Consult Clin Psychol*, 61:718–22.

Siegel, P.Z., Frazier, E.L., Mariolis, P, Brackbill, R.M., and Smith, C. (1993). Behavioral Risk Factor Surveillance, 1991: monitoring progress toward the nation's year 2000 health objectives. *Mor Mortal Wkly Rep CDC Surveill Summ*, 42:1–21.

Slovic, P. (1987). Perception of risk. *Science*, 236:280–5.

Sorensen, G., Pechacek, T., and Pallonen, U. (1986). Occupational and worksite norms and attitudes about smoking cessation. *Am J Public Health*, 76:544–9.

Sorensen, G., Rigotti, N., Rosen, A., Pinney, J., and Prible, R. (1991). The effects of a worksite nonsmoking policy: evidence for increased cessation. *Am J Public Health*, 81:202–4.

Sorensen, G., Stoddard, A., and Ockene, J. (1996). Worksite-based cancer prevention: primary results from the Working Well Trial. *Am J Public Health*, 86:939–47.

Sorensen, G., Emmons, K., Hunt, M.K., and Johnston, D. (1998). Implications of the results of community intervention trials. *Annu Rev Publ Health*, 19:379–416.

Stokols, D. (1992). Establishing and maintaining healthy environments: toward a social ecology of health promotion. *Am Psychol*, 47:6–22.

Stokols, D. (1996). Translating social ecological theory into guidelines for community health promotion. *Am J Health Promot*, 10:282–98.

Subar, A.F., Heimendinger, J., Krebs-Smith, S.M., Patterson, B.H., Kessler, R., and Pivonka, E. (1992). *Five a Day for Better Health: a baseline study of American's fruit and vegetable consumption*. Bethesda, MD: National Cancer Institute.

Subar, A.F., Heimendinger, J., Krebs-Smith, S.M., Patterson, B.H., Kessler, R., and Pivonka, E. (1995). Fruit and vegetable intake in the united states: the baseline survey of the Five a Day for Better Health Program. *Am J Health Promot*, 9:352–60.

Syme, S.L. (1997). Individual vs. community interventions in public health practice: some thoughts about a new approach. *Health Promotion Matters (VicHealth)* 2:2–9.

Tarlov, A.R. (1996). Social determinants of health, the sociobiological translation. In Blane, D., Brunner, E.J., and Wilkinson, R.G. (eds.), *Health and social organization*. London: Routledge, pp. 71–93.

Terborg, J., and Glasgow, R. (in press). Worksite interventions: a brief review of health promotion programs at work. In Baum, A., Newman, S., Weinman, J., West, R., and McManus, C. (eds.), *Cambridge handbook of psychology, health and medicine* (2nd ed.). London: Cambridge University Press.

Thomas, S.B., Quinn, S.C., Billingsley, A., and Caldwell, C. (1994). The characteristics of northern black churches with community health outreach programs. *Am J Public Health*, 84:575–9.

Tomatis, L. (1992). Poverty and cancer. *Cancer Epidemiol Biomarkers Prev* 1:67–175.

Troutt, D.D. (1993). *The thin red line: how the poor still pay more*. Oakland, CA: Consumers Union.

U. S. Department of Health and Human Services. (1990). *Healthy people 2000: national health promotion and disease prevention objectives*. (DHHS Pub. No. (PHS) 91-50212.) Washington, DC: U.S. Government Printing Office.

U.S. Department of Health and Human Services. (1996a). *Healthy people 2000 review, 1995–1996*. (DHHS Publication No. (PHS) 96-1256.) U.S. Department of Health and Human Services, Public Health Service, Centers for Disease Control and Prevention, National Center for Health Statistics, Washington, DC: U.S. Government Printing Office.

U.S. Department of Health and Human Services. (1996b). *Physical activity and health. A report of the Surgeon General*. Atlanta, GA: U.S. Department of Health and Human Services, Centers for Disease Control and Prevention, National Center for Chronic Disease Prevention and Health Promotion.

U.S. Preventive Services Task Force. (1996). *Guide to clinical preventive services* (2nd ed.). Baltimore, MD: Wiliams and Wilkins.

Velicer, W., Prochaska, J., and Bellis, J. (1993). An expert system intervention for smoking cessation. *Addict Behav,* 18:269–90.

Voorhees, C.C., Stillman, F.A., Swank, R.T., Heagerty, P.J., Levine, D.M., and Becker, D.M. (1996). Heart, body and soul: impact of church-based smoking cessation interventions on readiness to quit. *Prev Med,* 25: 277–85.

Wallack, L., and Wallerstein, N. (1987). Health education and prevention: designing community initiatives. *Int Q Community Health Educ,* 7:319–42.

Wallack, L., and Winkleby, M. (1986). Primary prevention: a new look at basic concepts. *Soc Sci Med,* 25:923–30.

Webber, D., Balsam, A., and Oehlke, B. (1995). The Massachusetts farmers' market coupon program for low income elders. *Am J Health Promot,* 9:251–3.

Weinstein, N. (1988). The precaution adoption process. *Health Psychol,* 7:355–86.

Wiist, W., and Flack, J. (1990). A church-based cholesterol education program. *Public Health Rep,* 105:381–7.

Wilkinson, R.G. (1992). Income distribution and life expectancy. *BMJ,* 304:165–8.

Willett, W.C., Colditz, G.A., and Mueller, N.E. (1996). Strategies for minimizing cancer risk. *Sci Am,* 275(3):88–91.

Williams, M.V., Parker, R.M., Baker, D.W., Parikh, N.S., Pitkin, K., Coates, W.C., and Nurss, J.R. (1995). Inadequate functional health literacy among patients at two public hospitals. *JAMA,* 274:1677–82.

Winkleby, M.A., Fortmann, S.P., and Barrett, D.C. (1990). Social class disparities in risk factors for disease: eight-year prevalence patterns by level of education. *Prev Med,* 19: 1–12.

12

Psychosocial Intervention

THOMAS A. GLASS

Within the larger field of social epidemiology, investigators are increasingly making the transition from observational studies to interventions designed to improve health and functioning. This transition has not, in all cases, been a smooth one. The design and evaluation of psychosocial interventions is an exceptionally challenging enterprise undertaken by practitioners forging what is still a relatively new field. In part, the difficulty of conducting intervention studies results from the need to modify existing study designs (most notably the randomized clinical trial) to fit the particular needs of psychosocial interventions. In addition, consensus has not been reached as to whether interventions should target individuals at high risk or entire communities. Further, debate continues as to whether health outcomes should be used or whether behavior change itself is a suitable end point for our investigations.

Early trials of psychosocial interventions have produced mixed results. Despite some early disappointments, progress in the development of new interventions and new

methodologies can now be seen. Psychosocial intervention studies are expensive, time-consuming, and complex undertakings that require careful planning and clear conceptualization. Well-executed psychosocial intervention studies can provide compelling evidence for a causal link between social factors and disease etiology. Further, they can help to identify the conditions under which candidate social factors are alterable, thereby offering hints as to the pathways through which social factors operate. Intervention studies also have an important policy role to play in deciding which programs will be deployed and which will join the legacy of demonstration projects that are never implemented. Three decades of experience have taught us that changing behavior is difficult and does not always lead to desired and anticipated improvements in health. With these challenges and promises in mind, the goals of this chapter are to:

1. Delineate the boundaries and characteristics of psychosocial interventions
2. Selectively highlight previous studies

3. Propose a series of theoretical tools to guide the next generation of intervention studies
4. Summarize the major methodological and conceptual pitfalls and some tentative ameliorative strategies
5. Suggest areas of future research

In addressing these goals, this chapter is guided by four propositions: Two are theoretical and conceptual, and two are methodological. These propositions summarize important lessons learned to date and are intended to guide researchers in the development of intervention studies in the future:

1. *Explicate the theoretical underpinnings of the intervention.* Detailed attention to problems of theory will guide the selection of variables, the choice of intervention strategies, and the design. The need for theory exists on several distinct levels. Previous research in this field has suffered from inattention to "upstream" factors through which the larger social context effects individual behavioral and psychological factors.

2. *Target a strategic psychosocial mechanism that has been shown to be related to the outcome.* Successful intervention designs focus on a circumscribed set of specific and strategically chosen mechanisms. If observational research has not demonstrated a link between the intended mechanisms and the outcome of interest, an intervention study is most likely premature.

3. *Choose a well-accepted and psychometrically sound measure of health or functioning as an outcome.* Psychosocial outcomes—such as coping, adjustment, and well-being—are important; however, they are far less compelling than are "hard" outcomes in which health or functioning is directly measured. In addition, previous research suggests that behavior change does not necessarily lead to changes in health. Therefore, behavior change itself may not be as compelling an outcome. Because psychosocial variables often rely on self-reports and are thus susceptible to various forms of bias, these variables are less attractive as outcome measures in studies of psychosocial intervention.

4. *Employ the strongest possible evaluation design.* Although the methodological challenges of pharmacological trials and psychosocial intervention trials are largely analogous, social epidemiologists can expect exceptional methodological scrutiny. For this reason, investigators should select the strongest possible designs. Sample sizes should be carefully considered, and when possible, randomized double-blind trials should be conducted. The unit of randomization can vary from individuals to more area-based units such as floors of a building, schools, work sites, and communities.

WHAT IS PSYCHOSOCIAL INTERVENTION?

The term *psychosocial intervention* is used widely in such fields as nursing, psychology, psychiatry, social work, sociology, and behavioral science. In its simplest meaning, the term refers to a systematic attempt to modify a psychosocial process. This can occur at the level of the individual, the family, the social network, the workplace, community, or at the population level. Defined in this way, changes in public policy designed to modify behavior, such as increased taxation of tobacco, constitute psychosocial interventions.

For the purposes of this chapter, however, the term will be used in a narrow way related to the mission of the field of social epidemiology. Since social epidemiology is the study of social and psychological factors as they relate to the etiology of disease, this means the chapter will focus on interventions aimed at changing some psychosocial process for the explicit purpose of modifying physical health or functioning. This includes the primary prevention of disease onset, recovery from illness, secondary prevention of disease, as well as modification of the course of disease. (For an introduction to the basic concepts of social epidemiology, see Kasl, 1983.) But it excludes psychiatric and psychological interventions that explicitly target mental health outcomes. It also excludes interventions designed to modify physiologic mechanisms. An example would be studies of the effect of relaxation techniques on blood pressure or cardiovascular reactivity (which are involved in the pathways of disease, but are not themselves physical health states). By extension, this also excludes those studies in which behavior change alone is the outcome, without explicit attention to the resulting health impact. Examples include interventions designed to result in smoking cessation, or the use of radon detection tests in the home. Another distinction is made between psychosocial interventions and health education efforts. In many respects, psychosocial intervention has much in common with health education at both the individual and community levels. Indeed, many of the interventions reviewed here involve education. To the extent that health education aims to modify health knowledge and attitudes alone, it falls outside of psychosocial intervention. (For excellent reviews of these studies see Abrams et al. 1997; Mullen et al. 1992; Sorensen et al. 1998.)

All four of these (excluded) intervention types are intended ultimately to modify health states or to alter the risk of disease in individuals or groups, but each constitutes a more fully elaborated field beyond the scope of this current chapter (see Chapter 11). Instead, the focus here will be on five types of psychosocial interventions and on the evaluation of intervention efficacy rather than design per se.

A TYPOLOGY OF PSYCHOSOCIAL INTERVENTIONS

There are several potential bases of organizing a typology of psychosocial interventions. One approach would be to emphasize the factors targeted for manipulation. Another would be to emphasize the desired outcome. A third approach would be to categorize interventions according to the intended target population (such as those afflicted with a disease or at high risk for that

disease). In this chapter, the first principle will be employed. Five types of intervention studies will be reviewed: (1) behavioral change interventions, (2) social support interventions, (3) disease management interventions, (4) distress mitigation interventions, and (5) control/efficacy enhancement interventions. This typology emphasizes the psychosocial mechanism targeted as well as whether the intervention is focused on prevention or alteration of the course of disease. The lines separating these three types are often blurred. This categorization is for heuristic purposes only as a way of describing the major studies that have been conducted to date. Table 12–1 lists some influential studies in each category. This is not intended to be an exhaustive list of studies. Many studies that lacked rigorous evaluation or which produced negative or inconclusive findings have been omitted. In the discussion below one or two examples of each intervention type will be given rather than a comprehensive review of all the studies that have been done.

Behavioral Change Interventions

The largest group of psychosocial intervention studies has been directed at the modification of specific behaviors that are risk factors for disease onset or recurrence. Most of these have been primary or secondary prevention efforts against cardiovascular disease. (For useful reviews, see Gyarfas 1992; Orth-Gomér and Schneiderman 1996; Razin 1982; Wenger et al. 1995.) Overall, the performance of population-based primary prevention trials designed to alter "lifestyle" factors has been mixed. Little or no benefit in long term follow-up has been observed in the Goteborg Primary Prevention Trial (Wilhelmsen et al. 1986), the Minnesota Heart Health Program (MHHP) (Luepker et al. 1994, 1996), and the Pawtucket Heart Health Program (Carleton et al. 1995). Disappointingly small changes in health behaviors have been observed in the Stanford Five-City Multi-Factor Risk Reduction Project (FCP) (Farquhar et al. 1990, 1985), and the WHO European Collabora-

Table 12-1. Selected list of psychosocial intervention studies by type

Principal Author/Publication	Study design	Intervention	Main results	General comments
Social Support Interventions				
"Psychosocial Benefits of a Cancer Support Group" (Cain et al. 1986)	Randomized controlled study of different support methods for women with gynecologic cancer. Standard counseling group ($n = 23$); Individual thematic counseling group ($n = 17$); group thematic counseling ($n = 20$)	Eight-session thematic counseling group focusing on information and coping techniques	Treatment groups (individual and group thematic counseling) significantly less depressed, less anxious, and more knowledgeable about their illness. Improved relationships with caregivers, fewer difficulties caregivers, fewer difficulties, and more participation in leisure activities	
"A Controlled Study of Respite Service for Caregivers of Alzheimer's Patients" (Lawton et al. 1989)	Randomized controlled trial. Control $n = 315$; treatment $n = 317$	One-year respite demonstration. Appealed to caregivers (not to respite seekers). Treatment groups offered formal respite care and were interviewed 1 year later	Families with respite care kept relative in the community significantly longer than did control group families. No significant relationship between change in well-being or caregiver burden, but satisfaction with program very high	
"A randomized Trial of Family Caregiver Support in the Home Management of Dementia" (Mohide et al. 1990)	Randomized controlled trial. Control $n = 30$ dyads, treatment $n = 30$ dyads	Six-month intervention period. Caregiver Support Program (CSP) for treatment group included weekly nurse visits initially, then as needed. Nurses assessed health of caregiver and encouraged them to seek medical attention if necessary. Caregivers received information and encouragement. Caregivers received 4-hour blocks of weekly in-home respite. Control group received care for patient only	No differences in depression and anxiety. Experimental group showed improvement in quality of life, found caregiver roles less problematic, and had greater satisfaction with nursing care	High attrition rate
"Exceptional Cancer Patient Program" (Morgenstern et al. 1984)	Nonrandomized retrospective follow-up. Control $n = 102$, treatment $n = 34$. Study included those who entered program between 1979 and 1981	Treatment group attended unstructured groups of 8–12 cancer patients plus invited relatives and friends. Discussed problems, engaged in mental imagery	Statistically significant beneficial effect of program on survival	May be due to selection bias—failure to match on duration of lag period between cancer diagnosis and program entry

Study	Design	Intervention	Results	Comments
"Behavioral Family Intervention with the Impaired Elderly" (Pinkston and Linsk, 1984)	Nonrandomized, no control group. Referred clients, n = 21.	Goal to increase positive behaviors of receivers and caregivers while decreasing behaviors considered to be "noxious." Employed reinforcement, prompts, and stimulus control	Mean scores for improvement on three target outcomes: self-care, social activities and positive behavior	No control group, small sample size
Home-based behavioral family treatment of the impaired elderly (Pinkston et al. 1988)	Nonrandomized, no control group. Design similar to 1984 study. N = 66	See 1984 study. Also targeting aggression and socialization	Case-by-case analysis, single subject designs. Improvement in targeted behavior (76%)	Varied illnesses and degrees of severity
"Effect of psychosocial treatment on survival of patients with metastatic breast cancer" (Spiegel et al. 1989)	Prospective group-intervention outcome study. Treatment group n = 50; control group n = 36. Random assignment?	Patients met in weekly psychological support groups	Tx group exhibited significantly less tension, fatigue, confusion, and more vigor than control group. Self-hypnosis led to significant decrease in pain. Trend toward less depression, fewer phobias, and fewer maladjusted coping responses. At 10-year follow-up, from entry to death, the study group lived twice as long as the controls (survival time ratio, control to study group, 18.9:36.6, $P < 0.0001$)	

Behavioral Change Interventions

Study	Design	Intervention	Results	Comments
"Multiple Risk Factor Intervention Trial (MRFIT)" (Anonymous,1982)	Randomized primary prevention trial of 12,866 high-risk middle-aged men recruited at 22 sites. Average duration of follow-up was 7 years. 361,662 men were screened, and 3.5% were enrolled/ Seven percent qualified on the basis of risk screening	Special intervention included stepped-care treatment for hypertension, counseling for cigarette smoking, dietary advice for lowering blood cholesterol	Risk factors decreased more for treatment group than control group, but differences were modest and may not have been sustained. Overall CHD mortality differences were nonsignificant. overall mortality rate 2% higher in treatment group	Trial criticized for not addressing social and environmental factors and for exclusive emphasis on high-risk individuals. Variation in risk reduction among high-risk individuals was high. Secular trends in risk factor reduction reduced statistical power from 90% to 60%. Demonstrates limitations of individually targeted "high-risk" approach

(*continued*)

Table 12-1. Selected list of psychosocial intervention studies by type—Continued

Principal Author/Publication	Study design	Intervention	Main results	General comments
"Community Intervention Trial for Smoking Cessation (COMMIT)," (Anonymous 1995; Royce et al. 1997)	Heavy smokers, $n = 10,019$; light-to-moderate smokers, $n = 10,328$	Community-level multichannel 4-year intervention designed to increase smoking cessation among 11 matched community pairs (10 in U.S., 1 in Canada)	Mean quit rate for heavy smokers who received intervention was 0.180. Mean quit rate for comparison group was 0.187; nonsignificant difference. Significant differences for light-to-moderate smokers in intervention (0.306) and comparison (0.275) communities	Women less likely than men to be heavy smokers but twice as likely to feel pressure to quit
"Pawtucket Heart Health Program" (Carleton et al. 1995)	Randomized community-based intervention	Community-wide education program applied to intervention city on three levels: risk factors, behavior change, and community activation	Statistically significant city decrease in projected cardiovascular disease rate for Pawtucket (16%) during peak intervention time. This decrease was not maintained after postintervention period	No long-term discernible effects on mortality or risk factors. Attributable to mass media messages to which both towns may have been exposed
"Stanford Five-City Multi-Factor Risk Reduction Project (FCP)" (Farquhar et al. 1990; Farquhar et al. 1985)	A 14-year trial of community-wide CVD risk reduction. Nonrandomized community level intervention in northern CA. Epidemiologic surveillance and measurement of health-related behaviors over 14-year period ($n = 122,800$ in treatment cities; $n = 197,500$ in control cities)	Community-wide organization and health education including media and "personal influence" in tx communities lasting 5 years. Targets included (1) lower plasma cholesterol through diet change, (2) reduced blood pressure, (3) weight control, and increased physical activity. Spanish language program also implemented	Net decrease in mean cholesterol level (2%), and mean blood pressure (4%) in both cohort and independent samples. These risk factor changes resulted in composite total mortality risk scores that were 15% lower in the intervention communities and CHD risk scores that were 16% lower	Positive intervention effect on risk factors. Results may not be generalizable since samples were not randomly chosen or assigned. Cities are intervention units. Results of independent samples differ from cohort samples. This may be due to less exposure to education (e.g. recent immigrants)
"Recurrent Coronary Prevention Project (RCCP)" (Friedman et al. 1984)	Postmyocardial infarction patients treated for 4.5 years, after which subjects were followed for additional 4 years. At beginning of trial control group $n = 270$, experimental group $n = 592$, comparison group $n = 151$	Control group received group cardiac counseling. Experimental group received group cardiac counseling plus type A behavioral counseling. Comparison group did not receive either type of counseling	At end of 4.5 years 35.1% of treatment group showed "markedly reduced" type A behavior. Control group decreased by 9.8%. Cumulative recurrence rate of MI of treatment group was 12.9% (compared with 21.2% cumulative recurrence rate of control group or 28.2% cumulative recurrence rate of comparison group)	

Study	Design	Intervention	Results	Comments
"HIV Risk Behavior Reduction Following Intervention with Key Opinion Leaders of Population: An Experimental Analysis" (Kelly et al. 1991)	One intervention city and two comparison cities (pop = 50,000–75,000 residents). Surveys of male patrons of clubs completed at baseline, 3 months (intervention n = 328; comparison n = 331), and 6 months after training period (intervention n = 278; comparison n = 330)	Key opinion leaders chosen by bartenders at clubs and were trained in HIV risk reduction behavior, strategies, and role-playing	Intervention city men who engaged in unprotected anal intercourse decreased (−25% from baseline), a reduction of unprotected receptive anal intercourse (−30%), an increase in condom use (16%) during anal intercourse, and a decrease in percentage of men with more than one sexual partner (−18%)	Generalizable to population but not to those who do not frequent clubs, nonwhites, and teens. Bias—self-reported results
"Modifying the Type A Coronary-Prone Behavior Pattern" (Levenkron et al. 1983)	Male volunteers (total n =38) between the ages of 25 and 50 received treatment. Comprehensive behavior therapy (CBT), n =12; group support (GS), n =13; brief information (BI), n = 13	CBT group received training in self-control and relaxation. GS group encouraged self-awareness of TABP, specification of Type-A behaviors, and "inducing change through non-specific support and exhortation of both therapist and group members"	CBT and GS groups showed decreases in TABP components (e.g., Jenkins Activity Survey, Hard driving, Job involvement factor, Framingham, and Type A Scale.) Trend in negative mean changes in plasma-free fatty acids for CBT and GS groups. CBT group exhibited significant decrease in triglyceride	Results may not be generalizable to population—subjects mainly from one corporation and were healthy, highly educated, and nondistressed males. Unexpected result: serum cholesterol increased across all groups
"Minnesota Heart Health Program (MHHP)" (Luepker et al. 1994; 1996)	13-year community-wide research and demonstration project	Three pairs of matched intervention and comparison communities received 5-year health education program. Program designed to improve health behaviors, lower blood cholesterol and blood pressure, and reduce cardiovascular disease morbidity and mortality	No discernible differences between intervention communities and comparison communities	Results attributed to secular trends of increasing health promotion and declining risk factors
"Lifestyle Heart Trial," (Ornish et al. 1990)	Randomized controlled clinical trial to test short-term effects of lifestyle on coronary heart disease	Intervention to teach lifestyle changes (low-fat vegetarian diet, smoking cessation, stress management, moderate exercise). $2 \times$ weekly group discussions provided social support to facilitate lifestyle changes. Discussions led by clinical psychologist; pro-	82% of experimental group had an average change toward regression of coronary artery lesion diameters. Greater changes were found in more severely stenosed lesions	Lifestyle changes may be effective without use of lipid-lowering drugs

(continued)

Table 12-1. Selected list of psychosocial intervention studies by type—Continued

Principal Author/Publication	Study design	Intervention	Main results	General comments
"The North Karelia Project." (Puska et al. 1989) See also (Jousilahti et al. 1994; Puska 1992; Puska et al. 1988, 1993; Salonen 1987; Salonen et al. 1989)	Comprehensive community-based health intervention launched in 1972. Results compiled through survey of representative samples of individuals in 3 communities—North Karelia (intervention) and Kuopio County and southwest Finland at 5-year intervals	moted adherence to program, communication skills, & expression of feelings Program targeted reductions in risk factors (smoking, serum cholesterol, and blood pressure). Comprehensive health education program to promote healthy lifestyles, taught practical skills, provided social support for change, and arranged environmental modifications. Unit of intervention was community	After 10 years, reductions in smoking (28%), hypertension (3%), and serum cholesterol levels (3%) were faster among men in intervention community than in comparison community or rest of Finland. Significant improvements in women observed only for blood pressure. Between 1974 and 1979, CHD mortality declined twice as fast in N. Karelia (22%) compared to reference community (12%) or rest of Finland (11%) ($p < 0.05$)	First large scale primary prevention demonstration (on which many other studies were based). Study launched in 1972 after public outcry over statistics showing that Finnish men had the highest rates of CHD mortality and risk factor prevalence in Europe. Study demonstrates importance of community approach as opposed to "high-risk" strategy (See Rose). Among the few studies that attempted environmental modifications along with traditional health education model. May have been effective because it predated onset of significant secular trend toward reductions in risk factors
"Washington Heights-Inwood Healthy Heart Program." (Shea et al. 1996)	Six-year community-based cardiovascular disease program in NYC, targeted urban, minority population	Program designed primarily to implement health education model rather than to evaluate its efficacy. High-fat diet, sedentary lifestyle, and smoking were primary risk factors targeted	Low-fat milk campaign, volunteer-led exercise club, and Spanish-language Smoking Cessation video were successful elements of campaign (as measured by potential for encouraging long-term behavioral change and for potential to transfer responsibility to community-based organizations.) School-based smoking prevention activities, cholesterol screening, and motivating	Community-based prevention program is feasible to prevent cardiovascular disease risk in low-income, minority, urban population. Evaluation of community health education is essential

Disease Management Interventions

<table>
<tr>
<td></td>
<td></td>
<td>community physicians to promote heart health were less successful</td>
<td></td>
</tr>
<tr>
<td>"Family Intervention after Stroke: Does Counseling or Education Help?" (Evans et al. 1988)</td>
<td>Randomized controlled trial. Control n = 63, education treatment n = 64, counseling and education treatment (n = 61)</td>
<td>Educational treatment consisted of two 1-hour sessions on basic stroke care. Counseling and educational treatment included seven 1-hour counseling sessions with a cognitive/behaviorally-trained social worker.</td>
<td>At 6 months and 1 year of follow-up, both treatments significantly improved caregivers' knowledge and stabilized some aspects of family function. Counseling treatment was more effective than education alone</td>
</tr>
<tr>
<td>"A Structured Psychiatric Intervention for Cancer Patients. I. Changes over Time in Methods of Coping and Affective Disturbance (Fawzy et al. 1990a); "A Structured Psychiatric Intervention for Cancer Patients. II. Changes over Time in Immunological Measures" Fawzy et al. 1990b)</td>
<td>Prospective longitudinal study of patients with early diagnosis of malignant melanoma with good prognosis. Subjects not randomized</td>
<td>Meetings included health education, problem-solving skills, stress management, and psychological support</td>
<td>Intervention group exhibited significantly lower rate of recurrence of disease and mortality than control group. Moderate to high levels of psychological turmoil followed diagnosis of cancer. Distress in experimental group decreased after intervention and increased use of adaptive coping strategies. Also increased positive, active coping methods and distraction strategies associated with decrease of negative mood</td>
</tr>
<tr>
<td>"Outcomes of Self-Help Education for Patients with Arthritis" (Lorig et al. 1985)</td>
<td>Randomized prospective longitudinal study. Control n = 65, treatment n = 134</td>
<td>Volunteers participated in 15–20 person groups (including family members) for 6 sessions over 4 months, facilitated by lay leaders. Course focused on nature of arthritis, appropriate use of medication, range of motion and isometric exercises</td>
<td>No conclusions of clinical significance. Conclusions about pain remain tentative. Increase in knowledge and recommended behaviors and lessened pain. Mid-severity-level arthritis sufferers. Pain scales subjective. Significant baseline differences were seen when measured with one of the pain scales. Self-reported data. Homogeneous sample—white, middle class, well-educated</td>
</tr>
<tr>
<td>"Long-Term Outcomes of an Arthritis Self-Management Study: Effects of reinforcement Efforts" (Lorig and Holman 1989)</td>
<td>Randomized controlled trial. Control n = 153, newletter n = 130, treatment n = 70</td>
<td>All participated in Arthritis Self-Management Course (ASMC), individually-designed exercise and relaxation programs, nutrition, medication usage, appropriate use of joints, patient/physician com-</td>
<td>Between baseline and 20 months all participants reduced their pain by 20%, depression by 14%, and physician visits by 35%. Course included significant others</td>
</tr>
</table>

(continued)

Table 12-1. Selected list of psychosocial intervention studies by type—Continued

Principal Author/Publication	Study design	Intervention	Main results	General comments
"Arthritis Self-Management: A Study of the Effectiveness of Patient Education for the Elderly" (Lorig et al. 1984)	200 participants (55–74 years old n = 151; 75–94 years old n = 43.) enrolled in a series of randomized controlled evaluation studies; questionnaires mailed out at 4, 8, and 20 months	munication, medical problem solving. One year after baseline, subjects were randomized and half were offered to take Arthritis Reinforcement Course. One group received four bi-monthly ARC newsletters; second group participated in course, third group did not participate. Twelve-hour community-based self-management course offered to two groups of people, stratified by age. Course taught by lay leaders of various age ranges	55–74 group maintained significant reduction in pain and gains in knowledge for 20 months. Also reductions in disability for 8 months. Older group, 75–94 increased knowledge for 20 months, decreased pain and increased number of visits to physician for 8 months	In some cases stronger results seen at 8 months than at 4 months. Difference if course had not been taught by layperson?
"Controlled Trial of Psychological Intervention in Myocardial Infarction" (Oldenburg et al. 1985)	Controlled trial. Standardized education treatment n = 16. standardized individualized counseling treatment n = 16, control group n = 14	Standardized education group listened to three audio tapes containing information about MI and relaxation training. Standardized individual counseling received educational component and 6–10 individual counseling sessions focusing on their fears and anxieties and other issues about their illness	At 3, 6, and 12 months, both intervention groups performed significantly better on measures of psychology and lifestyle functioning, and reported fewer symptoms of heart disease	Retrospective self-reporting. Low statistical power
"Behavioral Intervention with and Without Family Support for Rheumatoid Arthritis" (Radojevic et al. 1992)	Fifty-nine subjects with "definite" or classical rheumatoid arthritis randomly assigned to four treatment groups	Six-week treatment period. Behavior therapy group received four 90-minute sessions and 2 weeks of independent skill consolidation. Behavior Therapy Family Therapy group received	Behavioral interventions showed significantly greater improvement in joint exam pain at follow-up	Huge standard deviations for means—may not be good indicators of central tendency

"The Effect of Compliance with Treatment on Survival among Patients with Hematologic Malignancies" (Richardson et al. 1990)	same therapy with the inclusion of a family member. Education Family Support group included a family member in a presentation of videotaped educational information. Successive cohorts of newly diagnosed patients entered special educational groups (control n = 25; intervention with education and home visit n = 25; intervention with education and "shaping" n = 23; intervention with education, home visit and shaping n = 24). Three levels of disease severity or prognostic levels according to risk of death	High disease severity, high compliance with allopurinol and educational program cohort associated with increased survival	Links between compliance and survival are not clear

Distress Mitigation Interventions

"Stress Management and Exercise Training in Cardiac Patients with Myocardial Ischemia. Effects on Prognosis and Evaluation of Mechanisms (Blumenthal et al. 1997)	Non-randomized design using community controls (total n = 107). Patients with CAD and ischemia documented during stress testing were randomly assigned to either exercise (n = 34) or stress management training (n = 33). Annual patient follow-up continued for 5 years. Exercise group engaged in aerobic exercise 3 times per week for 16 weeks. Subjects monitored their heart rates. Stress-management intervention was based on "cognitive-social learning model of behavior." Program consisted of sixteen 1.5 hour sessions conducted in a group setting with 8 patients per group. Program modeled on the RCPP and Life Stress Monitoring Program using cognitive-behavioral principles	Stress management subjects experienced a lower relative risk of cardiac events compared to control subjects (RR = 0.26; P = 0.04). Patients in the exercise group showed a trend toward lower rates of cardiac events but the trend was not significant (RR = 0.68; P = 0.41)	
"Coping with Cancer during the First Year after Diagnosis: Assessment and Intervention" (Edgar et al. 1992)	Randomized controlled comparison study with follow-up (early intervention group n = 103; later intervention group n = 102) Coping-skills-based psychosocial intervention. Increase adaptation and coping skills of patients with newly-diagnosed cancer. Intervention administered immediately and four-months after diagnosis	Later-intervention group exhibited less depression, anxiety, and worry. In general, those with high baseline ego strength had lower distress	Results may be attributable to emotional distress of cancer diminishing over time. Patients may have mobilized resources better. Adherence may have been better

(continued)

Table 12-1. Selected list of psychosocial intervention studies by type—Continued

Principal Author/Publication	Study design	Intervention	Main results	General comments
"Ischemic Heart Disease Life Stress Monitoring Program" (Frasure-Smith and Prince 1989)	Long-term results of a 1-year randomized controlled trial involving 444 male patients. Treatment group $n = 222$; control group $n = 222$	Treatment group received standard care as well as stress monitoring and nurse intervention program. Control group received standard care	Results at 1-year: treatment patients ($n = 222$) had significantly reduced stress, and control patients ($n = 222$) twice as likely to die of cardiac causes as treatment patients. After end of 4th year, treatment group ($n = 176$) and control group ($n = 179$) exhibited statistically significant differences in MI recurrence	Weaknesses of study include substantial loss to follow-up. Subjects were eliminated from sample after randomization due to new information about eligibility and refusal. Our-of-hospital deaths may not be valid proxy of sudden death. Patients who experience second or subsequent MIs without complications are not represented.
"Effects of Individualized Breast Cancer Risk Counseling: A Randomized Trial" (Lerman et al. 1995); "A Randomized Trial of Breast Cancer Risk Counseling: Interacting Effects of Counseling, Educational level and Coping Style" (Lerman et al. 1996)	Evaluated the impact of individualized breast cancer risk counseling (BCRC) on breast-cancer-specific distress and general distress in 239 women with a family history of breast cancer. Following a baseline assessment of demographics, risk factors, coping styles, and distress, participants were assigned randomly to receive either BCRC or general health education (GHE; i.e., control group)	Standardized protocol for individualized breast cancer risk counseling	After controlling for education level, women who received BCRC had significantly less breast-cancer-specific distress at 3-month follow-up compared with women who received GHE. Also, women who received risk counseling were significantly more likely to improve their risk comprehension compared with women in the control condition (odds ratio [OR] = 3.5; 95% confidence interval [CI] = 1.3–9.5; $P = 0.01$)	A significant Education Level × Treatment Group interaction indicated that the psychological benefits of BCRC were greater for women with less formal education. In both the BCRC and GHE groups, participants who had monitoring coping styles exhibited increases in general distress from baseline to follow-up
"Randomized Trial of a Psychological Distress Screening Program after Breast Cancer: Effects on Quality of Life" (Maunsell et al. 1996)	Randomized controlled trial of newly diagnosed breast cancer patients. 200 women with localized or regional-stage disease randomized into control group and experimental group. Assessed at 3 and 12 months after initial surgical treatment $n = 123$; control group, $n = 127$	Control group received minimal psychosocial follow-up through already-existing clinic program. Experimental group received clinic services plus systematic screening of psychological distress plus telephone screening once every 28 days totaling to 12 calls	Overall psychological distress decreased for both groups. No significant differences between the two. Outcome measure is quality of life: physical health, functional status and psychosocial characteristics	Possible confounders: subjects may have enrolled in other treatment trials; met individually with a recovered breast cancer patient; consulted with a family physician, other physicians, someone practicing alternative medicine, psychiatrist or psychologist; sought help because of feeling depressed or sad; had a confi-

Study	Description	Results	Limitations
			dant; participated in activities to specifically aid or learn relaxation; made dietary changes; had breast cancer recurrence.
"Montreal Heart Attack Readjustment Trial" (Frasure-Smith 1995; Frasure-Smith et al. 1997)	Randomized controlled trial to reduce mortality in patients postmyocardial infarction (total n = 1376; 903 men; 473 women). Follow-up at 1 year	No significant differences in 1-year survival were observed. In preplanned analyses, an increase in cardiac and all-cause mortality among women in the PSI was seen	Intervention may have been underpowered. Average number of visits was 5–6. Nurses had little or no mental health training. Extension of the Ischemic Heart Disease Life Stress Monitoring Program
"Psychosocial Group Intervention and the Rate of Decline of Immunological Parameters in Asymptomatic HIV-Infected Homosexual Men" (Mulder et al. 1995)	Volunteers from a natural history study randomized into a cognitive–behavioral group (CBT) n = 14 and an experiential group therapy (ET) n = 12. Nonvolunteers used as controls	No positive differences. Men with largest reduction in psychological distress in both ET and CBT groups showed a smaller decline in CD4 cells	The comparison group was self-selected (not randomized). Sample size small. Relatively short follow-up period
"Group Coping Skills Instruction and Supportive Group Therapy for Cancer Patients: A Comparison of Strategies" (Telch and Telch 1986)	Randomized controlled trial. Coping skills instruction (n = 13); support group therapy (n = 14) and no-treatment control (n = 14). Six-weekly sessions of coping skills training and support group for clinically distressed cancer patients. Three groups: group coping skills instruction support group therapy and no-treatment control	Treatment group showed positive gains in affect, satisfaction, physical and social activities, cognitive distress, communication, and coping with medical procedures. Control group psychological functioning decreased	Sample included different cancer types
Control Interventions			
"Psychological, Sociological and Health Behavior Aspects of a Long-Term Activation Programme for Institutionalized Elderly People" (Arnetz and Theorell 1983)	Quasi-experimental design over a 6-month period. A program was devised in collaboration with residents of a senior apartment building and its staff. Aim of intervention was to increase social activation and to encourage enhanced control over daily life. Residents were given opportunities for self-directed activity planning. Staff were given a course on gerontology. The course stressed the importance of self-determination for the elderly	Social activity level increased 3-fold in intervention group at 6 months. Health differences were nonsignificant. Restlessness was decreased in intervention group	Small sample sizes makes conclusions difficult. Possibility of contamination from changes in the control floors

Table 12-1. Selected list of psychosocial intervention studies by type—Continued

Principal Author/Publication	Study design	Intervention	Main results	General comments
"Effects of Brief Psychotherapy during the Hospitalization Period on the Recovery Process in Heart Attacks" (Gruen 1975)	Hospitalized heart attack patients	Brief, cognitively oriented intervention designed to facilitate coping and to increase the subjects' sense of control	At 4 months, patients who received the intervention were less likely to have had arrhythmias, showed lower levels of depression and anxiety, and were more likely to return to normal levels of activity compared to matched controls.	
"Healthy Work: Stress, Productivity, and the Reconstruction of Working Life" (Karasek and Theorell 1990)	Employees in a nursing home. Experimental design	Workplace redesign to try to increase worker's sense of control, predictability and participation	Health care workers in the experimental group took fewer sick days and reported improved self-esteem	
"Transfer from a Coronary Care Unit" (Klein et al. 1968)		Modification of procedures in the coronary care unit including (1) preparing the patient for transfer, (2) continuity in doctors and nurses during ward transfers, (3) daily nurse visits to provide information and counseling	Intervention patients developed fewer cardiovascular complications and lower catecholamine excretion	Treatment and control groups differed on disease severity, which weakens overall findings
"The Effects of Choice and Enhanced Personal Responsibility for the Aged: A Field Experiment in an Institutional Setting" (Langer and Rodin 1976); "Long-Term Effects of a Control-Relevant Intervention with the Institutionalized Aged" (Rodin and Langer 1977)	Quasi-experimental trial conducted in a nursing home setting. Assignment by floors (total $n = 91$) 18-month follow-up. Treatment group $n = 20$; comparison group $n = 14$; control group $n = 9$	Residents in the experimental group were given a communication emphasizing their responsibility for themselves, whereas the communication given to the comparison group stressed the staff's responsibility for them. Intervention included houseplants that were either taken care of by the treatment residents or by the staff (comparison group)	Significant improvements were seen in activity, alertness, and general well-being. Also, differences in mortality rates between treatment group (15%) and comparison group (30%) were significant at 18 months	Possible biases—patients assigned throughout nursing home rather than by floor; patient–nurse interaction may have affected results (nurses may have reacted when patients began to improve)

tive Group Trial (World Health Organization 1986). Other trials aimed at high-risk individuals, including the Multiple Risk Factor Intervention Trial (MRFIT), observed small changes in health behaviors that did not translate into anticipated reductions in rates of morbidity or mortality (Anonymous 1982).

Numerous commentaries have been offered to explain why these large studies fell short of expectation, and the reader is referred to Mervyn Susser's exceptional summary editorial (1995). Among the points made by Susser is that many community-based trials have failed to overcome large-scale social movements, resulting in changes in the control subjects that in turn affected the power of the trial to detect real improvements. Or as Susser put it, the trials were *"outrun by the pace of social change"* (p. 157).

In most of these trials, the health behaviors that constitute risk factors for disease (diet, smoking, exercise) have been viewed as discrete, voluntary, and individually modifiable "lifestyle" choices, detached from the social context in which behaviors arise (Coreil et al. 1985). For this reason, many of these trials have been criticized for ignoring "upstream" social factors antecedent to behaviors at an individual level.

This tendency to ignore the social basis of behaviors is reflected in the theoretical foundations upon which many of the primary prevention trials have been formulated. In several cases, little evidence of a well-articulated theoretical framework can be found. Among those studies that have made their theoretical models explicit, most appear to have been influenced to varying degrees by some variant of social learning theory (see MacLean 1994). Like most psychological theories, social learning theory, to the extent that it emphasizes self-efficacy beliefs as properties of individuals, tends to shift the focus away from upstream factors related to the social context, toward more individually based models. The result is that the theories that have guided intervention research have contributed to the idea that health behaviors are discrete, atomized, and detached from larger social contexts.

A number of other trials did show evidence of risk factor reduction as well as declines in subsequent coronary heart disease (CHD) morbidity. In the Oslo trial, for example, 5-year CHD incidence was significantly reduced (by 47%) in the intervention group compared with the control group (Hjermann 1983). The first such community-based CHD prevention project was the North Karelia study, which involved a "comprehensive community organization for change" including individual behavior change interventions complemented by social supports and environmental modifications. This study was widely influential, in part because it demonstrated reductions in both risk factors (smoking, blood pressure, and serum cholesterol) and also reductions in both morbidity and mortality. The success of the first-generation studies, such as North Karelia, may have resulted from the accident of their timing: they began before large-scale secular trends toward increased exercise, dietary change, and smoking cessation had fully begun. Interestingly, in the aftermath of successful results in North Karelia, implementation of heart disease prevention efforts in the rest of Finland was slow to take root (Salonen 1991).

In contrast to the large-scale community interventions that targeted a wide range of health behaviors all at once, a series of more focused, theoretically grounded studies has sought to target a more narrow band of the behavioral spectrum. No domain of behavior has been more thoroughly subject to systematic investigation than type A behavior (TAB). Several large-scale attempts to alter TAB proved to be ineffectual in reducing subsequent recurrence rates (including the MRFIT study (Shekelle et al. 1985)). However, the most important intervention study in this area has been the Recurrent Coronary Prevention Project (RCPP) (Friedman et al. 1982, 1987; Powell et al. 1993). In that study, 1035 male and female subjects age 64 years or younger who had suffered their first or last documented acute myocardial infarction were enrolled in a 5-year study to determine the prevalence of TAB, the extent to which TAB itself is modifiable, and whether a program designed to alter TAB would result in lower rates of fatal and nonfatal coronary recurrence. After 1 year, results indicated that the prevalence of TAB was quite high (98%) and that rates of cardiovascular death and reinfarction were lower among subjects who received cardiologic and behavioral counseling compared to usual care controls (Friedman et al. 1982). In addition, the rate of cardiovascular death was lower among those who received counseling designed to reduce TAB even compared to those who received just cardiologic counseling. After 4.5 years of follow-up, 35% of the treatment group showed "markedly reduced TAB" compared with a decrease of 10% in the control group (Friedman 1986). Cumulative recurrence of MI was significantly lower (13% vs. 21%). The RCPP succeeded in showing that TAB could be modified and that the resulting change translated into fewer coronary events. It was also among the only studies that showed that the benefits of the intervention were persistent over at least 5.5 years (Friedman et al. 1987). Another feature of the RCPP worth mentioning is that the effects of counseling appeared to boost the benefits of educational interventions alone. Similar studies involving both educational interventions designed to alter TAB and that included an emotional support component have been conducted by Rahe and colleagues (Rahe et al. 1979).

Another important study involving a systematic attempt to alter risk-prone behavior was the Lifestyle Heart Trial conducted by Dean Ornish and colleagues (Ornish 1982; Ornish et al. 1983, 1990). In this randomized, controlled trial, 28 men were given a short-term, comprehensive, lifestyle intervention involving low-fat vegetarian diet, smoking cessation, stress management training, moderate exercise, and support group discussions led by a psychologist and were compared to a group of 20 usual care controls. Eighty-two percent of the experimental group showed evidence of regression of coronary artery lesions 1 year after intervention. Greater improvements were found in more severely stenosed lesions. The Lifestyle Heart Trial is notable as one of the first trials to demonstrate the benefits of a complex, multimodal behavioral intervention using a "hard" physiologic outcome. The success and visibility of Ornish's work have led to the widespread adoption of cardiac rehabilitation programs modeled on this work. The long-term benefits of these programs have not as yet been thoroughly evaluated, although a recent study using positron emission tomography (PET) has shown that the benefits of this intervention are detectable after 5 years (Gould et al. 1995).

Social Support Interventions

Social networks and support have been shown to be associated with mortality, with morbidity, with recovery, and with disease course in numerous previous studies (see Chapter 7 in this volume). Interventions designed to bolster support or to provide specialized types of support are a natural extension of these observational studies. While the exact mechanisms that underlie the association between social support and health are not known, the evidence is sufficient to warrant the development of innovative intervention strategies which are designed to impact particular pathways. Support interventions have been conducted primary at the individual level; however, several noteworthy programs have attempted to enhance the supportiveness of relationships in work sites (Heaney 1991) and in families (Gonzalez et al. 1989). Many of these support interventions have conceptual and methodological roots in the tradition of *network therapy* (Attneave 1978; Halevy-Martini et al. 1984; Speck and Attneave 1973). Typically, social support interventions have been conducted in populations previously afflicted with a major illness such as heart disease, stroke, cancer, or arthritis. Additional examples include treatment approaches for addictions (Galanter 1993;

Galanter et al. 1997) and schizophrenia (Garrison 1978; Lehtinen 1994; Wasylenki et al. 1992).

At least five modalities of support interventions can be distinguished: *(1)* professionally led support groups, *(2)* mutual support groups, *(3)* multifamily support groups, *(4)* support mobilization interventions, and *(5)* support substitution interventions. In various ways, and from various theoretical orientations, each attempts to bolster social support resources either by potentiating naturally occurring support systems or by utilizing what Gottlieb has termed "grafted support."[1] More extensive discussions of the conduct of support interventions can be found in overviews by Biegel et al. (1984) and Gottlieb (1985, 1988).

In general, the literature regarding support interventions has produced mixed results. This is the result, in part, of the methodological shortcomings of many of these studies, including small sample sizes and weak designs. For example, in a thoughtful review of support interventions in patients with rheumatoid arthritis, Lanza and Revenson (1993) argue that the failures of many support interventions may also be due to the lack of firm theoretical grounding. They also note that the issue of timing must be carefully considered when planning a network intervention. Because support is the product of relationships that develop and change slowly, the benefits of support interventions may be missed in short-term intervention studies. However, network mobilization must coordinate with the crisis phase of the illness or risk missing the window of opportunity for maximal efficacy. At least one network intervention effort appears to have failed because the intervention started too late (Friedland and McColl 1992).

Many interventions that do not identify themselves as support interventions nonetheless contain significant (and sometimes

---

[1]Gottlieb defines "grafted support" as support opportunities that are created by the intervention and are presumed to become efficacious sources of support over time (Gottlieb, 1988).

hidden) support components. This makes categorization of interventions difficult. For example, the studies by Ornish et al. (1990) of the impact of a "lifestyle" change intervention in men with heart disease is classified by the authors as a behavioral change intervention. Yet the support group organized as a vehicle to facilitate the behavioral intervention obviously provides an avenue for social support. It becomes difficult to separate the influence of this secondary support from the intended influence of the intervention on behavior. In other cases, interventions that are not intended to provide support but involve family and friends also create inadvertent opportunities for enhanced communication and support. For example, in an intervention to teach arthritis patients self-care behaviors in a group setting, participants cited the "feeling of knowing that everyone cared" as a benefit of the program (Knudson et al. 1981). The group leader also noted that participants "appeared to benefit psychologically from the emotional support given in the small-group setting" (Knudson et al. 1981, p. 81). These comments are noteworthy because the intervention itself was described as educational.

In many interventions that are described as health educational, social support is provided or facilitated as a secondary goal. (See, for example, the North Karelia study.) One important illustration is the Infant Health and Development Program, the most extensive comprehensive early intervention program yet to be evaluated for improving health and cognitive development among low-birth-weight and premature infants (Anonymous 1990; Brooks-Gunn et al. 1994). In that program, social support was provided both to families and to children attending clinics. As in most studies of this kind, few details are given about the nature of this support and its ultimate impact on outcome.

One intervention trial that has received much attention was conducted by Spiegel and colleagues (1989), who randomly assigned 86 patients with metastatic breast cancer to either a control group or a treatment group that received a 1-year intervention consisting of weekly supportive group therapy with self-hypnosis for pain. At 10-year follow-up, women in the treatment group on average had survived twice as long as those in the control group even after controlling for stage at diagnosis, treatment differences, and several other factors (mean of 36.6 months vs. 18.9 months, respectively). Although the treatment consisted of both support and disease management features, this study provides the most powerful evidence to date that a support-group model is associated with longer survival in critically ill patients.

Disease Management Interventions

A third cluster of interventions targets psychosocial aspects of the postonset phase of illness in an effort to enhance the patient's ability to cope with the disease or to prevent symptom recurrence. The emphasis in these studies is on providing specific coping strategies designed to address particular problems encountered in the course of the disease in question. One group of studies has focused on improving adherence to medical treatments. Perhaps the most important study of this types is by Richardson and colleagues (1990). In this study, 94 patients newly diagnosed with hematologic cancer were randomized to an intervention designed to improve compliance with chemotherapy or to a usual-care control group. Through education, home visits, and behavioral intervention, this study was able to show longer survival even after controlling for a variety of factors including compliance.

In another study, Fawzy and colleagues conducted a nonrandomized study to evaluate a disease management program in patients with early diagnosis of malignant melanoma with good prognosis (Fawzy et al. 1990a). The intervention included health education, problem-solving skills, stress management techniques, and psychological support. Results showed improvement in active coping skills; in significantly lower

depression, fatigue, confusion, and total mood disturbance; as well as higher vigor in the intervention group. Also important was the finding that the intervention was associated with beneficial changes in one aspect of immune system performance: the natural killer (NK) lymphoid cell system (Fawzy et al. 1990b). Long-term follow-up indicated that patients in the intervention group had longer survival (Fawzy et al. 1993). Other studies, including one which involved HIV-positive men, have failed to find improvement (or slower rates of deterioration) in immune parameters after psychosocial intervention (Mulder et al. 1995). This may have been the result of underpowered testing (n = 39).

Another group of studies has focused on improving self-management skills for patients suffering from chronic illness. An illustrative example comes from Lorig and colleagues, who evaluated the Arthritis Self-Management Program developed at the Stanford Arthritis Center (Lorig et al. 1985). This program included education, self-help groups, and home practice of self-management skills. The groups were led by a trained layperson with arthritis and included about 15 participants. Family involvement was optional. The intervention was associated with increased knowledge, improved self-care behaviors, and decreased pain. A follow-up study showed that these benefits were longlasting (Lorig and Holman 1989). Similar interventions have been launched in cardiac disease (Oldenburg et al. 1985), stroke (Evans et al. 1987), caregiving in dementia (Bourgeois et al. 1996; Lawton et al. 1989; Levy 1987a,b; Toseland and Rossiter 1989; Tune et al. 1988), and arthritis (Radojevic et al. 1992).

Distress Mitigation Interventions

A fourth type of psychosocial intervention that has shown considerable promise has been those interventions specifically designed to reduce or mitigate the distress associated with either the onset or treatment consequences of serious illness. These studies have employed a wide variety of techniques for reducing distress ranging from relaxation and education to careful screening and multimodal interventions that are tailored to particular patient needs. The most important characteristic of these interventions is that the primary target of change is the experience of distress. The majority of these studies have had improved coping skills or resources as a secondary goal.

One of the most important among this group of studies is the Ischemic Heart Disease Life Stress Monitoring Program (Frasure-Smith and Prince 1985, 1989). In this study, 461 male patients recovering from myocardial infarction were randomized to a usual-care condition or to a stress-monitoring intervention. The underlying hypothesis of this study was that targeting life stress through a coordinated program of screening and multimodal intervention would alter the risk of disease recurrence and death. Patients were interviewed over the phone to screen for signs of lifestress. Home-based nursing interventions were conducted in men who scored high on this screen. These interventions consisted of individually tailored combinations of education, support, and referral. One-year results showed that the program had significantly reduced stress symptoms and that control patients were about twice as likely to die of cardiac causes when compared to the intervention group (Frasure-Smith and Prince 1985). After 7 years of follow-up, the mortality differences were found to persist and appeared to be due primarily to sudden death of cardiac origin (Frasure-Smith and Prince 1989). Frasure-Smith's group has recently published results of a large-scale extension of the earlier intervention (the Montreal Heart Attach Readjustment Trial) designed to reduce life stress after myocardial infarction (MI) in a cohort of 1376 men and women. This newer trial showed no benefit although a significant increase in cardiac and all-cause mortality was observed in preplanned analyses among women in the intervention group (Frasure-Smith et al. 1997). Nevertheless, the influence of the Ischemic Heart

Disease Monitoring Program continues to be felt, due, in part, to pioneering innovations in two areas: (1) the concept of individually tailored interventions and (2) the importance of risk screening. Both techniques are now in use in the Enhancing Recovery in Coronary Heart Disease trial (EN-RICHD), a large multisite psychosocial intervention for post-MI patients funded by the National Heart Lung and Blood Institute (NHLBI) currently recruiting subjects in five sites. The ENRICHD project is one of the largest and most ambitious psychosocial intervention ever undertaken and is a major step forward in the evolution of the field of psychosocial intervention. The risk-screening methodology has also been extended to application among women newly diagnosed with breast cancer (Maunsell et al. 1996).

Control Interventions

Studies that have attempted to modify the individual's sense of control over stressful events constitute one additional type of study that deserves attention. In these studies, some attempt is made to affect the extent to which events are viewed as predictable and/or controllable. (For an excellent early review, see Krantz and Schulz 1980.) What makes these studies of particular interest for present purposes is that unlike the studies that focused on altering one or more characteristics of the individual, this group contains some of the best examples of attempts to modify the environment in order to induce an altered sense of mastery and control. These studies grew, in part, out of efforts to study ways in which the hospital environment could be modified to better prepare patients for surgery (Rodin et al. 1980). For example, in a classic study by Klein et al. (1968) environmental modifications were made in a coronary care unit that were designed to allow patients to feel more in control. The patients in that study who received the control-enhancing intervention evidenced fewer cardiovascular complications as well as lower catecholamine excretion. These studies, while smaller in number, are included in the present typology of psychosocial interventions because *(1)* they are explicitly theory-driven and *(2)* because they seek to target a particular psychosocial mechanism that has been linked to health. In addition, several of these studies have used health measures as outcomes.

Another early example of this type of study was conducted by Rodin and Langer (1977) to encourage elderly nursing home residents to make a greater number of choices and to feel more control and responsibility for their own lives. The goal of the intervention was to determine whether the declines in health and cognitive function often observed in institutionalized elderly patients could be slowed or reversed by modifying elderly residents' sense of control. Building on the tradition of environmental psychology, this study is among the few intervention designs that changed the physical and social environment in order to alter the targeted psychosocial factor. Residents in the intervention group were given a speech by the head administrator, who emphasized that residents were responsible for themselves. The comparison group was told that they would be taken care of by the staff. The treatment group was given houseplants and told that they must take care of them. The control subjects were given plants and told that the staff would water them. The responsibility-induced group became more active, showed better mood, and had fewer health declines. In a subsequent analysis of mortality patterns 18 months after the intervention, intervention subjects had significantly lower mortality rates (Rodin and Langer 1977).

In a series of studies, Karasek and Theorell have extended Rodin and Langer's model to workplace design (Karasek and Theorell 1990). These studies were explicitly guided by their demand–control model, which was later extended to include social support as a *mediating* variable. In another study mounted in a nursing home setting, they conducted an experiment in workplace redesign to try to increase worker's sense of control, predictability, and participation.

Health care workers in the experimental group took fewer sick days and reported improved self-esteem.

Having provided a brief and selective review of five types of intervention studies, we now turn to a review of the four main propositions suggested in the introduction. Readers may wish to review Table 12–1, which lists other notable examples of intervention studies not described in the text.[2]

PROPOSITION 1: EXPLICATE THE THEORY

Good intervention designs begin with strong theory. Although the role of theory has been recognized, substantial numbers of psychosocial interventions are performed and evaluated in the absence of a clearly articulated theoretical platform. Theory can be thought of on three distinct levels as it relates to intervention design. First, one can talk of a theory of theories, or stated differently, a broad-based set of assumptions and epistemological principles that guide the intervention at the highest level of abstraction. Second, it is important to specify a set of middle-level theoretical models that are useful in guiding the design of the intervention by providing an orientation to the psychosocial factors most likely to predict outcomes. These midlevel theoretical models also provide guidance as to the optimal intervention strategies. Although not an exhaustive list, three examples of midlevel theoretical approaches will be discussed: *social learning theory* (SLT), *transtheoretical models* (TTM), and *family systems theory* (FST). A third level of theory provides disease-specific insights into natural history; it views what role various psychosocial mechanisms may play and at what points in the disease course. A smaller-scale disease-specific theory is often essential for anchoring inter-

[2]In creating Table 12–1, we were careful to exclude studies in which methodological shortcomings were profound. Also, the review of behavior change interventions is quite limited. We emphasized those studies that were conducted using randomized control designs and which featured some health outcome.

vention strategies to the particular characteristics of a disease. Such small-scale theories guide the intervention by providing clues to the course of psychosocial challenges associated with each disease. For example, interventions designed for diseases of sudden onset require different strategies compared with those of diffuse onset (e.g., heart attack vs. arthritis). Illness situations involving an upward recovery trajectory are likewise different from those that are chronically degenerative (e.g., stroke vs. multiple sclerosis). A sound intervention design must attend to all three levels of theory. Each is discussed briefly in turn.

Metatheoretical Approaches

In a classic article the social anthropologist Roy D'Andrade proposed three tiers of general theory that apply to three distinct domains of scientific inquiry (D'Andrade 1986). The first domain is that of the *physical sciences,* in which all generalizations apply equally through all time and in which a few basic objects and forces operate and can be described in quantitative mathematical form by using a limited set of laws. These laws require a minimum set of qualifications or "boundary conditions." Second, is the domain of *natural sciences* that includes complex ecological and meteorological systems as well as biological systems. In contrast to the domain of physical sciences, this tier of scientific inquiry involves the explication of levels of complex systems, including their composition and their dynamics. At this level, finite and universal laws are not possible. Instead, general systems propositions are stated in probabalistic rather than deterministic form, or in what the author refers to as "natural language statements." Finally, D'Andrade calls the third domain *semiotic sciences.* These fields explain the nature of systems in which order is the consequence not of some finite set of universal laws or general systems propositions but of sentient actors engaged in a world of meaning they themselves help to create. With its root in the Greek *sema,* meaning sign or symbol, the semiotic sciences are the proper domain in which to gain an understanding of human consciousness and action. These three levels of scientific activity parallel those of the general systems theorist Ludwig von Bertalanffy, who differentiated among three tiers of systems (inanimate systems, living systems, and symbolic systems) (Bertalanffy 1952, 1975).

The field of social epidemiology lies within a paradoxical theoretical field, straddling the fence between a biomedical orientation to disease etiology that is grounded in the physical and natural sciences and a more humanistic conception rooted in the fields of anthropology, psychology, and sociology. The mission of social epidemiology requires an understanding of humans as biological entities as well as a view of patients as sense-making actors who operate in a semiotic system where that system itself is understood to have an independent influence on the etiology of disease.

In the writings of general systems theorists such as Bertalanffy and D'Andrade one can find a growing recognition that while these domains of scientific activity are to some degree separate, grand-scale theories are emerging which promise the possibility of synthesis across these levels. One example that has been promising is ecological theory, which attempts to specify nonlinear causal linkages across multiple levels of systems (Bronfenbrenner 1992, 1995; Levi 1997). Until such a synthesis is fully achieved, I would argue that social epidemiologists must be aware of this inherent tension. In an attempt to achieve legitimacy and acceptance within the dominant biomedical world, it is tempting for social epidemiologists to adopt a natural science perspective rather than work toward the challenging task of integrating natural and semiotic scientific concepts and theories. At the same time, social epidemiologists must come to terms with the inherent shortcomings of treating psychosocial phenomenon as though they obeyed finite and universal laws in the same sense that the objects of study of the physical sciences can be said to observe. Nowhere is this tension more troubling and obvious than in the domain of psychosocial intervention, in which the rules of research dictate a model of investigation which conforms to the rules of the natural and physical sciences, but where the design of the intervention itself must take into account the complexities of sentient human actors.

Midlevel Theoretical Approaches

Social learning theory

Most psychosocial interventions that explicitly articulate a theoretical starting point (and many that do not) are based on a general family of cognitive/behavioral paradigms. One of the best examples is social learning theory (SLT) as illustrated by Albert Bandura's seminal work on the concept of self-efficacy (Bandura 1982). In this model, self-efficacy is thought to be shaped by past and present behavior, as well as by the social environment via observation of behaviors in others and through verbal support and persuasion. Self-efficacy beliefs are thought to be domain-specific cognitive structures linked to health-promoting behaviors and to general well-being. Social learning theory principles have been employed in almost all of the intervention types described above. For example, numerous studies have employed SLT in the development of self-management programs aimed at minimizing the impact of chronic illnesses on functional capacity (Clark et al. 1988; Lorig, et al. 1984; Wilson and Pratt 1987). Social learning theory was also the central theoretical model guiding the development of the Stanford Five-City project (a behavior change intervention) (Farquhar et al. 1990). Social learning theory has also been influential in the development of social support interventions (Clark et al. 1992a). A fine discussion of theoretical issues in social learning theory and intervention design is found in Clark et al. (1992b).

Transtheoretical models

In the domain of behavior modification interventions, the transtheoretical model (TTM) of stages of change has emerged as a dominant theoretical force. According to this model, behavioral change unfolds over time in a series of stages from precontemplation, to contemplation, to preparation, to action, and finally to maintenance (Prochaska et al. 1997). Further, by studying behavior changes ranging from smoking cessation to mammography screening to condom use, TTM proponents have identified a finite set of processes of change that appear to be highly general. The model is *trans*theoretical because it assumes that no single theory can account for all the complexities of behavior change, and hence a synthesis on many smaller scale theories is proposed. This position parallels the one taken in this chapter: that multiple levels of theory are required to solve a series of general theoretical problems that face the intervention researcher.

The most important implication of the shift to what Prochaska calls the "stage paradigm" is the idea that different change processes are going on at each stage and therefore markedly different intervention strategies are needed. This concept of targeting the intervention to the stage of readiness for change has been implemented in very few intervention studies to date. However, TTM is potentially a rich and promising theoretical tool for the design of future interventions.

Family systems theory

Family systems theory grew out of the work of the sociologist Talcott Parsons; it also derives from general systems theorists, linguists, and communication theory. It is an alternative to individualistic explanations of psychopathology and treatment. The fundamental axiom of family systems theory is that all crisis events occur within an organic system of preexisting ties and that all coping and adaptation occurs within that same system context. (For an excellent general introduction to family systems theory, see Broderick 1993.) Systemic models of adaptation, also called ecological models (see, for example, Lanza and Revenson 1993), focus on the norms, values, rules, roles, and boundaries of the family system as opposed to the individual behaviors and attitudes of the patient. While cognitive–behavioral approaches focus on the individual patient as the object of intervention, the family systems perspective treats the larger social context in which the patient is lodged as the appropriate locus of treatment. Family systems theory views the family as a goal-seeking, self-regulating system that functions either adaptively or maladaptively in response to the crisis of illness. As such, family systems theory has been applied more frequently to disease-management interventions, although it has potential to yield important insights into disease etiology as well. Pioneering work in the application of family systems theory to intervention was done by Minuchin et al. (1978) and Rolland (1989). Family-systems-based interventions have seldom been rigorously evaluated, but they have been influential in the development of the multifamily disease-management interventions of Gonzales et al. (1989), as well as interventions in patients after stroke (Evans et al. 1988; Glass et al. in press).

Disease-Specific Theories

The final level of theory is perhaps the smallest in scale and pertains to disease-specific considerations of how the natural history of a disease relates to particular psychosocial risk factors or behavioral inputs. A disease-specific theory is an essential component of intervention design because just as any disease has a natural history at a physiologic level, so too do diseases follow a distinctive natural history at the psychosocial level. In the absence of an understanding of the sequence of psychosocial issues as they relate to disease etiology or course, interventions risk being improperly timed and sequenced (see Bloom and Kessler 1994 for a review). Some examples of this type of theory incorporate more general theoretical ideas. This is the case with work that has been done in the area of type A behavior (TAB). Initially identified in 1959, TAB has been extensively studied as a psychosocial precursor for heart disease (Friedman and Rosenman 1959). Type A behavior was the first behavioral factor convincingly shown to be independently associated with the risk of disease. After initial enthusiasm, interest in TAB has waned since the 1980s (Thoresen and Powell 1992). Interestingly, intervention trials have provided the strongest evidence for the importance of TAB in comparison to observational studies, where considerable confusion has emerged. In a comprehensive meta-analysis of 18 intervention studies in TAB, Nunes et al. (1987) concluded that psychosocial treatment resulted in significant reductions in TAB itself, as well as a lowered risk of 3-year mortality and a 50% reduction in coronary events. Type A behavior is a good example of the usefulness of small-scale theory, because it has all the requisite characteristics. First, it is grounded in a more general theoretical model (cognitive–behavioral theory). Second, it draws on knowledge of the natural history of a disease (atherosclerosis). Third, it yields specific hypotheses that link psychosocial mechanisms (hostility, impatience, and time urgency) to particular physiologic pathways (overstimulation of sympathetic nervous system leading to elevated catecholamines and corticosteroids).

The history of TAB research is also interesting for what it teaches the field of social epidemiology about the hazards of inadequate theoretical development and refinement. Initially, TAB was conceptualized as a complex behavioral response to external situations that challenge self-appraisals. Later, as TAB was adopted within biomedical research, the concept was transformed and simplified in order to fit an individualistic and mechanistic theoretical framework. Type A behavior was recast not as a complex interactional concept but as a lasting personality trait (Smith and Anderson 1986).[3]

---

[3]For an excellent and detailed discussion of theoretical issues as they relate to TAB, see Thoresen and Powell (Thoresen et al. 1992).

PROPOSITION 2: TARGET A SPECIFIC PSYCHOSOCIAL MECHANISM

The essential element of a psychosocial intervention is the systematic attempt to modify a psychosocial factor known to be associated with the desired outcome. The implication of this observation is that intervention design and testing should always follow a sequence of earlier steps in which observational studies have documented the relevance of some specified set of psychosocial factors which mediate or moderate the etiological pathways leading to the disease in question. As noted earlier, the development of a coherent theoretical model which provides a rationale for the link between the psychosocial mechanism and the end points of interest is a prerequisite. The greater the level of specificity and detail regarding the proposed mechanism of action, the more likely the results of the intervention will have meaning and interpretability. Unlike observational studies in which hypothesis generation and other exploratory goals may be useful, *an intervention study must be hypothesis-driven*. Failure to specify a set of specific hypotheses leads to a muddled design and to uninterpretable results.

One common weakness of intervention designs is the failure to specify the psychosocial target clearly enough. Some investigators have used a "shotgun" approach in which a wide range of conceptually unrelated interventions are designed to improve overall well-being, quality of life, or adjustment. An example is the randomized study by Cain et al. (1986) in which women with gynecologic cancer were given "counseling designed in response to the needs of women with gynecologic cancer" whose aim was to reduce "long-term psychosocial distress." In this trial, which also suffered from small sample sizes, the results would have been uncompelling even if the trial had achieved positive results, because the interventions were too numerous and poorly described.

Many community-based primary prevention trials designed to modify behaviors shown previously to be associated with risk of coronary artery disease were launched in the 1970s including the WHO collaborative trials (World Health Organization 1986), the Oslo trial (Hjermann 1983), the Göteborg trial (Wilhelmsen et al. 1986), the Stanford three- and five-city trials (Farquhar et al. 1985, 1990), and the MRFIT trial (Benfari 1981). As has been suggested previously, the results of these trials have been mixed. As the field has come to grips with the results of these trials, it is now clear that targeting high-risk individuals for behavior change interventions is not as simple as it was once thought to be. Although these trials are considered by many to be the flagship intervention studies within the field of social epidemiology, disappointing results may have arisen from too much *epidemiology* and not enough *social*.

While all of these trials featured strong designs with ample power, most were not thoroughly grounded in theory. In this tradition, lifestyle and behaviors have not been conceptualized within larger psychosocial contexts. Rather, these trials illustrate the biomedicalization of behavior, in which smoking, diet, and other risk behaviors are viewed within a narrowly individualistic framework. (For a thoughtful elaboration of this point, see McMichael 1989.) It is essential that intervention planners recognize that behaviors and lifestyles are themselves products of particular social contexts and that simplistic thinking at the service of brutally simple but powerful experimental designs is not likely to be successful.

Social Networks and Support: One Example

It is a central premise of this chapter that particular psychosocial factors with a strong track record of association with the desired health outcome should be targeted for intervention guided by a clear theory of how that variable operates and how it is related to the outcome. The failure to adequately ground an intervention in this level of specificity can lead to poor intervention design and lack of coherent findings. Consider social networks and support as an example.

Viewed broadly, the concept of social networks and support encompasses a wide range of psychosocial processes involving kin-based and non-kin-based relationships. A crucial distinction must be made between the structural characteristics of an individual's social ties and connections, called *social networks,* and the functional consequences of those ties, called *social supports* (Berkman 1985; Seeman and Berkman 1988). For purposes of intervention design, this distinction is crucial because it is clear from the observational literature that short-term outcomes are more sensitive to social support, while longer-term outcomes (including survival) appear to be most powerfully impacted by social networks. Moreover, within the domain of social networks and support, more fine-tuning is required in the selection of the target for intervention.

It is furthermore essential to distinguish between the concept of support as a characteristic of the individual as opposed to a characteristic of environments (Rook and Dooley 1985). This distinction has important implications for intervention because the former view leads to interventions that target individuals, while the latter view leads to interventions designed to facilitate interactions and support through environmental influences.

Another example of the importance of having a clearly defined theory of social support and its relationship to health can be found by examining the debate regarding the relative importance of support as a main effect or a buffering effect. As has been pointed out by, among others Gesten and Jason (1987), the implications of this are far-reaching. If support operates mainly through direct channels, a population-based intervention might be expected to succeed. If the benefits of support accrue primarily through its ability to buffer the deleterious effects of particular stressors, however, focusing on high-risk populations is the preferred approach. While empirical evidence from the observational literature can be found for both types of effects, researchers interested in conducting social support interventions should be clear at the outset that their theory fits the intended population.

PROPOSITION 3: IDENTIFY AN APPROPRIATE HEALTH OR FUNCTIONAL OUTCOME

In designing a psychosocial intervention, one of the most crucial decisions that must be made is what outcome to study and how it should be measured. There are two crucial considerations that must be addressed in the selection of a suitable outcome. First, is this outcome likely to be viewed as relevant, well accepted, and reliably measured by the larger audience to whom this trial is directed? Second, is this outcome likely to be a sensitive marker of the beneficial impact of the intervention as planned?

Relevance of the Outcome

It is an accepted canon of clinical trial research that while the intervention itself can be controversial, the primary outcome measure used to judge its effectiveness cannot. In a methodological manifesto written by the National Institute of Health (NIH)'s Office of Alternative Medicine, this observation was worded in the following succinct way: "alternative treatments, yes; alternative outcomes, no" (Levin 1996). Despite this observation, a large proportion of psychosocial intervention trials have been conducted using measures that are not regarded by the wider audience as valid, reliable, and relevant to health care decision-makers. Examples include trials that examine perceived distress, well-being, or psychosocial adjustment. The measurement problems in each of these areas are well known and general consensus on the optimal measurement approach is lacking. Other researchers have erred by using newly designed instruments as outcome measures. In the absence of strong evidence on the reliability and validity of an outcome measure, the use of new, poorly accepted, or untested measures is to be strongly avoided.

The question as to what should be measured is a also controversial one. Any psychosocial intervention trial involves a targeted psychosocial mechanism that is, *a priori*, assumed to be related to a health or functional outcome. Some investigators have opted for the measurement of those mechanisms as the primary outcome of interest. For example, Prochaska has argued that interventions that measure behavioral change as their primary outcome (e.g., smoking or condom use) are more compelling because the risky behavior in question may be implicated in many diseases (Prochaska et al. 1997). Although this argument is compelling for many, it is also true that the interventions that have had the greatest impact have been those that have employed a "hard" outcome involving some health state or functional status. Prominent examples include studies by Ornish (reduction in sclerotic plaque), Spiegel (longer survival), and Frasure-Smith (fewer recurrent MIs). Countless numbers of psychosocial intervention trials have demonstrated changes in mechanisms but have failed to demonstrate that these changes translate into the expected health benefits. As social epidemiologists, we must attend to the dual challenges of demonstrating efficacy and testing etiological hypotheses. In that sense, a strong argument can be made for the selection of "harder" health and functional outcomes. Otherwise, proponents of psychosocial intervention are "preaching to the choir."

PROPOSITION 4: CHOOSE A STRONG DESIGN

The central point of this chapter is to argue that psychosocial intervention, because it operates in the murky waters of soft science and biopsychosocial metaphysics, must overachieve methodologically. A sizable proportion of research conducted under the rubric of psychosocial intervention has been methodologically (if not theoretically) sub-

standard. Literally hundreds, if not thousands, of studies have been done using samples that were too small to detect meaningful differences, using nonrandomized and uncontrolled designs, and using outcome measures that are either not well accepted or are insensitive to the influences of the treatment. The legacy of this large body of work is that the vast majority of these studies have no impact on clinical practice. Perhaps worse, many biomedical researchers do not fully recognize the fact that exquisitely done studies do exist. The antidote to this problem is the recognition that social epidemiologists cannot afford the luxury of weak study designs despite substantial limitations in time, expertise, and resources. Although, as will be argued, the randomized clinical trial (RCT) design is not the only game in town, the RCT is a well-accepted standard of intervention evaluation that offers the most powerful evidence of both efficacy and etiological significance. In what follows, I hope to lay out a selection of the most important methodological issues faced by investigators in this field in an attempt to head off the most common methodological shortcomings that lead to inconclusive or uninterpretable results.

Standardization of Interventions

In a classically designed RCT designed to test a pharmacological treatment, both the active agent and the placebo are standardized both for content and dosage. Standardization of psychosocial interventions is obviously substantially more difficult. Any intervention which involves talking is likely to vary both across subjects and across interventionists. Some would argue that the problems associated with standardization of interventions constitute a fatal flaw. While this is an extreme view, investigators are obligated to take steps in the design of the intervention to maximize the degree of standardization. The key to standardization is to develop a thorough and detailed intervention protocol prior to launching the study. The intervention protocol describes the procedures and policies of the intervention *a priori*. Interventionists should be trained and tested to insure that the intervention is being implemented reliably across interventionists.

Investigators must balance the need for standardization against the problems associated with an overly rigid and structured protocol. One approach to standardization is the use of scripted presentations. These are useful for educational interventions involving homogeneous populations but may be overly structured in other settings. An alternative model has been developed for the Families in Recovery from Stroke Trial (FIRST).[4] In this approach, we recognize the need to shape the content of the intervention to the particular psychosocial needs of the each family (Glass et al. in press). Balance is achieved across these competing goals through the use of an instrument designed to record the content of individual intervention sessions. This instrument is comprised of a matrix with each session in the columns and each of 16 primary content domains in the rows. Interventionists record the extent to which each content domain is discussed in each of 15 intervention sessions. In the early phase of the intervention, the content of the sessions is dictated by the needs of each stroke survivor. Toward the end of the 15 sessions, the interventionist addresses any content areas that have not been previously discussed. Using this tool, it becomes possible to both track the particular content of the intervention as delivered and to insure that some attention is paid to all content domains while at the same time allowing for the flexibility to tailor the intervention content to the needs of individual families.

In summary, standardization of the interventionist is an important issue that requires

planning and balance. The benefits of standardization go beyond the technical virtues of study design. Previous reports suggest that more tightly structured interventions improve attendance and satisfaction (Taylor et al. 1988). One promising new methodology for standardizing interventions involves using computer-based expert-systems programming to create individually tailored informational and feedback interventions. This technique has been used extensively by Prochaska and colleagues in work on smoking cessation (Prochaska et al. 1993). Not only can expert-systems-based interventions be highly standardized using data-derived algorithms, but it becomes possible to record the content of the intervention sessions precisely.

Blinding

The cardinal virtues of the RCT design are randomization and blinding (sometimes called masking). The former assures that any differences seen between the two groups after intervention can be reliably attributed to the intervention. Blinding is a procedure which further strengthens our confidence in the internal validity of the results by removing (or minimizing) several potential sources of bias. In the typical pharmacological trial, the gold-standard practice is to conduct a triple-blinded study in which the subject, the investigator (the physician) and the evaluator are all blinded as to treatment status. In a psychosocial intervention, blinding the participant is normally both ethically and practically impossible. By virtue of the nature of psychosocial intervention, the active engagement of the intellectual and emotional faculties of the patient is a prerequisite to the success of the intervention. This creates logistic problems in a study design that benefits from maximal blinding. It is my contention that the crucial issue in psychosocial intervention is how to insure that the outcome assessor is blinded. Efforts to approximate the RCT ideal of the blinded subject normally backfire. Having made this concession, the additional peril of contagion between the

---

[4]The FIRST study is a randomized clinical trial designed to test the efficacy of a family support intervention in elderly stroke patients. The study is funded by the National Institute of Neurological Diseases and Stroke and the National Institute on Aging and is currently recruiting subjects in multiple sites in the Boston area. It is expected that 290 subjects will be randomized in that trial (Glass et al. in press).

outcome assessor and the unblinded subject becomes apparent. In our own study, we have worked hard to create a system in which the outcome assessor is maximally insulated from opportunities to become unblinded. The project director calls each subject prior to their follow-up interview to remind them not to reveal their treatment status. The interview is carefully scripted to include a disclaimer to remind subjects not to make reference to any other study staff members they may have encountered. Despite working with elderly brain injured patients, our experience is that these efforts are effective in minimizing the occurrence of unblinding. One general procedure that has been used in several other trials is to ask staff members who assess outcomes to guess the treatment status of each subject. Our experience in the FIRST study is that assessors are often wrong.However, guessing allows the investigators to quantify the effectiveness of blinding by statistically testing whether the assessors are "guessing" correctly more often than would be expected by chance. If they are not, this becomes compelling evidence even for the harshest critic.

The Selection of the Control Groups

In addition to random assignment, the strength of the clinical trial derives from the ability to compare the effects in the treatment group to a control condition. To the extent that the treatment and control groups are similar at baseline, differences between these groups can be attributed to the effect of the intervention. In pharmacological trials, the control group is given a sham treatment to which they are blinded. In psychosocial intervention, sham treatments are unfeasible for both technical and ethical reasons. Alternatively, four approaches have been used: *(1)* usual care controls, *(2)* attentional controls, *(3)* information-only controls, and *(4)* waiting list controls. In the first case, care is taken to insure that control-group subjects receive identical medical and social services. This approach can be especially problematic in disease-management interventions in which

the target of the intervention is often the removal of barriers to increased medical utilization. While it is nearly impossible to insure that the two groups differ only on exposure to the intervention, the best approach to achieving a clean design is to institute a process assessment strategy in order to monitor health care access, differences in screening, and greater levels of attention. Primary care providers who are aware that a given patient is in the intervention arm of a trial may be more likely to follow a patient aggressively. For this reason, it is advisable to minimize communication between the intervention staff and adjacent usual care providers.

In order to insure that treatment differences are not the result of the expectancy effects engendered by enhanced attention, some trials have employed attentional controls. This is more common in psychiatric trials. Attentional controls in psychosocial intervention are highly problematic in my view because they add considerable expense to the intervention design and they are likely to backfire. It is very difficult to train an attentional control provider to remain inert in the course of interacting with ill patients. In the aftermath of serious illness, any attempt to engage patients and families in discussion that is not in some way therapeutic violates social norms and can damage rapport between the study and its participants. Control subjects who see through the blatant attempt to provide inert attentional controls are likely to withdraw from the study—a methodological disaster.

An additional approach to the control condition has been to utilize information-only controls. In this method, control subjects are given written educational materials or are provided with informational sessions by study staff. The latter example is a special case of an attentional control. While easy to standardize, the provision of information without a context or the opportunity to ask questions is a nearly empty gesture. Providing enriched educational control conditions risks biasing the results of the trial toward the null. The use of an educational control condition is a common feature of multiarm trials in which the main intervention is tested against a usual-care control and an educational control to see whether the addition of the main intervention is of benefit. This multicontrol design should be avoided in circumstances in which the addition of a separate treatment arm would reduce the power of the study to detect reasonably small effect sizes in the other two arms.

One final method is the use of the waiting-list controls, in which the intervention is offered to volunteers on a first-come basis until the desired sample size is achieved (see, for example, Mulder et al. 1994). Subsequent volunteers are used as control subjects. This design is often used as a precursor to a crossover design in which the control subjects are offered the intervention at the end of the evaluation period. The use of waiting-list controls is controversial. If intervention timing is critical, this approach is clearly inferior to other models. Also, care must be taken to insure that those who volunteer first are not systematically different in motivation, level of access to information about the study, or in illness severity as compared to later volunteers.

Subject Recruitment and Enrollment

The strength of RCT studies is the extent to which internal validity is maximized by study design. The weakness, as has been observed, is the significant threats that exist to external validity. Any clinical trial is, by definition, a study of volunteers. This is because all clinical trials are subject to rigorous human-subjects-review processes that require extensive disclosure of study hypotheses and design features prior to enrollment. The limitations of volunteer subject recruitment are not insubstantial. In the randomized trial methodology, random assignment and blinding are strong features.

Subject recruitment takes place within an institutional setting (e.g., a hospital, a work site, a community clinic) or via community outreach. In the case of institutional recruitment, it is extremely important to standardize recruitment and screening procedures to the greatest extent possible. Care

must be taken to insure that screeners are not sifting through potential candidates looking for those that might benefit most from the intervention. Another potential strategy for participant recruitment is through the media. Newspaper, radio, and organizational newsletters can be used to disseminate information about the availability of an intervention trial. This approach has serious limitations. As illustrated by the experience of the Family Support Project, media outreach tends to select persons who are either acutely in crisis or who have waited too long after the onset of a crisis for the intervention to be maximally effective (Montgomery and Borgatta 1985). This and other opportunistic methods of recruitment create excessive heterogeneity in the timing of intervention startup. The negative consequences of volunteer bias are thus heightened.

Subject Retention and Follow-up

Sample attrition is a major problem in clinical trial designs. Because clinical trials are by nature studies of volunteers, the external validity of these trials is suspect. However, the internal validity can only by assured if a high proportion of subjects who are randomized complete the trial and are included in the analysis. A strong design feature in this regard is the use of the intention-to-treat rule (ITT), which requires that all patients who are randomized be included in the analysis regardless of their postrandomization status. This is a conservative but promising strategy that has rarely been employed in psychosocial intervention studies to date. (For further information, see Gibaldi and Sullivan 1997; Hogan and Laird 1996; Newell 1992.)

While the general problem of losses to follow-up is of grave concern for the investigator, perhaps an even greater problem arises when the rates of sample attrition differ by treatment status. There are several reasons to worry that differential losses to follow-up may occur. First, subjects randomized into the control group may be more likely to withdraw from the study, feeling that they had been denied an exciting intervention program. Alternatively, subjects who are randomized into the intervention group may be overly challenged by the intervention or may express their resistance to behavioral modification by withdrawal from the study. Either scenario is drastic because it dramatically decreases the power of the test to detect real differences. Investigators must carefully consider the possibility of factors that might impact the probability of a subject completing the trial and adjust by including inflation factors to the power calculations. As an example, Mohide et al. (1990) conducted a randomized trial of a family caregiver support program for the home management of patients with dementia. Although underpowered at the outset with only 30 subjects in the treatment and control group, the study was devastated by a loss-to-follow-up of 30% due mostly to subjects being transferred to long-term care. This study is an unfortunate example of how the intervention itself can predispose subjects to be more likely to withdraw in favor of alternative, more accepted modes of intervention.

Reactivity and Contamination Effects

More than pharmacological trials, tests of psychosocial interventions are susceptible to the influence of reactivity and contamination effects that can bias the results of the study toward the null. The risks of contamination are particularly acute when the randomization unit is some location in sociogeographic space (such as floors of a buildings, work sites, or even neighborhoods). If individuals in the intervention group have contact with subjects in the control group, they may discuss aspects of the intervention causing crossover influences. Although more difficult to detect, this may also produce demoralization in the control subjects, which can lead to early withdrawal or nonadherence to follow-up observations. Building insulation between intervention and control groups is an important aspect of intervention design when groups are to be the units of randomization.

The influence of contamination from secular trends should also be strongly consid-

ered. As has been argued, many of the most famous public health interventions have been crippled because policy changes or natural trends cause substantial improvements in control subjects. It may also be prudent to measure contamination through the use of process variables to measure the extent to which the intervention or other external processes are effecting the control subjects. Most importantly, it is crucial that power calculations be conducted with conservative estimates of how much improvement can be expected in the unexposed (control) group.

Another seldom-appreciated aspect of reactivity effects is the impact of social comparison processes within support groups (Lanza et al. 1993). In a support-group context, subjects who judge themselves to be doing better than other members of the support group are likely to feel positively about the intervention. However, those individuals who are doing worse may be negatively impacted, resulting in paradoxical effects. The same problem exists within behavioral training interventions when group education and feedback are used. At the same time, when the intervention is designed to target individuals at increased risk for a particular disease outcome, substantial reactivity effects can occur if members of the control group change their behavior simply because they are eligible to participate.

Finally, lessons learned from high-visibility community risk-reduction trials aimed at high-risk subjects point to the substantial potential for contamination of study results. In the most notable example, meaningful evaluation of treatment benefits in the MRFIT trial was compromised because many of the men voluntarily reduced their risk-factor exposure as a result of being labeled "high risk" (The Multiple Risk Factor Intervention Trial Group 1982).

Alternatives to Clinical Trials

It has been argued that clinical trials offer the most compelling evidence in favor of the benefits of psychosocial intervention, but the clinical trial is not the only useful evaluation tool. One of the most important criticisms of the RCT methodology is that marginalized groups tend to be excluded from participation disproportionately. This is a significant threat to the external validity of these studies. Among the implications of this is that minority groups are less likely to participate in RCTs, making alternative designs important to verify the usefulness of psychosocial interventions in diverse populations. A number of alternative designs have merit and should be encouraged. Investigators must balance the relative costs and complexities of the clinical trial design against those benefits. One lower-cost alternative is the use of single-group designs in particular populations in which each subject is used as their own control. This design is useful in circumstances in which the outcome of interest is assumed to be rapidly responsive to intervention effects. This way, baseline, preintervention assessments can be assumed to be reliable and valid. An example is the home-based intervention to train caregivers to manage behavior problems in cognitively impaired elderly persons conducted by Pinkston and colleagues at the University of Chicago (1988). This trial was solidly grounded in behavioral theory and used preintervention interviews with both elderly clients and their caregivers as control conditions. Although improvements in the targeted behaviors were seen in 76% of the dyads, the absence of a distinct control group limits the internal validity of this design.

SUMMARY

To summarize this discussion of methodological issues, one might profitably ask: What are the things most likely to go wrong in a psychosocial intervention trial? A review of hundreds of studies in the course of preparing this chapter leads one to believe that there are three general methodological flaws that have, more than all others, led to poor research and inconclusive findings. The leading cause of faulty methodology is the use of underpowered tests. Of the dozens of intervention trials that report negative or inconclusive findings, the vast majority failed to adequately consider the sample sizes that would be required to ade-

quately detect benefit. More than half the studies I reviewed had sample sizes of fewer than 30 cases per treatment condition. It is impossible to conclude much of anything from trials of this size. Many of these trials are testing complex multiarm treatment conditions without understanding that the complexity of the design has compromised the study's ability to adequately test even the first-order hypothesis.

The second major methodological weakness of these studies is the selection of inappropriate or inconsequential outcome measures. In this era of managed care, a golden opportunity exists for social epidemiologists to develop and test low-cost, low-impact interventions that have real consequences for health and well-being. To the extent that researchers fail to pick outcome measures that are relevant to larger policy and practice questions, or pick outcomes that are not sensitive to the impact of the intervention planned, negative results are certain to occur.

Finally, many high-visibility intervention trials have failed to take account of the substantial complexities associated with changing behavior. In part, this is due to a lack of a coherent conceptual grounding which places health behaviors within a broader biopsychosocial context. In other cases, it involves a failure to maintain the intervention duration or intensity sufficiently to allow the flower of behavioral change to bloom (another point made by Susser 1995). And in still other cases, it has resulted from a failure to adequately account for the contaminating influences of secular trends and crossover effects.

CONCLUSION AND FUTURE RESEARCH DIRECTION

The field of psychosocial intervention is currently in an awkward stage of growth. On the one hand, many individual-level psychosocial interventions have produced mixed or negative results. In their review of the best trials of primary prevention of coronary heart disease (including both psychosocial and pharmacological interventions) McCormick and Skrabanek (1988) conclude that no improvement in total mortality has been achieved. On the other hand, investigators are becoming more sophisticated in the design and testing of psychosocial interventions, which raises hopes for the future. Moreover, the time is right for a reevaluation of methods and priorities. This chapter concludes with two observations about the future of psychosocial intervention. At first glance, it may appear that these observations are antithetical to one another. If one accepts the need to be both practical and forward thinking, the apparent paradox is diminished. On the one hand, I argue that intervention researchers must think in new ways about how to contextualize health behaviors by moving from individually focused interventions to interventions that are aimed at the social environments in which behaviors are lodged (including families, work groups, neighborhoods, and communities). On the other hand, I would argue that maintaining the highest possible standards of methodology using well-accepted methods is the optimal strategy to insure forward movement.

Thinking New: Beyond Individual-Level Interventions

In light of the shortcomings of some individually targeted interventions, many of which have not been well guided by sound theory, several leading figures have called for the emergence of a "new" public health which emphasizes population-level interventions and a focus on upstream causes of health and well-being (Anonymous 1994; Kaplan 1995; McKinlay 1995; Rose 1985, 1992). A leading proponent of such a shift, John McKinlay, observes that

Changing reimbursement policies for just one drug (Haladol), used primarily by older people, is likely to produce a greater reduction in falls and hip fractures than the costly and generally futile individualized approaches to improve muscle strength and bone density. Adding only 8 cents to U.S. cigarette taxes apparently caused 2 million adults to stop smoking and prevented 600,000 teenagers from starting. (McKinlay 1993, p. 113)

The details of the "new" public health are beginning to take shape. A general trend can be seen toward health-promotion efforts targeted at organizations, communities, and entire populations (for an excellent recent review, see Sorensen et al. 1998). Health service researchers have shown repeatedly that experiments to modify public policies, particularly those that regulate what is and is not reimbursed, can have dramatic impact on health outcomes (for a review see Terris 1980). Consensus has not yet been reached on how population-level and community-based interventions are best evaluated, but several promising strategies have been developed. In one example, community outreach was used to recruit African-American women into a study to test a multimodal intervention to reduce HIV risk and to promote condom use. The intervention emphasized ethnic and gender pride, HIV risk-reduction information, sexual self-control, sexual assertiveness and communication skills, proper condom use skills, and developing partner norms supportive of consistent condom use (DiClemente and Wingood 1995). This study illustrates the importance of building gender and cultural competence into interventions.

Another innovative example is work by Kelly and colleagues (1991) in which popular opinion leaders were recruited and trained to modify community norms around HIV risk behaviors. This study attempted to move beyond the focus on individuals by targeting community norms. The design was evaluated by conducting interviews among randomly selected persons in both intervention and control cities.

Finally, there are several areas in which promising intervention models have been developed, but little evaluation research has been conducted. Examples include neighborhood interventions for violence prevention or helping to maintain the elderly in their homes. As epidemiologic evidence mounts as to the importance of diet and nutrition, innovative interventions aimed at communities and work sites will be needed. Promising examples include the five-a-day initiative at a community level (Havas et al.

1995) and the Working Well study aimed at work sites (Kristal et al. 1995). While several useful policy interventions designed to reduce access barriers to underserved populations have been mounted, one additional area that appears to be promising is the use of community empowerment and social network mobilization concepts to reduce access barriers. Previous examples, including the Tenderloin project involving community mobilization among poor urban elderly persons, have not been well evaluated with respect to health outcomes (Minkler 1985). As observational studies accumulate, and more is known about the ways in which social environments and other upstream factors shape the psychosocial processes that influence health, intervention models will be further enriched.

Thinking Old: Sticking to what Works

In conjunction with the call for a shift from individual- to community-level interventions has come a parallel challenge to expand the range of evaluation methodologies to include "interpretive" and "qualitative" designs (McKinlay 1995; Sorensen et al. 1998). McKinlay invokes the language of Thomas Kuhn, whose classic work *The Structure of Scientific Revolutions* (1962) described the changes over time in scientific "paradigms." According to McKinlay, an essential part of the "new" paradigm of public health is a critique of positivism and a move to accept alternative systems of evidence (McKinlay 1995). This argument fails to distinguish between *ontology* and *epistemology*.[5] As Kuhn argued, in order for the cracks and fissures that inevitably exist within any single paradigm to accumulate

to a critical mass (at which point they become the impetus for a paradigm revolution) they must be articulated in a language that is common and acceptable to those on both sides of the paradigmatic divide. For example, observations about the retrograde motion of mercury helped bring down Newtonian physics and usher in the now established Einsteinian paradigm. The methods and procedures used to document and describe that phenomenon were (roughly) consistent with the rules of knowledge acquisition within the Newtonian paradigm (epistemology) even though they sharply contradicted that paradigm's ontology. Otherwise, it would have been easy for the practitioners of the established paradigm to dismiss such revolutionary observations out of hand. Moreover, if indeed a new paradigm, characterized by an increasing awareness of extraindividual, upstream factors in health is in ascendance, the use of "interpretive" and "qualitative" designs for the documentation of anomalies may be precariously premature. For these reasons, it has been a central theme of this chapter that psychosocial interventions, while attempting to identify the impact of social and psychological phenomenon on disease etiology (paradigmatic anomalies), must nevertheless recognize the practical necessity of methodological overachieving within the framework of a noncontroversial science of evaluation. Otherwise, we are doing little more than "preaching to the choir."

REFERENCES

Abrams, D.B., Emmons, K.M., and Linnan, L.A. (1997). Health behavior and health education: the past, present, and future. In Glanz, K., Lewis, F.M., and Rimer, B.K. (eds.), *Health behavior and health education: theory, research, and practice.* San Francisco, CA: Jossey-Bass, pp. 453–78.

Anonymous. (1982). Multiple risk factor intervention trial. Risk factor changes and mortality results. Multiple Risk Factor Intervention Trial Research Group. *J Am Med Assoc*, 248:1465–77.

Anonymous. (1990). Enhancing the outcomes of low-birth-weight, premature infants. A multisite, randomized trial. The Infant Health

[5] I recognize that philosophers of science will not like the distinction I am suggesting. Indeed, most philosophers of sciences appear to agree that Kuhn's ideas of change in science are out of date. To some extent Kuhn lives on among nonphilosophers because the concept of a paradigm has become an inkblot onto which any argument can be projected. For the present purposes, I mean to suggest only that from a strategic point of view, advocates of a new theory of health and disease (ontology) should recognize the need to differentiate that new theory from any single set of rules of knowledge (epistemology).

and Development Program. *J Am Med Assoc*, 263:3035–42.

Anonymous. (1994). Population health looking upstream (editorial). *Lancet*, 343:429–30.

Anonymous. (1995). Community Intervention Trial for Smoking Cessation (COMMIT): I. Cohort results from a four-year community intervention. *Am J Public Health*, 85:183–92.

Arnetz, B.B., and Theorell, T. (1983). Psychological, sociological and health behavior aspects of a long-term activation programme for institutionalized elderly people. *Soc Sci Med*, 17:449–56.

Attneave, C.L. (1978). Therapy in tribal settings and urban network intervention. *Fam Proc*, 8:192–210.

Bandura, A. (1982). Self-efficacy mechanisms in human agency. *Am Psychol*, 37:122–47.

Benfari, R.C. (1981). The Multiple Risk Factor Intervention Trial (MRFIT) III The model for intervention. *Prev Med*, 10:426–42.

Berkman, L.F. (1985). The relationship of social networks and social support to morbidity and mortality. In Cohen, S., and Syme, S.L. (eds.), *Social support and health*. Orlando, FL: Academic Press, pp. 241–62.

Bertalanffy, L.v. (1952). Theoretical models in biology and psychology. In Krech, D., and Klein, G.S. (eds.), *Theoretical models and personality theory*. Durham, NC: Duke University Press, pp. 24–38.

Bertalanffy, L.v. (1975). *Perspectives on general systems theory: scientific-philosophical studies*. New York: George Braziller.

Biegel, D.E., Shore, B.K., and Gordon, E. (1984). *Building support networks for the elderly: theory and applications*. Beverly Hills, CA: Sage.

Bloom, J.R., and Kessler, L. (1994). Risk and timing of counseling and support interventions for younger women with breast cancer. *J Nat Cancer Institute Monographs*, 16:199–206.

Blumenthal, J.A., Jiang, W., Babyak, M.A., Krantz, D.S., Frid, D.J., Coleman, R.E., Waugh, R., Hanson, M., Appelbaum, M., O'Connor, C., and Morris, J.J. (1997). Stress management and exercise training in cardiac patients with myocardial ischemia. Effects on prognosis and evaluation of mechanisms. *Arch Intern Med*, 157:2213–23.

Bourgeois, M.S., Schulz, R., and Burgio, L. (1996). Interventions for caregivers of patients with Alzheimer's disease: a review and analysis of content, process, and outcomes. *Int J Aging Hum Dev*, 43:35–92.

Broderick, C.B. (1993). *Understanding family process: basics of family systems theory*. Newbury Park: Sage.

Bronfenbrenner, U. (1992). Ecological systems theory. In Vasta, R. (ed.), *Six theories of child development: Revised formulations and current issues*. London, England: Jessica Kingsley, pp. 187–249.

Bronfenbrenner, U. (1995). Developmental ecology through space and time: a future perspective. In Moen, P., and Elder, G.H.J. (eds.), *Examining lives in context: perspectives on the ecology of human developmen*. Washington, DC: American Psychological Association, pp. 619–47.

Brooks-Gunn, J., McCarton, C.M., Casey, P.H., McCormick, M.C., Bauer, C.R., Bernbaum, J.C., Tyson, J., Swanson, M., Bennett, F.C., and Scott, D.T. (1994). Early intervention in low-birth-weight premature infants. Results through age 5 years from the Infant Health and Development Program. *J Am Med Assoc*, 272:1257–62.

Cain, E.N., Kohorn, E.I., Quinlan, D.M., Latimer, K., and Schwartz, P.E. (1986). Psychosocial benefits of a cancer support group. *Cancer*, 57:183–9.

Carleton, R.A., Lasater, T.M., Assaf, A.R., Feldman, H.A., and McKinlay, S. (1995). The Pawtucket Heart Health Program: community changes in cardiovascular risk factors and projected disease risk. *Am J Public Health*, 85:777–85.

Clark, N.M., Rakowski, W., Wheeler, J.R., Ostrander, L.D., Oden, S., and Keteyian, S. (1988). Development of self-management education for elderly heart patients. *Gerontologist*, 28:491–4.

Clark, N.M., Janz, N.K., Becker, M.H., Schork, M.A., Wheeler, J., Liang, J., et al. (1992a). Impact of self-management education on the functional health status of older adults with heart disease. *Gerontologist*, 32:438–43.

Clark, N.M., Janz, N.K., Dodge, J.A., and Sharpe, P.A. (1992b). Self-regulation of health behavior: the "take PRIDE" program. *Health Educ Q*, 19:341–54.

Coreil, J., Levin, J.S., and Jaco, E.G. (1985). Life style—an emergent concept in the sociomedical sciences. *Cult Med Psychiatry*, 9:423–37.

D'Andrade, R. (1986). Three scientific world views and the covering law model. In Fiske, D.W., and Shweder, R.S. (eds.), *Metatheory in social science*. Chicago, IL: University of Chicago Press, pp. 19–41.

DiClemente, R.J., and Wingood, G.M. (1995). A randomized controlled trial of an HIV sexual risk-reduction intervention for young African-American women. *J Am Med Assoc*, 274:1271–6.

Edgar, L., Rosberger, Z., and Nowlis, D. (1992). Coping with cancer during the first year after diagnosis. Assessment and intervention. *Cancer*, 69:817–28.

Evans, R.L., Bishop, D.S., Matlock, A.L., Stranahan, S., Smith, G.G., and Halar, E.M. (1987). Family interaction and treatment adherence after stroke. *Arch Phys Med Rehabil*, 68:513–7.

Evans, R.L., Matlock, A.-L., Bishop, D.S., Stranahan, S., and Pederson, C. (1988). Family intervention after stroke: does counseling or education help? *Stroke*, 19:1243–9.

Farquhar, J.W., Fortmann, S.P., Maccoby, N., Haskell, W.L., Williams, P.T., Flora, J.A., Taylor, C.B., Brown, B.W. Jr., Solomon, D.S., and Hulley, S.B. (1985). The Stanford Five-City Project: design and methods. *Am J Epidemiol*, 122:323–34.

Farquhar, J.W., Fortmann, S.P., Flora, J.A., Taylor, C.B., Haskell, W.L., Williams, P.T., Maccoby, N., and Wood, P.D. (1990). Effects of communitywide education on cardiovascular disease risk factors. The Stanford Five-City Project. *J Am Med Assoc*, 264:359–65.

Fawzy, F., Cousins, N., Fawzy, N., Kemeny, M., Elashoff, R., and Morton, D. (1990a). A structured psychiatric intervention for cancer patients. I. Changes over time in methods of coping and affective disturbance. *Arch Gen Psychiatry*, 47:720–5.

Fawzy, F.I., Kemeny, M.E., Fawzy, N.W., Elashoff, R., Morton, D., Cousins, N., and Fahey, J.L. (1990b). A structured psychiatric intervention for cancer patients. II. Changes over time in immunological measures. *Arch Gen Psychiatry*, 47:729–35.

Fawzy, F.I., Fawzy, N.W., Hyun, C.S., Elashoff, R., Guthrie, D., Fahey, J.L., and Morton, D.L. (1993). Malignant melanoma. Effects of an early structured psychiatric intervention, coping, and affective state on recurrence and survival 6 years later. *Arch Gen Psychiatry*, 50:681–9.

Frasure-Smith, N. (1995). The Montreal Heart Attack Readjustment trial. *J Cardiopulmonary Rehab*, 15:103–6.

Frasure-Smith, N., and Prince, R. (1985). The Ischemic Heart Disease Life Stress Monitoring Program: impact on mortality. *Psychosom Med*, 47:431–45.

Frasure-Smith, N., and Prince, R. (1989). Long-term follow-up of the Ischemic Heart Disease Life Stress Monitoring Program. *Psychosom Med*, 51:485–513.

Frasure-Smith, N., Lesperance, F., Prince, R.H., Verrier, P., Garber, R.A., Juneau, M., Wolfson, C., and Bourassa, M.G. (1997). Randomised trial of home-based psychosocial nursing intervention for patients recovering from myocardial infarction. *Lancet*, 350:473–9.

Friedland, J.F., and McColl, M. (1992). Social support intervention after stroke: results of a randomized trial. *Arch Phys Med Rehabil*, 73:573–81.

Friedman, M., Thoresen, C.E., Gill, J.J., Ulmer, D., Powell, L.H., Price, V.A., Brown, B., Thompson, L., Robin, D.D., and Breall, W.S. (1986). Alteration of type A behavior and its effects on cardiac recurrences in post myocardial infarction patients: summary results of the Recurrent Coronary Prevention Project. *Am Heart J*, 112:653–65.

Friedman, M., and Rosenman, R.H. (1959). Association of a specific overt behavior pattern with increase in blood cholesterol, blood clotting time, incidence of arcus senilis, and clinical coronary arterery disease. *J Am Med Assoc*, 112:653–65.

Friedman, M., Thoresen, C.E., Gill, J.J., Ulmer, D., Thompson, L., Powell, L., Price, V., Elek, S.R., Rabin, D.D., Breall, W.S., Piaget, G., Dixon, T., Bourg, E., Levy, R.A., and Tasto, D.L. (1982). Feasibility of altering type A behavior pattern after myocardial infarction: Recurrent Coronary Prevention Project study: methods, baseline results and preliminary findings. *Circulation*, 66:83–92.

Friedman, M., Thoresen, C.E., Gill, J.J., Powell, L.H., Ulmer, D., Thompson, L., Price, V.A., Rabin, D.D., Breall, W.S., and Dixon, T. (1984). Alteration of type A behavior and reduction in cardiac recurrences in postmyocardial infarction patients. *Am Heart J*, 108:237–48.

Friedman, M., Powell, L.H., Thoresen, C.E., Ulmer, D., Price, V., Gill, J.J., Thompson, L., Rabin, D.D., Brown, B., and Breall, W.S. (1987). Effect of discontinuance of type A behavioral counseling on type A behavior and cardiac recurrence rate of post myocardial infarction patients. *Am Heart J*, 114:483–90.

Galanter, M. (1993). *Network therapy for alcohol and drug abuse: a new approach in practice*. New York, NY: Basic Books.

Galanter, M., Keller, D.S., and Dermatis, H. (1997). Network therapy for addiction: assessment of the clinical outcome of training. *Am J Drug Alcohol Abuse*, 23:355–67.

Garrison, V. (1978). Support systems of schizophrenic and nonschizophrenic Puerto Rican migrant women in New York City. *Schizophr Bull*, 4:561–96.

Gesten, E.L., and Jason, L.A. (1987). Social and community interventions. *Annu Rev Psychol*, 38:427–60.

Gibaldi, M., and Sullivan, S. (1997). Intention-to-treat analysis in randomized trials: who gets counted? *J Clin Pharmacol*, 37:667–72.

Glass, T., Dym, B., Greenberg, S., Rintell, D., Roesch, C., and Berkman, L.F. (in press). Psychosocial intervention in stroke: The Families in Recovery from Stroke Trial (FIRST). *Am J Orthopsychiatry.*

Gonzalez, S., Steinglass, P., and Reiss, D. (1989). Putting the illness in its place: discussion groups for families with chronic medical illnesses. *Fam Process,* 28:69–87.

Gottlieb, B. (1985). Theory into practice: issues that surface in planning interventions which mobilize support. In Sarason, I.G., and Sarason, B.R. (eds.), *Social support: theory, research, and application.* The Hague: Martinus Nijhoff, pp. 417–37.

Gottlieb, B.H. (1988). Marshalling social support. *Beverly Hills,* CA: Sage.

Gould, K.L., Ornish, D., Scherwitz, L., Brown, S., Edens, R.P., Hess, M.J., Mullani, N., Bolomey, L., Dobbs, F., and Armstrong, W.T. (1995). Changes in myocardial perfusion abnormalities by positron emission tomography after long-term, intense risk factor modification. *J Am Med Assoc,* 274:894–901.

Gruen, W. (1975). Effects of brief psychotherapy during the hospitalization period on the recovery process in heart attacks. *J Consult Clin Psychol,* 43:232–3.

Gyarfas, I. (1992). Review of community intervention studies on cardiovascular risk factors. *Clin Exp Hypertens [A]* 14:223–37.

Halevy-Martini, J., Hemley-van der Velden, E.M., Ruhf, L., and Schoenfeld, P. (1984). Process and strategy in network therapy. *Fam Process,* 23:521–33.

Havas, S., Heimendinger, J., Damron, D., Nicklas, T.A., Cowan, A., Beresford, S.A., Sorensen, G., Buller, D., Bishop, D., and Baranowski, T. (1995). 5 A Day for better health—nine community research projects to increase fruit and vegetable consumption. *Public Health Rep,* 110:68–79.

Heaney, C.A. (1991). Enhancing social support at the workplace: assessing the effects of the caregiver support program. *Health Educ Q,* 18:477–94.

Hjermann, I. (1983). A randomized primary preventive trial in coronary heart disease: the Oslo study. *Prev Med,* 12:181–4.

Hogan, J.W., and Laird, N.M. (1996). Intention-to-treat analyses for incomplete repeated measures data. *Biometrics,* 52:1002–17.

Jousilahti, P., Tuomilehto, J., Korhonen, H.J., Vartiainen, E., Puska, P., and Nissinen, A. (1994). Trends in cardiovascular disease risk factor clustering in eastern Finland: results of 15-year follow-up of the North Karelia Project. *Prev Med,* 23:6–14.

Kaplan, G.A. (1995). Where do shared pathways lead? Some reflections on a research agenda. *Psychosom Med,* 57:208–12.

Karasek, R., and Theorell, T. (1990). *Healthy work: stress, productivity, and the reconstruction of working life.* New York: Basic Books.

Kasl, S. (1983). Social and psychological factors affecting the course of disease: an epidemiological perspective. In Mechanic, D. (ed.), *Handbook of health, health care and the health professions.* New York: The Free Press, pp. 683–708.

Kelly, J.A., St Lawrence, J.S., Diaz, Y.E., Stevenson, L.Y., Hauth, A.C., Brasfield, T.L., Kalichman, S.C., Smith, J.E., and Andrew, M.E. (1991). HIV risk behavior reduction following intervention with key opinion leaders of population: an experimental analysis. *Am J Public Health,* 81:168–71.

Klein, R.F., Kliner, V.A., Zipes, D.P., Troyer, W.G., and Wallace, A.G. (1968). Transfer from a coronary care unit. *Arch Intern Med,* 122:104–8.

Knudson, K.G., Spiegel, T.M., and Furst, D.E. (1981). Outpatient educational program for rheumatoid arthritis patients. *Patient Counseling Health Educ,* 3:77–82.

Krantz, D.S., and Schulz, R. (1980). A model of life crisis, control, and health outcomes: cardiac rehabilitation of relocation of the elderly. In Baum, A., and Singer, J.E. (eds.), *Advances in environmental pyschology: applications of personal control.* Hillsdale, NJ: Lawrence Erlbaum, pp. 23–57.

Kristal, A.R., Patterson, R.E., Glanz, K., Heimendinger, J., Hebert, J.R., Feng, Z., and Probart, C. (1995). Psychosocial correlates of healthful diets: baseline results from the Working Well Study. *Prev Med,* 24:221–8.

Kuhn, T.S. (1962). *The structure of scientific revolutions.* Chicago, IL: University of Chicago Press.

Langer, E.J., and Rodin, J. (1976). The effects of choice and enhanced personal responsibility for the aged: a field experiment in an institutional setting. *J Pers Soc Psychol,* 34:191–8.

Lanza, A.F., and Revenson, T.A. (1993). Social support interventions for rheumatoid arthritis patients: the cart before the horse? *Health Educ Q,* 20:97–117.

Lawton, M.P., Brody, E.M., and Saperstein, A.R. (1989). A controlled study of respite service for caregivers of Alzheimer's patients. *Gerontologist,* 29:8–16.

Lehtinen, K. (1994). Need-adapted treatment of schizophrenia: family interventions. *Br J Psychiatry Suppl,* 23:89–96.

Lerman, C., Lustbader, E., Rimer, B., Daly, M., Miller, S., Sands, C., and Balshem, A. (1995). Effects of individualized breast cancer risk counseling: a randomized trial. *J Nat Cancer Inst,* 87:286–92.

Lerman, C., Schwartz, M.D., Miller, S.M., Daly, M., Sands, C., and Rimer, B.K. (1996). A randomized trial of breast cancer risk counseling: interacting effects of counseling, educational level, and coping style. *Health Psychol*, 15:75–83.

Levenkron, J.C., Cohen, J.D., Mueller, H.S., and Fisher, E.B. Jr. (1983). Modifying the type A coronary-prone behavior pattern. *J Consult Clin Psychol*, 51:192–204.

Levi, L. (1997). A biopsychosocial approach to etiology and pathogenesis. *Acta Physiol Scand Suppl*, 640:103–6.

Levin, J.S., Glass, T.A., Kushi, L.H., Schuck, J.R., Steele, L., and Jonas, W.B. (1997). Quantitative methods in research on complementary and alternative medicine. A methodological manifesto. NIH Office of Alternative Medicine. *Med Care*, 35:1079–94.

Levy, L.L. (1987a). Psychosocial intervention and dementia: I. State of the art, future directions. *Occup Ther Ment Health*, 7:69–107.

Levy, L.L. (1987b). Psychosocial intervention and dementia: II. The cognitive disability perspective. *Occup Ther Ment Health*, 7:13–36.

Lorig, K., and Holman, H.R. (1989). Long-term outcomes of an arthritis self-management study: effects of reinforcement efforts. *Soc Sci Med*, 29:221–4.

Lorig, K., Laurin, J., and Holman, H.R. (1984). Arthritis self-management: a study of the effectiveness of patient education for the elderly. *Gerontologist*, 24:455–7.

Lorig, K., Lubeck, D., Kraines, R.G., Seleznick, M., and Holman, H.R. (1985). Outcomes of self-help education for patients with arthritis. *Arch Rheumatol*, 28:680–5.

Luepker, R.V., Murray, D.M., Jacobs, D.R. Jr., Mittelmark, M.B., Bracht, N., Carlaw, R., Crow, R., Elmer, P., Finnegan, J., and Folsom, A.R. (1994). Community education for cardiovascular disease prevention: risk factor changes in the Minnesota Heart Health Program. *Am J Public Health*, 84:1383–93.

Luepker, R.V., Rastam, L., Hannan, P.J., Murray, D.M., Gray, C., Baker, W.L., Crow, R., Jacobs, D.R. Jr., Pirie, P.L., Mascioli, S.R., Mittelmark, M.B., and Blackburn, H. (1996). Community education for cardiovascular disease prevention. Morbidity and mortality results from the Minnesota Heart Health Program. *Am J Epidemiol*, 144:351–62.

MacLean, D.R. (1994). Theoretical rationale of community intervention for the prevention and control of cardiovascular disease. *Health Rep*, 6:174–80.

Maunsell, E., Brisson, J., Deschenes, L., and Frasure-Smith, N. (1996). Randomized trial of a psychologic distress screening program after breast cancer: effects on quality of life. *J Clin Oncol*, 14:2747–55.

McCormick, J., and Skrabanek, P. (1988). Coronary heart disease is not preventable by population interventions. *Lancet*, 2(8615): 839–42.

McKinlay, J.B. (1993). The promotion of health through planned sociopolitical change: challenges for research and policy. *Soc Sci Med*, 36:109–17.

McKinlay, J.B. (1995). The new public health approach to improving physical activity and autonomy in older populations. In Heikkinen, E., Kuusinen, J., and Ruoppila, I. (eds.), *Preparation for Aging*. New York: Plenum Press, pp. 87–103.

McMichael, A.J. (1989). Coronary heart disease: interplay between changing concepts of aetiology, risk distribution, and social strategies for prevention. *Community Health Studies*, 13:5–13.

Minkler, M. (1985). Building supportive ties and sense of community among the inner-city elderly: the Tenderloin Senior Outreach Project. *Health Educ Q*, 12:303–14.

Minuchin, S., Rosman, B.L., and Baker, L. (1978). *Psychosomatic families*. Cambridge, MA: Harvard University Press.

Mohide, E.A., Pringle, D.M., Streiner, D.L., Gilbert, J.R., Muir, G., and Tew, M. (1990). A randomized trial of family caregiver support in the home management of dementia. *J Am Geriatr Soc*, 38:446–54.

Montgomery, R.J.V., and Borgatta, E.F. (1985). *Family support project: final report to the administration on aging*. Seattle, WA: Universtiy of Washington, Institute on Aging/Long-Term Care Center.

Morgenstern, H., Gellert, G.A., Walter, S.D., Ostfeld, A.M., and Siegel, B.S. (1984). The impact of a psychosocial support program on survival with breast cancer: the importance of selection bias in program evaluation. *J Chron Dis*, 37:273–82.

Mulder, C.L., Emmelkamp, P.M., Antoni, M.H., Mulder, J.W., Sandfort, T.G., and de Vries, M.J. (1994). Cognitive-behavioral and experiential group psychotherapy for HIV-infected homosexual men: a comparative study. *Psychosom Med*, 56:423–31.

Mulder, C.L., Antoni, M.H., Emmelkamp, P.M., Veugelers, P.J., Sandfort, T.G., van de Vijver, F.A., and de Vries, M.J. (1995). Psychosocial group intervention and the rate of decline of immunological parameters in asymptomatic HIV-infected homosexual men. *Psychother Psychosom*, 63:185–92.

Mullen, P.D., Mains, D.A., and Velez, R. (1992). A meta-analysis of controlled trials of cardiac patient education. *Patient Educ Couns*, 19:143–62.

Newell, D.J. (1992). Intention-to-treat analysis: implications for quantitative and qualitative research (see comments). *Int J Epidemiol*, 21:837–41.

Nunes, E.V., Frank, K.A., and Kornfeld, D.S. (1987). Psychological treatment for type-A behavior pattern: a meta-analysis of the literature. *Psychosom Med,* 48:159–73.

Oldenburg, B., Perkins, R.J., and Andrews, G. (1985). Controlled trial of psychological intervention in myocardial infarction. *J Consult Clin Psychol,* 53:852–9.

Ornish, D. (1982). *Stress, diet, and your heart.* New York: Holt, Rinehart and Winston.

Ornish, D., Scherwitz, L.W., Doody, R.S., Kesten, D., McLanahan, S.M., Brown, S.E., DePuey, E., Sonnemaker, R., Haynes, C., Lester, J., McAllister, G.K., Hall, R.J., Burdine, J.A., and Gotto, A.M. Jr. (1983). Effects of stress management training and dietary changes in treating ischemic heart disease. *J Am Med Assoc,* 249:54–9.

Ornish, D., Brown, S.E., Scherwitz, L.W., Billings, J.H., Armstrong, W.T., Ports, T.A., McLanahan, S.M., Kirkeeide, R.L., Brand, R.J., and Gould, K.L. (1990). Can lifestyle changes reverse coronary heart disease? *Lancet,* 336:129–33.

Orth-Gomér, K., and Schneiderman, N. (1996). *Behavioral medicine approaches to cardiovascular disease prevention.* Mahway, NJ: Lawrence Erlbaum Associates.

Pinkston, E.M., and Linsk, N.L. (1984). Behavioral family intervention with the impaired elderly. *Gerontologist,* 24:576–83.

Pinkston, E.M., Linsk, N.L., and Young, R.N. (1988). Home-based behavioral family treatment of the impaired elderly. *Behav Ther,* 19:331–44.

Powell, L.H., Shaker, L.A., Jones, B.A., Vaccarino, L.V., Thoresen, C.E., and Pattillo, J.R. (1993). Psychosocial predictors of mortality in 83 women with premature acute myocardial infarction. *Psychosom Med,* 55: 426–33.

Prochaska, J.O., DiClemente, C.C., Velicer, W.F., and Rossi, J.S. (1993). Standardized, individualized, interactive, and personalized self-help programs for smoking cessation. *Health Psychol,* 12:399–405.

Prochaska, J.O., Redding, C.A., and Evers, K.E. (1997). The transtheoretical model and stages of change. In Glanz, K., Lewis, F.M., and Rimer, B.K. (eds.), *Health behavior and health education: theory, research, and practice.* San Francisco, CA: Jossey-Bass, pp. 60–84.

Puska, P. (1992). The North Karelia Project: nearly 20 years of successful prevention of CVD in Finland. *Hygie,* 11:33–5.

Puska, P., Niemensivu, H., Puhakka, P., Alhainen, L., Koskela, K., Moisio, S., and Viri, L. (1988). Results of a one-year worksite and mass media based intervention on health behaviour and chronic disease risk factors. *Scand J Soc Med,* 16:241–50.

Puska, P., Tuomilehto, J., Nissinen, A., Salonen, J.T., Vartiainen, E., Pietinen, P., Koskela, K., and Korhonen, H.J. (1989). The North Karelia Project: 15 years of community-based prevention of coronary heart disease. *Ann Med,* 21:169–73.

Puska, P., Korhonen, H.J., Torppa, J., Tuomilehto, J., Vartiainen, E., Pietinen, P., and Nissinen, A. (1993). Does community-wide prevention of cardiovascular diseases influence cancer mortality? *Eur J Cancer Prev,* 2:457–60.

Radojevic, V., Nicassio, P.M., and Weisman, M.H. (1992). Behavioral intervention with and without family support for rheumatoid arthritis. *Behav Ther,* 23:13–30.

Rahe, R.H., Ward, H.W., and Hayes, V. (1979). Brief group therapy in myocardial infarction rehabilitation: three- to four-year follow-up of a controlled trial. *Psychosom Med,* 41:229–42.

Razin, A.M. (1982). Psychosocial intervention in coronary artery disease: a review. *Psychosom Med,* 44:363–87.

Richardson, J.L., Shelton, D.R., Krailo, M., and Levine, A.M. (1990). The effect of compliance with treatment on survival among patients with hematologic malignancies. *J Clin Oncol,* 8:356–64.

Rodin, J., and Langer, E.J. (1977). Long-term effects of a control-relevant intervention with the institutionalized aged. *J Pers Soc Psychol,* 35:897–902.

Rodin, J., Rennert, K., and Solomon, S.K. (1980). Intrinsic motivation for control: fact or fiction. In Baum, A., and Singer, J.E. (eds.), *Advances in environmental pyschology: applications of personal control.* Hillsdale, NJ: Lawrence Erlbaum, pp. 131–48.

Rolland, J. (1989). Chronic illness and the family life cycle. In Carter, B., and McGoldrick, M. (eds.), *The changing family life cycle.* Boston: Allyn and Bacon, pp. 433–56.

Rook, K.S., and Dooley, D. (1985). Applying social support research: theoretical problems and future directions. *J Soc Issues,* 41: 5–28.

Rose, G. (1985). Sick individuals and sick populations. *Int J Epidemiol,* 14:32–8.

Rose, G.A. (1992). *The strategy of preventative medicine.* Oxford: Oxford University Press.

Royce, J.M., Corbett, K., Sorensen, G., and Ockene, J. (1997). Gender, social pressure, and smoking cessations: the Community Intervention Trial for Smoking Cessation (COMMIT) at baseline. *Soc Sci Med,* 44:359–70.

Salonen, J.T. (1987). Did the North Karelia project reduce coronary mortality? (letter). *Lancet*, 2:1.

Salonen, J.T. (1991). Prevention of coronary heart disease in Finland—application of the population strategy. *Ann Med*, 23:607–12.

Salonen, J.T., Tuomilehto, J., Nissinen, A., Kaplan, G.A., and Puska, P. (1989). Contribution of risk factor changes to the decline in coronary incidence during the North Karelia project: a within-community analysis. *Int J Epidemiol*, 18:595–601.

Seeman, T.E., and Berkman, L.F. (1988). Structural characteristics of social networks and their relationship with social support in the elderly: who provides support. *Soc Sci Med*, 26:737–49.

Shea, S., Basch, C.E., Wechsler, H., and Lantigua, R. (1996). The Washington Heights–Inwood Healthy Heart Program: a 6-year report from a disadvantaged urban setting. *Am J Public Health*, 86:166–71.

Shekelle, R.B., Hulley, S.B., Neaton, J.D., Billings, J.H., Borhani, N.O., Gerace, T.A., Jacobs, D.R., Lasser, N.L., Mittlemark, M.B., and Stamler, J. (1985). The MRFIT behavior pattern study. II. Type A behavior and incidence of coronary heart disease. *Am J Epidemiol*, 122:559–70.

Smith, T.W., and Anderson, N.B. (1986). Models of personality and disease: an interactional approach to Type A behavior and cardiovascular risk. *J Pers Soc Psychol*, 50: 1166–73.

Sorensen, G., Emmons, K., Hunt, M.K., and Johnston, D. (1998). Implications of the results of community intervention trials. *Ann Rev Public Health*, 19:379–416.

Speck, R., and Attneave, C. (1973). *Family networks*. New York: Vintage.

Spiegel, D., Bloom, J.R., Kraemer, H.C., and Gottheil, E. (1989). Effect of psychosocial treatment on survival of patients with metastatic breast cancer. *Lancet*, 14:888–91.

Susser, M. (1995). The tribulations of trials—intervention in communities. *Am J Public Health*, 85:156–8.

Taylor, S.E., Falke, R.L., Mazel, R.M., and Hilsberg, B.L. (1988). Sources of satisfaction and dissatisfaction among members of cancer support groups. In Gottlieb, B.H. (ed.), *Marshalling social support: Formats, processes, and effects*. Newbury Park, CA: Sage, pp. 187–208.

Telch, C.F., and Telch, M.J. (1986). Group coping skills instruction and supportive group therapy for cancer patients: a comparison of strategies. *J Consult Clin Psychol*, 54:802–8.

Terris, M. (1980). Epidemiology as a guide to health policy. *Annu Rev Public Health*, 1:323–44.

The Multiple Risk Factor Intervention Trial Group. (1982). Multiple risk factor intervention trial: risk factor changes and mortality results. *J Am Med Assoc*, 248:1465–77.

Thoresen, C.E., and Powell, L.H. (1992). Type A behavior pattern: new perspectives on theory, assessment, and intervention. *J Consult Clin Psychol*, 60:595–604.

Toseland, R.W., and Rossiter, C.M. (1989). Group interventions to support family caregivers: a review and analysis. *Gerontologist*, 29:438–48.

Tune, L.E., Lucas-Blaustein, M.J., and Rovner, B.W. (1988). Psychosocial interventions. In Jarvik, L.F., and Winograd, C.H. (eds.), *Treatments for the Alzheimer patient: the long haul*. New York, NY: Springer, pp. 123–36.

Wasylenki, D., James, S., Clark, C., Lewis, J., Goering, P., and Gillies, L. (1992). Clinical issues in social network therapy for clients with schizophrenia. *Community Ment Health J*, 28:427–40.

Wenger, N.K., Froelicher, E.S., Smith, L.K., Ades, P.A., Berra, K., Blumenthal, J.A., Certo, C.M.E., Dattilo, A.M., Davis, D., DeBusk, R.F., Drozda, J.P., Fletcher, B.J., Franklin, B.A., Gaston, H., Greenland, P., McBride, P.E., McGregor, C.G.A., Oldridge, N.B., Piscatella, J.C., and Rogers, F.J. (1995). *Cardiac Rehabilitation*. Clinical Practice Guideline No. 17, *AHCPR Publication No. 96-0672*. Rockville, MD: Department of Health and Human Services, Public Health Service, Agency for Health Care Policy and Research and the National Heart Lung and Blood Institute.

Wilhelmsen, L., Berglund, G., Elmfeldt, D., Tibblin, G., Wedel, H., Pennert, K., Vedin, A., Wilhelmsson, C., and Werko, L. (1986). The multifactor primary prevention trial in Göteborg, Sweden. *Eur Heart J*, 7:279–88.

Wilson, W., and Pratt, C. (1987). The impact of diabetes education and peer support upon weight and glycemic control of elderly persons with noninsulin dependent diabetes mellitus (NIDDM). *Am J Public Health*, 77:634–5.

World Health Organization. (1986). European Collaborative Trial of Multifactorial Prevention of Coronary Heart Disease: final report on the 6-year results. *Lancet*, 1(8486):869–72.

13

Toward a New Social Biology

ERIC J. BRUNNER

Many categories of morbidity and mortality exhibit an inverse social gradient. In the United Kingdom there are higher death rates in lower social classes for almost all major causes, including deaths due to most cancers, circulatory diseases, many infectious diseases, and accidents and violence (Drever and Whitehead 1997). The important exceptions are HIV, colon cancer, and brain cancer, which do not show inverse social gradients. The purpose of this chapter is to examine some of the biological processes that underlie social gradients in health. My intention is not explain away the phenomena, but to describe pathways by which social structures may plausibly operate, and to examine some of the evidence that such pathways do in fact operate.

Why should we study the social–biological interface? First, evidence obtained in different populations provides useful insights for etiological research. The fact that the Japanese have low serum cholesterol levels and a very low rate of coronary disease indicated that diet is probably an important cause of the disease. Related to this, Japan-

ese migrants to the United States after World War II rapidly developed American levels of coronary disease, particularly if they adopted a local way of life, pointing to cultural determinants of health (Marmot and Syme 1976). Second, basic research in biology and physiology provides good evidence that environmental stressors may be responsible for acute and chronic disease via stress mechanisms such as the fight-or-flight response. The application of this body of knowledge in studies of the social determinants of health has begun to yield important results. For example, there appear to be socially patterned differences in cortisol secretion that correspond to income, to social isolation and depression, and to prevailing differences in coronary death rates (Kristenson et al. 1998).

The study of social and biological variables at the same time is intrinsically valuable because we are, as humans, both social and biological. There are public health gains to be made when we approach health and ill-health from this perspective. Beyond the intellectual project to test the stress hypothesis, for example, lies the potential to inform the debate about social conditions and health; in what ways can we organize ourselves to make life less difficult, more rewarding, and healthier for a larger proportion of the people?

THEORETICAL FRAMEWORK

The proposition that social factors are key determinants of health is not new. It is widely accepted that a primary social determinant is level of economic development. In the long period before population health went through the transition away from the predominance of epidemic infection, material conditions were manifestly critical to the survival of infants, children, and adults alike. During the Industrial Revolution living standards rose rapidly and unevenly, producing our modern socially and economically stratified towns and cities. Writing about the new urban poverty in London, Manchester, Birmingham, and Leeds in the 1840s, Engels described its health impact starkly:

The number of people who die from causes attributable to inadequate nourishment is far greater than the number of those who die of actual starvation. A continual lack of sufficient food leads to illnesses which prove fatal. An illness from which a well-fed person would speedily recover soon carries off those who are hopelessly undernourished. The English workers call this "social murder." (1848)

Mortality differentials related to socioeconomic position were documented in official statistics (Table 13–1). Though not the subject of this chapter, the biological explanation of the health effects of social conditions in the 19th century would clearly begin with undernutrition and susceptibility to infection (McKeown 1979). The dry, warm, hygienic housing and plentiful supply of fresh food available to the middle classes and capitalists, but not yet to the laboring classes, produced conditions under which life expectancy and infant mortality improved dramatically.

During the 20th century, average living

Table 13–1. Death rates in the Manchester suburb of Chorlton-on-Medlock according to three categories of streets and houses, 1844.

Class of streets*	Class of houses	Rate of mortality
1st	1st	1 in 51
	2nd	1 in 45
	3rd	1 in 36
2nd	1st	1 in 55
	2nd	1 in 38
	3rd	1 in 35
3rd	1st	not given
	2nd	1 in 35
	3rd	1 in 25

Source: P.H. Holland (surgeon), Report of the Commission of Enquiry into the state of large towns and populous districts, 1844. Cited in Engels 1958.

* 1st, highest category, 3rd, lowest category.

standards in the industrialized countries rose substantially and, where there has been adequate welfare provision, the majority do not live in poverty. Increases in average income in such countries do not lead to corresponding gains in average life expectancy. The data point not to average gross national product (GNP) per capita but to income distribution within the population as the important determinant. The smaller the gap between rich and poor, the lower are the mortality rates and the greater is the gain in overall life expectancy (Wilkinson 1996). It appears that relative rather than absolute living standards may be crucial determinants of health. These findings pose a challenge to social epidemiologists and policymakers because they imply that social organization has an influence on health at every level of status and income.

The task for social epidemiologists thus is to develop a robust theoretical view that explains social inequalities in health within and between countries. Psychosocial influences, in particular social cohesion and exclusion, material insecurity, and working conditions and their psychological correlates at individual level, are proposed to explain health differences associated with relative as opposed to absolute income in affluent but unequal societies. But there is not yet enough evidence to go beyond the general point that "social and economic in-

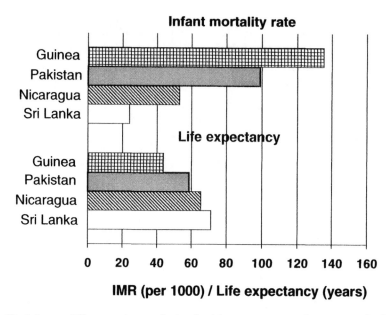

Figure 13–1. Large differences in population health status are seen between underdeveloped nations. All four countries have a GNP per capita in the range $400–$500 (1991–1992). Source: UNDP 1994.

fluences on health are not confined to developing countries, nor are they encapsulated by measures of mean income alone" (Marmot 1996). In fact, the mean income–health association is not very strong even among the poorest nations (Fig. 13–1), which is consistent with the view that multiple explanations are likely to be found. Social structure, historical and current living and working conditions, social cohesion and other psychosocial phenomena, and health-related behaviors are each potentially important. Their relative contributions will depend on the particular society and the particular time period being investigated. The difficult theoretical and empirical problem we are faced with is how we are to reconcile material, behavioral, and psychosocial explanations for health inequalities at population level.

Biology, as the common pathway by which each of the above factors must work, may help in these investigations. Two paradigms that have recently emerged provide a useful framework. Both address the weakness of research models that attempt to ex-

plain social and geographical inequalities in health exclusively on the basis of adult exposures. Both recognize the potential importance of processes that take place before adulthood. Barker and co-workers' biological programming concept (Barker 1992) emphasizes the links between poor development in utero and infancy and later chronic disease. Recognition of such processes has generated a second way to link early life with adult disease: the lifecourse approach (Kuh and Ben-Shlomo 1997). A key concept of the lifecourse perspective is accumulation of risk throughout an individual's lifetime, taking account of social and environmental influences on biological processes.

THE EARLY LIFE HYPOTHESIS

"Programming" is seen to account for the associations of low birth weight and thinness or shortness at birth with adult risk of cardiovascular disease and non-insulin-dependent diabetes in several cohorts (Barker et al. 1993). Undernutrition and other environmental insults may occur at critical periods of early development, producing lasting organ impairments and metabolic and endocrine abnormalities. Low growth rates up to 1 year are thus related to several cardiovascular risk factors: raised adult blood pressure, plasma glucose, insulin, fibrinogen, and apolipoprotein B. Among men born in Hertfordshire in 1911–1930, death rates from heart disease were almost three times higher for those weighing 8 kg or less at age 1, compared to those weighing 12 kg or more. The size of these effects implies that a biological time bomb may be set during early life. In addition, there is evidence that adult factors add to programmed risk. For instance, particularly high rates of non-insulin-dependent diabetes are seen among those who were small in infancy and are obese as adults.

THE LIFECOURSE PERSPECTIVE

The lifecourse perspective (Kuh and Ben-Shlomo 1997) admits the possibility of critical periods and programming but emphasizes the accumulation of risk resulting from exposure to adverse environments and illness during childhood, adolescence, and adulthood.

This view sees the influences of the intervening years between early life and the onset of disease to be essential in a full account of health determinants. Longitudinal study designs, with their associated costs and slowness, are needed to explore questions of latency, interaction, and reversibility. With respect to the relative importance of childhood vs. adult factors for specific disease outcomes, there is only limited evidence currently available from longitudinal studies which include repeated measures of socioeconomic position (Davey Smith 1997). These studies suggest that risk of premature cardiovascular disease is sensitive to early disadvantage, while many cancers depend to a large degree on adult circumstances. Smoking rates, interestingly, tend to be more strongly associated with adult than with childhood social position.

RESEARCH METHODS

Data implicating psychological and social factors in health come from observational epidemiology and from short-term laboratory and field investigations. Long-term and acute studies each have their strengths and weaknesses, and integrating findings from each reduces difficulties in interpretation and helps to realise the potential of the evidence.

Epidemiology is increasingly giving attention to social factors as exposures of interest, rather than as confounders, though social classifications need considerable further development (Krieger et al. 1997), particularly in cross-cultural comparisons (Whitty et al. 1999). Epidemiological cohort studies which include biological measures perform well against Hill's criteria for causal inference because they allow the evaluation of observed associations in terms of strength, consistency, temporality, dose–response gradient, and biological plausibility. Nevertheless, distinguishing between confounders and mediators in observational studies is not straightforward because many variables can be related both to the exposure and to the outcome of interest. For example, income, lifestyle, and psychosocial characteristics of work are each related to employment grade, and in turn to coronary risk, in the Whitehall cohort (Brunner 1996). The collinearity problem can be tackled by examining evidence drawn from diverse populations, when it may be possible, by design, to separate the exposures of interest. The availability of biological data within a study may also help to resolve such problems by providing opportunities for investigating mechanisms of action. An example is given in Panel 13–1 for the case of hostility as a cause of coronary disease.

The weakness of the epidemiological approach lies in the need for substantial resources, in particular because cohort studies typically require a decade or more of follow-up, and large study samples are needed to demonstrate interactions when relatively rare clinical disease is the out-

PANEL 13-1. HOSTILITY AND HEART DISEASE: WHAT IS THE MEDIATOR?

It has been proposed that hostility may contribute to the socioeconomic gradient in coronary disease through its effect on cardiovascular reactivity. The blood pressure reaction to Raven's Matrices, a nonverbal mental stress test, was obtained on 1091 male civil servants (Carroll et al. 1997). All subjects completed the Cook-Medley/MMPI hostility questionnaire. The results are shown in the bar graph, which uses employment grade to stratify subjects according to socioeconomic position.

Socioeconomic position, hostility and blood pressure reactions to mental stress in the Whitehall II study

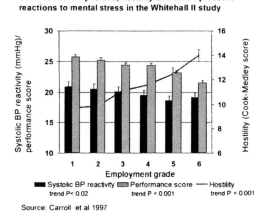

Source: Carroll et al 1997

Hostility was strongly linked with lower grade, consistent with a psychosocial explanation for the link between socioeconomic position and coronary risk. Hostility was however *inversely* related to systolic blood pressure reactivity ($P < 0.05$), such that a large pressor reaction was associated with low hostility, and with higher grade. We can conclude that the hostility–coronary disease association, shown in prospective and ecological studies, seems unlikely to be mediated by blood pressure reactivity. This interpretation would be strengthened if other types of psychosocial stress, such as interpersonal challenges, produced similar results.

Performance scores were directly related to grade and inversely related to hostility scores ($P < 0.001$), but performance was not associated with blood pressure reactivity. Perhaps higher grade subjects were more positively engaged with the stress task. Speculatively, the rewards of occupying a higher status position may include greater stress tolerance (apparently regardless of performance). The capacity for flexible arousal, to respond to psychological demands with a large pressor reaction and then to return rapidly to a resting state, may be a desirable product of social conditioning. Unless it is possible to demonstrate a biological pathway linking hostility to coronary risk we cannot dismiss the possibility that hostility, as measured, is a covariate of social position without a causal role in coronary disease.

come. The collection of biological measures of risk and subclinical markers of disease development, if available, may overcome both of these problems by permitting studies with shorter follow-up time and smaller sample sizes. Sub–study designs may also be useful. For instance, intensive investigations have been embedded within the Whitehall II cohort study to test hypotheses about neuroendocrine mechanisms in cardiovascular disease, and to study determinants of endothelial dysfunction, an early subclinical marker of atherosclerosis (Sorensen et al. 1995; Anderson et al. 1995).

Behavioral medicine, psychophysiology, and related disciplines provide methods for studying the effects of psychosocial and short-term stress on biology which complement epidemiology (Steptoe 1998). Psychobiologists have tended to emphasize individual differences, but there is growing awareness (Ockenfels et al. 1995; Seeman et al. 1995; Hellhammer et al. 1997) that social factors are among the most powerful influences on physical and mental health (Blane et al. 1996).

One approach is to show biological effects independent of health behaviors. The well-known study by Friedman and Rosenman, for example, showed a sharp rise in serum cholesterol and a fall in blood clotting time among accountants as the April 15th U.S. tax deadline approached, neither of which effects could be explained by changes in weight, exercise, or diet (Friedman et al. 1958). The extrapolation of such findings to the pathogenesis of disease depends on the assumption that effects accumulate. Here the evidence is incomplete, but we will see later in the chapter that recent research points to such cumulative effects in relation to cardiovascular disease. Further, it appears that chronic stress, like acute stress, may lead to immunosuppression with possible increases in vulnerability to a range of diseases (Cohen and Herbert 1996).

Investigation of short-term effects can add to our understanding of endocrine and metabolic mechanisms when large-scale epidemiology may be too blunt an instrument. These approaches can show the complexity of the mind–body interface, provided that care is taken in extrapolating short-term stress experiments to the effects of psychosocial factors on health over the lifetime. Thus, experimentally, acute psychological stress in humans is associated with hemoconcentration, and it appears that acutely raised lipid and clotting factor levels may primarily be due to this reversible and nonspecific process (Muldoon et al. 1995). Causal inferences about degenerative disease will therefore usually need evidence from population studies as well as from acute investigations.

This section has outlined some broad methodological approaches to health research which utilize social, psychological and biological variables simultaneously. It is far from comprehensive, and important omissions include the study of common genetic polymorphisms (Masters and Beyreuther 1998), which are likely to contribute to the social distribution of disease through gene–environment interactions (Fig. 13–2), and animal studies, which can provide insights, for example, into the biologi-

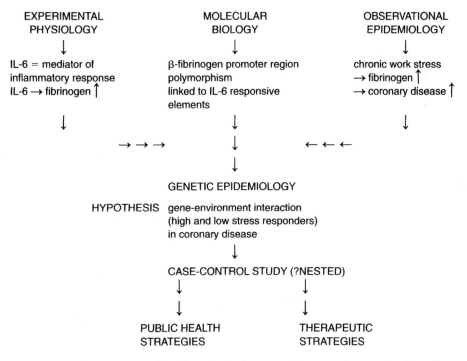

Figure 13–2. Schematic example of hypothetical gene–environment interaction. Beta-fibrinogen polymorphism and stress response phenotype. IL-6, interleukin-6. See text for related evidence.

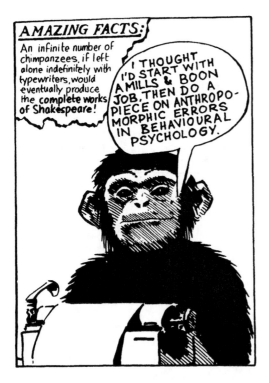

cal consequences of natural and manipulated social structures (see Chapter 15). Such studies fortunately lack many of the confounding problems produced by the human tendency to indulge in health-damaging behaviors. As is the case with acute psychophysiological experiments and long-term stress effects, analogies between animal and human society are best approached with caution (Cartoon 13–1).

The rest of this chapter presents evidence for biological mechanisms by which social and psychological factors can influence health, and which may mediate contemporary social inequalities in health. Psychosocial influences may be seen to act in two distinct ways. They may directly cause biological changes which predispose to disease, or they may, indirectly, influence behaviors such as smoking and diet which are themselves determinants of risk.

SOCIAL AND PSYCHOLOGICAL FACTORS IN HEALTH INEQUALITIES

One question, referred to above, is whether we are able to separate the effects of relative deprivation from those of material circumstances. If psychosocial exposures contribute to the explanation of the continuous gradient in health inequalities, which extends into the highest social strata (Marmot et al. 1984), we need to identify the important factors involved. Two necessary conditions are that their prevalence is linked with lower socioeconomic position and that the exposure of interest is associated with disease or disease markers.

Childhood

Emotional deprivation in childhood is linked to poor educational attainment and behavioral problems such as hyperactivity and other conduct disorders which may be precursors of a lifetime of material and emotional insecurity. Studies of the attachment patterns of parents and their children suggest early caregiver experiences may contribute to the intergenerational transmission of physical and psychological vulnerability (Fonagy 1996). Such childhood disadvantage may interact with other early factors such as low birth weight which are associated with lower parental social class to produce adverse effects on later health (Power and Hertzman 1997). Acquisition of health capital (constitution) in childhood, often indexed by height, appears to be important for the cohort now in their fifth and sixth decades. Extensive literature (Rona 1981) shows a strong link between adult height and socioeconomic position in childhood, with factors such as economic hardship, large family, and family conflict all linked to short stature in adulthood (Nystrom Peck and Lundberg 1995; Montgomery et al. 1997). These early life influences do not necessarily imply an irreversible trajectory. Studies with young rhesus monkeys suggest the consequences of experimental social isolation can be modified with timely intervention and that long-term effects are most likely to be seen under stress conditions in adulthood (Suomi 1997).

Psychogenic dwarfism is an extreme syndrome associated with severe childhood deprivation. Psychosocial growth retardation of a less dramatic nature was documented in Widdowson's study of orphaned children in postwar Germany (Widdowson 1951). Under identical food rationing regimes, those who lived in the Bienenhaus orphanage initially under the control of the stern and forbidding Fraülein Schwarz gained less weight and grew more slowly than children cared for by the affectionate Fraulein Grün at the Vogelnest orphanage. By chance, Schwarz replaced Grün during the study and the growth rates reversed, despite the provision of extra food at Vogelnest. This controlled crossover study provides evidence that adverse psychosocial circumstances in childhood can influence growth. The extent to which this is a "direct" psychosocial effect or one mediated by appetite loss is open to speculation.

Results from a more recent study suggest long-term effects on health can result from early material deprivation, although the mechanisms are again not clear. Self-rated health at age 33 in the National Child Development Study (the U.K. 1958 birth cohort) was poorer among those of lower current occupational status, and parental social class at birth accounted for part of this difference (Power et al. 1998).

Adulthood

On the basis of current evidence, key health-related psychosocial factors linked to the income gradient in adult life include perceived financial strain (Ullah 1990), job insecurity (Gallie and Vogler 1994; Bartley 1994), low control and monotony at work (Karasek et al. 1981; Marmot et al. 1997), stressful life events and poor social networks (Berkman and Syme 1979; Rosengren et al. 1993; Stansfeld et al. 1998; Ruberman et al. 1984), low self-esteem (Brown 1986), hostility (Williams 1991), and fatalism (Eaker et al. 1992). Depression and anxiety are not included in this list because they are themselves measures of health; however, there is growing evidence that minor psychiatric morbidity plays a mediating role between social circumstances and physical illness such as cardiovascular disease (Stansfeld et al. 1993, 1997).

There was a stepwise relationship between Civil Service employment grade (1992 salary range £6483–£87,620, roughly $11,000–$150,000) and the prevalence of several of the psychosocial factors listed above at the baseline of the Whitehall II study (Marmot et al. 1991). Low control and variety at work, relatively little social contact with friends, higher frequency of stressful life events, difficulty paying bills, higher Cook-Medley hostility scores, and external health locus of control were all associated with a lower position in the occupational hierarchy. These relationships were evident even before employment security in the British Civil Service was systematically reduced in the late 1980s (Ferrie et al. 1995).

The contribution of psychosocial conditions at work to the inverse occupational gradient in coronary heart disease is a key observation from Whitehall II. Utilizing Karasek and Theorell's self-report questionnaire, analysis of 5-year disease incidence rates shows that low job control is associated with increased coronary risk regardless of employment grade (Bosma et al. 1997) and that this measure of job strain explains, statistically, much of the occupational gradient in coronary disease (Marmot et al. 1997). While the specific role of work characteristics needs futher research, these findings support the general point that psychosocial factors are important in understanding the social distribution of coronary heart disease.

The etiological role of psychosocial factors in coronary heart disease has recently been reviewed (Hemingway and Marmot 1999). The evidence from cohort studies of healthy subjects ($n \geq 500$) is strongest for low social supports, low control at work, and depression and anxiety. For only one other factor, hostility, is there sufficient evidence available to provide an overview. Three of the five studies, the Western Electric (Shekelle et al. 1983), MRFIT (Dembroski et al. 1989), and Normative Aging (Kawachi et al. 1996), provided evidence for causation. A study of Danish men (Barefoot et al. 1995) was equivocal, and a 33-year follow-up of Minnesota students

(Hearn et al. 1989) observed no association. If the "hostility complex" consists of behaviors (aggression), emotions (anger), and attitudes (cynicism) it may be that the Cook-Medley questionnaire, frequently used in these studies, indexes cynicism well, but not aggression and anger. In summary, the review shows that psychosocial influences are predictors of coronary heart disease in a number of different populations, and it highlights the lack of larger studies in the field.

NEUROENDOCRINE PATHWAYS

Turning to the question of mechanism, it is certainly plausible that chronic stresses may be translated into modified neuroendocrine and physiological functioning with later consequences for disease susceptibility. From an evolutionary standpoint, humans are adapted to meet the challenge of external, potentially lethal, but short-term threats, perhaps from wild animals or from one another. Frequent and prolonged activation of the fight-or-flight and other endocrine responses appears to be maladaptive (Sapolsky 1993) and may prove to be central in understanding the social distribution of cardiovascular, infectious, and other diseases.

The main axes of neuroendocrine response appear to be the sympatho–adrenal and hypothalamic–pituitary–adrenal systems. Walter Cannon (professor of physiology at Harvard 1906–1942) elucidated the role of the sympathetic branch of the autonomic nervous system and circulating catecholamines in the dynamic process of metabolic self-regulation, coining the term homeostasis to refer to the feedback mechanisms which maintain constant internal conditions, such as body temperature, in the face of environmental change. Hans Selye, a Czech-Canadian physician, focused on the corticosteroids, which like catecholamines have widespread effects both centrally and peripherally. He proposed a three-stage nonspecific stress response: first, the alarm reaction, when the body responds to danger; second, resistance, when the body attempts to restore itself; and third, if the stress continues, exhaustion, with the risk of stress-related disorder (1956). Evidence for the third of these stages is comparatively weak.

The allostatic load hypothesis (McEwen 1998) links the psychosocial environment to physical disease via the two neuroendocrine pathways above and adds the cardiovascular, metabolic, and immune systems to its key mechanisms. Allostatic load, or stress-induced damage, is considered relevant in cardiovascular disease, cancer, infection, and cognitive decline and has been described as a sign of accelerated aging. The related concept of allostasis—the ability to achieve stability through change—extends Canon's notion of homeostasis to include physiological systems such as that controlling blood glucose, which is less tightly regulated than, for example, body temperature. The price of adaptation to external and internal stress may be wear and tear on the organism, the result of chronic over- or underactivty of allostatic systems to produce allostatic load. The challenge is to identify suitable markers of the accumulation of damage. A 3-year longitudinal study of older Americans (Seeman et al. 1997) utilized measures of five established cardiovascular risk factors plus urinary catecholamines and cortisol and serum dehydroepiandrosterone sulfate (an adrenal androgen). Subjects with lower baseline allostatic load scores had better physical and mental functioning. Over the follow-up period the same group showed less decline in these measures and they were less likely to develop cardiovascular disease.

The Sympatho–Adrenal System

Rapid release of adrenaline from the adrenal medulla and noradrenaline from sympathetic nerve endings produces cognitive arousal, sensory vigilance, bronchodilation, tachycardia, alteration of organ blood flows, raised blood pressure, hemoconcentration, and energy mobilization. The precise nature of the activation varies according to the stressor and its duration, but its function is essentially to prepare for or maintain physical exertion. Wide between-person variation in the size and duration of endocrine responses is attributed to individual differences in psychological coping resources (Grossman 1991). Laboratory animals have very different physiological responses to a given stressor, reflecting differences in prior stress history (McCarty and Gold 1996). There is potential for interactions between immediate and chronic psychosocial adversity, and protective factors, each of which may be determined by social status.

The measurement problems associated with the use of catecholamines in stress research have been discussed (Baum and Grunberg 1995). The half-life of some 2 minutes makes circulating levels volatile, and heart rate or blood pressure readings are often preferable for reasons of reproducibility in acute studies. Urinary catecholamine output is of interest as a measure of stress responsiveness because it is an integrated measure of sympatho–adrenomedullary activity. A pilot study (White et al. 1995) suggests that a 24-hour collection is probably desirable, at least in smaller studies. Comparison of overnight collections with concurrent 24-hour samples showed that while more convenient, the overnight sample produces considerably less information. For estimating long-term mean adrenaline output, a sample size some threefold larger is required to achieve the same power as a 24-hour collection.

Heart-rate variability is a novel method for characterizing autonomic influences on the heart (Kawachi et al. 1995). Power spectral density analysis of heart-rate variability yields low-frequency (0.04–0.15 Hz) and high-frequency (0.18–0.4 Hz) components (Bigger et al. 1992). Total variability is reduced by sympathetic activation and increased by vagal activity. The low frequency component is increased by mental stress and moderate exercise. The high frequency component is abolished by atropine and therefore appears to index vagal activity.

An increase in low frequency and in the low:high frequency ratio and a reduction in total power indicate sympathetic predominance.

The Hypothalamic–Pituitary–Adrenal System

The second and less rapid adrenocortical component of the stress response results in cortisol release. There are several feedback loops (Fig. 13–3) which regulate the activity of the hypothalamic–pituitary–adrenal (HPA) axis. The control system, involving each of the three hormones, corticotropin-releasing factor (CRF), adrenocorticotropic hormone (ACTH), and cortisol itself, provides sensitive mechanisms for adjustment of the circulating cortisol level during everyday life and in stress situations. Like the sympatho–adrenal system, the HPA axis appears to be conditioned by psychosocial factors (Seeman et al. 1995; Ockenfels et al. 1995; Kirschbaum et al. 1995; Hellhammer et al. 1997) which are associated with lower social position. Prolonged elevations or blunted responses from a raised baseline seem to be characteristic of an actual or projected failure to cope with challenge. These patterns of cortisol secretion differ from the normal sharp response and rapid return to a low baseline and correspond to Selye's proposed nonspecific stress mechanism (1956).

Glucocorticoids such as cortisol have many metabolic and psychological effects. They play a key role in the maintenance of basal and stress-related metabolic homeostasis. As insulin antagonists they mobilize energy reserves by raising blood glucose and promoting fatty acid release from adipose tissue. In the physically inactive situation these superfluous energy substrates will lead to increased hepatic lipoprotein output. The potent immunosuppressive action of glucocorticoids is well known. Activation of the HPA axis appears to protect the individual from the potentially malign effects of inflammation and infection, and the resulting host response. Using the mitogen-stimulated lymphocyte proliferation assay, leukocytes from patients with sepsis were more

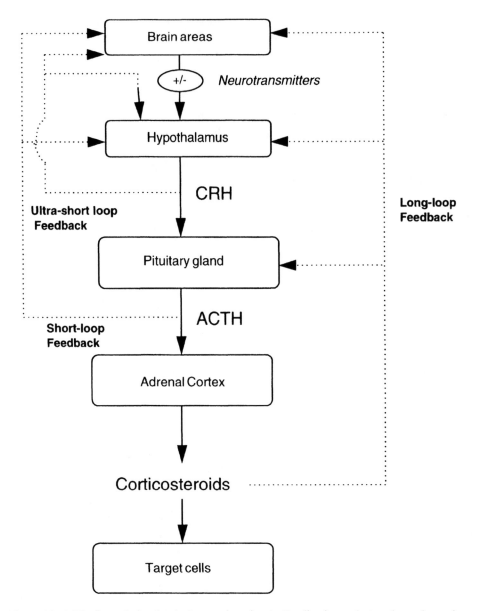

Figure 13–3. The hypothalamic–pituitary–adrenal axis. Feedback regulation depends on the levels of intermediate hormones. CRH, corticotropin releasing hormone; ACTH, adrenocorticotropic hormone. Redrawn from Brown 1994.

sensitive to the antiproliferative action of dexamethasone than those of controls. During recovery, sensitivity declined. Cytokines antagonize the glucocorticoid effect, thus providing a means by which a systemic inhibition of immune response may be accompanied by an appropriate local reaction (Molijn et al. 1995).

Within the brain the hippocampus is a target for glucocorticoids; they promote vigilance in the short term (Grossman 1991). Prolonged high levels of cortisol, such as in Cushing's Syndrome, may provoke paranoia or depression. Some depressed patients respond to metyrapone, an inhibitor of cortisol biosynthesis (Checkley

1996). Restraint stress in rats is associated with reversible hippocampal neurone loss, probably as a result of high glucocorticoid levels. Aspects of aging may be connected with related irreversible processes (Sapolsky et al. 1986) but evidence is scant in humans. Glucocorticoids are implicated in learning and memory formation (Rose 1995), and in the mode of action of memory-enhancing (nootropic) drugs of the acetam family. Centrally administered glucocorticoids enhance retention in experimental animals, consistent with the adrenocortical response to training challenges and the ability of glucocorticoid receptor antagonists to reduce memory formation. At higher glucocorticoid levels, however, learning is reduced. Speculatively, there may be an association between functioning of HPA axis and development of Alzheimer's disease.

Controls on cortisol secretion are complex. There is evidence that the feed-forward effect of sympatho–adrenal activity is countered by other neuroendocrine mechanisms to determine the pattern of the stress response. In a study (Delitala et al. 1991) where an acute cortisol response was obtained by administration of the adrenergic agonist methoxamine, the rise could be blocked by giving subjects a synthetic endorphin, which mimics the effect of endogenous opioids. These peptides appear to inhibit pituitary release of adrenocorticotropic hormone. The adverse effects of psychological stress, mediated by cortisol, may thus be limited by a sense of well-being, as a consequence of factors such as self-perception (Seeman et al. 1995; Kirschbaum et al. 1995) or exercise conditioning.

The precise arousal patterns linked with social subordination are as yet unclear. Among captive rhesus monkeys those with heightened stress responses tend to occupy lower positions in the dominance hierarchy (Suomi 1997). This contrasts with the autonomic (blood pressure) reactivity findings in Whitehall II study (Panel 13–1), which showed that higher-grade men had larger reactions to experimental stress. In a study utilizing 12 salivary cortisol samples given over 2 days, unemployed and employed subjects did not differ in their cortisol reactivity to acute daily stressors but did show differences in diurnal rhythm. The unemployed group had relatively higher morning and lower evening levels (Ockenfels et al. 1995). A comparison of Swedish and Lithuanian men given a stress test revealed higher morning cortisols and blunted reactivity among the low-income group drawn from the higher coronary risk Lithuanian population (Kristenson et al. 1998).

These studies illustrate novel approaches to the assessment of HPA axis functioning. Blood cortisol has a half-life of about 1 hour, and there is a marked and pulsatile diurnal pattern with significant day-to-day variability, all of which pose challenges to the study designer. The relatively invasive venipuncture method of sampling is being replaced by saliva collections in the laboratory or as subjects participate in their usual daily activities (Kirschbaum and Hellhammer 1994; Van Eck et al. 1996). Urinary output of a range of adrenal steroids and their metabolites can be measured to obtain integrated measures of secretion. For example, we are using urinary output to investigate the suggestion of a social gradient in serum dehydroepiandrosterone sulfate (DHEAS) which is evident in a subsample of men in the Whitehall II study (high employment grades: 2.5, 95% CI 2.2–2.8 vs. low grades: 2.1, 1.9–2.4 μmol/l, $P = 0.07$, unpublished data). Dehydroepiandrosterone sulfate is an androgen which antagonizes some of the effects of cortisol. Recent findings suggest HPA axis function may depend as much on tissue responsiveness as on secretion of cortisol. For instance, subjects with a family history of essential hypertension (Walker et al. 1996a) and subjects with insulin resistance (Walker et al. 1996b) show increased sensitivity to glucocorticoids.

Neuroendocrine Mechanisms in Cardiovascular Disease

It is a plausible but unproved hypothesis that direct neuroendocrine mechanisms are involved in the production of social inequalities in coronary heart disease. Reduced heart rate variability, indicating predominance of sympathetic over parasympathetic activity, has been linked with adverse work characteristics, depression, hostility, and anxiety, and separately with increased risk of sudden death (Algra et al. 1993). Depression, which is linked with excessive glucocorticoid production (Checkley 1996), predicts future coronary disease (Hemingway and Marmot, 1999). Cushing's syndrome is characterized by central obesity and increased risks for hypertension, diabetes, and coronary disease. Central obesity is linked with these diseases and is a feature of low socioeconomic status in many healthy populations (Brunner et al. 1998).

The neuroendocrine hypothesis (Bjorntorp 1991) proposes that chronic stress drives susceptible individuals toward the metabolic syndrome pattern of abnormalities (Reaven 1993) (central obesity, glucose intolerance, insulin resistance, lipoprotein disturbances, and reduced fibrinolysis). In other words, the brain, via the HPA axis and other neuroendocrine pathways, is able to push the body into a pathological state. This can be seen as an example of allostatic load (McEwen 1998).

The alternative behavioral explanation for the observed associations among HPA and metabolic syndrome variables (Hautanen and Adlercreutz 1993) is perhaps equally plausible. In this case, inappropriate diet and physical inactivity lead to central obesity among those predisposed. The increased mass of abdominal fat tissue, with its high concentration of glucocorticoid receptors, pulls cortisol out of the circulation and thereby alters feedback to the pituitary and hypothalamus. Here, modified neuroendocrine function is the consequence, and behavioral and consitutional factors are the causes. Psychosocial factors over the lifecourse are likely to be related to predisposition, as is fetal programming.

Early influence on HPA axis functioning in adulthood has recently been identified by Barker's group. Lower birth weight was associated with higher morning plasma cortisol level among men 59–70 years old (Phillips et al. 1998). Their related findings give evidence that plasma cortisol levels within the normal range are among the determinants of blood pressure and glucose tolerance. In this group of men fetal programming of the HPA axis was more important than the effect of current socioeconomic position. While it seems likely that both fetal growth and experiences during the lifecourse will turn out to be of importance in shaping neuroendocrine function in later life, an outstanding question is whether apparently adverse cortisol responses are directly responsible for future ill-health or merely markers of psychological state. Related to this is the issue of reversibility. Longitudinal studies are needed to clarify the relative importance of the neuroendocrine, behavioral, and early life hypotheses.

Stress, Infection, and Immunity

Infectious disease contributes to social differences in morbidity in countries such as Britain, and though evidence is lacking (Cohen and Herbert 1996), infection and immunity may be implicated a variety of conditions such as peptic ulcer; gastric, cervical, and other cancers; and possibly coronary disease (Danesh and Appleby 1998; Vallance et al. 1997). Interest in inflammatory processes in heart disease was reinforced in 1994 with the publication of a study showing an association between coronary events and chronic gastric *Helicobacter pylori* infection (Mendall et al. 1994). Such asymptomatic infections, acquired in childhood and linked with deprivation and overcrowded housing, may produce a long-term low level systemic inflammatory response which enhances atherogenesis. Supporting this, a meta-analysis (Danesh et al. 1998) found consistently moderate to high prospective associations between levels of the inflammatory markers fibrinogen, C-reactive protein, albumin and leucocyte count, and risk of coronary disease. Against the infection–inflammation hypothesis, a further systematic review from the same group (Danesh and Peto 1998) found no consistent link between *H. pylori* seropositivity and the same group of inflammatory markers.

Although the link between chronic infection and coronary disease appears weak, the strength of the prospective associations between inflammatory markers and coronary disease suggests that stress mechanisms may

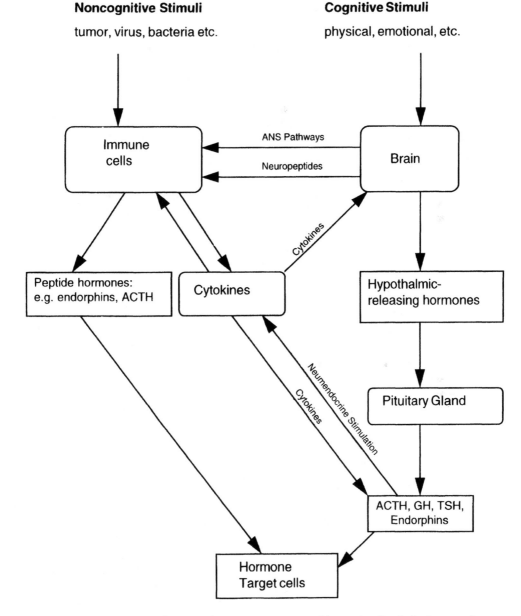

Figure 13–4. Communication between the neural, endocrine, and immune systems. Schematic diagram. The brain perceives cognitive stimuli which can influence immune function via neuropeptides, the autonomic nervous system, and the HPA axis. The immune system responds to noncognitive stimuli (infection and tumor growth) by secreting cytokines (immune messengers) and peptide hormones which act on the brain and neuroendocrine system. The immune system thus has a sensory function. Redrawn from Brown 1994.

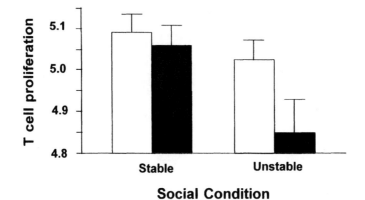

Social Condition

Figure 13–5. Social instability, affiliative behavior, and immune function in macaque monkeys. The high affiliation group (open bars) appears to be protected from the stress of social instability. Evidence for a stress-buffering effect of social affiliations on cell-mediated immune function comes from Cohen's studies of captive macaque monkeys (Cohen 1992). Animals were randomized for 2 years either to stable social groups or to groups which were altered every month. Repeated observations established levels of affilia-tive behavior based on grooming, passive physical contact, or close proximity with others in the group. Against the measure of mitogen-stimulated T-cell proliferation the high-affiliation group appeared to be protected from the stress of social instability. Although such effects are of unknown significance for health, the same research group has shown that social status predicts susceptibility to influenza virus (Cohen 1997). Redrawn from Cohen et al. 1992.

be involved, via effects on inflammation. Consistent with this suggestion, the brain is able to influence immune function. There is autonomic innervation of the relevant tissues (bone marrow, thymus, spleen, and lymph nodes), there are neuroendocrine controls on inflammatory mechanisms, and glucocorticoids have large effects on the immune system (Fig. 13–4). In Whitehall II, employment grade and chronic low control at work were linked to raised fibrinogen (Brunner et al. 1996), suggesting that inflammatory processes may mediate the effect of psychosocial circumstances on disease risk. Animal studies show it is plausible that immune function may be protected by social factors (Fig. 13–5).

One proposed link between both cognitive and noncognitive stimuli (such as infection) and inflammation is the cytokines. The cytokines are a group of inflammatory mediators which may contribute to atherogenesis. Tumor necrosis factor-α has been shown to be a trigger for the production of interleukin-6 (IL-6) by many cell types, and is implicated in the development of obesity-linked insulin resistance. Interleukin-6 appears to be a major regulator of C-reactive protein and fibrinogen synthesis in the liver. Both cytokines have been shown to be raised among heart disease cases (Mendall et al. 1997). The possibility of a psychosocial trigger is suggested by a study of astronauts (Stein and Schluter 1994). Spaceflight evoked raised urinary IL-6 and cortisol on the first day, but not on other days before or after launch, consistent with a psychological explanation, since infection would not appear to be implicated. Mechanistically, cytokine expression due to psychosocial stimuli seems possible, as there is evidence for expression of IL-6 messenger RNA within the brain and for the existence of IL-6 receptors on human adrenal cells.

EVIDENCE FROM THE WHITEHALL STUDIES

In the first Whitehall study there was a threefold excess in coronary death rate in the lowest compared to the highest Civil Service employment grade, and a continuous inverse risk gradient across the grades (Marmot et al. 1978). The three classic risk factors—plasma cholesterol, smoking, and blood pressure—accounted for around only a quarter of the gradient in incident premature heart disease across employment grades (Marmot et al. 1978). This surprising finding is partly explained by problems of measurement. The proportion accounted for would have been considerably larger if repeated rather than single measurements had been made, in view of the biological variability of blood pressure and the difficulty in determining accurate smoking histories. Despite this caveat, the conventional risk factor model was seen to be inadequate: quantitatively because it could not explain variations in risk well enough, and qualitatively because it did not tackle the upstream structural and psychological aspects of health differences.

The Whitehall II Study

In response to the limitations of the original Whitehall study, a younger cohort of Civil Servants is now being followed. Repeated measurements are being made of a much expanded set of biological markers, dietary habits, and psychosocial variables. The Whitehall II study of 10,308 male and female civil servants working in London began in 1985–1988 (Marmot et al. 1991). The questionnaire and medical examination were repeated, in modified form, at the second follow-up in 1991–1993, and results from these two phases are presented below. Anthropometric and biochemical data were collected at both phases of the study. Self-report questionnaires provide data on social, economic, psychological, and behavioral factors.

The British Civil Service provides a valuable population for studying the determinants of health. Within one set of institutions, where broad similarities in the environment might be expected to minimize differences in health, quite the reverse is found to be true. Salary levels in 1992 reveal marked differentials in income across employment grades (Brunner 1996) (clerical staff salary range £6483–£11,917, roughly $11,000–$20,000 professional and executive staff £8517–£25,554, roughly $14,000–$43,000 senior administrative staff £25,330–£87,620, roughly $43,000–$150,000). The grade classification identifies a clear hierarchy in the material circumstances of the men and women in the Civil Service. More than 97% of those in the higher administrative grades owned their own homes in 1987 compared with some 60% in clerical and office support jobs. Similarly, a car was available to some 90% of senior staff but to 60% in the lowest employment grade. Notably, all study participants were employed at the time of the baseline survey, and none was in absolute poverty.

Social Inequality, Central Obesity, and the Metabolic Syndrome

In order to test the hypothesis that the metabolic syndrome contributes to the explanation of social inequalities in coronary risk, the second medical examination of the Whitehall II cohort included a 2-hour 75 g oral glucose tolerance test and measurements of waist and hip circumferences (Brunner et al. 1997a). Prevalence of the metabolic syndrome was defined on the basis of a clustering of risk factors according to their sex-specific distributions. Individuals were considered to have the metabolic syndrome when three or more of the following were in the adverse quintile: 2-hour glucose, systolic blood pressure, fasting triglycerides, high-density lipoprotein (HDL) cholesterol, and waist–hip ratio. Subjects taking hypotensive medication were assigned to the highest blood pressure quintile and known diabetics to the highest 2-hour glucose quintile. Clustering of unfavorable levels of these variables was demonstrated with multivariate statistical analysis (grade of membership models and principal components analysis). In both sexes, these methods identified two risk factor subclusters: glucose/insulin/blood pressure and triglycerides/HDL cholesterol/waist–hip ratio.

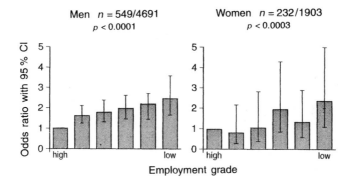

Figure 13–6. Prevalence of the metabolic syndrome by employment grade in the Whitehall II study. Odds ratios and 95% confidence interval adjusted for age and, in women, menopausal status. *P* values are for trend test across grades. See text for definition of metabolic syndrome. Source: Brunner et al. 1997a.

The metabolic syndrome pattern was strongly associated with lower grade (Fig. 13–6) in both men (odds ratio = 2.2) and women (odds ratio = 2.8). For comparison, 10-year coronary mortality in the first Whitehall study in the clerical grade was 2.3-fold greater than that among administrators (Marmot et al. 1984). In the absence of marked differentials in serum total cholesterol or blood pressure, the findings suggest a biological explanation for the social gradient in risk of coronary disease in this group of European ethnicity (Davey Smith et al. 1996). This proposition awaits incident disease analysis. Our use of sex-specific quintiles for the component variables constrains women to have approximately the same prevalence of "abnormality" as men. If, in fact, the syndrome is less prevalent in women (Larsson et al. 1992) our definition may misclassify more women than men. It may be for this reason that the association between metabolic syndrome and employment grade is less linear among women than men. It may also be that the influence of social position on coronary risk is mediated by different factors among women and men (Bullers 1994).

The inverse occupational gradient in the metabolic syndrome was little altered by taking account of current reported health behaviors (Table 13–2). Degree of obesity was highly associated with prevalence of the metabolic syndrome, but smoking status and physical activity level were weakly or not at all associated. Among women, low/moderate alcohol consumers (1–14 units/week) had a lower probability of exhibiting the syndrome than nondrinkers. Logistic regression analysis was performed with the metabolic syndrome as the dependent variable and employment grade as the predictor variable. Adjustment for the behavioral factors had little effect on the grade gradient, reducing it by 11% in men and 9% in women. Adjustment for body-mass index as well as behavioral factors produced attenuations of a further 22% in men and 1% in women.

The weakness of the behavioral explanation is consistent with psychosocial effects. One possibility is that this cluster of risk factors may in part be the product of altered neuroendocrine activity, of the HPA axis in particular, in response to long-term exposure to adverse psychosocial circumstances (Bjorntorp 1991; McEwen 1998) associated with low social status. For example, financial problems and hostility, as assessed by the Cook-Medley/MMPI questionnaire, were found to be associated with central obesity (a component of the metabolic syndrome) in each of the four race/sex groups in the Coronary Artery Risk Development in Young Adults (CARDIA) study of young adults (Kaye et al. 1993).

Table 13–2. Odds ratios for metabolic syndrome according to body mass index and health related behaviours*

Variable	Men	P value	Women	P value
Body-Mass Index (kg/m^2)				
<24.9	1	<0.0001	1	<0.0001
25–29.9	4.95		5.70	
≥30	15.8		18.9	
Smoking Status				
Never smoker	1	<0.05	1	NS
Ex-smoker	1.27		1.14	
Current smoker	1.35		1.13	
Alcohol Intake				
None	1		1	
Low/moderate	0.81	NS	0.61	<0.005
High	1.00	NS	0.64	NS
Physical Activity				
None–Mild	1	<0.005	1	NS
Moderate	0.88		0.97	
Vigorous	0.65		0.64	

Source: Brunner et al. 1997a.

*Adjusted for age, and menopausal status in women.

Chi-square tests for trend, except for alcohol, for which heterogeneity test was utilized.

Lifecourse Behavioral and Psychosocial Determinants of Fibrinogen

The soluble protein fibrinogen is the precursor of fibrin, the structural component of blood clots. Fibrinogen is raised in inflammatory states and circulating levels predict future coronary disease and stroke. It may thus be a biological mediator contributing, along with the metabolic syndrome, to the high rates of coronary disease experienced by people in unfavorable socioeconomic circumstances (Markowe et al. 1985). As is the case with coronary risk, smoking accounts for some but not all of the social gradient in fibrinogen (Brunner et al. 1993). Adverse factors in early life, manifested as poor growth in infancy, have also been linked to a high adult fibrinogen level (Barker et al. 1992), and it may be that fibrinogen is a mediating factor between experiences early in the lifecourse and later coronary disease.

Associations between plasma fibrinogen and factors operating throughout the lifecourse, including the psychosocial characteristics of work, were analyzed cross-sectionally among 2095 men and 1202 women aged 45–55 years who provided blood samples at the Whitehall II study baseline (Brunner et al. 1996). Lower socioeconomic status, indexed by employment grade, was associated with higher fibrinogen with marked and linear differences from top to bottom grade of 0.22 g/l in men and 0.37 g/l in women (Fig. 13–7). Measures of childhood environment—adult height, father's social class and level of education—were inversely associated with adult plasma fibrinogen level in both sexes (Table 13–3).

Low control over work was inversely related to fibrinogen in both sexes when assessed by personnel managers (Table 13–3). A similar association between fibrinogen and self-rated control (Karasek et al. 1981) was seen among men but not women. Men in the top tertile of both self-rated and ex-

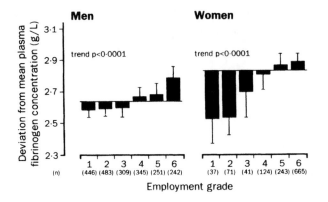

Figure 13–7. Plasma fibrinogen by employment grade in the Whitehall II study. Data given as deviations in fibrinogen from the overall mean for men or women (2.64, 2.84 g/l) with 95% CI. Means are adjusted for age and ethnic origin, and menopausal status in women. Employment grade is stratified into 6 levels (1 = highest, 6 = lowest). Source: Brunner et al. *Lancet* 1996. Reproduced with permission.

ternally assessed control over work had lower fibrinogen levels than those in the bottom tertile of both measures (−0.16, 95% CI −0.07, −0.26) g/l, P < 0.001). There was no difference across these extremes among women (−0.02, 95% CI −0.19, 0.16 g/l, NS). These paradoxical findings may be due to gender differences in perception and reporting of the psychosocial environment, which require further investigation.

Employment grade differences in fibrinogen concentration must reflect employment grade differentials in determinants of fibrinogen. Smoking and alcohol consumption are clearly important, as may be psychosocial factors. Here, externally assessed low control was related to higher fibrinogen to a similar extent in men and women. The inverse job strain–fibrinogen relationships are much attenuated by adjustment for employment grade, reflecting the strong association between low employment grade and low control over work. This finding is analogous to that obtained in the Chicago Western Electric study (Alterman et al. 1994). The adjusted relative risk of coronary disease mortality among subjects with high job strain was 1.40, falling to 1.03 on adjustment for occupational class. Ideally, it would be desirable to show an "independent" relationship between job strain and

fibrinogen in order to exclude the possibility of confounding. If, however, job strain is in itself a determinant, or mediator, of the employment grade differentials in fibrinogen, such statistical adjustments are inappropriate. Thus, after adjustment for alternative socioeconomic measures (Table 13–3) the job control–fibrinogen association persisted to a greater extent than when adjustment was based on occupational status.

The explanatory power of low job control for the employment grade differential in 5-year self-reported heart disease incidence is, in fact, substantial. Compared with social support, height, and standard coronary risk factors, low control made the largest contribution to the socioeconomic gradient (Marmot et al. 1997). In view of the observed associations between low control and fibrinogen, a mediating role for haemostatic and inflammatory processes seems plausible.

Dietary Habits Are Socially Patterned

Patterns of food consumption are the product of a combination of economic, cultural, and personal factors. Developed countries have adopted a high-fat-food culture which appears to be resistant to change. Major social differences in nutrient intake, and thus diet-related diseases, among British adults

Table 13–3. Percent difference in fibrinogen concentration associated with unit differences in measures of childhood circumstances, socioeconomic position, height, and work characteristics, with various adjustments for related variables: Whitehall II study

Adjustments	% difference in fibrinogen concentration associated with unit difference in:						
	Employment grade (6 grades)	Education (3 categories)	Father's social class (manual/non-manual)	Housing status (tenant/owner)	Height*	Self-rated control at work*	Externally assessed control at work*
Men (n = 1570)							
Age, ethnic origin only (A/E)	−1.6% (p<0.0001)	−1.4% (p<0.05)	−2.8% (p<0.05)	−9.3% (p<0.0001)	−1.5% (p<0.005)	−1.6% (P<0.005)	−1.7% (P<0.005)
A/E plus employment grade	—	−0.2%	−2.0% (p<0.05)	−6.7% (p<0.005)	−1.2% (p<0.05)	−0.7%	−0.6%
A/E plus SES†	1.2% (p<0.005)	—	—	—	−1.2% (p<0.05)	−1.0% (P<0.05)	−1.0%
A/E plus BMI, health behaviors, and symptoms‡	−0.8% (p<0.005)	−0.5%	−1.8%	−6.0% (p<0.005)	−0.9%	−0.9%	−1.0%
Women (n = 791)							
Age, ethnic origin, menopause (A/E/M)	−1.9% (p<0.005)	−2.9% (p<0.05)	−2.9% (p<0.05)	−3.9% (p<0.05)	−1.1%	0.8%	−2.0% (P<0.05)
A/E/M plus employment grade	—	−1.7%	−1.3%	−2.7%	−0.7%	2.1% (p<0.005)	−1.1%
A/E/M plus SES†	−1.2%	—	—	—	−0.9%	1.5% (p<0.05)	−1.2%
A/E/M plus BMI, health behaviors, and symptoms‡	0.8%	−1.5%	−0.5%	−2.3%	−0.4%	1.4% (p<0.05)	−1.1%

Source: Brunner et al. 1996.

A 1% difference in fibrinogen corresponds to 0.025 g/L.

*Standardized measurements, scaled to mean = 0, standard deviation = 1.

†SES = alternative measures of socioeconomic status: access to car, housing status, years of education, father's social class.

‡Health behaviors = cigarettes (n/day), alcohol (units/week), vigorous exercise (h/week). BMI = body-mass index.

are seen in minerals (iron, magnesium, potassium and calcium), vitamins (retinol, B vitamins including folate, and ascorbic acid) and other antioxidants, while mean total and saturated fat intake shows relatively little systematic social variation (Gregory et al. 1990; Stallone et al. 1997). These data on the social patterning of nutrition—similar fat intakes, but large differentials in micronutrient density—point to systematic social differences in food sources as an important issue for public health.

Income is a determinant of dietary intake that is usually studied in the context of developing nations. It is evident, however, that polarization of income levels has taken place in developed countries to the extent that food poverty may be a major problem. Childhood poverty, defined as residence in a household with an income on or below state income support level, was experienced by 29% of children in the United Kingdom in 1992 (Harker 1996). The consequences of low family income may be transmitted across the lifecourse because dietary patterns are initially acquired in childhood and may be resistant to later change. The sustained influence of childhood dietary pattern into adulthood has been shown among men in Kuopio, Finland (Lynch et al. 1997). In this group, poor childhood socioeconomic circumstances were associated with lower consumption of fruit and vegetables and with lower vitamin C intakes as adults. A survey of British children conducted in the immediate pre–Second World War period showed that adverse conditions, marked by overcrowding and low per capita food expenditure, were linked with reduced growth in general and shorter leg length in particular (Davey Smith and Brunner 1997). Mortality follow-up (Gunnell et al. 1998) shows that long-term health effects of poor nutrition in childhood are evident in higher rates of adult coronary disease. However, in line with evidence from animal studies and some epidemiological findings, males (but not females) who had more favorable nutrition and longer leg length as children appeared to have a higher cancer risk. These findings emphasize the need for lifecourse studies to understand the lifetime health effects of nutrition and related factors.

The psychosocial determinants of dietary patterns in adulthood are being investigated in the Whitehall II study. Such effects are

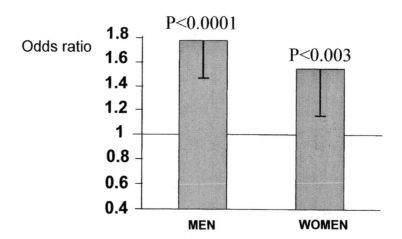

Figure 13–8. Health control beliefs and diet. Odds ratios for men and women, adjusted for age and employment grade, for the likelihood of meeting a healthy eating criterion (fresh fruit/ vegetables daily or more and usually eat wholemeal/brown bread and drink reduced fat milk) according to perceived level of control over heart attack risk. Whitehall II study 1991–1993.

important because healthy adults appear to be quite resistant to health-oriented dietary advice (Brunner et al. 1997b). We analyzed the relation between health locus of control and health-related dietary pattern (Brunner 1997). The diet variable was constructed using self-report food type and frequency data. Subjects indicated their sense of fatalism in relation to heart attack risk on a three-point scale. The composite diet variable was constructed to summarize reported dietary pattern with reference to positive healthy eating messages: reported consumption of reduced fat milk, fresh fruit and vegetables, and higher-fiber breads. If all of these three criteria were met, the subject was defined as a healthy eater or vice versa. Logistic regression analysis shows that the likelihood of being a healthy eater, as defined, is related to perception of control over heart attack risk independently of employment grade (Fig. 13–8). These results illustrate the indirect pathway by which psychosocial factors may be linked to health outcomes via behavioral factors.

CONCLUSION

Shigechiyo Izumi, born in 1865 on the Japanese island of Tokunoshima, was at age 118 credited as the oldest person alive. He gave his secret of long life as "not worrying" (Morris 1983). While this cohort study of a single individual tells us nothing about the population determinants of longevity, it suggests that life span is as much as 40 years longer than the current average life expectancy. It also points to the widespread belief that coping and adaptation are key determinants of a long and happy life, though it is evident that human physiology has a finite capacity to deal with the slings and arrows of misfortune (Seeman et al. 1997). This chapter has attempted to show that progress is being made toward understanding social influences on accumulation of disease risk by means of a variety of biologically oriented approaches. Though the science has a long way to go, there is considerable evidence that the social environment is as important to human biology today as it was in the days of Queen Victoria and President Lincoln.

REFERENCES

Algra, A., Tijssen, J.G.P., Roelandt, J.R.T.C., Pool, J., and Lubsen, J. (1993) Heart rate variability from 24-hour electrocardiography and the 2-year risk for sudden death. *Circulation*, 88:180–5.

Alterman, T., Shekelle, R.B., Vernon, S.W., and Burau, K.D. (1994) Decision latitude, psychologic demand, job strain, and coronary heart disease in the Western Electric study. *Am J Epidemiol*, 139:620–7.

Anderson, T.J., Uehata, A., Gerhard, M.D., Meredith, I.T., Knab, S., Delagrange, D., Lieberman, E.H., Ganz, P., Creager, M.A., Yeung, A.C., and Selwyn, A.P. (1995). Close relation of endothelial function in the human coronary and peripheral circulations. *J Am Col Cardio*, 26:1235–41.

Barefoot, J.C., Larsen, S., von der Lieth, L., and Schroll, M. (1995). Hostility, incidence of acute myocardial infarction and mortality in a sample of older Danish men and women. *Am J Epidemiol*, 142:477–84.

Barker, D.J.P. (1992). *Fetal and infant origins of adult disease*. London: British Medical Journal.

Barker, D.J.P., Meade, T.W., Fall, C.H.D., Lee, A., Osmond, C., Phipps, K., and Stirling, Y. (1992). Relation of fetal and infant growth to plasma fibrinogen and factor VII concentrations in adult life. *BMJ*, 304:148–52.

Barker, D.J.P., Hales, C.N., Fall, C.H.D., Osmond, C., Phipps, K., and Clark, P.M.S. (1993). Type 2 (non-insulin-dependent) diabetes mellitus, hypertension and hyperlipidaemia (syndrome X): relation to reduced fetal growth. *Diabetologia*, 36:62–7.

Bartley, M. (1994). Unemployment and ill health: understanding the relationship. *J Epidemiol Community Health*, 48:333–7.

Baum, A., and Grunberg, N. (1995). Measurement of stress hormones. In Cohen, S., Kessler, R.C., and Gordon, L.U. (eds.), *Measuring stress: a guide for health and social scientists*. New York: Oxford University Press, pp. 175–92.

Berkman, L.F. and Syme, S.L. (1979). Social networks, host resistance and mortality: a nine-year follow-up of Alameda County residents. *Am J Epidemiol*, 109:186–204.

Bigger, J.T., Fleiss, J.L., Steinman, R.C., Rolnitzky, L.M., Kleiger, R.E., and Rottman, J.N. (1992). Frequency domain measures of heart period variability and mortality after my-ocardial infarction. *Circulation*, 85:164–71.

Bjorntorp, P. (1991). Visceral fat accumulation: the missing link between psychosocial factors and cardiovascular disease? *J Int Med*, 230:195–201.

Blane, D., Brunner, E.J., and Wilkinson, R.G. (1996). *Health and social organization: towards a health policy for the 21st century*. London: Routledge.

Bosma, H., Marmot, M.G., Hemingway, H., Nicholson, A., Brunner, E.J., and Stansfeld, S. (1997). Low job control and risk of coronary heart disease in the Whitehall II (prospective cohort) study. *BMJ*, 314:558–65.

Brown, G.W. (1986). Social support, self esteem and depression. *Psychol Med*, 16:813–31.

Brown, R.E. (1994). *An introduction to neuroendocrinology*. Cambridge, UK: Cambridge University Press.

Brunner, E.J. (1996). The social and biological basis of cardiovascular disease in office workers. In Blane, D., Brunner, E., and Wilkinson, R. (eds.), *Health and social organization: towards a health policy for the 21st century*. London: Routledge, pp. 272–313.

Brunner, E.J. (1997). Inequalities in diet and health. In Shetty, P., and McPherson, K. (eds.), *Diet, nutrition and chronic disease: lessons from contrasting worlds*. Chichester, UK: Wiley, pp. 77–97.

Brunner, E.J., Davey Smith, G., Marmot, M.G., Canner, R., Beksinska, M., and O'Brien, J. (1996). Childhood social circumstances and psychosocial and behavioural factors as determinants of plasma fibrinogen. *Lancet*, 347:1008–13.

Brunner, E.J., Juneja, M., and Marmot, M.G. (1998). Abdominal obesity and disease are linked to social position (letter). *BMJ*, 316:508–9.

Brunner, E.J., Marmot, M.G., Nanchahal, K., Shipley, M.J., Stansfeld, S.A., Juneja, M., and Alberti, K.G.M.M. (1997a). Social inequality in coronary risk: central obesity and the metabolic syndrome. Evidence from the Whitehall II study. *Diabetologia*, 40:1341–9.

Brunner, E.J., Marmot, M.G., White, I.R., O'Brien, J.R., Etherington, M.D., Slavin, B.M., Kearney, E.M., and Davey Smith, G. (1993). Gender and employment grade differences in blood cholesterol, apolipoproteins and haemostatic factors in the Whitehall II study. *Atherosclerosis*, 102:195–207.

Brunner, E.J., White, I.R., Thorogood, M., Bristow, A., Curle, D., and Marmot, M.G. (1997b). Can dietary interventions change diet and cardiovascular risk factors? A meta-analysis of randomized controlled trials. *Am J Public Health*, 87:1415–22.

Bullers, S. (1994). Women's roles and health: the mediating effect of perceived control. *Women Health*, 22:11–30.

Carroll, D., Davey Smith, G., Marmot, M.G., Canner, R., Beksinska, M., and O'Brien, J. (1997). The relationship between socio-economic status, hostility, and blood pressure reactions to mental stress in men: data from the Whitehall II study. *Health Psychol*, 16:131–6.

Checkley, S. (1996). The neuroendocrinology of depression and chronic stress. *Br Med Bull*, 52:597–617.

Cohen, S., and Herbert, T.B. (1996). Health psychology: psychological factors and physical disease from the perspective of human psychoneuroimmunology. *Annu Rev Psychol*, 47:113–42.

Cohen, S., Kaplan, J.R., Cunnick, J.E., Manuck, S.B., and Rabin, B.S. (1992). Chronic social stress, affiliation, and cellular immune response in nonhuman primates. *Psychol Sci*, 3:301–4.

Cohen, S., Doyle, W.J., Skoner, D.P., Rabin, B.S., and Gwaltney, J.M. (1997). Social ties and susceptibility to the common cold. *JAMA*, 277:1940–4.

Danesh, J., and Appleby, P. (1998). Persistent infection and vascular disease: a systematic review. *Exp Opin Invest Drugs*, 7:691–713.

Danesh, J., and Peto, R. (1998). Risk factors for coronary heart disease and infection with *Helicobacter pylori*: meta-analysis of 18 studies. *BMJ*, 316:1130–2.

Danesh, J., Collins, R., Appleby, P., and Peto, R. (1998). Association of fibrinogen, c-reactive protein, albumin, or leukocyte count with coronary heart disease. *JAMA*, 279:1477–81.

Davey Smith, G. (1997). Socioeconomic differentials. In Kuh, D., and Ben-Shlomo, Y. (eds.), *A life course approach to chronic disease epidemiology*. Oxford: Oxford University Press, pp. 242–73.

Davey Smith, G., and Brunner, E.J. (1997). Socioeconomic differentials in health: the role of nutrition. *Proc Nutr Soc*, 56:75–90.

Davey Smith, G., Neaton, J.D., Wentworth, D., Stamler, R., and Stamler, J. (1996). Socioeconomic differentials in mortality risk among men screened for the Multiple Risk Factor Intervention Trial: I. White men. *Am J Public Health*, 86:486–96.

Delitala, G., Palermo, M., Tomasi, P., Besser, M., and Grossman, A. (1991). Adrenergic stimulation of the human pituitary-adrenal axis is attenuated by an analog of met-enkephalin. *Neuroendocrinology*, 53:41–6.

Dembroski, T.M., MacDougall, J.M., and Costa, P.T. Jr. (1989). Components of hostility as predictors of sudden death and myocardial infarction in the Multiple Risk Factor Intervention Trial. *Psychosom Med* 51:514–22.

Drever, F., and Whitehead, M. (1997). *Health inequalities.* (Decennial Supplement Series DS No.15, 1–257.) London: Her Majesty's Stationery Office, Office for National Statistics.

Eaker, E.D., Pinsky, J., and Castelli, W.P. (1992). Myocardial infarction and coronary death among women: psychosocial predictors from a 20 year follow-up of women in the Framingham study. *Am J Epidemiol,* 135:854–64.

Engels, F. (1848). *The condition of the working class in England* (tr. Henderson, O.W., and Chaloner, W.H., 1958). New York: Macmillan.

Ferrie, J.E., Shipley, M.J., Marmot, M.G., Stansfeld, S., and Davey Smith, G. (1995). Health effects of anticipation of job change and nonemployment: longitudinal data from the Whitehall II study. *BMJ,* 311:1264–9.

Fonagy, P. (1996). Patterns of attachment, interpersonal relationships and health. In Blane, D., Brunner, E.J., and Wilkinson, R.G. (eds.), *Social organization and health: towards a health policy for the 21st century.* London: Routledge, pp. 125–51.

Friedman, M., Rosenman, R.H., and Carrol, V. (1958). Changes in the serum cholesterol and blood clotting time in men subjected to cyclic variation of occupational stress. *Circulation,* 17:852–61.

Gallie, D., and Vogler, C. (1994). Labour market deprivation, welfare, and collectivism. In Gallie, D., Marsh, C., and Vogler, C. (eds.), *Social change and the experience of unemployment.* Oxford: Oxford University Press, pp. 299–317.

Gregory, J., Foster, K., Tyler, H., and Wiseman, M. (1990). *The Diet and Nutrition Survey of British adults.* London: Her Majesty's Stationery Office.

Grossman, A.B. (1991). Regulation of human pituitary responses to stress. In Brown, M.B., Koob, G.F., and Rivier, C. (eds.), *Stress: neurobiology and neuroendocrinology.* New York: Marcel Dekker, pp. 151–71.

Gunnell, D.J., Davey Smith, G., Frankel, S., et al. (1998). Childhood leg length and adult mortality: follow up of the Carnegie (Boyd Orr) survey of diet and health in pre-war Britain. *J Epidemiol Community Health,* 52:142–52.

Harker, L. (1996). *Key poverty statistics.* London: Child Poverty Action Group.

Hautanen, A., and Adlercreutz, H. (1993). Altered adrenocorticotropin and cortisol secretion in abdominal obesity: implications for the insulin resistance syndrome. *J Int Med,* 234:461–9.

Hearn, M., Murray, D.M., and Luepker, R.B. (1989). Hostility, coronary heart disease and total mortality: a 33 year follow up study of university students. *J Behav Med,* 12: 105–21.

Hellhammer, D.H., Buchtal, J., Gutberlet, I., and Kirschbaum, C. (1997). Social hierarchy and adrenocortical stress reactivity in men. *Psychoneuroendocrinology,* 22:643–50.

Hemingway, H., and Marmot, M. (1999). Psychosocial factors in the aetiology and prognosis of coronary heart disease: a systematic review of prospective cohort studies. *BMJ,* 318:1460–7.

Karasek, R., Baker, D., Marxer, F., Ahlbom, A., and Theorell, T. (1981). Job decision latitude, job demands and cardiovascular disease: a prospective study of Swedish men. *Am J Public Health,* 71:694–705.

Kawachi, I., Sparrow, D., Vokonas, P.S., and Weiss, S.T. (1995). Decreased heart rate variability in men with phobic anxiety (data from the normative aging study). *Am J Cardiol,* 75:882–5.

Kawachi, I., Sparrow, D., Spiro, A., Vokonas, P.S., and Weiss, S.T. (1996). A prospective study of anger and coronary heart disease. *Circulation,* 94:2092–5.

Kaye, S.A., Folsom, A.R., Jacobs, D.R., Hughes, G.H., and Flack, J.M. (1993). Psychosocial correlates of body fat distribution in black and white young adults. *Int J Obes,* 17: 271–7.

Kirschbaum, C., and Hellhammer, D. (1994). Salivary cortisol in psychoneuroendocrine research: recent developments and applications. *Psychoneuroendocrinology,* 19:313–33.

Kirschbaum, C., Prussner, J.C., Stone, A.A., Federenko, I., Gaab, J., Lintz, D., Schommer, N., and Hellhammer, D.H. (1995). Persistent high cortisol responses to repeated psychological stress in a subpopulation of healthy men. *Psychosom Med,* 57:468–74.

Krieger, N., Williams, D.R., and Moss, N.E. (1997). Measuring social class in U.S. public health research: concepts, methodologies and guidelines. *Annu Rev Public Health,* 18:341–78.

Kristenson, M., Kucinskiene, Z., Bergdahl, B., and Orth-Gomer, K. (1998). Risk factors for ischaemic heart disease in different socioeconomic groups of Lithuania and Sweden: the Livicordia study. Linköping, Sweden: Linköping University Medical Dissertations no. 547.

Kuh, D., and Ben-Shlomo, Y. (1997). *A life course approach to chronic disease epidemiology.* Oxford: Oxford University Press.

Larsson, B., Bengtsson, C., Bjorntorp, P., Lapidus, L., Sjostrom, L., Svardsudd, K., Tibblin, G., Wedel, H., Welin, L., and Wilhelmsen, L. (1992). Is abdominal body fat distribution a major explanation for the sex difference in the incidence of myocardial infarction? *Am J Epidemiol*, 135:266–73.

Lynch, J.W., Kaplan, G.A., and Salonen, J.T. (1997). Why do poor people behave badly? Variation in adult health behaviours and psychosocial characteristics by stages of the socioeconomic lifecourse. *Soc Sci Med*, 44:809–19.

Markowe, H.L.J., Marmot, M.G., Shipley, M.J., Bulpitt, C.J., Meade, T.W., Stirling, Y., Vickers, M.V., and Semmence, A. (1985). Fibrinogena: possible link between social class and coronary heart disease. *BMJ*, 291:1312–4.

Marmot, M.G. (1996). The social pattern of health and disease. In Blane, D., Brunner, E., and Wilkinson, R. (eds.), *Health and social organisation: towards a health policy for the 21st century*. London: Routledge, pp. 42–67.

Marmot, M.G., and Syme, S.L. (1976). Acculturation and coronary heart disease in Japanese Americans. *Am J Epidemiol*, 104:225–47.

Marmot, M.G., Rose, G., Shipley, M., and Hamilton, P.J.S. (1978). Employment grade and coronary heart disease in British civil servants. *J Epidemiol Community Health*, 32:244–9.

Marmot, M.G., Shipley, M.J., and Rose, G. (1984). Inequalities in death: specific explanations of a general pattern. *Lancet*, 1:1003–6.

Marmot, M.G., Davey Smith, G., Stansfeld, S.A., Patel, C., North, F., Head, J., White, I., Brunner, E.J., and Feeney, A. (1991). Health inequalities among British Civil Servants: the Whitehall II study. *Lancet*, 337:1387–93.

Marmot, M., Bosma, H., Hemingway, H., Brunner, E.J., and Stansfeld, S.A. (1997). Contribution of job control and other risk factors to social variations in coronary heart disease incidence. *Lancet*, 350:235–9.

Masters, C.L., and Beyreuther, K. (1998). Science, medicine and the future: Alzheimer's disease. *BMJ*, 316:446–8.

McCarty, R., and Gold, P.E. (1996). Catecholamines, stress, and disease: a psychobiological perspective. *Psychosom Med* 58:590–7.

McEwen, B.S. (1998). Protective and damaging effects of stress mediators. *N Engl J Med*, 338:171–9.

McKeown, T. (1979). *The role of medicine: dream, mirage or nemesis?* Oxford: Basil Blackwell.

Mendall, M.A., Goggin, P.M., Molineaux, N., Levy, J., Toosy, T., Strachan, D., Camm, A.J., and Northfield, T.C. (1994). Relation of *Helicobacter pylori* infection and coronary heart disease. *Br Heart J*, 71:437–9.

Mendall, M.A., Patel, P., Asante, M., Ballam, L.,

Morris, J., Strachan, D.P., Camm, A.J., and Northfield, T.C. (1997). Relation of serum cytokine concentrations to cardiovascular risk factors and coronary heart disease. *Heart*, 78:273–7.

Molijn, G., Spek, J.J., and van Uffelen, J.C. (1995). Differential adaptation of glucocorticoid sensitivity of peripheral blood mononuclear leukocytes in patients with sepsis or septic shock. *J Clin Endocrinol Metab*, 80:1799–803.

Montgomery, S., Bartley, M., and Wilkinson, R.G. (1997). Family conflict and slow growth. *Arch Dis Child*, 77:326–30.

Morris, D. (1983). *The book of ages*. London: Jonathan Cape.

Muldoon, M.F., Herbert, T.B., Patterson, S.M., Kameneva, M., Raible, R., and Manuck, S.B. (1995). Effects of acute psychological stress on serum lipid levels, hemoconcentration, and blood viscosity. *Arch Intern Med*, 155:615–20.

Nystrom Peck, M., and Lundberg, O. (1995). Short stature as an effect of economic and social conditions in childhood. *Soc Sci Med*, 41:733–8.

Ockenfels, M.C., Porter, L., Smyth, J., Kirschbaum, C., Hellhammer, D.H., and Stone, A.A. (1995). Effect of chronic stress associated with unemployment on salivary cortisol: overall cortisol levels, diurnal rhythm and acute stress reactivity. *Psychosom Med*, 57:460–7.

Phillips, D.I.W., Barker, J.P., Fall, C.H.D., Seckl, J.R., Whorwood, C.B., Wood, P.J., and Walker, B.R. (1998). Elevated plasma cortisol concentrations: a link between low birth weight and insulin resistance syndrome? *J Clin Endocrinol Metab*, 83:757–60.

Power, C., and Hertzman, C. (1997). Social and biological pathways linking early life and adult disease. *Br Med Bull*, 53:210–21.

Power, C., Matthews, S., and Manor, O. (1998). Inequalities in self-rated health: explanations from different stages of life. *Lancet*, 351:1009–14.

Reaven, G.M. (1993). Role of insulin resistance in human disease (syndrome X): an expanded definition. *Annu Rev Med*, 44:121–31.

Rona, R.J. (1981). Genetic and environmental factors in the control of growth in childhood. *Br Med Bull*, 37:265–72.

Rose, S.P.R. (1995). Cell-adhesion molecules, glucocorticoids and long-term-memory formation. *Trends Neurosci*, 18:502–6.

Rosengren, A., Orth-Gomer, K., Wedel, H., and Wilhelmsen, L. (1993). Stressful life events, social support, and mortality in men born in 1933. *BMJ*, 307:1102–5.

Ruberman, W., Weinblatt, E., Goldberg, J.D.,

and Chaudhary, B.S. (1984). Psychosocial influences on mortality after myocardial infarction. *N Engl J Med*, 311:552–9.

Sapolsky, R.M. (1993). Endocrinology alfresco: psychoendocrine studies of wild baboons. *Recent Prog Horm Res*, 48:437–68.

Sapolsky, R.M., Krey, L.C., and McEwen, B.S. (1986). The neuroendocrinology of stress and aging: the glucocorticoid cascade hypothesis. *Endocr Rev*, 7:284–301.

Seeman, T.E., Singer, B., and Charpentier, P. (1995). Gender differences in patterns of HPA axis response to challenge: MacArthur Studies of Successful Aging. *Psychoneuroendocrinology*, 20:711–25.

Seeman, T.E., Singer, B.H., Rowe, J.W., Horwitz, R.I., and McEwen, B.S. (1997). Price of adaptation: allostatic load and its health consequences. *Arch Intern Med*, 157:2259–68.

Selye, H. (1956). *The Stress of life.* New York: McGraw-Hill.

Shekelle, R.B., Gale, M., Ostfeld, A.M., and Paul, O. (1983). Hostility, risk of coronary heart disease and mortality. *Psychosom Med*, 45:109–14.

Sorensen, K.E., Celermajer, D.S., Spiegelhalter, D.J., Georgakopoulos, D., Robinson, J., Thomas, O., and Deanfield, J.E. (1995). Non-invasive measurement of human endothelium dependent arterial responses accuracy and reproducibility. *Br Heart J*, 74: 247–53.

Stallone, D.D., Brunner, E.J., Bingham, S.A., and Marmot, M.G. (1997). Dietary assessment in Whitehall II. The influence of reporting bias on apparent socioeconomic variation in nutrient intakes. *Eur J Clin Nutr*, 51:815–25.

Stansfeld, S.A., Davey Smith, G., and Marmot, M.G. (1993). Association between physical and psychological morbidity in the Whitehall II Study. *J Psychosom Res*, 37:227–38.

Stansfeld, S.A., Fuhrer, R., Head, J., Ferrie, J., and Shipley, M. (1997). Work and psychiatric disorder in the Whitehall II study. *J Psychosom Res*, 43:73–81.

Stansfeld, S.A., Head, J., and Marmot, M.G. (1998). Explaining social class differences in depression and well-being. *Soc Psychiatry Psychiatr Epidemiol*, 33:1–9.

Stein, T.P., and Schluter, M.D. (1994). Excretion of IL-6 by astronauts during spaceflight. *Am J Physiol*, 266:E448–E552.

Steptoe, A. (1998). Psychophysiological bases of disease. In Johnston, D.W., and Johnston, M. (eds.), *Comprehensive clinical psychology*, vol. 8: *Health psychology.* New York: Pergamon, pp. 39–78.

Suomi, S.J. (1997). Early determinants of behaviour: evidence from primate studies. *Br Med Bull*, 53:170–84.

Ullah, P. (1990). The association between income, financial strain and psychological well-being among unemployed youths. *J Occup Psychol*, 63:317–30.

United Nations Development Programme (UNDP). (1994). *Human Development Report 1994.* New York: Oxford University Press.

Vallance, P., Collier, J., and Bhagat, K. (1997). Infection, inflammation, and infarction: does acute endothelial dysfunction provide a link? *Lancet*, 349:1391–2.

Van Eck, M., Berkhof, H., Nicolson, N., and Sulon, J. (1996). The effects of perceived stress, traits, mood states and stressful daily events on salivary cortisol. *Psychosom Med*, 58: 447–58.

Walker, B.R., Best, R., Shackleton, C.H.L., Padfield, P.L., and Edwards, C.R.W. (1996a). Increased vasoconstrictor sensitivity to glucocorticoids in essential hypertension. *Hypertension*, 27:190–6.

Walker, B.R., Seckl, J.R., and Phillips, D.I.W. (1996b). Increased dermal glucocorticoid sensitivity is associated with insulin resistance and related cardiovascular risk factors (abstract). *J Hypertens*, 14:142.

White, I.R., Brunner, E.J., and Barron, J.L. (1995). A comparison of overnight and 24 hour collection to measure urinary catecholamines. *J Clin Epidemiol*, 48:263–7.

Whitty, C.J.M., Brunner, E.J., Shipley, M.J., Hemingway, H., and Marmot, M.G. (1999). Differences in biological risk factors for cardiovascular disease between three ethnic groups in the Whitehall II study. *Atherosclerosis*, 142:279–86.

Widdowson, E.M. (1951). Mental contentment and physical growth. *Lancet* 1:1316–8.

Wilkinson, R.G. (1996). *Unhealthy societies: the afflictions of inequality.* London: Routledge.

Williams, R.B. (1991). A relook at personality types and coronary heart disease. *Prog Cardiol*, 4:91–7.

14

Ecological Approaches: Rediscovering the Role of the Physical and Social Environment

SALLY MACINTYRE AND ANNE ELLAWAY

> Ecology: *a branch of biology dealing with living organisms' habits, modes of life, and relationships to their surroundings.*
> *Concise Oxford Dictionary*, Fifth Edition, (1964), p. 386

THE ECOLOGICAL FALLACY

Ecological approaches have received a bad press within sociology and epidemiology. For the last 50 or so years, analysis at the ecological level has been regarded as suspect and inherently inferior to individual-level analysis. For example:

> epidemiology texts offer a consistent appraisal of ecological studies: they are crude attempts to ascertain individual-level correlations. The flaws in such studies limit their usefulness to "hypothesis generation," leaving the more esteemed process of "hypothesis testing" to individual level data. The problems are generally attributed to the "ecological fallacy," a logical fallacy inherent in making causal inference from group data to individual behaviours. (Schwartz 1994, p. 819)

The "ecological fallacy" involves inferring individual-level relationships from relationships observed at the aggregate level. In an influential paper Robinson illustrated why such inferences can be fallacious via observed correlations between skin color and illiteracy in the United States. Using exactly the same data, he showed that the correlation between color and illiteracy was 0.203 for individuals, 0.773 when data were aggregated to the state level, and 0.946 when data were aggregated to the level of nine geographical divisions of the United States. He pointed out that ecological and individual correlations between the same variables can differ and need not even have the same sign. For instance, an individual-level correlation between foreign birth and illiteracy was 0.118, but the same data produced a correlation of −0.619 when aggregated to the level of states (Robinson 1950).

There are numerous examples of the lack of correspondence between individual level associations and group-level associations of the same or similar variables. Within countries, smokers are more likely to die prematurely than nonsmokers. However, countries with high smoking rates (such as Japan or France) do not necessarily have high premature death rates. At a country level the association observed at an individual level between low socioeconomic status (SES) and coronary heart disease (CHD) may appear to reverse, with more affluent countries having higher rates of CHD. This does not mean that smoking does not predispose to premature death, or that one has to choose between a model of CHD as being either a disease of affluence or of poverty; rather it means that one has to be clear about the appropriate level of analysis and measurement and careful about extrapolating from one level to another (in either direction). A hung jury can be characterized as being indecisive, but this does not mean that the individual jurors composing it are indecisive; indeed, it probably means they are each extremely decided, which is why they are unwilling to compromise (Schwartz 1994). The ecological fallacy consists of inferring that because there is a certain size and direction of relationship between two variables when measured at an aggregate level, the same relationship will be observed at the individual level, which, as the above examples show, is not always the case.

The size of the correlation coefficient between two variables tends to be related to the size of the grouping (area, region, country) to which the data are aggregated. A statistician has demonstrated this point by showing how the values of a correlation between two variables can be increased from 0.54 to 0.95 simply by grouping the areas into larger units (Blalock 1961). Kasl argued that: "Ecological analyses can produce correlations as high as the mid 0.90s with variables which to the best of our knowledge are likely to reflect spurious associations only" (1979, p. 785) and suggested that "when facing the results of a macro-social or ecological analysis, the safest attitude for the reader to adopt is one of profound scepticism" (1979, p. 784).

In 1970 Hauser published a "cautionary tale," presenting an analysis which appeared to show that students in schools with high sex ratios had higher educational aspirations than students in schools with low sex ratios. This effect of school context (sex ratio) persisted when sex, intelligence, and father's education were all taken into account, and Hauser suggested that this "consexual effect" was a consequence of antici-patory socialization. However, he then went on to show that this contextual interpretation was "speculative, artifactual, and substantively trivial" and to argue against the use of contextual analysis (1974). Damning critiques of the ecological approach and illustrations of its statistical basis have been published not only within sociology (Hauser 1974) but also within epidemiology (Piantadosi et al. 1988).

Such critiques have been commonly interpreted to mean that one should always avoid an ecological approach. We would like to argue that although scepticism is to be encouraged in science, it may be misplaced, and that in this case it is usually based on a confusion between the improper use of aggregate data as proxy for individual data (the "ecological fallacy") and the analysis of the effects of the social and physical environment on the health of individuals or populations (an ecological perspective). We believe that the disdain for ecological analysis is based on an overgeneralization from the problems of incorrect inference from aggregate to individual levels and that this has led to an avoidance of ecological data even when it would be appropriate. In this chapter we argue for the importance of an ecological perspective that would take into account humans' "*habits, modes of life, and relationships to their surroundings*" (see dictionary definition of ecology above) and suggest that there is much interesting and important work to be done to explore the potential influence of the physical and social environment on human health or health behaviors. Such work should contribute both to our fundamental understanding of processes that shape individual and population health and provide pointers to possible loci for interventions to improve human health.

OVERGENERALIZATION FROM THE CRITIQUE OF THE ECOLOGICAL FALLACY

The appropriateness or otherwise of an ecological approach depends on the purpose of the study and the logical status of interpretations made from the measure. If one's personal or family socioeconomic status is hypothesized to be a possible determinant of mental illness, it is invalid to test this relationship on the basis of ecological correlations between rates of incidence of mental illness and aggregate socioeconomic measures. But if one is postulating that the segregation of populations on economic grounds leads to local subcultural factors implicated in the incidence of mental illness, an ecological correlation may be the best way of assessing which clusters of factors are related to incidence. The socioeconomic composition of the neighborhood could be used in this fashion as a contextual variable, with no inferences being made about its individual relationship to mental illness (Clausen and Kohn 1959). Ecological correlations may be valuable even if they do not reflect individual correlations, particularly in research concerned with group processes; Robinson's correlation at the state level of percentage black and percentage illiterate is a substantively interesting sociological finding, irrespective of the fact that the individual correlation is lower, and it might be interesting to look at the historical and economic factors leading to some states both importing large black populations and neglecting their school systems (Menzel 1950).

If one is interested in groups then it may be inappropriate to focus only on individuals. The "atomistic" (Riley 1963) or "individualistic" (Scheuch 1969) fallacy involves incorrectly inferring information about the environment from data on individuals (for example, that the combination of many decided electors will produce a decisive election result). An individual analysis may show that married women have more friends than widows, and it might be inferred from this that marriage is the mechanism promoting friendship. However, this may only be true in settings in which the majority are married; the important factor may be the proportion of women of different marital statuses in the immediate environment (widows might have more friends in homes for the elderly containing a high proportion of widows), and this proportion is a property of the setting (Riley 1963). This type of fallacy has received much attention and criticism in the field of environmental studies. Indeed a recent paper stated: "It could be considered a scientific disgrace that 25 to 30 years later some environmental researchers still make the error of using the individual as the unit of analysis when they want to make inferences about settings" (Richards 1996, p. 223). We thus need to be aware that the fallacy of the wrong level can apply in both directions.

Schwarz (1994, p. 819) has argued that emphasis on the ecological fallacy encourages three equally fallacious notions:

1. That individual-level models are more perfectly specified than ecological-level models
2. That ecological correlations are all substitutes for individual-level correlations
3. That group level variables do not cause disease

These fallacies tend to encourage researchers to overvalue individual-level data (and by implication, individual-level models or theories) and conversely to undervalue group-level or contextual-level data (and by implication, models or theories which take the social or physical environment into account). Although social epidemiology and medical sociology purport to take seriously in their theorizing contextual factors (families, peer groups, workplaces, neighborhoods, subcultures, etc.), the overgeneralization of the problem of the ecological fallacy has led to overconcentration on individual-level models and measures. This individual focus may arise from a confusion between a *methodological* issue (the validity of inferring from one level to another) and a *conceptual* issue (what sorts of factors influence health or behaviors). In the remainder of this chapter we illustrate these general points with particular reference to the literature on SES and health and on the spatial patterning of health.

CONFUSION OF CONCEPTS, METHODS, AND LEVELS

The field of research on SES and health is replete with conceptual confusions about appropriate levels of analysis. As we have noted before, much research in Britain using ecological-level data on social class and mortality uses area data as a proxy for individual data (Macintyre et al. 1993). For example, the Townsend and Carstairs indices of social deprivation correctly characterize local areas, being based on the proportions of residents with certain characteristics (unemployment, car ownership, overcrowding, and housing tenure in the Townsend index and male unemployment, overcrowding, car ownership, and low social class in the Carstairs index) (Townsend et al. 1988; Carstairs and Morris 1991). Their use is thus appropriate for resource allocation based on the proportion of deprived people in an area or for characterizing the social composition of the local population. However, such indices are often incorrectly used to infer the level of deprivation of an individual or family, as if living in an area with many unemployed people or high rates of non car ownership means that one is unemployed or does not own a car.

The deprivation score of the area of residence is frequently attached to individuals in epidemiological analysis as if it characterizes the person. If the interest is in whether living in an area with many poor people has some effect on health this is legitimate, but it is rarely explicit whether this is the underlying hypothesis or whether ecological characteristics are uncritically being applied as if they automatically pertain to individuals. Such indices are also used for sampling in order to achieve a study population with particular socioeconomic characteristics. At the extremes of deprivation scores this might be reasonable on probabilistic grounds, but in areas with middling ecological deprivation scores there may be a mix of people at all points in a continuum of social or material deprivation, and it is therefore illegitimate to assume that all residents are of middling socioeconomic status (McLoone and Boddy 1994). It is also illegitimate to infer that because there are multiple indicators of deprivation present in an area (for example, poverty, lone parenthood, unemployment, overcrowding), the people in the area are all multiply deprived (for example, poor, unemployed lone parents living in overcrowded accommodation (Holterman 1975)).

Many analyses using area-based SES measures do not make it clear whether these are being conceptualized as being true ecological measures, i.e., as measuring something about the local social or physical environment, or as characteristics of the individual. It is often not specified whether SES is being conceptualized as being a property of the individual, the household, or the neighborhood or larger area, and any mechanisms potentially linking area SES and individual health or behavior are left unstated or simply assumed.

For example, an analysis in Britain examined premature mortality in relation to social deprivation in the local area (measured by rates of unemployment, no car access, non ownership of homes, and employed people in the lowest two occupational social classes), and to personal deprivation, measured by individual or household counterparts of these area variables. The authors concluded that: "the excess mortality associated with residence in areas designated as deprived by aggregate census based indicators is wholly explained by the concentration in those areas of people with adverse personal or household socio-economic factors." (Sloggett and Joshi 1994, p. 1470)

Further, they suggest that "the evidence does not confirm any social miasma whereby the shorter life expectancy of disadvantaged people is further reduced if they live in close proximity to other disadvantaged people" (Sloggett and Joshi 1994, p. 1473). Their reference to "social miasma" is the only mention in this paper of any theory about the potential mechanisms which might link either local or personal levels of deprivation to premature mortality. It at least suggests some underlying assumptions about possible pathways, which many papers do not, but this is only one of many possible mechanisms, and it is not spelled out why this particular pathway is the one the authors think might explain any potential effect on health of area-level social deprivation. Living in an area characterized by high unemployment, low social class, etc., could equally well be hypothesized to effect health adversely because such areas are more likely to attract chemical dumping or have high levels of air pollution, or because the industries typically located in such places involve hazardous operations (Bullard and Wright 1993; Northridge and Shepard 1997). However, many papers do not specify any clear hypotheses about the possible pathways by which area or household socioeconomic deprivation might influence health; individual-, household-, or area-level indicators of SES are often used interchangeably and without specifying the underlying causal model.

Similarly, different investigators, and investigators in different countries, may have entirely different assumptions about what it is that "type of place" might be measuring and what possible pathways might be involved in observed associations between place of residence and health. For example, a paper on place of birth and premature mortality for circulatory disease among blacks in the United States found that those born in the South had higher mortality than those born in the Midwest, Northeast, or West (wherever the place of death). This was interpreted as suggesting that childhood adversity (mainly poverty and poor nutrition) is related to premature mortality and as possibly confirming a recent hypothesis that exposures in early life may trigger biological programming which can influence mortality risks in adulthood (Barker 1992, 1994). This interpretation is based on "the fact that southern blacks historically suffered from abject poverty with nutritional deprivation" (Schneider et al. 1997, p. 800). But there are many other ways in which the South might differ from other regions of the United States, and without any controls for individual childhood adversity, there is no way of deciding whether it is poverty and nutritional deprivation rather than climatic, gene pool, or other possible features of the South which lead to excess mortality. This particular interpretation relies on a whole chain of taken-for-granted assumptions about the social meaning of "being born in the South," and about mechanisms relating these to later health.

RENEWED INTEREST IN AREA ANALYSIS

Since the early 1990s there has been some rehabilitation of an ecological perspective within social epidemiology, medical geography, and medical sociology and a resurgence of interest in the effects on health of residence in different types of neighborhoods, localities, and regions.

Within epidemiology there has been something of a backlash against the apparent individualism of chronic disease epidemiology and a call for a return to a more traditional focus both on the health of populations and on cultural, social structural, group-level, and environmental influences on health (Kaplan 1996; Schwartz 1994; Susser 1994). It has been argued for example that even health behaviors displayed by individuals cannot be understood without taking into account the characteristics of, and processes occurring at, the levels of both the immediate and broader environment. Von Korff et al. point out that the risk of initiation of tobacco use is associated with attributes of the child (e.g., self-esteem, academic achievement, refusal skills); attributes of the child's family (e.g., parental attitude toward smoking); general characteristics of the community (e.g., ease of minors' access to cigarettes, school policies regarding smoking); and wider social factors (e.g., economic policies influencing the price of cigarettes) (Von Korff et al. 1992, p. 1078). Diet is similarly likely to be influenced not only by personal tastes, cognitions, and beliefs but also by the local social context (family, peer group, subculture, workplace, neighborhood) and by larger social factors such as the cuisine of the culture and the system of food production and distribution (Macintyre et al. 1998; Mennell et al. 1992).

Recently within medical geography there has been a call to return to an earlier emphasis on "place." Kearns has described how challenges from within and outside geography have led to a revived interest in localities. He identified three major challenges: justice-oriented critiques of ill-health and health service delivery systems, innovative thinking about health philosophy by bodies such as the World Health Organization, and the structure/agency debate within contemporary social theory; "implicit within all these developments is the traditional geographical concern of place, the local context of health, disease, and social process" (Kearns 1993, p. 140). He argues for a renewed focus on places as actually experienced by people and as a context for their lives, rather than on statistical analysis of spatial relationships between individuals, places, and institutions. Jones and Moon have argued that, despite the existence of many published studies based in specific localities: "Seldom . . . does location itself play a real part in the analysis; it is the canvas on which events happen but the nature of the locality and its role in structuring health status and health related behaviour is neglected" (Jones and Moon 1993, p. 515).

In similar vein, we have previously argued that although there is a long tradition in Britain of research on area of residence and health: "Rarely has this involved investigating socio-economic or cultural features of areas that might influence health; usually studies use area level data, for example about specific pathogens or about levels of deprivation, as surrogates for individual level data, rather than being interested in the areas themselves." We argued further that there should be more research "directly studying features of the local social and physical environment which might promote

or inhibit health" (Macintyre et al. 1993, p. 213).

Interestingly, in the light of what Susser and others have suggested is the traditional concern of epidemiology with population health and with the environment, some have argued that one reason for the neglect of studies of localities and health within sociology has been the dominance of an individualistically oriented epidemiological paradigm within the sociological study of inequalities in health. Phillimore argues that developments in the field of social inequalities in health have been shaped and confined by the health and population data sets available, largely derived from censuses, rather than being driven by sociological theory (Phillimore 1993).

The essence of these recent pleas from epidemiologists, geographers, and sociologists is that the fear of the ecological fallacy and an overreliance on individual-level data and measurements have tended to lead to an overindividualistic approach to determinants of health. Despite lip service frequently being paid to the importance of contextual or environmental ("upstream") influences on health, very little research has been done on the health-promoting or health-damaging characteristics of such contexts; most research has focused on their expression in individual life circumstances and health.

Another factor leading to the possible rehabilitation of an ecological perspective has been recent empirical work on income distribution in relation to mortality. Wilkinson has argued that the level of income inequality in a society influences mortality rates independently of the absolute level of mean income of that society (Wilkinson 1996). Research examining the income distribution and mortality rates in U.S. states has confirmed a relationship between income inequality and mortality, with higher death rates in those states with the most unequal distribution of income, adjusted for state median income (Kaplan et al. 1996; Kennedy et al. 1996). Similarly, a study in Britain found that mortality rates were positively associated with the variation in deprivation between small areas within larger administrative areas (Ben-Shlomo et al. 1996).

One way in which community income distribution has been hypothesized to influence health has been via social cohesion or social capital (Wilkinson 1996, 1997). Work by Putnam on social participation has been used to suggest that community levels of social cohesion may influence mortality (Putnam 1993), and this has rekindled interest in the concept of social capital first introduced by Coleman (1988). Social capital is an inherently ecological concept and so has focused attention on properties of communities and the processes by which social capital is maintained or diminished (Lasker et al. 1994).

It should, however, be noted in this case that the explanation may lie not in contextual features such as social cohesion or social capital, as is often suggested, but in the fact that in places where there is more income inequality, there will be more poor people, and it may be among them that the higher mortality is concentrated. Gravelle has argued that associations between unequal income distribution and population health may be a statistical artefact resulting from the use of aggregate rather than individual data and describes this as an example of the "ecological fallacy" (1998). A similar point was made by the authors of a paper which found that survival, controlling for sex, age, and family size, was related to income inequality in the local area even after adjusting for mean community income, but that after adjusting for household income this association was no longer significant (Fiscella and Franks 1997). They suggest that the previously reported ecological associations between income inequality and mortality may reflect confounding between individual family income and mortality. This particular debate highlights the importance of our earlier arguments about the need for clarity in thinking about what the indicators used in research are actually measuring and what pathways are being assumed or measured.

COMPOSITIONAL AND CONTEXTUAL EXPLANATIONS

An important distinction underlying much thinking in this field is between *compositional* and *contextual* explanations for spatial variations in outcomes such as mortality, health, health risk, and health behaviors. A compositional explanation for area differences would be that areas include different types of individuals, and that differences between these individuals account for the observed difference between places. For example, it might be argued that poor people die earlier than rich people, so it is not surprising that areas with lots of poor people have low average life expectancy: Poor people would die early wherever they live and rich people live longer wherever they live, so any observed spatial patterning in life expectancy is purely due to the spatial concentration of poor or rich people in different sorts of areas, and life expectancy is therefore a property of the individual, not of areas.

A contextual explanation would be that there are features of the social or physical environment which influence the health of those exposed to it (either in addition to or in interaction with individual characteristics). People of whatever levels of personal poverty or affluence might live longer if they lived in nonpolluted areas with a pleasant climate and an excellent range of services and amenities; or, rich people might live just as long wherever they live because they have the personal resources to cope with a range of environments, but poor people might die particularly early in underresourced neighborhoods (Congdon 1995; Jones and Duncan 1995; Langford and Bentham 1996; Macintyre 1986, 1997b; Shouls et al. 1996). An interesting and useful set of graphical representations of the logically possible relationships between individual and contextual characteristics, and interactions between them, is provided in Jones and Duncan (1995).

It is important to keep in mind the distinction between these *compositional* and *contextual* models because in the field of area variations in health they are often confused. Moreover, much research seeking to unpack the relative importance of people's personal characteristics as compared with the characteristics of the places where they live ignores possible interactions between these levels and treats individual characteristics as being independent of the local environment. Yet one of the most obvious consequences of being personally deprived (e.g., having low income and little education) is that you may have to end up living in the type of place which is in itself health damaging (e.g., with substandard housing, no opportunities for employment, and high levels of hazardous pollution). Conversely, having high income and good education allows one to move to salubrious leafy suburbs with plenty of opportunities for a healthy lifestyle and protection from stresses and hazards. Similarly, if you live in a place with a booming manufacturing industry (for example, shipbuilding) you are much more likely to receive the job and training opportunities that mean you end up in a skilled blue collar occupation, and command a reasonable income, than if you live in an area with a depressed industrial base and no training opportunities. Your SES and income are thus partly a product of your place of upbringing, rather than being intrinsically personal attributes (and indeed can change over time when your industry goes into recession). Thus in terms of lived social processes, the distinction between personal disadvantage and levels of disadvantage in the locality may be somewhat artificial.

However, much recent research, in Britain at least, has tried to unravel the question of whether observed differences in health or health behaviors between areas have purely compositional explanations or require additional contextual explanations.

Multivariate analysis and, more recently, multilevel modeling, have increasingly been used to examine the relative importance of individual and local factors or the interaction between individual and local factors. New statistical approaches have permitted several levels of analysis to be taken into account simultaneously (Jones 1991; Jones et al. 1992; Keithley et al. 1984; Von Korff et al. 1992).

What is the evidence so far? Some investigators have concluded that compositional effects explain apparent spatial patterning in a range of outcomes. Sloggett and Joshi, as noted above, reported that the excess mortality associated with areas of residence designated as deprived by census-based indicators in Britain was wholly explained by the concentration in those areas of people with adverse personal or household socioeconomic factors (1994). Multilevel modeling of regional variation of psychiatric morbidity in the United Kingdom found that neither the type of local neighborhood nor the region had much effect on rates once individual characteristics were taken into account (Duncan et al. 1993). The same authors also reported that "place, expressed as regional differences, may be less important than previously implied" for smoking and drinking behavior and that contextual effects previously reported from a British U.K. national health and lifestyle survey (Blaxter 1990) were an artefact of the aggregate data she had used (Duncan et al. 1993). A Dutch study of mental disorders also found little evidence that contextual effects explained the high rates of poorer mental health in deprived urban areas, most of this higher prevalence being due to a higher concentration of people of lower SES in these areas (Reijneveld and Schene 1998). All these papers suggest that what at first sight might look like contextual, area, differences are really compositional differences.

Other work has, however, found that compositional effects cannot entirely explain variations in health or health behaviors. An important paper from the Alameda County study in California showed that residents in a federally designated poverty area in Oakland experienced a 45% higher age-, race-, and sex-adjusted mortality over a 9-year follow-up period compared with those not resident in the poverty area. This increased risk of death persisted when there was multivariate adjustment for baseline health status, race, income, employment status, education, access to medical care, health insurance coverage, and a whole range of behavioral factors often assumed to be the link between socioeconomic status and health. The authors conclude that "these results support the hypothesis that properties of the sociophysical environment may be important contributors to the association between low socio-economic status and excess mortality, and that this contribution is independent of individual behaviours" (Haan et al. 1987, p. 989).

A more recent study using the National Longitudinal Mortality Study (a large national database of the U.S. noninstutionalized population assembled from survey data collected from 1978 to 1985, followed up using the National Death Index for 1979–1989) examined the power of median census tract income and family income to predict mortality over an 11-year period. Both median census tract income and family income predicted mortality, lower income being associated with higher mortality. The effect of family income was not much reduced when median census tract income was taken into account; when family income was taken into account, the effect of median census tract income was reduced but still present, especially among those under 65, and among black people. After taking family income into account black men and women aged 25–64 living in low-income areas had, respectively, 40% and 30% higher mortality than those living in higher SES areas. Although family income had a stronger association with mortality than median census tract income, these results were interpreted as suggesting that "area socio-economic status makes a unique and substantial contri-

bution to mortality and should be explored in health policy and disease prevention research" (Anderson et al. 1997, p. 42).

A multilevel modeling analysis of three different health outcomes in Britain found significant contextual effects for death and long-term illness at middle age; infant mortality was less strongly related to deprivation at the individual level and showed less evidence of contextual variance (Congdon 1995). A more detailed multilevel analysis of self-reported chronic illness used individual data derived from the 1% sample of anonymized records (SARs) from the 1991 British census combined with area data from this census. This found evidence for both compositional and contextual effects and showed that the former were larger than the latter. All individuals living in areas with high levels of illness (which tend to be more deprived areas) show greater morbidity, even after allowing for their individual characteristics. However, within affluent areas, where morbidity was generally lower, the differences in health between rich and poor individuals was particularly large (Shouls et al. 1996). Another study using the SARs data found that geographical differences in limiting long-term illness remain substantial even when individual level sociodemographic variables such as age, sex, ethnicity, housing tenure, social class, and car ownership are taken into account (Gould and Jones 1996).

Recent work on the patterning of cardiovascular disease risk factors and outcomes has reported differences between areas that are not completely accounted for by individual characteristics. A study using data from a cardiovascular risk survey of adults in Scotland used multilevel modeling to examine predictors of diastolic blood pressure, cholesterol, alcohol consumption, and smoking. Although much of the variance was present at the individual level, the existence of significant additional variance at the district level in blood pressure, cholesterol, and alcohol led the authors to conclude that places may have a role in the distribution of CHD risk (Hart et al. 1997). A study in the West of Scotland found that both area-based and individual-based socioeconomic indicators made independent contributions to cardiovascular risk factors and mortality (Davey Smith et al. 1998). A study of individuals in four communities in the United States used multilevel models to estimate associations with neighborhood variables after adjustment for individual-level indicators of SES. Living in deprived neighbourhoods was associated with increased rates of coronary heart disease and of CHD risk factors, with associations generally persisting after adjustment for individual-level variables (Diez-Roux et al. 1997).

Recently Duncan and colleagues have suggested that they may have been too swift in their earlier rejection of the role of contextual variables in the patterning of health behaviors. In a subsequent multilevel analysis of smoking in Britain they concluded:

see pg 339

there does seem to be some contextual variation between electoral wards in terms of the log-odds of an individual being a smoker controlling for compositional make-up.

It would appear, therefore, that smoking cultures develop in local neighbourhoods whereby the co-presence of similarly behaving people influences the number of times people practice that behaviour. In places where there are few smokers consumption is discouraged; where there are many it is stimulated. (Duncan et al. 1996, page 827)

Other studies have likewise detected area differences in health-related behaviors. A study in 15 communities in the United States showed significant variation between them in smoking, fat and alcohol consumption, and use of seatbelts and found that these differences persisted after control for demographic, health status, and other health behavioral characteristics of the people in the communities. The authors argued that unique features of communities may influence health behaviors and suggested that the results confirm the potential importance of contextual effects on individual health behavior (Diehr et al. 1993). A study of Finnish adolescents, which linked individual data to information about socioeconomic characteristics of municipalities, found that drinking alcohol and use of high-fat milk products were related to socioregional context as well as to the socioeconomic background of the adolescents. Gender modified this relationship: "even within the same socio-regional context boys may be subjected to different kinds of environmental pressures than girls" (Karvonen and Rimpela 1996, p. 1473). Similar conclusions were reached in an analysis of alcohol use in the same study, the authors concluding that "variation in alcohol use among Finnish adolescents is related to where they live, and not simply to demographics" (Karvonen 1995, p. 57). We have found that diet, smoking, and exercise differed between four socially contrasting neighbourhoods in Glasgow, Scotland, even after taking into account individual predictors of these behaviors (Ellaway and Macintyre 1996; Forsyth et al. 1994).

Other measures of health and functioning such as waist–hip ratio and reaction times (Ecob 1996), respiratory volume and reported symptoms of heart disease, high blood pressure, and stroke (Jones and Duncan 1995), and body size and shape (Ellaway et al. 1997) have also been shown to vary between small areas after adjustment for individual predictors.

Thus more recent studies using multivariate techniques have tended to suggest that mortality, health, health risks, and health behaviors may vary between areas (measured at various scales from small neighborhoods to regions or provinces) in ways that are not completely explicable by individual characteristics such as age, sex, and socioeconomic status. Although many authors caution that the finding of apparent contextual effects may be due to unmeasured individual characteristics, imprecision of measurement, misspecification of models or residual confounding (Davey Smith et al. 1998; Diez-Roux et al. 1997; Hart et al. 1997; Humphreys and Carr Hill 1991), most conclude that contextual influences may be real and not simply statistical artifacts.

A lot of effort has, therefore, been devoted to the examination, via multivariate analysis, of whether or not there are area effects on health within countries. Some scholars have been reluctant to accept that differences between regions or neighborhoods might be generated by contextual effects. This is perhaps surprising given that few people would bother to examine whether differences in mortality, health, or health risks between nations are due to compositional or contextual effects. We tend to take it for granted that persons of similar sex, age, occupation, and income would have different health and health behavior experiences according to whether they lived in Japan, France, or the United States, because of differing cultural, economic, political, climatic, historical, or geographical contexts.

EXPLANATIONS FOR AREA DIFFERENCES

As the above review indicates, a considerable amount of effort has recently been invested in examining whether apparent area differences in health are due to compositional or contextual effects. Much less energy has been devoted to investigating possible explanations for any observed contextual effects. Little explicit attention has been given to the meaning of area-level socioeconomic status and to how aggregate indices of SES might translate into pathways through which people's health might be promoted or damaged by their local area.

Apart from studies of particular environmental toxins, there is very little research on what environmental or cultural features of local areas or regions in contemporary societies might promote or damage health. This lack may be because we tend to think that characteristics of the people living in the area—the sociodemographic composition of the area—actually describe the area, or because we tend to assume that "we all know what different sorts of areas are like"

and therefore do not need to study them. As we have noted before:

The problem with these sorts of reactions is firstly that they treat 'social class' and 'area' as if they are explanations in themselves, rather than attributes whose links to health need further clarification; and secondly they do not give any suggestions for policy other than trying to make people of low social class more like higher social class people (either by changing their behaviours or by changing their socio-economic circumstances—actions which may be either ineffective or not politically feasible). (Macintyre 1997b, p. 4)

In our own work in the West of Scotland, we have been trying to look directly at features of local areas that might be health promoting or health damaging. We have been using as an organizing framework the following five types of features of local areas which might influence health:

1. *Physical features of the environment shared by all residents in a locality.* These include the quality of air and water, latitude, climate, etc., and are likely to be shared by neighbourhoods across a wide area. In Glasgow, for example, all the drinking water for a city of nearly a million comes from the same loch, so the two-and-a-half-fold differences in death rates between neighbourhoods cannot be explained by variations in drinking water.

2. *Availability of healthy environment at home, work, and play.* Areas vary in their provision of decent housing, secure and nonhazardous employment, safe play areas for children, etc. These environments may not affect everyone living in an area in the same way that air and water quality do; they may affect the employed more than the unemployed, families with children more than elderly people, and so on.

3. *Services provided, publicly or privately, to support people in their daily lives.* These include education, transport, street cleaning and lighting, policing, health, and welfare services. Again, how these affect people may depend on personal circumstances. Public transport may matter more if you do not have a car.

4. *Sociocultural features of a neighbourhood.* These include the political, economic, ethnic, and religious history of a community: norms and values, the degree of community integration, levels of crime, incivilities and other threats to per-

sonal safety, and networks of community support.

5. *The reputation of an area.* How areas are perceived—by their residents, by service or amenity planners and providers, by banks and investors—may influence the infrastructure of the area, the self-esteem and morale of the resident, and who moves in and out of the area. (Macintyre 1997b, pp. 4–5)

These categories are not mutually exclusive and may well interact with each other, and their health effects may vary by people's personal resources. More broadly, we conceptualize features such as these as "opportunity structures," that is, socially constructed and socially patterned features of the physical and social environment which may promote or damage health either directly or indirectly through the possibilities they provide for people to live healthy lives.

We selected two socially contrasting localities (comprising four socially more homogeneous neighborhoods) in Glasgow City in 1987 in order to study the impact of local opportunity structures on people's health (Macintyre et al. 1989). All individuals in three target age groups (15, 35, and 55) were approached for interview in 1987/8 and were resurveyed in 1992/3 and again in 1997 in a 10-year follow-up. The face-to-face interviews, mostly conducted in the respondents' homes, collected a wide range of data on personal and social circumstances, health knowledge, health beliefs and values, health-related behavior, and past and present health. We have also been gathering data from a range of sources about the social and physical environments in the localities, using the framework above as a guide.

We have shown that opportunity structures, as defined above, were less conducive to health or health-promoting activities in the poorer area than in the better-off area. We demonstrated that access to healthy recreation was more limited in the poorer area, as was the provision of public transport and retail outlets (facts made more significant because car ownership was 33% lower in this area) (Macintyre et al. 1993).

In addition, there were lower levels of provision of some aspects of primary health care in the poorer than the richer area (e.g., more patients per doctor, less equipment such as electrocardiographs, and less time available per patient) (Wyke et al. 1992).

We have found marked differences between neighborhoods in the reported consumption of "healthy" foods (Forsyth et al. 1994), smoking and participation in sport (Ellaway and Macintyre 1996), and body size and shape (Ellaway et al. 1997) after controlling for known predictors of these (sex, age, and socioeconomic status). This may be related to our findings that in the more deprived neighborhoods, the price of certain "healthy foods" is higher, the availability and quality of fruit and vegetables are lower, and the price differential between a "healthy food basket" and "less healthy food basket" is greater (Sooman et al. 1993); and that the ways in which people make use of their local neighborhood for health-promoting activities such as socializing, taking exercise, and shopping differs between these socially contrasting localities (Macintyre and Ellaway 1998).

Housing conditions and housing-related stressors (cold, damp, noise, overcrowding, vibration, accident risks) were related to area of residence, and we found that these in turn were related at the individual level, after taking income, age, and sex into account, to longstanding illness and depression (Ellaway and Macintyre 1998). We have also shown that perceptions of the local environment such as levels of amenities, problems, crime, neighborliness, and the reputation of the area differ between our study areas, and at an individual level they are associated with health (controlling for age, sex, SES, and area of residence, negative perceptions of the local area were significantly associated with poorer self assessed health and with anxiety) (Sooman and Macintyre 1995).

We have thus shown that many aspects of local areas which might be related to people's health, or access to opportunities to live healthily, are systematically poorer in a more socially disadvantaged area. We are extending this work by gathering further information about community resources and activities, job vacancies, public and private investment, urban planning policies, and other features of the physical and social environment. We advocate similar attempts to examine, directly, features of local communities which might promote or damage health rather than further work simply using aggregate census-type data to characterize neighborhoods.

We stress the need to study these features directly, rather than through the views of residents, because of the methodological problem of contamination between health measures (particularly mental health measures) and perceptions of the environment (Stansfield et al. 1993) and possible confounding of area and individual characteristics. Depressed people might, for example, be more likely to report negative features of their environment. However, we have found that, in general, "objective" measures of features of areas demonstrate sharper differences between areas than do "subjective" measures. For example, when measured by dividing the number of rooms per household by the number of persons in the household, we found a significant difference in overcrowding between our areas; however, there was no difference between them in the prevalence of perceived overcrowding in the home. When we studied public transport provision in our two study localities we did so by examining bus and train timetables and the provision of shoppers' and hospital buses, and we found markedly better provision in the more affluent area. When we asked residents about how they felt about public transport in their locality the differences between the two areas were not nearly so great. We interpret this disjunction between the "objective" and "subjective" measurement of overcrowding and public transport provision as stemming from the higher expectations of higher SES households in the better-off area and lower expectations and lifelong experience of poor services among lower SES households in the

poorer area (Macintyre 1997b; Macintyre et al. 1993).

CONCLUSION

Ecological approaches were disfavored for many years in social epidemiology and medical sociology. This disdain was associated with a focus on individual, and a neglect of contextual, determinants of health. More recently there has been a partial rehabilitation of an ecological perspective, triggered in part by the ability of new statistical techniques such as multilevel modeling to disentangle compositional and contextual effects and in part because of converging theoretical trends within geography, epidemiology, and sociology.

The idea that the social or physical environment might influence health would be regarded as a commonplace within other branches of medicine or social science. The influence of the social environment on biological measures was shown years ago (Schottstaedt et al. 1958, 1959; Wolf 1993), and in fields such as crime (Donnelly 1988; Stark 1987), child and adolescent development (Aneshensel and Sucoff 1996; Coulton et al. 1996; McLeod and Edwards 1995), welfare of the elderly (Krause 1996), educational performance (Barber and Olsen 1997; Brooks-Gunn et al. 1993), and urban planning (Blackman et al. 1989; McCarthy et al. 1985), the study of the impact of settings on human behavior and performance has been standard and uncontroversial for decades. In all these fields attention is paid to features of the settings which might influence outcomes and to the mechanisms by which they do so.

Public health practitioners and researchers in the 19th and early 20th centuries focused on threats to health in the immediate environment by dealing with sewage, the provision of clean water, legislation against the sale of adulterated foods, and housing and working conditions (Chadwick 1842; Engels 1848, 1969). With the decline in infectious diseases and the lessening of such obvious objective threats to health as contaminated food and water or overcrowded housing, public health interest in the role of place declined. With the rediscovery of social inequalities in health, during the 1980s in Europe and the 1990s in the United States, attention focused mainly on chronic diseases such as heart disease, respiratory disease, and cancer, and on the role of the class structure, and of material circumstances in generating and maintaining inequalities in health (Macintyre 1997a). Perhaps surprisingly, given the interest in material circumstances and exposures, the role of the local physical and social environment in generating inequalities in health has largely been neglected in favor of the role of individual attributes such as education, income, employment, and psychosocial resources.

Although much of the recent work examining the relative importance of compositional vs. contextual explanations for area variations in health has been methodologically and technically very sophisticated, it has been less conceptually and theoretically sophisticated. There has been little explicit theorizing about the causal processes that might be involved in the association between either individual socioeconomic status or local socioeconomic conditions and mortality or health; there has been an overreliance on data that happen to be available (for example, from censuses) rather than on measures chosen as best representing the underlying construct implicated in a causal model; and there has been a recourse to taken-for-granted assumptions about the meaning and significance of SES whether measured at an individual, household, or area level. Some indicators used have a rather remote connection with hypothesized constructs, and there is often little attempt to measure features of the environment directly.

Despite this rather negative evaluation of some features of recent work, we would endorse the rehabilitation of an ecological perspective, not only because it is likely to help produce better causal models of determinants of health but also because it may provide information on possible points of lever-age to improve population health. An emphasis on compositional explanations for patterns of population health tends to imply that policies should be directed toward people (for example, by individually focused health education messages). A recognition that contexts may influence health may help to balance this individual focus by redirecting attention to interventions at the environmental level (for example, by improving housing stock and public transport, providing green spaces for healthy recreation, or regulating workplace hazards).

REFERENCES

Anderson, R.T., Sorlie, P., Backlund, E., Johnson, N., and Kaplan, G.A. (1997). Mortality effects of community socioeconomic status. *Epidemiology*, 8:42–7.

Aneshensel, C.S., and Sucoff, C.A. (1996). The neighborhood context of adolescent mental health. *J Health Soc Behav*, 37:293–310.

Barber, B.K., and Olsen, J.A. (1997). Socialization in context: connection, regulation, and autonomy in the family, school, and neighborhood, and with peers. *J Adolesc Res*, 12:287–315.

Barker, D. (1992). *The fetal and infant origins of adult disease*. London: BMJ.

Barker, D. (1994). *Mothers, babies and disease in later life*. London: BMJ.

Ben-Shlomo, Y., White, I.R., and Marmot, M. (1996). Does the variation in the socioeconomic characteristics of an area affect mortality? *BMJ*, 312:1013–4.

Blackman, T., Evason, E., Melaugh, M., and Woods, R. (1989). Housing and health: a case study of two areas in West Belfast. *J Soc Policy*, 18:1–26.

Blalock, H. (1961). *Causal inferences in non-experimental research*. Chapel Hill: University of North Carolina Press.

Blaxter, M. (1990). *Health and lifestyles*. London: Tavistock/Routledge.

Brooks-Gunn, J., Duncan, G.J., Klebanov, P.K., and Sealand, N. (1993). Do neighborhoods influence child and adolescent development? *Am J Sociol*, 99:353–95.

Bullard, R., and Wright, B. (1993). Environmental justice for all: community perspectives on health and research needs. *Toxicol Ind Health*, 9:821–41.

Carstairs, V., and Morris, R. (1991). *Deprivation and health in Scotland*. Aberdeen: Aberdeen University Press.

Chadwick, E. (1842). *Report of an enquiry into the sanitary conditions of the labouring population of Great Britain.* London: Poor Law Commission.

Clausen, J., and Kohn, M. (1959). The relation of schizophrenia to the social structure of a small city. In Pasamanick, B. (ed.), *Epidemiology of mental disorder.* (Pub. No. 60.) Washington, DC: American Association for the Advancement of Science.

Coleman, J. (1988). Social capital in the creation of human capital. *Am J Sociol,* 94 Suppl 95:S95–120.

Congdon, P. (1995). The impact of area context on long-term illness and premature mortality; an illustration of multilevel analysis. *Reg Stud,* 29:327–44.

Coulton, C., Korbin, J., and Su, M. (1996). Measuring neighbourhood context for young children in an urban area. *Am J Community Psychol,* 24:5–32.

Davey Smith, G., Hart, C., Watt, G., Hole, D., and Hawthorne, V. (1998). Individual social class, area-based deprivation, cardiovascular disease risk factors, and mortality: the Renfrew and Paisley study. *J Epidemiol Community Health,* 52:399–405.

Diehr, P., Koepsell, T., Cheadle, A., Psaty, B., Wagner, E., and Curry, S. (1993). Do communities differ in health behaviours? *J Clin Epidemiol,* 46:1141–9.

Diez-Roux, A.V., Nieto, F.J., Muntaner, C., Tyroler, H.A., Comstock, G.W., Shahar, E., Cooper, L.S., Watson, R.L., and Szklo, M. (1997). Neighborhood environments and coronary heart disease: a multilevel analysis. *Am J Epidemiol,* 146:48–63.

Donnelly, P. (1988). Individual and neighbourhood influences on fear of crime. *Sociolog Focus,* 22:69–85.

Duncan, C., Jones, K., and Moon, G. (1993). Do places matter: a multilevel analysis of regional variations in health related behaviour in Britain. *Soc Sci Med,* 37:725–33.

Duncan, C., Jones, K., and Moon, G. (1996). Health related behaviour in context—a multi level modelling approach. *Soc Sci Med,* 42:817–30.

Ecob, R. (1996). A multilevel modeling approach to examining the effects of area of residence on health and functioning. *J R Stat Soc A,* 159:61–75.

Ellaway, A., and Macintyre, S. (1996). Does where you live predict health related behaviours? a case study in Glasgow. *Health Bull,* 54:443–6.

Ellaway, A., and Macintyre, S. (1998). Does housing tenure predict health in the UK because it exposes people to different levels of housing related hazards in the home or its surroundings? *Health Place,* 4:141–50.

Ellaway, A., Anderson, A., and Macintyre, S. (1997). Does area of residence affect body size and shape? *Int J Obes,* 21:304–8.

Engels, F. (1848, 1969). *The conditions of the working classes in England 1844–45.* Frogmore, UK: Panther Books.

Fiscella, K., and Franks, P. (1997). Poverty or income inequality as a predictor of mortality: a longitudinal cohort study. *BMJ,* 314:1724–8.

Forsyth, A., Macintyre, S., and Anderson, A. (1994). Diets for disease? intraurban variation in reported food consumption in Glasgow. *Appetite,* 22:259–74.

Gould, M.I., and Jones, K. (1996). Analyzing perceived limiting long-term illness using UK census microdata. *Soc Sci Med,* 42:857–69.

Gravelle, H. (1998). How much of the relation between population mortality and unequal distribution of income is a statistical artifact? *BMJ,* 316:382–5.

Haan, M., Kaplan, G., and Camacho, T. (1987). Poverty and health; prospective evidence from the Alameda county study. *Am J Epidemiol,* 125:989–98.

Hart, C., Ecob, R., and Davey Smith, G. (1997). People, places and coronary heart disease risk factor: a multilevel analysis of the Scottish Heart Health Study archive. *Soc Sci Med,* 45:893–902.

Hauser, R. (1974). Contextual analysis revisited. *Sociolog Methods Res,* 2:365–75.

Holterman, S. (1975). Areas of deprivation in Great Britain: an analysis of 1971 Census data. *Soc Trends,* 6:33–47.

Humphreys, K., and Carr Hill, R. (1991). Area variations in health outcomes—artifact or ecology. *Int J Epidemiol,* 20:251–8.

Jones, K. (1991). Specifying and estimating multilevel models for geographical research. *Trans Inst Br Geographers,* 16:148–59.

Jones, K., and Duncan, C. (1995). Individuals and their ecologies: analysing the geography of chronic illness within a multilevel modelling framework. *Health Place,* 1:27–40.

Jones, K., and Moon, G. (1993). Medical geography: taking space seriously. *Prog Hum Geography,* 17:515–24.

Jones, K., Johnston, R., and Pattie, C.J. (1992). People, places and regions: exploring the use of multilevel modeling in an analysis of electoral data. *Br J Polit Sci,* 22:343–80.

Kaplan, G. (1996). People and places: contrasting perspectives on the association between social class and health. *Int J Health Serv,* 26:507–19.

Kaplan, G.A., Pamuk, E.R., Lynch, J.W., Cohen,

R.D., and Balfour, J.L. (1996). Inequality in income and mortality in the United States: analysis of mortality and potential pathways. *BMJ*, 312:999–1003.

Karvonen, S. (1995). Regional differences in drinking among Finnish adolescents. *Addiction*, 90:57–64.

Karvonen, S., and Rimpela, A. (1996). Socio-regional context as a determinant of adolescents' health behavior in Finland. *Soc Sci Med*, 43:1467–74.

Kasl, S. (1979). Mortality and the business cycle: some questions about research strategies when utilizing macro-social and ecological data. *Am J Public Health*, 69:784–8.

Kearns, R.A. (1993). Place and health: towards a reformed medical geography. *Professional Geographer*, 45:139–47.

Keithley, J., Byrne, D., Harrisson, S., and McCarthy, P. (1984). Health and housing conditions in public-sector housing estates. *Public Health*, 98:344–53.

Kennedy, B.P., Kawachi, I., and Prothrow-Stith, D. (1996). Income distribution and mortality: cross sectional ecological study of the Robin Hood index in the United States. *BMJ*, 312:1004–7.

Krause, N. (1996). Neighborhood deterioration and self-rated health in later life. *Psychol Aging*, 11:342–52.

Langford, I., and Bentham, G. (1996). Regional variations in mortality rates in England and Wales: an analysis using multi level modelling. *Soc Sci Med*, 42:897–908.

Lasker, J.N., Egolf, B., and Wolf, S. (1994). Community social change and mortality. *Soc Sci Med*, 39:53–62.

Macintyre, S. (1986). The patterning of health by social position in contemporary Britain: directions for sociological research. *Soc Sci Med*, 23:393–415.

Macintyre, S. (1997a). The Black Report and beyond: what are the issues? *Soc Sci Med*, 44:723–45.

Macintyre, S. (1997b). What are spatial effects and how can we measure them? In Dale, A. (ed.), *Exploiting national survey data: the role of locality and spatial effects*. Manchester, UK: Faculty of Economic and Social Studies, University of Manchester, pp. 1–17.

Macintyre, S., and Ellaway, A. (1998). Social and local variations in the use of urban neighbourhoods: a case study in Glasgow. *Health Place*, 4:91–4.

Macintyre, S., Annandale, E., Ecob, R., Ford, G., Hunt, K., Jamieson, B., Maciver, S., West, P., and Wyke, S. (1989). The west of Scotland Twenty-07 study: health in the community. In Martin, C., and McQueen, D. (eds.), *Read-*

ings for a new public health. Edinburgh: Edinburgh University Press, pp. 56–74.

Macintyre, S., Maciver, S., and Sooman, A. (1993). Area, class and health: should we be focusing on places or people? *J Soc Policy*, 22:213–34.

Macintyre, S., Reilly, J., Miller, D., and Eldridge, J. (1998). Food choice, food scares, and health: the role of the media. In Murcott, A. (ed.), *The nation's diet: the social science of food choice*. London: Longman, pp. 228–49.

McCarthy, P., Byrne, D., Harrison, S., and Keithley, J. (1985). Housing type, housing location and mental-health. *Soc Psychiatry*, 20:125–30.

McLeod, J., and Edwards, K. (1995). Contextual determinants of children's responses to poverty. *Soc Forces*, 74:1487–516.

McLoone, P., and Boddy, F.A., (1994). Deprivation and mortality in Scotland 1981 and 1991. *BMJ*, 309:1465–70.

Mennell, S., Murcott, A., and Van Otterloo, A. (1992). *The sociology of food: eating, diet and culture*. London: Sage.

Menzel, H. (1950). Comment on Robinson's "Ecological correlations and the behaviour of individuals." *Am Sociol Rev*, 15:674.

Northridge, M., and Shepard, P. (1997). Environmental racism and public health. *Am J Public Health*, 87:730–2.

Phillimore, P. (1993). How do places shape health? Rethinking locality and lifestyle in North-East England. In Platt, S., Thomas, H., Scott, S., and Williams, G. (eds.), *Locating health: sociological and historical explorations*. Aldershot, UK: Avebury.

Piantadosi, S., Byar, D., and Green, S. (1988). The ecological fallacy. *Am J Epidemiol*, 127:893–904.

Putnam, R. (1993). *Making democracy work: civic traditions in modern Italy*. Princeton, NJ: Princeton University Press.

Reijneveld, S., and Schene, A. (1998). Higher prevalence of mental disorder in socioeconomically deprived urban areas in the Netherlands: community or personal disadvantage? *J Epidemiol Community Health*, 52:2–7.

Richards, J.M. (1996). Units of analysis, measurement theory, and environmental assessment: a response and clarification. *Environ Behav*, 28:220–36.

Riley, M. (1963). *Sociological research 1: a case approach*. New York: Harcourt Brace.

Robinson, W. (1950). Ecological correlations and the behaviour of individuals. *Am Sociol Rev*, 15:351–7.

Scheuch, E. (1969). Social context and individual behaviour. In Dogan, M., and Rokkan, S.

(eds.), *Quantitative ecological analyses in the social sciences.* Cambridge, MA: MIT Press.

Schneider, D., Greenberg, M.R., and Lu, L.L. (1997). Region of birth and mortality from circulatory diseases among black Americans. *Am J Public Health,* 87:800–4.

Schottstaedt, W., Pinsky, R., Mackler, D., and Wolf, S. (1958). Sociologic, psychologic and metabolic observations on patients in the community of a metabolic ward. *Am J Med,* 25:248–57.

Schottstaedt, W., Pinsky, R., Mackler, D., and Wolf, S. (1959). Prestige and social interaction on a metabolic ward. *Psychosom Med,* 21:131–41.

Schwartz, S. (1994). The fallacy of the ecological fallacy: the potential misuse of a concept and the consequences. *Am J Public Health,* 84:819–24.

Shouls, S., Congdon, P., and Curtis, S. (1996). Modelling inequality in reported long term illness in the UK: combining individual and area characteristics. *J Epidemiol Community Health,* 50:366–76.

Sloggett, A., and Joshi, H. (1994). Higher mortality in deprived areas: community or personal disadvantage? *BMJ,* 309:1470–4.

Sooman, A., and Macintyre, S. (1995). Health and perceptions of the local environment in socially contrasting neighbourhoods in Glasgow. *Health Place,* 1:15–26.

Sooman, A., Macintyre, S., and Anderson, A. (1993). Scotland's health: a more difficult challenge for some? The price and availability of healthy foods in socially contrasting localities in the West of Scotland. *Health Bull,* 51:276–84.

Stansfield, S.A., Davey Smith, G., and Marmot, M. (1993). Association between physical and psychological morbidity in the Whitehall II Study. *J Psychosom Res,* 37:227–38.

Stark, R. (1987). Deviant places: a theory of the ecology of crime. *Criminology,* 25:893–909.

Susser, M. (1994). The logic in ecological: I. The logic of analysis. *Am J Public Health,* 84: 825–9.

Townsend, P., Phillimore, P., and Beattie, A. (1988). *Health and deprivation: inequality and the North.* London: Routledge.

Von Korff, M., Koepsell, T., Curry, S., and Diehr, P. (1992). Multi level analysis in epidemiologic research on health behaviours and outcomes. *Am J Epidemiol,* 135:1077–82.

Wilkinson, R.G. (1996). *Unhealthy societies: the afflictions of inequality.* London: Routledge.

Wilkinson, R. (1997). Health inequalities: relative or absolute material standards? *BMJ,* 314:591–4.

Wolf, S. (1993). Social environment and health: the struggle to document a truism. *Integr Physiol Behav Sci,* 28:115–7.

Wyke, S., Campbell, G., and McIver, S. (1992). The provision of primary care services in a working class and middle class locality in Glasgow. *Br J Gen Pract,* 42:271–5.

15

Multilevel Approaches to Understanding Social Determinants

MICHAEL MARMOT

A subtitle for this chapter might well consist of a series of questions. How might cortisol levels in anesthetized baboons relate to government policy? Should decisions about public health strategy take into account data on Kyoto-Wistar rats? Is a death from alcoholic cirrhosis in Hungary relevant to improving health in Manchester in the north of England? Why should the fibrinogen level of a clerical assistant in the British Civil Service be an important piece of the puzzle in understanding social determinants of health? How does Nathan Detroit's girlfriend help in illuminating the mind–body problem?

This chapter attempts to sketch out preliminary answers to these questions. I start from the view that by attempting to answer questions such as these we gain a better chance of understanding how social forces act on individuals to affect their biological processes and change disease risk. Such questions also lead to an exploration of how biology shapes behavior, which may in turn affect both social processes and disease risk. Although I shall be more concerned with the

first of these, how social processes affect biology, the second is also clearly relevant to an understanding of how biological and social processes interact to affect susceptibility to disease.

The message of the chapter is that to understand the social determinants of health we have to use data from international comparisons, from within-country differences, from studies of individuals, and from studies of biological processes in animals and humans.

INTRODUCTION

The following topics may help to amplify the questions set out in the subtitle of this chapter and by so doing pose the problems that require explanation.

The Social Gradient in Disease

What started out as "good housekeeping" in the first Whitehall study of British civil servants has shaped 20 subsequent years of research. Initially, when we noted that coronary heart disease mortality was higher in the lower echelons of the British Civil Service than among the top grades we were somewhat surprised. The 25-year follow-up of the Whitehall I participants confirms the original finding of an inverse gradient in mortality: the lower the grade the higher the mortality (Marmot and Shipley 1996). Figure 15–1 shows this by age at death (Marmot and Shipley, unpublished). At younger ages the relative mortality differential between bottom and top grades is fourfold. The relative difference declines somewhat at older ages but the absolute difference is increased. Any potential explanation for this finding has to deal with the issue of the gradient. As so often, when examining environmental risks we do not appear to be dealing with a threshold, i.e., a division between those in poverty and others. The issue here is, in a sense, whether grade of employment is a proxy for how much "exposure" an individual has had.

Table 15–1 shows that what was true at 10 years of follow-up (Marmot et al. 1984) is still the case at 25 years: The social gradient in mortality is observed for most of the major causes of death. The challenge for explanation is not only to explain the gradient but also to have an account of why there

should be a gradient in so many different causes of death.

The relevance to policy flows from the proposition that, in principle, it should be possible for everyone below the top grade of the Civil Service to have health status approximating that of the top grade. We know that the slope of the social gradient in mortality can change. In England and Wales for example it increased quite sharply over the period 1971–1991 (Drever et al. 1996). If it is possible for the slope of the gradient to increase, it should be possible to achieve a narrowing of the social differential. The limits to such an achievement are likely to be social, political, and economic. However, to move in the direction of such progress we need to understand the causes of this gradient in health.

European East–West Differences in Health

In Europe during the postwar period, health as measured by life expectancy paid little respect to political boundaries. Figure 15–2 shows data for three countries from the former Austro-Hungarian Empire for life expectancy at age 15. Removing the effects of infant mortality, between 1950 and 1970 the three countries differed little (Chewe

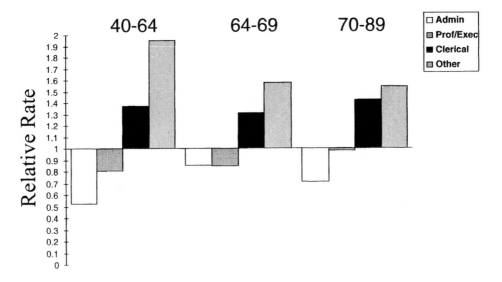

Figure 15–1. All-cause mortality by grade and age—Whitehall men 25-year follow-up (Marmot and Shipley, unpublished).

Table 15–1. Whitehall 25 year mortality (rate ratios and number of deaths) by Civil Service grade and cause of death

Cause of death (ICD code)	Rate ratio				
	Administrative	Professional/ Executive	Clerical	Other	χ^2 test for trend (1 df)
Lung cancer (162.1)	0.6 (16)	1.0 (348)	1.9 (159)	2.5 (135)	102.77
Other cancer (140–239, excluding 162.1)	0.8 (71)	1.0 (1063)	1.1 (279)	1.2 (182)	11.47
CHD (410–414)	0.8 (102)	1.0 (1628)	1.3 (517)	1.4 (332)	52.39
Cerebrovascular disease (430–438)	0.9 (26)	1.0 (361)	1.3 (119)	1.1 (68)	3.72
Other cardiovascular (404, 420–429, 440–458)	0.7 (23)	1.0 (374)	1.5 (138)	1.5 (92)	24.28
Chronic bronchitis (491–492)	0.6 (2)	1.0 (40)	4.3 (47)	4.8 (35)	54.30
Other respiratory (460–490, 493–519)	0.7 (20)	1.0 (322)	2.0 (162)	2.5 (129)	94.19
Gastrointestinal disease (520–577)	0.9 (7)	1.0 (92)	1.3 (28)	2.0 (27)	9.20
Genitourinary disease (580–607)	0.9 (4)	1.0 (50)	1.4 (18)	2.5 (22)	10.58
Accident and violence (800–949, 960–978)	0.7 (3)	1.0 (51)	1.5 (16)	1.6 (10)	3.09
Suicide (950–959, 980–989)	0.5 (2)	1.0 (45)	1.3 (12)	1.2 (6)	0.95
Other deaths	0.6 (11)	1.0 (201)	1.2 (58)	1.1 (33)	2.71
Causes not related to smoking*					
Cancer	0.9 (52)	1.0 (719)	1.0 (174)	1.2 (118)	3.37
Noncancer	0.8 (47)	1.0 (732)	1.4 (250)	1.6 (173)	43.92
All causes**	0.8 (290)	1.0 (4586)	1.4 (1557)	1.5 (1073)	260.54

*Includes men whose specific cause of death was not known.

**All causes less 140–141, 143–149, 150, 157, 160–163, 188–189, 400–404, 410–414, 426, 491, 492, 430–438, 440–448, 480–486, 531–534.

Network 1996). From around 1970 on, the figures diverge. Typical of the countries of "western" Europe, Austria showed a clear improvement in life expectancy in the subsequent 25 years, whereas there was stagnation or even decline in Czechoslovakia (later the Czech Republic) and Hungary. This was even more marked in the countries of the former Soviet Union. In Russia, life expectancy at age 15 for men declined from 52 years in 1987 to less than 45 years in 1994.

Overall, in the 1990s there was a 6-year gap in life expectancy between countries of eastern and western Europe. Of this 6 years slightly more than 3 years was due to cardiovascular mortality, 1.2 years to external causes of death (i.e., accidents and violence), and slightly under 1 year to infant mortality. The mortality crisis in eastern Europe has predominantly affected middle-aged men. There is much interest in the effects on chronic disease of factors operating during fetal development, infancy, and childhood (Barker 1992; Kuh and Ben-Shlomo 1997). If the worsening of the health situation in the countries of central and eastern Europe was a result of circumstances of early life, one might expect mortality patterns to show a cohort effect. There is in fact no evidence of a cohort effect (Marmot and Bobak, unpublished). This suggests that the health situation in the countries of central and eastern Europe relates to conditions in

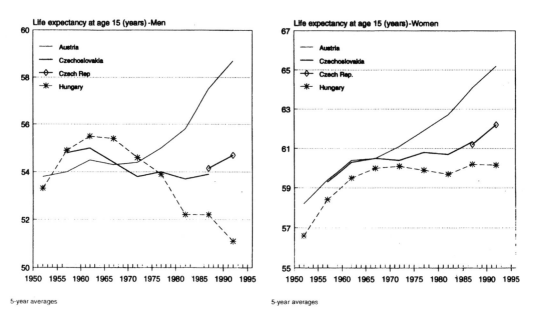

Figure 15–2. Life expectancy at age 15 in Austria, Hungary and Czechoslovakia 1950–94 (men and women) (Chewe Network 1996).

those countries operating during the 1970s and beyond.

We have hypothesized that the causes of the socioeconomic differences in disease within a country such as Great Britain may be similar to the causes of the east–west differences in mortality.

Learning from Nonhuman Primates

Evans drew parallels between what he termed long-term studies of free-living primates: Sapolsky's studies of baboons in the Serengeti ecosystem and our studies of civil servants in the Whitehall ecosystem (Evans 1996). His point was that social animals such as baboons form into hierarchies, as do human primates, and indicators of ill-health appear to follow a similar social gradient. Similarly the studies of other primate colonies may illuminate biological underpinnings of psychosocial influences on disease.

The Mind–Body Problem

In considering social influences, we should recognize that an important gateway to health is through the mind (A. Tarlov, personal communication). This is not a proposition that is doubted as a result of people's everyday experience. An old lady dies the day after her 100th birthday; a man dies within weeks of the death of his wife of 50 years; Damon Runyon's Adelaide develops a cold wondering if Nathan Detroit will turn their 14-year engagement into marriage (Runyon 1997); people succumb to a variety of disorders after stressful life changes or chronic difficulties.

There has been no difficulty imagining that stress is related to disease. Perhaps the reason why pioneers such as Selye (1956, 1978) did not gain ready acceptance is that the concept was seen as not sufficiently scientific. The scientific challenge has been conception, definition, and measurement of psychosocial factors and examination of the pathways by which they operate.

Genes, Early Life, Lifecourse, and Adult Social Circumstances

Many of us study the influence of current circumstances on disease risk. We do this for several reasons. First, the evidence suggests that current social circumstances are important determinants of disease risk. Second, there are practical difficulties in mounting studies that trace influences through a whole life on subsequent disease. Third, while it is important to understand that policies for today's children may improve health for the next generation of adults, we also wish to find ways of improving the health of today's adults.

That said, people do not arrive into their social positions in adulthood by chance. Their social position is affected by what they bring with them from earlier life, as is their response to social circumstances. We need to have a way of thinking about the interactions between genetic endowment and experiences from early life and adult social circumstances.

MODELS

Einstein has been reported to have said something along the lines of: *Our scientific view of the universe should be as simple as possible but not more simple than that.* A model that showed all the possible ways that all the possible social influences might affect the variety of diseases would be impossibly complex. Further, its complexities would be such that it would not be a useful guide to scientific study.

At the other extreme a model along the lines of "poverty causes disease" is likely to be too simple for scientific understanding, although it might be argued it is sufficient for policy, if alleviation of poverty reduces disease rates. Perhaps. But what if the model were "inequality is associated with disease"? Here, the policy options are not so clear. Which inequality? Income? Wealth? Social status? Social capital? Even if the evidence were that it was income inequality that was driving the health inequalities, then what? Fiscal policy can effect post-tax income inequalities but has no impact on pretax inequalities. If the source of these were understood better, we might conclude

that they were not within easy grasp of government policy.

To reduce inequalities in health, we do need to understand better the mediators. Further, a case can be made that in order to demonstrate that a particular psychosocial factor is both a cause of ill-health and a contributor to social inequalities in health, an understanding of biological mechanisms is important.

This suggests that we need simplified models of how these different levels of cause operate. Figure 15–3 presents a version of the model that helps guide our research. A caricature of some social epidemiology would be that it has spent too much time relating an indicator of social structure, such as income, education, or occupation, to mortality or other health outcome without asking why. The research task is to give an account of what links social structure to health outcomes—to ask, what are the intermediary steps? Without difficulty one could add categories and several more arrows to this sketch, but we have seen our task as putting in notional path coefficients to this diagram. We want therefore to know how potential causal factors relate to social structure, and we want to understand how they relate to health behaviors or to more direct psychological processes that influence the body's psycho–neuro–endocrine–immune pathways.

This model helps not only to understand how potential causal factors may interrelate, it also provides a guide to potential intervention points. To illustrate, let us consider the example of plasma fibrinogen level. Plasma fibrinogen has been shown to be a risk factor for cardiovascular disease. We have shown that plasma fibrinogen is related to low control in the workplace, to health behaviors such as smoking and exercise, to height and father's social class, and it follows an inverse social gradient in that the lower grades of the British Civil Service have higher levels (Markowe et al. 1985; Brunner et al. 1996). There is a trial currently underway testing the efficacy of war-

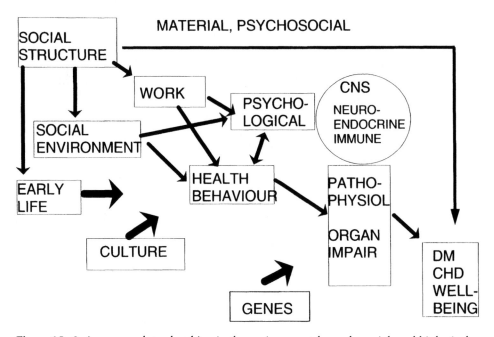

Figure 15–3. An approach to sketching in the environmental, psychosocial, and biological pathways linking socioeconomic status to diabetes mellitus (DM), coronary heart disease (CHD), and well-being.

farin, which lowers plasma fibrinogen level, in reducing cardiovascular disease. If this proves efficacious one potential point of intervention might be medical care. A second point of intervention may be attempts to change smoking and exercise, i.e., influence individual behaviors. A third point of intervention might be attention to work environments that might create more control for a higher proportion of employees. A fourth might be attention to childhood socioeconomic environment given the association between fibrinogen level and father's social class. If such interventions were successful there would be a reduction in the social gradient in plasma fibrinogen level. However, our analyses suggest that these factors do not explain all of the social gradient in fibrinogen. This exposes ways in which the model needs to be enriched.

Rather than construct one megamodel to take into account all possible strands of the causal web, it is almost certainly more use-

ful to construct different models for different purposes. For example, Kuh and colleagues are concerned with chains of risk linking factors that operate at various points of the lifecourse to adult health. They have put forward Figure 15–4 as a guide to their research (1997). This does not replace the model in Figure 15–3 but is complementary to it.

We are collaborating with Andrew Steptoe, a psychologist. He is studying psychobiological processes in disease etiology. This requires more detail than is given in Figure 15–3, and different detail than that in Figure 15–4. His outline is in Figure 15–5 (Steptoe 1998). It reflects the need for better specification of which psychological and which biological factors are involved in, for example, cardiovascular disease.

To delve further into biological mechanisms, will, again, require further specification. For example, Lightman is concerned with neuroendocrine and immune mecha-

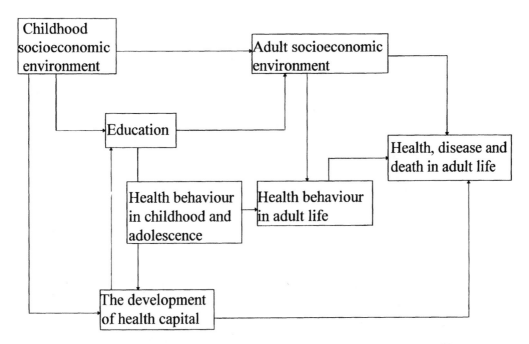

Figure 15–4. Examples of chains of risk (Kuh et al. 1997).

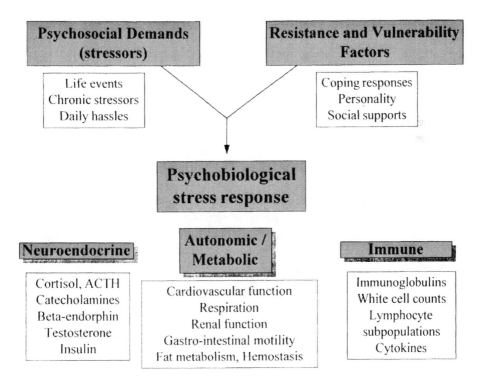

Figure 15–5. Outline of the major physiological elements of the psychobiological stress response (Steptoe, 1998).

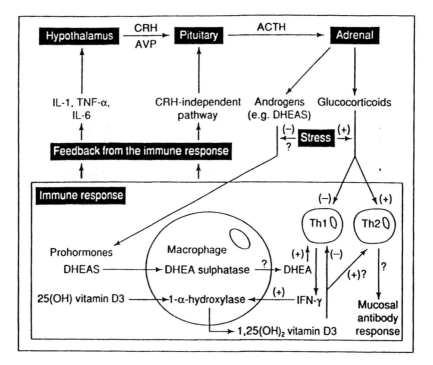

Figure 15–6. Neuroendocrine and immune mechanisms in response to stress (Rook et al. 1994).

nisms in disease. An example of a model guiding his research is Figure 15–6 (Rook et al. 1994).

The choice between these models is not one of aesthetics; the models serve different purposes. They complement each other. Figure 15–3 attempts to give the social epidemiological perspective; Figure 15–4 takes a lifecourse approach; Figure 15–5 is psychobiological; and Figure 15–6 explores endocrine and immune mechanisms. There should, in addition, be one or more models that explicate social and economic processes. The point here is not whether each of these models is precisely correct. Each is susceptible to criticism and no doubt could or should change. However, if our aim is to understand how social influences affect health, and in particular cause social inequalities in health, we will need models such as these that illustrate the various levels at which responsible factors may operate, and the pathways involved.

INTEGRATING LEVELS

As stated above, the purpose of this chapter is to make the case that we need to integrate research from different levels of inquiry. This is not to argue that any single piece of research needs to be integrated. In fact, one could almost argue the contrary. The more specific and focused the research the greater the likelihood of providing a useful answer to a question. The point of integration is to put the specific questions in a context so that they may help provide answers to the broad question related to the social determinants of health in populations. Further, by having the broader question in mind to provide context, the nature of the specific questions might change. It is not therefore a matter of choosing between specific focus or integration: both are required.

This sets the theme for the next section, in which a number of pairs of alternatives are listed. In each case, the answer I shall offer to the question of which of the pair is more important will be: both. Both are important to gaining a full picture of the social determinants of health. The attempt here is to be illustrative rather than exhaustive.

Study Animals or Humans?

Reference was made above to Sapolsky's studies of baboons. Figure 15–7 reproduces Sapolsky's finding that high-density lipoprotein (HDL) cholesterol was lower in low-status than high-status baboons, but there was no difference in low-density lipoprotein (LDL) cholesterol (Sapolsky and Mott 1987). Figure 15–7 shows findings for these biochemical variables from Whitehall II by grade of employment. It shows, similarly that low-status civil servants have lower HDL cholesterol than high-status ones. Low HDL cholesterol is part of the metabolic syndrome of insulin resistance which shows an inverse social gradient: higher prevalence in lower grades (Brunner et al. 1997). Sapolsky has evidence that plasma cortisol is associated with the status differential in lipid disturbances. This suggests that activity of the hypothalamic–pituitary–adrenal axis is involved in mediating the link between social status and metabolic disturbances.

Studies of nonhuman primates also illustrate the importance of the sympathetic–adrenomedullary system. The Bowman Gray studies of cynomolgus monkeys are classics in the field. They have demonstrated that low-status females and males have more atherosclerosis than those of high status (Shively and Clarkson 1994; Shively et al. 1994). However, this can be changed, at least in males. In one experiment, males from different social groupings were intermingled. Under these circumstances of social instability, high-status males developed more atherosclerosis, thus reversing the pattern seen in stable groups. This reversal can be abolished by prior treatment with propanolol, which is a beta sympathetic blocker. It thus implicates the sympathoadrenomedullary pathway in the reversal of the social gradient under conditions of acute stress for high-status males (Manuck et al. 1995).

It may be argued that although we share more than 90% of our genes in common

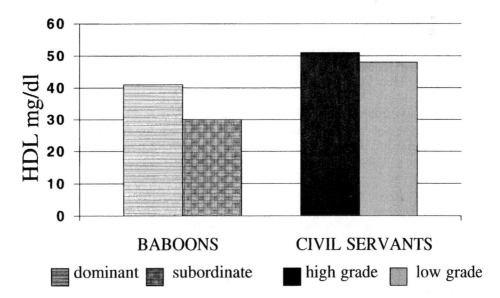

Figure 15–7. High-density lipoprotein (HDL) cholesterol in high- and low-status male baboons and male civil servants (Sapolsky and Mott 1987; Brunner et al. 1997).

with other primate species, psychosocial processes in humans are not the same as in apes and monkeys. This argument would say that we, therefore, have little to learn from the study of nonhuman primates, let alone from rodents or other animals. If only because of human language, if for no other reason, human's social and psychological interaction is a good deal more subtle and complex than that of other animals. These animal studies do tell us, however, about biological pathways that are plausible links between psychosocial factors and disease processes.

It is tempting to think that there may be other lessons, as well. For example, we may learn about the potential importance of both genetic predisposition and patterns of upbringing to frequency of health problems. Suomi's long-term elegant studies (1997) among rhesus monkeys (*Macaca mulatta*) show that about 20% of any troop are high reactors. They are more likely than others to exhibit depressive responses to maternal separation with greater and more prolonged activation of the hypothalamic–pituitary–adrenal axis, more dramatic sympathetic arousal, more rapid central norepinephrine turnover, and greater selective immunosuppression. These differential responses remain quite stable throughout development. Evidence suggests that the pattern of high reaction is genetically determined but it can be reproduced in nongenetically predisposed animals by raising them without their mothers. Interestingly these high reactors tend to end up at the bottom of the social hierarchy. There is also potential intergenerational transmission, nongenetic, of this tendency. Females raised without their mothers are likely to be abusive or neglectful of their first born offspring.

This genetic high-reactor destiny can be interrupted by changing the environment. When animals genetically predisposed to become high reactors were cross fostered with especially nurturant mothers they showed no signs of the behavioral disorders usually associated with being a high reactor. Rather they showed signs of precocious be-

havioral development and rose to the top of the hierarchy as adults. When the females among them became mothers they showed the maternal style typical of their especially nurturant foster mothers.

One further example may provide a caution to those who view genetic predisposition as some sort of irreversible genetic destiny. One animal model, much used for studying hypertension, is that of the spontaneously hypertensive rat (SHR). An experiment in cross-fostering, however, showed the importance of early environment in expressing this characteristic (Cierpial and McCarthy 1987). When pups of SHR rats were cross fostered with Kyoto-Wistar mothers they did not develop hypertension as they matured. This "pure" genetic characteristic could not manifest itself as the phenotype of hypertension without the appropriate environmental stimulus.

Individual or Population Risks

Epidemiology grows out of at least two distinct traditions: public health and clinical medicine. The public health tradition emphasizes the environmental causes of illness. Practitioners who come to epidemiology out of clinical medicine tend to be concerned, as clinical medicine is, primarily with the individual. In the end, it is the individual who gets sick; indeed it is his coronary arteries, her kidneys, or his gastrointestinal tract that becomes afflicted. Therefore medicine's concern with epidemiology is to help understand individual risks or indeed risks to parts of individuals. Without some focus on the individual, we could not understand mechanisms of disease. If we focus only on individuals, we cannot obtain the perspective on social influences that provides the integration that this chapter is calling for.

Geoffrey Rose argued that the determinants of variations between individuals within a population may be different from the determinants of variations between populations. Put differently, he suggested that one type of question is, where do individuals lie on the population distribution of a

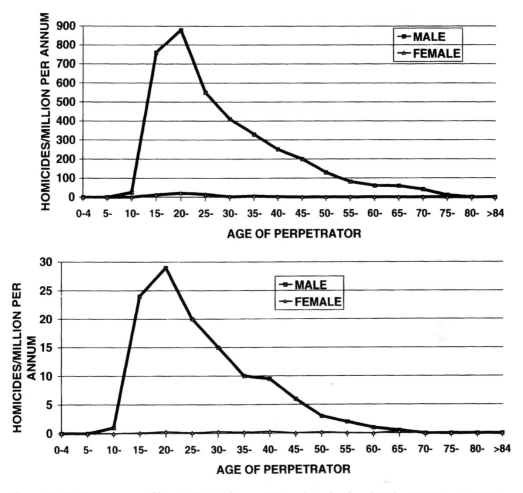

Figure 15–8. Perpetrators of homicide in Chicago (A), and England and Wales (B) (Cronin 1991).

characteristic. A second type of question is, what is the position of the distribution, for example the mean, which may vary between populations (1992)?

Figure 15–8 illustrates this in a surprising way. (This is taken from a discussion of Rose's work [Marmot 1998].) It shows that the age/sex distribution of the perpetrators of homicide does not differ at all between Chicago and England and Wales. The rates are much higher for males between ages 15 and 30 than for any other group, with a peak in both cases at ages 20 to 24. This has been interpreted as a clear example of an evolved propensity of males to react to environmental challenges in violent ways

(Cronin 1991). Just as striking as the identity of the age/sex distributions is the difference in scale. The homicide rate in Chicago is 30 times that of England and Wales: At its peak, 900 per million compared to 30 per million. There may indeed be an evolved tendency that determines a constancy of the shape of the age/sex distribution. The position of the distribution, the 30-fold higher rate in Chicago is, however, determined by the social environment. There may be, therefore, two types of question. The first relates to individual differences. Why is it that within Chicago some people commit homicide and others do not? A second type of question is why there are such gross differences in rates between Chicago and England and Wales? The division between individual risks and population risks is not only a division between Chicago and England and Wales. Within Chicago, there are neighborhood differences in rates of violent crime that are related to properties of those neighborhoods (Sampson et al. 1997). Nevertheless, the individual difference question is why some individuals within a disordered neighborhood commit homicide, where the majority do not.

If we wish to prevent homicides, we could perhaps have a strategy that sought out high risk individuals and attempted to intervene. Alternatively, we could accept the homicide rate for what it is—namely, a reflection of a disordered society—and ask the appropriate question of how to improve that society. If the homicide rate is high, it is almost certain that a range of other social pathologies are also highly prevalent.

This argues for analyses of environmental-level characteristics. Such analyses at the environmental level are usually criticized for being subject to the ecological fallacy: i.e., it is incorrectly assumed that correlations that apply to groups will apply to individual risks. Perhaps we should turn this fallacy on its head and argue that analyses of individual risks may be subject to the atomistic fallacy: i.e., analyses at the individual level may be inappropriate if we are seeking to determine social environmental causes of illness (Marmot 1998).

As one approach, individual characteristics may, on aggregate, characterize an environment. We have been studying the relation between perceived control and markers of ill-health in a number of eastern European populations (Marmot and Bobak in press; Bobak et al. 1998; Bobak et al. submitted). We asked whether it was perhaps possible to characterize degree of control for a whole population. We therefore plotted mean of perceived control over health for seven eastern European populations against CHD mortality rates and found a strong inverse association (Figure 15–9), (Bobak, unpublished).

These are individual characteristics summed up to apply to whole populations. The question is whether there are environmental characteristics independent of the properties of individuals who live in those areas. A study of the health effects of air pollution is likely to start by looking at areas of high exposure and low exposure, rather than individual differences in exposure. Similarly, those arguing on the side of an area effect might argue that a polluted water supply is a characteristic of an area. On the other side, one could point to John Snow's classic studies of cholera (1855). Part of the compelling evidence for the importance of water in cholera transmission was the observation of individual differences in risk. Within one street some households were affected and others not. This related to the source of their domestic water. The Alameda County study showed that mortality rates were higher in poverty areas independent of a wide range of individual characteristics, including income (Haan et al. 1987). This argued for an area effect. Alternatively, it could be posited that the individual characteristics of people living in different areas were incompletely characterized.

One way of settling the argument as to whether there is an area effect over and above the characteristics of individuals is to discuss range of exposure. Thus, there appears to be an area effect for pollution because within an area there is comparatively narrow range of exposure compared to the variation in exposure between areas. There is not some emergent property of areas—simply individuals who are exposed or not exposed. According to this line of reason, the question is simply a practical one of designing a study with sufficient range of variation. There are no group effects because in the end it is individuals who get sick.

This is not a wholly satisfactory answer. Rereading Durkheim (1897, 1997) and Geoffrey Rose (1992), I asked, why are death rates relatively so fixed? In the United Kingdom there are 152,000 deaths a year from coronary heart disease. Next year there may be a few less because, happily,

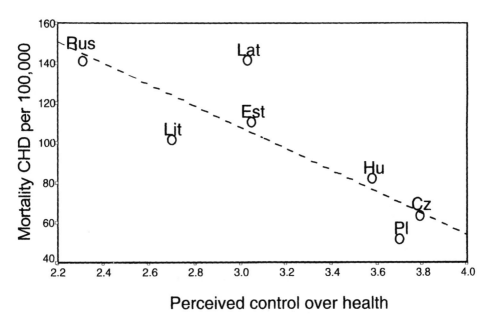

Figure 15-9. Ecological analyses of relation between mean of perceived control from sample surveys in each of Russia (Rus), Lithuania (Lit), Latvia (Lat), Estonia (Est), Hungary (Hu), Czech Republic (Cz), and Poland (Pl), and CHD mortality rates in those countries (Bobak, unpublished).

there is a long-term secular decline in CHD and because the aging of the population makes little year on year impact. There may be a few less but it will not be as few as 100,000 deaths or even 130,000. It will turn out to be very close to a rate of 186/100,000. Similarly, next year the rate in Hungary will be higher than the United Kingdom, close to 250/100,000 (Marmot 1998).

Cause-specific death rates are characteristics of societies. There must be determinants of these patterns. If we start with characteristics of individuals we ask, did the individuals who died smoke, or did they have high cholesterol? But the individuals who died this year will not contribute to next year's death rate. These are characteristics of societies, over and above the characteristics of individuals, that determine the death rate. Similarly for more than a century, areas in the north of England (including Manchester) have had higher mortality rates than areas in the south.

The question then is whether there are emergent properties of societies that are not simply the sum of individual characteristics. Might the unemployment rate have an effect on the health of a population not only because individuals who are unemployed have worse health than others? Social integration and social capital might be candidates for such emergent properties. This is discussed in Chapter 8 of this volume. In the end, of course, it is individuals who do or do not succumb to disease. However, if the primary determinants of disease are mainly economic and social, its remedies must also be economic and social (Rose 1992).

This takes us back to the hypotheses stated above: that the causes of social variations within a society may be similar to the causes of the east–west differences in mortality. Consider the hypotheses of control and health. Perceived control is an individual-level characteristic: people perceive they have control over aspects of their lives or they do not. It may also be a characteristic of the environment. There are work environments that allow people varying degrees of control (Karasek and Theorell 1990). Control can therefore be seen as a characteristic of the environment which may contribute to social inequalities in cardiovascular disease (Bosma et al. 1997; Marmot et al. 1997). It may also be a characteristic of a population, as illustrated above for the countries of central and eastern Europe.

As this "control" example illustrates, it is not possible to make a categorical statement that causes of individual differences *are* distinct from the causes of population differences. It may be the case. There are likely to be a large number of cases that fit with Suomi's studies of rhesus monkeys or the studies of SHR rats described above. These illustrate that there are genetic predispositions to disease that will account, to some extent, for individual differences, but these interact with or are modified by influences from the environment.

Such differences in susceptibility need not, of course, be genetic. Barker (1997) and Hales (1997) emphasize that in utero exposures may condition risks of subsequent development of diabetes. They emphasise that low birth weight, followed by development of obesity in adulthood, puts an individual at particularly high risk.

Psychosocial or Material Factors?

This question became a particular debating topic after *the Black Report* on inequalities in health (Black et al. 1988; MacIntyre 1997). It became related to the question of absolute vs. relative deprivation. One version of the argument is that social factors cause illness through an effect of poverty on ill-health. Poverty is, almost by definition, a reflection of absolute deprivation. Here, absolute deprivation means lack of the material necessities of life. The link between poverty and ill-health could also be the result of increased exposure to material hazards.

We have argued that the Whitehall gradient in morbidity and mortality is consistent with the effect of relative rather than absolute deprivation (Marmot et al. 1995). People second from the top in the British

Civil Service have worse health than those at the top. People third from the top have worse health than those above them in the hierarchy. It is difficult to think of this as material deprivation. It is the case that Civil Service employment grade is correlated with income. Hence, the lower the grade the less the access to material resources. Nevertheless, most civil servants are above the poverty threshold below which the obvious causes of material deprivation operate.

Wilkinson, from a different perspective, has also argued the case for relative deprivation. He points out that within a society income is related to mortality. Among rich countries, however, there is little relation between mean income and mortality. He finds the relation is with income inequality (1996). His explanation is that within a society income maps onto social status. This is why it is related to mortality, not because of income level per se. Between countries, income level is not an important predictor because social status of countries is a less meaningful concept to individuals within countries. Income inequality is a predictor because it indicates other social features of a society. Wilkinson therefore emphasizes psychosocial explanations of inequalities in health.

As the model, reproduced as Figure 15–3 should make clear, pursuing a psychosocial explanation does not negate the importance of material factors. Such material factors may be influenced by psychosocial factors. For example, the persistence of smoking in low-income women may relate to the psychosocial factors operating on those women (Graham 1994). Alternatively, they may provide the substrate on which psychosocial factors operate. For example, the health record of Albania has inspired some comment. Unique among the countries of central and eastern Europe, its health record continued to improve, despite one of the more restrictive and repressive political regimes. One explanation for this apparent paradox is that Albania is, in essence, a Mediterranean country. The Mediterranean diet may be an important factor in keeping rates of coronary heart disease low and hence improving overall life expectancy (Gjonca and Bobak 1997).

One cannot avoid the concept of multiple causation. This is not unique to the study on noninfectious disease. The tubercle bacillus is the specific cause of tuberculosis. Without infection with the tubercle bacillus people cannot get tuberculosis. But most people infected with the tubercle bacillus do not have clinical tuberculosis. Other factors—for example, those associated with poverty and nutrition—influence susceptibility. Similarly, it is rare for a nonsmoker to suffer from lung cancer. But a lower-grade civil servant who smokes has a higher risk of lung cancer than a higher-grade civil servant with a similar smoking history (Marmot et al. 1984; van Rossum submitted).

The evidence reviewed in this book makes the case that psychosocial factors are important intermediaries between social influences and disease. This does not mean that psychosocial factors determine which disease people get or that they operate in isolation from other causes of disease.

Where malnutrition is rife and mean plasma cholesterol levels of the population are low, no amount of stress associated with poverty will lead to epidemic coronary heart disease. Where overnutrition is the problem and mean plasma cholesterol levels of the population are high, as in Britain, coronary heart disease rates of the population are high. This does not, however, explain the social gradient in Whitehall. Figure 15–10 from the 25-year follow-up of the Whitehall study confirms the findings of the 10-year follow-up: i.e., smoking, cholesterol, blood pressure, sedentary lifestyle, and height explain no more than a third of the gradient in coronary heart disease mortality. Other factors act on the substrate provided by these risk factors. Our evidence from the Whitehall II study is that the psychosocial work environment, in particular low control, may make an important contribution to accounting for the gradient in coronary heart disease (Marmot et al. 1997).

In trying to distinguish between psychosocial and other explanations for the social gradient in disease (see Figure 15–3),

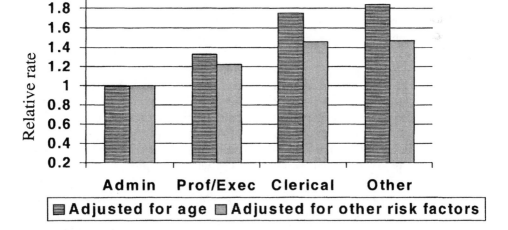

controlling for (a) age, and (b) age, smoking systolic blood pressure, plasma cholesterol concentration, height and blood sugar

Figure 15–10. Whitehall CHD mortality—25-year follow-up adjusted for risk factors (Marmot and Shipley, unpublished).

there is a potential measurement issue. It has been suggested that low control in the workplace appears to account for much of the social gradient in cardiovascular disease only because it is a measure of social status (Davey Smith and Harding 1997). Hence in a multivariate statistical model, one measure of social status "accounts" for the association with disease of another measure of social status. Taken to its logical conclusion this line of argument suggests that we can never "account" for the association between socioeconomic position and disease risk. Any potential intermediary must be associated with socioeconomic position. Hence it could be argued that smoking appears to account for some of the social gradient in disease simply because it is a marker of socioeconomic status. This line of reasoning suggests that one should be cautious in concluding that any indicator of social status has a causal relation with disease.

The view argued in this chapter is that the enterprise of attempting to explain the reasons for the socioeconomic gradient in health and disease is not fatally flawed. It must, however, go beyond simple correlations. Many factors are associated with socioeconomic position. The choice of which is important in the causal link with disease will depend on its performance in models such as those presented in Figures 15–3 through 15–6. Thus, one would not argue that low control might be an important link between socioeconomic status and ill-health simply on the basis of one multivariate analysis of civil servants. Quite apart from epidemiological replication, one should look at psychobiological studies of the links between low control and potential biological pathways and at animal studies.

So far, I have avoided the issue of causation of specific diseases as against general susceptibility to disease. In the Whitehall study the social gradient in mortality cut across most of the major causes of death. Men in the lower grades of the British Civil Service had higher mortality rates from heart disease, stroke, respiratory diseases, gastrointestinal diseases, cancers linked to smoking, cancers not linked to smoking, and external causes of death (Marmot et al. 1984). One approach to explanation is that there are specific explanations for each of these. Lower social status may be associated with more smoking, crowding, damp houses, infections, poor nutrition, air pollution, and other specific noxious influences. An alternate explanation is that susceptibility to disease varies with social status. The specific disease depends on other exposures. This idea of general susceptibility goes back to Selye (1956, 1978) and the early work of Syme (Syme and Berkman 1976) and Cassel (1976). We lack good models of general susceptibility. It may be that the current interest in psychoneuroimmunology may address this lack.

Early Life or Current Circumstances

In a series of studies Barker has produced strong evidence that exposures in early life have a powerful influence on the risk of developing chronic disease in adulthood (1992). In particular, he suggests that there are critical periods of development. If the fetus is exposed to maternal malnutrition during one of these critical periods it will have increased risk of diabetes or cardiovascular disease in later life. In his model, although a "once-off" exposure has a permanent effect in setting risk, it does not act to the exclusion of subsequent influences. His data suggest that people with low birth weight who subsequently become obese are at particularly high risk of diabetes (Lithell et al. 1996). Wadsworth, following the 1946 birth cohort has shown similar results for hypertension (1997).

Power and Hertzman considered two types of effect of early life on adult health: latency and pathway models. The latency model is the effect that Barker describes. Exposure in utero during a critical period can program the individual to susceptibility to subsequent disease risk. In the pathway model, people who are exposed to adverse circumstances early in life are exposed to adverse circumstances later (Power and Hertzman 1997). This is the type of model laid out in Figure 15–4.

Consideration of the lifecourse thus suggests three possible ways early experiences can affect adult disease risk. First, there may be latent effects consequent upon the exposure during a critical period. Second, there may be cumulation of advantage and disadvantage through the lifecourse which affect disease risk. Third, childhood experiences may have a determining effect on the circumstances in which an individual finds her- or himself during adulthood. It may be these circumstances in adulthood that affect risk, rather than the cumulation of experiences that preceded them. In practice all three processes are likely to be operative and their relative importance will vary depending both on the disease and on the circumstance (Kuh and Ben-Shlomo 1997).

Barker's body of evidence points clearly to an effect of critical periods. Power's studies of people followed to age 33 in the 1958 British birth cohort point to the effect on health of cumulation of advantage and disadvantage acting throughout the lifecourse (Power et al. 1998). She shows that at age 33 people whose social class, based on their occupation, was IV and V (semiskilled and unskilled) were more than twice as likely to be in poor health as those in social classes I and II. This excess risk of poor health in both men and women could be largely explained by a combination of influences from preschool, school age, and working life. The major factors identified were:

1. Socioeconomic environment at birth and (for women) in childhood
2. Socioemotional adjustment in adolescence (age 16)
3. Qualifications achieved at the end of school
4. Adult smoking at ages 23 to 33 (men)
5. Psychosocial job strain at age 33

Circumstances from early life cannot be the whole story. The increase in mortality in the countries of eastern Europe does not show a cohort pattern. It affects men of different ages in the middle-age range all at about the same time. The 7-year decline in life expectancy in Russia in less than a decade shows how powerful the effect of current social and economic circumstances can be. We know that not all groups in the countries of central and eastern Europe were affected equally by the mortality crisis. There are marked social gradients in mortality in these countries (Bobak and Marmot 1996). It may well be that people were rendered susceptible to the dramatic affects of altered social and economic circumstances by their earlier life experiences. Both are likely to be important "causes" of high rates of morbidity and mortality.

CONCLUSIONS

This chapter started with some apparently random questions. The intention of the chapter was to show that answers to questions about baboons, rats, Hungary, civil servants, the north of England, and Nathan Detroit's girlfriend are indeed relevant to understanding of the social determinants of health. Leonard Syme taught that when a problem is difficult it may have to be approached from several directions. Paraphrasing Medawar, we need to break up the scientific question of the social determinants of health into manageable pieces. There is no point in being lost in battle with problems that are too difficult to solve (Medawar 1967). We must not, however, focus on the manageable pieces to the exclusion of the larger picture.

The enterprise of understanding the social determinants of health entails an understanding of how society operates, an appreciation of the major causes of diseases under study, an understanding of psychological processes and how they may interact with relevant biological mechanisms, and a readiness to learn from animal models. On its own, without collaboration with these other disciplines, social epidemiology can progress only part of the way.

This chapter has argued the case for models that help us understand how the different levels interact. Any model is at best a simplification of a hypothesis, and at worst misleading. Nevertheless, such models may be a necessary faltering step on the way to understanding how the social determinants of health operate, and hence what can be done about them.

ACKNOWLEDGMENTS

Michael Marmot is supported by a Medical Research Council Research Professorship.

REFERENCES

Barker, D.J.P. (1992). *Fetal and infant origins of adult disease*. London: British Medical Journal.

Black, D., Morris, J.N., Smith, C., Townsend, P., and Whitehead, M. (1988). *Inequalities in health: the Black Report; the health divide*. London: Penguin.

Bobak, M., and Marmot, M.G. (1996). East–West mortality divide and its potential explanations: proposed research agenda. *BMJ*, 312:421–5.

Bobak, M., Marmot, M., Pikhart, H., Rose, R., Hertzman, C. (Submitted). Socioeconomic factors, material inequalities, and perceived control in self-rated health: cross-sectional data from seven post-communist countries.

Bobak, M., Pikhart, H., Hertzman, C., Rose, R., and Marmot, M. (1998). Socioeconomic factors, perceived control and self-reported health in Russia. A cross-sectional survey. *Soc Sci Med*, 47:269–72.

Bosma, H., Marmot, M.G., Hemingway, H., Nicholson, A., Brunner, E.J., and Stansfeld, S. (1997). Low job control and risk of coronary heart disease in the Whitehall II (prospective cohort) study. *BMJ*, 314:558–65.

Brunner, E., Davey Smith, G., Marmot, M., Canner, R., Beksinska, M., and O'Brien, J. (1996). Childhood social circumstances and psychosocial and behavioral factors as determinants of plasma fibrinogen. *Lancet*, 34:1008–13.

Brunner, E.J., Marmot, M.G., Nanchahal, K., Shipley, M.J., Stansfeld, S.A., Juneja, M., and Alberti, K.G.M.M. (1997). Social inequality in coronary risk: central obesity and the metabolic syndrome. Evidence from the Whitehall II study. *Diabetologia*, 40:1341–9.

Cassel, J.C. (1976). The contribution of the so-cial environment to host resistance. *Am J Epidemiol*, 104:107–23.

CHEWE network (1996) Explaining socioeconomic variations in coronary heart disease across eastern and western Europe. London: International Centre for Health and Society, University College London.

Cierpial, M.A., and McCarthy, R. (1987). Hypertension in SHR rats: contribution of maternal environment. *Am J Physiol*, 253:H980–4.

Cronin, H. (1991). *Ant and the peacock*. Cambridge, UK: Cambridge University Press.

Davey Smith, G., and Harding, S. (1997). Is control at work the key to socio-economic gradients in mortality? *Lancet*, 350:1369–70.

Drever, F., Whitehead, M., and Roden, M. (1996). Current patterns and trends in male mortality by social class (based on occupation). *Popul Trends*, 86:15–20.

Durkheim, É. (1897, 1997). *Suicide: a study in sociology*, ed. Simpson, G. (tr. Spaulding, J.A., and Simpson, G., 1951). New York: Free Press.

Evans, R.G. (1996). Health, hierarchy and hominids. In Culyer, A.J., and Wagstaff, A. (eds.), *Reforming health care systems: experiments with the NHS*. (Proceedings of the Annual Meetings of the British Association of the Advancement of Science (Section F), 1994.) Aldershot, UK: Edward Elgar, pp. 35–64.

Gjonca, A., and Bobak, M. (1997). Albanian paradox: another case of the protective effect of the Mediterranean lifestyle? *Lancet*, 350:1815–17.

Graham, H. (1994). Gender and class as dimensions of smoking behavior in Britain: insights from a survey of mothers. *Soc Sci Med*, 38:691–8.

Haan, M., Kaplan, G.A., and Camacho, T. (1987). Poverty and health: prospective evidence from the Alameda County study. *Am J Epidemiol*, 125:989–98.

Hales, C.N. (1997). Non-insulin-dependent diabetes mellitus. *Br Med Bull*, 53:109–22.

Karasek, R., and Theorell, T. (1990). *Healthy work: stress, productivity, and the reconstruction of working life*. New York: Basic Books.

Kuh, D., and Ben-Shlomo, Y. (1997). *A lifecourse approach to chronic disease epidemiology*. New York: Oxford University Press.

Kuh, D., Power, C., Blane, D., and Bartley, M. (1997). Social pathways between childhood and adult health. In Kuh, D., and Ben-Shlomo, Y. (eds.). *A lifecourse approach to chronic disease epidemiology*. New York: Oxford University Press, pp. 169–98.

Lithell, H.O., McKeigue, P.M., Berglund, L.,

Mohsen, R., Lithell, U.B., and Leon, D.A. (1996). Relation of size at birth to non-insulin dependent diabetes and insulin concentrations in men aged 50–60 years. *BMJ*, 312:406–10.

Macintyre, S. (1997). The Black Report and beyond: what are the issues? *Soc Sci Med*, 44:723–45.

Manuck, S.B., Marsland, A.L., Kaplan, J.R., and Williams, J.K. (1995). The pathogenicity of behavior and its neuroendocrine mediation: an example from coronary artery disease. *Psychosom Med*, 57:275–83.

Markowe, H.L.J., Marmot, M.G., Shipley, M.J., Bulpitt, C.J., Meade, T.W., Stirling, Y., Vickers, M.V., and Semmence, A. (1985). Fibrinogena: possible link between social class and coronary heart disease. *BMJ*, 291: 1312–4.

Marmot, M. (1998). Improvement of social environment to improve health. *Lancet*, 351: 57–60.

Marmot, M., and Bobak, M. (In press). Psychosocial and Biological Mechanisms Behind the Recent Mortality Crisis in Central and Eastern Europe. In Cornia, A.G. and Panicci, R. (eds.) *The Mortality Crisis in Transitional Economies*. Oxford University Press.

Marmot, M.G., and Shipley, M.J. (1996). Do socioeconomic differences in mortality persist after retirement? 25 year follow up of civil servants from the first Whitehall study. *BMJ*, 313:1177–80.

Marmot, M.G., Shipley, M.J., and Rose, G. (1984). Inequalities in death: specific explanations of a general pattern. *Lancet*, 1: 1003–6.

Marmot, M.G., Bobak, M., and Davey Smith, G. (1995). Explanations for social inequalities in health. In Amick, B.C., Levine, S., Tarlov, A.R., and Chapman Walsh, D. (eds.), *Society and health*. New York: Oxford University Press, pp. 172–210.

Marmot, M., Bosma, H., Hemingway, H., Brunner, E.J., and Stansfeld, S.A. (1997). Contribution of job control and other risk factors to social variations in coronary heart disease incidence. *Lancet*, 350:235–9.

Medawar, P.B. (1967). *The art of the soluble*. London: Methuen.

Power, C., and Hertzman, C. (1997). Social and biological pathways linking early life and adult disease. *Br Med Bull*, 53:210–22.

Power, C., Mathews, S., and Manor, O. (1998). Inequality in self-rated health: explanations from different stages in life. *Lancet*, 351: 1009–14.

Rook, G.A.W., Hernandez-Pando, R., and Lightman, S.L. (1994). Hormones, peripherally activated prohormones and regulation of the Th1/Th2 balance. *Immunol Today*, 15:301–3.

Rose, G. (1992). *The strategy of preventive medicine*. Oxford: Oxford University Press.

Runyon, D. (1997). *Guys and dolls and other stories*. London: Penguin.

Sampson, R.J., Raudenbush, S.W., and Earls, F. (1997). Neighborhoods and violent crime: a multilevel study of collective efficacy. *Science*, 277:915–24.

Sapolsky, R.M., and Mott, G.E. (1987). Social subordinance in wild baboons is associated with suppressed high density lipoprotein-cholesterol concentrations: the possible role of chronic social stress. *Endocrinology*, 121:1605–10.

Selye, H. (1956, 1978). *The stress of life* (rev. ed.). New York: McGraw-Hill.

Shively, C.A., and Clarkson, T.B. (1994). Social status and coronary artery atherosclerosis in female monkeys. *Art Thromb*, 14:721–6.

Shively, C.A., Adams, M.R., Kaplan, J.R., Williams, J.K., and Clarkson, T.B. (1994). Social stress, ovarian function, and coronary artery atherosclerosis in primates. In Czaikowski, S.M., Hill, D.R., and Clarkson, T.B. (eds.), *Proceedings of conference on women, behavior and cardiovascular disease, Bethesda, MD, Sept. 25–27, 1994*. Washington, DC: U.S. Government Printing Office, pp. 127–144.

Snow, J. (1855). *On the mode of communication of cholera* (2nd ed.). London: Churchill.

Steptoe, A. (1998). Psychophysiological bases of disease. In Johnston, M., and Johnston, D. (eds.), *Comprehensive clinical psychology*, vol. 8: *Health psychology*. New York: Elsevier Science, pp. 39–78.

Suomi, S.J. (1997). Early determinants of behavior: evidence from primate studies. *Br Med Bull*, 53:170–84.

Syme, S.L., and Berkman, L.F. (1976). Social class, susceptibility, and sickness. *Am J Epidemiol*, 104:1–8.

Van Rossum, C., Shipley, M., Van de Mheen, H., Grobbee, D., and Marmot, M.G. (Submitted). Employment grade differences in cause specific mortality. 25 year follow-up of civil servants from first Whitehall study.

Wadsworth, M.E.J. (1997). Changing social factors and their long-term implications for health. *Br Med Bull*, 53:198–209.

Wilkinson, R.G. (1996). *Unhealthy societies: the afflictions of inequality*. London: Routledge.

16

Health and Social Policy

S. JODY HEYMANN

The evidentiary base for social determinants of health has grown increasingly strong. The evidence shows that people living in poverty have poorer health, even when controlling for exposure to other known risk factors for disease (VanLoon et al. 1995; Fiscella and Franks 1997; Montgomery et al. 1996; Issler et al. 1996; Starfield 1992; Wise and Meyers 1988). Mortality rates are higher in states and countries where economic inequalities are greater (Adler et al. 1994; Ben-Shlomo et al. 1996). Job insecurity, job strain, and job loss lead to poorer health outcomes (Bosma et al. 1997; Brenner 1983; Haan 1985; Hinkle et al. 1968; House et al. 1986; Karasek 1979; Mattiasson et al. 1990), as do inadequate social supports (Johnson and Hall 1988; Berkman et al. 1992, 1993; Seeman et al. 1994; Berkman 1995). Racial discrimination contributes to a series of poorer health outcomes including high blood pressure and cardiac disease (Jones et al. 1991; Krieger and Sidney 1996).

These findings are a critically important start but their ultimate value will be determined by our ability to address the problems they underscore. Addressing social inequalities, discrimination, poor work and other social conditions presents new and different challenges than past public health problems.

When it was found that high cholesterol contributed to heart disease, recommendations that could be followed by individuals were made. Individuals could change their diet, exercise, take medication. Major social change was not believed to be necessary to address the risks associated with elevated cholesterol.

When smoking was found to be linked to a wide range of cancers and heart disease, again the approach began with individual recommendations. Smoking cessation programs that individuals could sign up for and pharmaceutical products to assist with nicotine withdrawal were developed. Social change was not initially believed to be necessary to address the effects of first-hand smoke, although recently it has played a crucial role. How essential social change was to a solution only became apparent when the cardiac, respiratory, and other effects of secondary smoke were found. Making areas smoke-free in restaurants, public transportation, and other settings has played an invaluable role in efforts to curb the ill effects of smoking. However, getting these societal changes passed was far more difficult than initiating the individual programs.

Immunizations to prevent infectious diseases likewise could be implemented both on an individual and social scale. Individuals receiving immunizations benefit, but to eradicate the threat of different diseases, widespread immunization are necessary. While a variety of barriers to implementation has made mounting successful immunization programs challenging nationally and internationally, a series of factors has facilitated these programs. Most immunizations in childhood series are highly effective and inexpensive. While complex, providing immunizations is nowhere near as complex as addressing social inequalities, discrimination, or poor working conditions.

Social determinants of poor health can only be addressed by societal solutions. If we are to succeed in addressing the social determinants of health highlighted in this book, we must begin by learning from the many who have tried before us. Long before there was evidence that poverty and social inequalities led to poor health outcomes, there were people who sought to eliminate poverty and decrease social inequalities. The same is true for racial discrimination, poor working conditions, and a number of the other social determinants of health discussed. Yet, success has often been elusive.

This chapter first highlights some of the experiences others have had in trying to address these problems. The chapter will then go on to examine what we need to know and do to make a difference.

CHALLENGES IN SUCCESSFULLY ADDRESSING PROBLEMS DISCUSSED IN THIS BOOK

- Major social change requires sustained public support and political will.
- We still have a great deal to learn about

how to effectively combat poverty, social inequalities, and discrimination.
- Programs often don't receive a sufficient amount or duration of support to determine if they could succeed.
- Even successful programs do not necessarily receive sustained support.
- When problems are inadequately addressed because of insufficient knowledge of how to address them, or limitations in implementation, the public often becomes skeptical of future attempts.

While the majority of the cases below will be taken from the United States, a review of social policy over the past half-century in many European countries would also yield examples of partial successes and partial failures in addressing income inequalities, discrimination, and achieving and sustaining political support for effective programs. For those unfamiliar with the examples discussed below, a brief Glossary of program terms is provided.

Combating Poverty and Decreasing Economic Inequalities

Earlier chapters in this book have documented the extensive evidence that poverty and economic inequalities contribute significantly to poor health. Yet, successfully combating poverty and decreasing economic inequalities has been far from straightforward.

In 1935, when Aid to Dependent Children (ADC) was passed as part of the sweeping reforms of the New Deal, the country had decided that it was impossible for single mothers, most of whom were single because of the death of or abandonment by a spouse, to support themselves economically and still provide adequate care for their children. But support for the program flagged. From 1975 to 1990, the percent of Americans who believed that governments should help the poor was below 40%. While the percent of Americans who believed the government should work to decrease income inequalities was higher than the percent of Americans who believed that the government should help the poor, less than 50% of most Americans during that period believed that the government should work to decrease income inequalities (Bobo and Smith 1994).

By 1996, a fundamental shift in the public debate over single parents living in poverty had taken place. The public had changed from believing it was impossible for most single women to care for their children while earning enough money to subsist to buying that there was nothing other than willpower stopping single parents living in poverty from working full time and caring for their children.

During the recent period of shifting political views, politicians led the charge to change Aid to Families with Dependent Children (AFDC), the program which succeeded ADC. Many factors contributed to the change in popular opinion, including the increase in middle-class women working, the political stereotyping of those receiving welfare, a decrease in public confidence that government could solve problems, and creation of a public belief that the program was perpetuating a culture of poverty (Heclo 1994; Marmor et al. 1990; Lehman 1991).

In August 1996, the United States Congress repealed AFDC and the federal promise of income for parents and children living in poverty. They passed The Personal Responsibility and Work Opportunity Reconciliation Act of 1996, which imposed a 5-year lifetime limit on income assistance. Parents who are unemployed and without any source of income after 5 years will receive no benefits; their children are to receive no financial support. Food stamps also are to be eliminated for those who do not return to work within the time limits (Congressional Research Service 1996; U.S. Congress 1996).

During this same period, public support also dwindled for federal tax and spending programs aimed at minimizing inequality. The post-transfer income inequalities increased more between 1980 and 1990 than the pretransfer inequalities (Gramlich et al. 1993).

The United States was not the only country to be losing the war against poverty in the 1980s. Poverty increased among families with children in Europe as well (McFate et al. 1995). Social insurance programs in the United States which are targeted at the poor have not been sustained as effectively as universal social insurance programs—undoubtedly in part because of the difference in political support. During the past two decades, the increased spending on non-means-tested programs including Social Security and Medicare has been greater than the total spending on all means-tested programs (programs targeting low-income recipients) (Burtless 1994). Yet these programs have maintained more public support (Lomax-Cook 1990) even in an era of intense debate over what to cut to eliminate the deficit. During the same period, AFDC benefits, which were means-tested, did not keep pace with inflation (Gramlich et al. 1993).

Building Human Capital

Earlier chapters in this book have suggested the potential importance of increasing human capital. Human capital has been shown to directly impact health outcomes. Investments in human capital have also been raised as one way to decrease social inequalities. To date, a wide range of initiatives have been aimed at increasing human capital. These initiatives have ranged from Head Start, targeted at preschool children, to the Job Training Partnership Act, aimed at those ready for employment.

Preschool programs for children living in poverty have been shown to have long-term benefits including decreasing school dropout rates, unemployment, teen pregnancy, and juvenile delinquency (Murnane 1994).

The Comprehensive Employment and Training Act (CETA) of 1973 led to 25%–75% gains in the wages of adult women who received training and work experience (Burtless 1994).

Unfortunately, the human capital programs reveal that even programs demonstrated to be effective at reaching their goals are not guaranteed either sufficient or sustained federal support. While federal support continues for low-income preschool children in the Head Start program, there has never been sufficient support so that there were enough spaces for all children who are eligible for the program. In the 1980s, overall spending on education and training programs for the poor was decreased (Burtless 1994).

Despite Congressional Budget Office estimates that it led to significant increases in annual real wages of women who participated, CETA was discontinued in 1982. When political movements pressed for privatization, CETA was replaced by the Job Training Partnership Act (JTPA). The JTPA places participants in private sector jobs and is run by "private industry councils" (Blank 1994). While JTPA showed gains in wages, it showed smaller gains in wages than CETA (Bloom et al. 1993).

Other programs have had mixed results. The National Supported Work Demonstration Program of the late 1970s was able to improve outcomes for AFDC recipients but not for ex-convicts. Programs that provide public sector employment may have led to displacement of other workers outside the program (Blank 1994; Lehman 1994).

Improving Conditions of the Working Poor

Policy experts concerned with poverty and social inequality in the United States have increasingly focused on the work lives of the poor. Programs that aimed at helping the working poor have had both successes and limitations. The Targeted Jobs Tax Credit was designed to encourage employers to hire workers designated as disadvantaged. The tax credit effectively subsidized wages. However, few employers took advantage of the Targeted Jobs Tax Credit, and concerns were raised that employees eligible for the credit were stigmatized (Burtless 1985).

Minimum wage laws have been used as part of the Fair Labor Standards Act to increase standards of living. Minimum wage laws have sparked debate among researchers, policymakers, and the public regarding the extent to which increasing the minimum wage decreases the number of people hired at the minimum wage. If this were the case, then increases in minimum wage would benefit those who kept their job and who received the increase but be to the detriment of minimum wage earners who lost their job. In addition, the minimum wage increases have also been critiqued for not adequately targeting low-income families (Horrigan and Mincy 1993). Minimum wage increases benefit all those who are earning the minimum wage including both workers in low-income families and youth who may come from middle- or upper-income families but have their first job at the minimum wage. Finally, minimum wage increases—reflective of the political will to increase them—have not kept up with either mean family income increases or inflation.

An alternative approach has been the Earned Income Tax Credit (EITC). Under the EITC, low-income working families receive tax credits. The program is targeted at low-income families. As a federal tax credit, the EITC effectively increases the earned wages without providing an incentive for employers to hire fewer people. The EITC increases have been politically easier to pass than AFDC increases, both because EITC rewards those who work and because the EITC shows up as foregone tax revenue as opposed to dollars paid out in the federal budget (Blank 1994). The latter difference reflects how significant political differences can be, even when they are economically equivalent. Limitations of the EITC include the fact that it provides little assistance to low-income single earners without children and it provides no benefit for those who are unable to find a job.

The success and failure of initiatives have been influenced by external conditions as well as by programs' inherent characteristics and by the presence or absence of sufficient political will to sustain the initiatives.

Social policy changes do not have the protection that occurs in a controlled medical research environment. The context and outcome of welfare-to-work initiatives provide just one example. California's GAIN program was successful in increasing employment, earnings, and decreasing welfare use. A similarly designed federal initiative, the Family Support Act and JOBS program passed in 1988, began as the country entered a recession and was far less successful (Blank 1994).

Combating Discrimination

Previous chapters in this book have underscored the serious impact of discrimination on health. Yet the results of public policy initiatives during the past four decades to combat discrimination have been mixed, just as the results of initiatives targeting economic inequalities have been mixed.

Civil rights legislation passed in 1964 made it illegal to discriminate in employment on the basis of race in firms that received federal funding. The Civil Rights Act of 1991 expanded the ban on discrimination to include all workplaces (Lehman 1994).

This legislation has led to marked decreases in employment-based discrimination (Jaynes and Williams 1989). While antidiscrimination legislation has clearly had an important impact, it is equally clear that it has not eliminated employment and other discrimination based on race (Alenikoff 1992). Furthermore, legislation alone could not address the impact of past discrimination, which had led to lower school completion rates, less access to college, and fewer mentors in leadership positions in industry and government, among many other things.

Whereas the Civil Rights Act of 1964 *sought to eliminate ongoing* discrimination in schools and in the workplace, subsequently developed affirmative action policies sought to remedy the long-term effects of past discrimination (Wilson 1996). Yet,

affirmative action policies were no more a magic bullet for discrimination than the Civil Rights Act. As William Julius Wilson has noted, affirmative action policies by and large provided opportunities for the more advantaged minority individuals, not the more disadvantaged (1996).

These successes and limitations are not unique to the United States. In 1968, antidiscrimination legislation was passed in a race-relations act in Great Britain which also addressed employment and housing. Research supports the notion that discrimination decreased after the passage of the act, but it is equally clear that discrimination in these areas continues in Great Britain (Brown 1995). In the 1970s, France implemented a series of policies aimed at integrating areas of cities that had become immigrant ghettos. These policies, however, often resulted in immigrants living in overcrowded conditions in adjacent neighborhoods with poor housing (Body-Gendrot 1995). In the 1980s, public–private partnerships were developed in France to improve the quality of the neighborhoods where immigrants were living. Nonetheless, the targeted neighborhoods remained isolated, with poor transportation and degraded buildings (Body-Gendrot 1995).

To maintain policies, political will behind them must be maintained. In the United States, since the 1970s, public opinion—and the political will it helped shape—has been mixed regarding affirmative action. The support for programs which "compensated" for past wrongs was greater than the support for programs which gave "preferential" treatment for minorities. The support for affirmative action in hiring was often less than the support for affirmative action in training or education (Lipset and Schneider 1978; Bobo and Smith 1994). In 1990, the majority of white Americans opposed preferential hiring of black Americans (Wilson 1996). Local policies developed to address racial disparities have faced just as many problems as national policies. When individual cities have developed plans to integrate housing, they have faced public opposition and litigation (Husock 1989, 1990).

MAKING A DIFFERENCE

Social epidemiologic research has made important headway in understanding the societal correlates and causes of many health problems. Yet, much remains to be done in the areas of developing policy responses that will effectively address these root causes and building the political support necessary to make changes.

The importance of political will and social strategies, in addition to a knowledge base, has been raised for the case of health promotion in general, and tobacco control in particular (Atwood et al. 1997; Richmond and Kotelchuck 1991).

To develop policy initiatives which are as successful at addressing the social determinants of poor health as smoking cessation programs and policies aimed at decreasing smoking have been at breaking the link between smoking and cancer, several steps must be taken. Successful policy formation will need to rely not only on understanding the problems targeted by social epidemiologic research but on developing meaningful policy responses and building political support for these responses (see Table 16–1).

The Role of Research in Developing Policy Responses

Research can contribute significantly to the development of policy initiatives. Intervention research can provide crucial information on what may be effective methods of addressing problems.

Policy research can play a critical role in examining the costs and benefits of public policies. Just as medications treating childhood cancer have side effects, policies addressing social determinants of health are likely to have side effects.

Presumed costs and benefits in policy changes can play as big a role in political decisions as do known consequences. As a result, research into the assumptions underlying political rhetoric is often crucial. For example, while there is no strong evidence supporting the rhetoric that welfare benefits

Table 16–1. Ingredients for Developing Successful Programs

Understanding the problem	Developing policy responses	Building political support
Understanding the cause of the problem • including understanding what are the precipitates as opposed to the correlates of the problem	Programs that are effective in a range of political settings and in the context of a range of other initiatives • the other initiatives which will be passed or repealed will be unpredictable	Sufficient political support to pass programs in a form that they are viable • with compromises that will not compromise the effectiveness of the policies • without changes that will undermine the policy
Understanding what needs to be changed to address the problem • mediating factors may be more feasible to address than ultimate causes—it is important to understand when it is necessary to address the ultimate causes	Programs that are effective in a range of economic situations • in the long run it is inevitable that any program that is sustained will exist against a backdrop of both strong and weak economic conditions	Sufficient political support to sustain the initiative over the time necessary for its effectiveness to become clear
	Programs that are effective in a range of demographic settings • Federal programs need be effective in each state. State programs need to be effective in a wide range of localities	

have led to increased childbearing among welfare recipients, this misperception has driven such policies as family caps.

Social epidemiologic research can provide important insights into the salience of the social context of problems and the interventions used to address them. Welfare-to- work programs and programs for children with learning disabilities provide two examples of the importance of social context in policy formation. Programs designed to increase the numbers of mothers on welfare entering the work force may be effective in a strong economy with record low unemployment but disastrous in a recession. Programs aimed at addressing the special needs of children with learning disabilities may be highly politically successful and effective when schools have adequate budgets and yet be political pariahs when legislation cutting property taxes highly constrains local school dollars.

New research methods need to be developed to address many of the relevant research questions. A number of differences exist between the approach frequently taken by researchers and social policymakers. Six examples follow.

1. Multivariate regression analysis answers the question: Holding everything else equal, if we change this one variable, what will happen? However, in the policy sphere, rarely is just one change made.

Horsetrading may result in health insurance for children in exchange for a deal with the tobacco industry. Changes in policy which affect the economic cycle may simultaneously affect programs for the poor. A senator from a state with a strong gun lobby may sign on to a crime bill that contains antidiscrimination language only if the bill eliminates gun control measures.

2. It is difficult to convince a legislature to conduct a randomized clinical trial of social policy.

How can they justify in "soundbites" to their constituents spending money on something that is likely to fail? If they're sure that it will work, how can they justify not making it available to everyone? Randomized

trials are often double blinded—impossible in the public policy sphere. Furthermore, a randomized clinical trial often examines whether an intervention works well in one setting. However, when federal legislation is passed, the policy needs to be effective in a wide range of settings across the country. The program which succeeds in some areas but fails in others is likely to be revoked or go underfunded because of its failures, with little attention to its successes.

3. Many research methods are designed to look at means or other measures of central tendency and not at distributions. Yet, in terms of political support, the distribution of effects may be equally or more important.

4. In calculating the mean effects of a program, researchers may eliminate "outliers"—individuals whose experience is so extreme that the researchers worry the experience may have nothing to do with the program. Yet in policy spheres, where individual stories can be used to capture media attention and symbolize programs, "outliers" can drive the debate.

5. Public health researchers often spend time examining how services can be most cost-effectively targeted. They look at which subpopulations, which small groups, would benefit the most from a particular intervention. Yet not uncommonly, the questions posed by public discourse can be the opposite. In order to pass a piece of legislation, a senator must get at least half of all senators to agree. To avoid or break a filibuster, that senator may need 60% of votes. In order to get his or her colleagues' agreement, the senator must make a compelling case that the service or program will have widespread benefits and impact people in each colleagues' states—not have targeted benefits.

The political advantage of widespread benefits gained support for and underpinned the continued success of Medicare, which offers universal coverage for the elderly, in contrast to Medicaid, which targets the poor (Scott 1995).

An untargeted program, Social Security,

is touted for its impacts not on inequality, but on increasing the income of all elderly, including the poor. Yet, as a result of Social Security, 83% of elderly Americans who would otherwise be living in poverty have incomes above the poverty line (Danziger and Weinberg 1994). In contrast, unemployment and workers' compensation bring less than 1% of poor families out of poverty; AFDC and other means-tested benefits bring only 28% of families with children out of poverty (Danziger and Weinberg 1994).

6. Long-term effectiveness is the gold standard for researchers. A medication whose best results are in the first 3 months and not in the long term is not regarded nearly as highly as a treatment that may show little benefit in the short run but is highly effective in the long run. While long-term effectiveness is the theoretical gold standard in policy programs as well, the practical reality is far different.

For policies to be passed, leaders must believe that the impact will be felt rapidly— within the time frame of a political cycle— so that the benefits of the program will be seen before the next budget battle, before the next election, and certainly before the policy is reviewed again. For programs to receive continued funding, they must show their effectiveness early on. Policies that take a long time to show results do not last. They are altered or repealed. They simply do not stay in place long enough to demonstrate their effectiveness.

For their results to be more useful in the policy sphere, epidemiologists need to spend more time with methods which seek:

- To understand the distribution of experiences as well as the average impact
- To understand uncommon experiences as well as common experiences, the experience of those who are "outliers" as well as modal experiences
- To examine the extent to which social and economic contexts make a difference to problems and their causes
- To examine the extent to which interven-

tions and policy solutions are effective under a wide range of social and economic conditions
- To document the effects of interventions on the general population and not just targeted populations

Political Support

Public opinion critically influences policy formation (Page and Shapiro 1983). In policies designed to decrease discrimination, public opinion has been shown to play an important role both in what public policies get adopted (Burstein 1979) and in how they are implemented (Burstein 1985). Public opinion has played an equally critical role in the formulation, maintenance, and repeal of policy initiatives targeted at poverty and inequalities in income distribution (Shapiro and Young 1989).

It is important for social epidemiologists to understand what shapes public opinion on issues critical to public health if they hope to see changes in social policies impacting on health. Moneyed interests have long influenced public opinion through paid media. More recently they have influenced politicians and public opinion through "Astroturf" organizations in which they use money to pay to create "grass roots" movements (Smith 1988; Youngclaus 1998). The candidates with the most money to spend on campaigns won over 90% of the elections in 1996 (Common Cause 1996). In-state referenda designed to be more accessible to the public, corporations, and interest groups with more money have also had greater influences. In the state of Massachusetts, every ballot initiative with more resources to spend than the opposition won in 1996 (Anand 1998).

Nonetheless, there are clearly important examples where policy changes have taken place against moneyed interests. Policy initiatives to decrease smoking in certain areas and to decrease the advertising and sales of cigarettes to youth provide one recent important example.

Academics need to spend more time thinking about how their work reaches the

Branches of Government

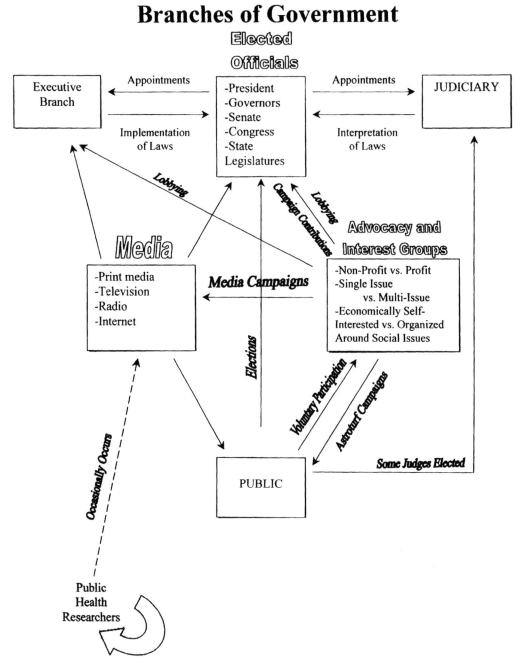

Figure 16–1. Web of influence.

public sphere. Clearly, few among the groups who have the potential to either initiate policy change or support it or block its path read the epidemiologic literature. That is not to say that the literature does not influence public opinion, values, or policy. However, it is to say that stopping with writing an article in an academic journal and neither formulating policy recommendations nor making efforts to have those recommendations reach those who can act on them is like throwing seeds into the wind. They may land, they may bear fruit, but taking the time to till the land and to plant them is far more likely to reap results.

Rarely does research magically enter the public debate on its own. Researchers who are concerned with having an impact on the health of communities need to spend time thinking about how their research will go from bookshelf or journal archive to program or public policy. Each of us needs to think about which participants in the democratic process will learn about the results of our studies, how they will learn about them, and how to get useful information to participants. Researchers also need to think about how to hear back from community members and others active in the political process regarding ways to make research more relevant.

To effectively influence policy making in a democracy, researchers need to know what information is compelling to the electorate, what information is compelling to those in power, how the information will get to each participant, and what information will make those who are politically unsympathetic respond.

In the past, public health researchers have often felt their work would be effective so long as it is published and, perhaps, presented to reporters (Fig. 16–1). Sometimes this has worked. Other times it has resulted in research that contributes far less than it should. Studies of what has shaped public opinion on social policy issues show that media influences public perception of policy issues through its method of presenting material as well as through the content (Iyengar 1987, 1990). Iyengar has demonstrated that when the media presents policy issues through the stories of individual lives, those who watch are more likely to attribute the cause of the problems to individuals than to social problems (1987, 1990). This difference is particularly important in an era when the media principally presents social problems through descriptions of individual lives and when researchers are often called on to give information on individual lives as a means of stories attracting public interest

and television programs receiving higher ratings.

Public health researchers increasingly need to work directly with all branches of the government and with the public.

CONCLUSION

The science of social epidemiology has markedly advanced in making a compelling case that social conditions are a major determinant of health. But, at the turn of the millenium, we still have a lot further to go to answer the "So what?" question or, better phrased, "What now?"

If we are to address the causes of health problems that social epidemiology highlights, we will need to go beyond individuals' health care practices. Neither individual interventions nor pharmaceutical products will be able to address social determinants of health. Neither poverty nor economic inequalities, neither racial discrimination nor issues of job loss and insecurity can be addressed by the health care system. Each is influenced by social policy, not health policy.

While it is an essential first step, determining that poverty, social inequalities, discrimination, poor social networks, and the like are bad for health will not be enough. Even if they weren't bad for health, most people would agree that poverty is bad for the lives of those affected, as is discrimination, job loss, and job insecurity. Yet, achieving effective change in these areas has often been elusive.

Intervention studies have begun to show important results—for example, that early education programs can have a significant impact on the health and lifecourse of children, that social conditions affect individuals' health initiatives, such as ceasing smoking. But these are only the beginnings of what we need to know to effectively address the social conditions that have been shown in this volume to have significant negative effects on the health and well-being of populations. Addressing these issues will require developing different research tools, allowing wider participation in determining what research questions are asked, and making sure that the results are debated in wider circles than purely academic ones.

Epidemiology has always been a practical science. The goal has always been to use what we learn to improve public health. Given that goal, it is crucial that we better understand the challenges that need to be met if we are to address the social determinants of health.

GLOSSARY

INCOME SUPPORT/REDUCTION IN INCOME SUPPORT PROGRAMS

Aid to Dependent Children (ADC)

Established by the Social Security Act of 1935 as a cash grant program to enable states to aid low-income children without fathers. Specifically designed to support widows so they would not have to leave their children and go to work. Replaced by AFDC in 1950.

Aid to Families with Dependent Children (AFDC)

Formerly called ADC. Provided income support to low-income families. Individual states defined "need" and set benefit levels within federal limitations. All 50 states and the District of Columbia operated AFDC programs. Federal government paid from 50% to 80% of the AFDC benefit costs in a state. Provided Food Stamp subsidies. Replaced by TANF in 1996.

Temporary Assistance to Needy Families (TANF)

In 1996, TANF replaced AFDC with capped block grants. Eliminates entitlement to aid. Requires work in order to receive benefits after 2 years and imposes a 5-year time limit on duration of family cash welfare. By 2002, states are required to have half of their single-parent welfare recipients working at least 30 hours per week.

Family Caps

Policy which denied additional welfare benefits to women who had children while on welfare. Under waivers to the Family Support Act of 1988, 20 states had taken steps to impose family caps by late 1995 in spite of the fact that research found that "variations in welfare benefit levels and the incremental benefit have no statistically significant impacts on the subsequent childbearing decisions of young mothers in general, nor on the subsequent childbearing decisions of women who received welfare in particular" (Acs 1996).

TRAINING AND EMPLOYMENT PROGRAMS

Manpower Development Training Act (MDTA)

Began in 1962 as a classroom training program for unemployed skilled workers. Rapidly evolved into a program focused on low-skilled and minority workers. Included programs aimed at disadvantaged youth. Replaced by CETA in 1973.

Comprehensive Employment and Training Act (CETA)

Designed to provide on-the-job training for less-skilled workers. Funded temporary public sector employment with the hope of encouraging workers to find private sector jobs. Reached its height in 1977–1978 when it placed over 1 million people in public sector jobs and provided training assistance to another 1.3 million workers (Blank 1994). Terminated in 1982 and replaced by JTPA.

Job Training Partnership Act (JTPA)

Designed to offer job training and search assistance to disadvantaged workers. Less funding and fewer placements than CETA. Also differs from CETA in that there are no funds for public sector job creation and it is run by local "private industry councils" (PICs) rather than by local governments.

National Supported Work Demonstration Program

Run from 1975 to 1979 at 15 locations throughout the United States. Found employment for roughly 10,000 people (ICPSR

1998). Geared toward "extremely disadvantaged workers," including ex–drug addicts, ex-convicts, long-term AFDC recipients, and disadvantaged youth (considered the least "work-ready" populations). Provided participants with group counseling and placed participants into structured work settings that generally included job training. Has been linked to significant gains for long-term AFDC recipients, some small gains for ex–drug addicts, but negligible gains within other groups (Blank 1994).

Greater Avenues for Independence (GAIN)
Begun in 1985, this program located in California served as the leading model for the Family Support Act's combination of education, job training, and graduated work requirements in the JOBS program.

Job Opportunities and Basic Skills Training (JOBS)
On October 13, 1988, Congress passed the Family Support Act, which required all states to create mandatory work–welfare programs and specifically required states to create JOBS program. The JOBS program required states to provide education, job skills training, job readiness, job development, and job placement as well as help with job search, on-the-job training, work supplementation, and community work experience. Required states to spend 55% of their funds on recipients who had received AFDC for any 36 of the last 60 months, for parents under age 24 who had not completed high school or had little or no work experience in the last year, and for members of families whose youngest child was within 2 years of being ineligible for AFDC.

EARLY EDUCATION

Head Start
Began in 1965 in the Office of Economic Opportunity as a way to serve children of low-income families (now administered by the Administration for Children and Families). National program which provides comprehensive developmental services for low-income, preschool children ages three to five and social services for their families. In 1994, the federal government established Early Head Start, which serves low-income pregnant women and families with infants and toddlers.

TAX CREDITS

Targeted Jobs Tax Credit (TJTC)
Enacted in 1978. Federal income tax credit available to employers who hired low-income workers from certain target groups. Advertised to employers that their taxes could be reduced by up to $2400 per worker, essentially subsidizing their wages and theoretically making it more attractive for employers to hire them. Very low participation rates and some evidence that eligibility for program stigmatized workers in the labor market rather than helped them (Blank 1994; Lehman 1994). The TJTC expired for individuals hired after June 30, 1992. Renamed the Work Opportunity Tax Credit (WOTC) in 1994.

Work Opportunity Tax Credit (WOTC)
Provides same tax credit for employers as TJTC for up to 40% of the first $6000 paid for new employees who work 400 or more hours during first 12 months of employment. Credit for new hires employed 120 to 400 hours is 25%. Reauthorized through July 1, 1998, and amended by the Taxpayer Relief Act signed August 1997. Amended to target eight groups: welfare recipients; 18- to 24-year-old food stamp recipients; veterans; vocational rehabilitation referrals; 18- to 24-year-old residents of one of the 105 federally designated urban or rural Empowerment Zones or Enterprise Communities (EZ/EC); 16- to 17-year-old EZ/EC residents hired as Summer Youth Employees; ex-felons who are members of a low-income family; and SSI recipients.

Welfare-to-Work Tax Credit
Federal tax credit of 35% of qualified wages for the first year of employment (if employed at least 400 hours or 180 days) and 50% for the second year. Applies to long-

term family assistance recipients who received Aid to Families with Dependent Children (AFDC) or Temporary Assistance to Needy Families (TANF) for at least 18 consecutive months or whose AFDC or TANF eligibility expired under federal or state law. The maximum Welfare-to-Work Tax Credit is $3500 the first year and $5000 the second year of employment, for a maximum tax savings of $8500 per new hire.

Earned Income Tax Credit (EITC)

Enacted in 1975 as first legislation to use tax system as a way to provide resources for the poor. Specifically designed to supplement earnings of low-income families with children through tax reductions and refundable tax credits. The amount of EITC a family can receive depends on household income and number of children in the household. In 1996, a family with two or more children was allowed to earn up to $28,495 a year and qualify for the EITC. Taxpayers who have qualifying children and earn between $6350 and $11,650 could get up to the maximum credit ($2152 if they have one qualifying child or $3556 if they have two or more qualifying children). People who had no qualifying children and earned between $4200 and $5300 were eligible for a maximum credit of $323 (Missouri Department of Social Services 1998; Georgia Department of Family and Children's Services 1998).

ACKNOWLEDGMENTS

This work was made possible by generous support as a Seagram's Associate of the Canadian Institute for Advanced Research. I would like to thank Cara Bergstrom for developing the glossary, both Christine Kerr and Cara Bergstrom for their invaluable research and staff assistance, and Eijean Wu for her excellent assistance with the literature review.

REFERENCES

Acs, G. (1996). The impact of welfare on young mothers' subsequent childbearing decisions. *J Hum Resources*, 31:898–915.

Adler, N.E., Boyce, T., Chesney, M.A., Cohen, S., Follman, S., Kahn, R,L., and Syme, S.L. (1994). Socioeconomic status and health. The challenge of the gradient. *Am Psychol*, 49:15–24.

Alenikoff, A.F. (1992). The constitution in context: the continuing significance of racism. *Univ Colorado Law Rev*, 63:325–72.

Anand, G. (1998). Massachusetts ballot initiatives paying off for business. *Boston Globe*, March 9, p. B1.

Atwood, K., Colditz, G.A., and Kawachi I. (1997). From public health science to prevention policy: placing science in its social and political contexts. *Am J Public Health*, 87:1603–5.

Ben-Shlomo, Y., White, I.R., and Marmot, M. (1996). Does the variation in the socioeconomic characteristics of an area affect mortality? *BMJ*, 312:1013–4.

Berkman, L.F. (1995). The role of social relations in health promotion. *Psychosom Med*, 57:245–54.

Berkman, L.F., Leo-Summers, L., and Horwitz, R.I. (1992). Emotional support and survival after myocardial infarction: a prospective, population-based study of the elderly. *Ann Int Med*, 117:1003–9.

Berkman, L.F., Seeman, T.E., Albert, M., Blazer, D., Kahn, R., Mohs, R., Finch, C., Schneider, E., Cotman, C., McClearn, G., Nesselroade, J., Featherman, D., Garmezy, N., McKhann, G., Brim, G., Prager, D., and Rowe, J. (1993). High, usual and impaired functioning in community-dwelling older men and women: findings from the MacArthur Foundation Research Network on Successful Aging. *J Clin Epidemiol*, 46:1129–40.

Blank, R.M. (1994). The employment strategy: public policies to increase work and earnings. In Danziger, S.H., Sandefur, G.D., and Weinberg, D.H. (eds.), *Confronting poverty: prescriptions for change*. New York: Russell Sage Foundation, pp. 365–95.

Bloom, H.S., Orr, L.O., Cave, G., Bell, S., and Doolittle, F. (1993). *The national JTP study: report to the U.S. Department of Labor*. Bethesda, MD: Apt.

Bobo, L., and Smith, R.A. (1994). Antipoverty policy, affirmative action, and racial attitudes. In Danziger, S.H., Sandefur, G.D., and Weinberg, D.H. (eds.), *Confronting poverty: prescriptions for change*. New York: Russell Sage Foundation, pp. 365–95.

Body-Gendrot, S. (1995). Immigration, marginality, and French social policy. In McFate, K., Lawson, R., and Wilson, W.J. (eds.), *Poverty, inequality, and the future of social policy: Western states in the new world order*. New York: Russell Sage Foundation, pp. 571–83.

Bosma, H., Marmot, M.G., Hemingway, H., Nicholson, A.C., Brunner, E., and Stansfeld,

S.A. (1997). Low job control and risk of coronary heart disease in Whitehall II (prospective cohort study). *BMJ*, 314:558–65.

Brenner, M.H. (1983). Unemployment and health in the context of economic change. *Soc Sci Med*, 17:1135–8.

Brown, C. (1995). Poverty, immigration, and minority groups: policies toward minorities in Great Britain. In McFate, K., Lawson, R., and Wilson, W.J. (eds.), *Poverty, inequality, and the future of social policy: Western states in the new world order*. New York: Russell Sage Foundation, pp. 585–605.

Burstein, P. (1979). Public opinion, demonstrations, and the passage of antidiscrimination legislation. *Public Opin Q*, 79:157–72.

Burstein, P. (1985). *Discrimination, jobs, and politics*. Chicago: University of Chicago Press.

Burtless, G. (1985). Are targeted wage subsidies harmful? evidence from a wage voucher experiment. *Ind Labor Relations Rev*, 39:105–13.

Burtless, G. (1994). Public spending on the poor: historical trends and economic limits. In Danziger, S.H., Sandefur, G.D., and Weinberg, D.H. (eds.), *Confronting poverty: prescriptions for change*. New York: Russell Sage Foundation, pp. 51–84.

Common Cause. (1996). *Campaign finance activities of 1996*. Washington, DC: Common Cause.

Congressional Research Service. (1996). *New welfare law: the personal responsibility and work opportunity reconciliation act of 1996*. (CRS Report for Congress, EPW.) Washington, DC: Library of Congress, pp. 96–687.

Danziger, S.H., and Weinberg, D.H. (1994). The historical record: trends in family income, inequality, and poverty. In Danziger, S.H., Sandefur, G.D., and Weinberg, D.H. (eds.), *Confronting poverty: prescriptions for change*. New York: Russell Sage Foundation, pp. 18–50.

Fiscella, K., and Franks, P. (1997). Poverty or income inequality as predictor of mortality: longitudinal cohort study. *BMJ* 314:1724–8.

Georgia Department of Family and Children's Services. (1998). Web site. Earned Income Tax Credit (EITC) page. <http://www. chatham dfcs.org/workfirst/eitc.html>.

Gramlich, E. M., Kasten, R., and Sammartino, F. (1993). Growing inequality in the 1980s: the role of federal taxes and cash transfers. In Danziger, S., and Gottschalk, P. (eds.) *Uneven tides: rising inequality in America* New York: Russell Sage Foundation, pp. 251–75.

Haan, M. (1985). Job strain and cardiovascular disease: a ten-year prospective study. *Am J Epidemiol*, 122:532–40.

Heclo, H. (1994). Poverty politics. In Danziger, S.H., Sandefur, G.D., and Weinberg, D.H. (eds.), *Confronting poverty: prescriptions for change*. New York: Russell Sage Foundation, pp. 396–437.

Hinkle, L.E., Whitney, L.H., Lehman, E.W., Dunn, J., Benjamin, B., King, R., Plakun, A., and Flehinger, B. (1968). Occupation, education, and coronary heart disease. *Science*, 161:238–48.

Horrigan, M.W., and Mincy, R.B. (1993). The minimum wage and earnings and income inequality. In Danziger, S., and Gottschalk, P. (eds.), *Uneven tides: rising inequality in America* New York: Russell Sage Foundation, pp. 251–75.

House, J.S., Strecher, V., Metzner, H.L., and Robbins, C. (1986). Occupational stress and health among men and women in the Tecumseh Community Health Study. *J Health Soc Behav*, 27:62–77.

Husock, H. (1989). *Integration incentives in suburban Cleveland*. Case Program Series (#C16-89-877.0). Cambridge, MA: Kennedy School of Government, Harvard University.

Husock, H. (1990). *Occupancy controls and racial integration at Starrett City* (A, B, C, and Epilogue). Case Program Series (#C16-90-962.0). Cambridge, MA: Kennedy School of Government, Harvard University.

Inter-university Consortium for Political and Social Research (ICPSR) Archive. <http://www. icpsr.umich.edu/cgi/ab.prl?file=7865>.

Issler, R.M.S., Giugliana, E.R.J., Krutz, G.T., Menese, C.F., Justo, E.B., Kreutz, V.M., and Pires, M. (1996). Poverty levels and children's health status: study of risk factors in an urban population of low socioeconomic level. *Rev Saude Publica*, 30:506–11.

Iyengar, S. (1987). Television news and citizens. Explanations of national issues. *Am Polit Sci*, 81:815–32.

Iyengar, S. (1990). Framing responsibility for political issues. The case of poverty. *Polit Behav*, 12:19–40.

Jaynes, G., and Williams, R. (eds.). (1989). *A common destiny: blacks in American society*. Washington, DC: National Academy Press.

Johnson, J.V., and Hall, E.M. (1988). Job strain, workplace social support and cardiovascular disease: a cross-sectional study of a random sample of the Swedish working population. *Am J Public Health*, 78:1336–42.

Jones, C., LaVeist, T.A., and Lillie-Blanton, M. (1991). "Race" in the epidemiologic literature: an examination of the American Journal of—Epidemiology, 1921–1990. *Am J Epidemiol*, 134:1079–84.

Karasek, R.A. (1979). Job demands, job decision

latitude, and mental strain: implications for job redeisgn. *Admin Sci Q* 24:285–307.

Krieger, N., and Sidney, S. (1996). Racial discrimination and blood pressure: the CARDIA study of young black and white adults. *Am J Public Health,* 86:1370–8.

Lehman, J.H. (1991). To conceptualize, to criticize, to defend. *Yale Law J,* 101:685–727.

Lehman, J. S. (1994). Updating urban policy. In Danziger, S.H., Sandefur, G.D., and Weinberg, D.H. (eds.), *Confronting poverty: prescriptions for change.* New York: Russell Sage Foundation, pp. 226–52.

Lipset, S.M., and Schneider, W. (1978). The Bakke case: how would it be decided at the bar of public opinion? *Public Opinion,* March/April:38–48.

Lomax-Cook, F. (1990). Congress and the public: convergent opinions on social security. In Aaron, H.J. (ed.), *Social security and the budget:* Proceedings of the First Conference of the National Academy of Social Insurance, Washington, DC. New York: University Press of America, pp. 79–107.

Marmor, T.R., Mashaw, J.L., and Harvey, P.L. (1990). *America's misunderstood welfare state: persistent myths, enduring realities.* New York: Basic Books.

Mattiasson, I., Lindgarde, F., Nilsson, J.A., and Theorell, T. (1990). Threat of unemployment and cardiovascular risk factors: longitudinal study of quality of sleep and serum cholesterol concentrations in men threatened with redundancy. *BMJ,* 301:461–6.

McFate, K., Smeeding, T., and Rainwater, L. (1995). Market and states: poverty trends and transfer system effectiveness in the 1980s. In McFate, K., Lawson, R., and Wilson, W.J. (eds.), *Poverty, inequality, and the future of social policy: Western states in the new world order.* New York: Russell Sage Foundation, pp. 29–66.

Missouri Department of Social Services. (1998). Web site. Earned Income Tax Credit (EITC) page. <*http://www.dss.state.mo.us/wreform/taxcred.htm*>.

Montgomery, L.E., Kiely, J.L., and Pappas, G. (1996). The effects of poverty, race and family structure on U.S. children's health: data from the NHIS, 1978 through 1980 and 1989 through 1991. *Am J Public Health,* 86:1401.

Murnane, R.J. (1994). Education and the well-being of the next generation. In Danziger, S.H., Sandefur, G.D., and Weinberg, D.H. (eds.), *Confronting poverty: prescriptions for change.* New York: Russell Sage Foundation, pp. 289–307.

Page, B.J., and Shapiro, R.Y. (1983). Effects of public opinion on policy. *Am Polit Sci Rev,* 77:175–90.

Richmond, J.B., and Kotelchuck, M. (1991). Coordination and development of strategies and policy for public health promotion in the United States. In Holland, W.W., Detels, R., and Knox, G., (eds.), *Oxford textbook of public health* Volume 1. Oxford: Oxford Medical Publications, pp. 441–54.

Scott, E. (1995). *Catastrophic health insurance for the elderly.* Case Program Series (#1278.0). Cambridge, MA: Kennedy School of Government, Harvard University.

Seeman, T.E., Berkman, L.F., Blazer, D., and Rowe, J.W. (1994). Social ties and support and neuroendocrine function: the MacArthur Studies of Successful Aging. *Ann Behav Med,* 16:95–106.

Shapiro, R.Y., and Young, J.T. (1989). Public opinion and the welfare state: the United States in comparative perspective. *Polit Sci Q,* 104:59–87.

Smith, H. (1988). *The power game.* New York: Random House.

Starfield, B. (1992) Effects of poverty on health status. *Bull N Y Acad Med,* 68:16–24.

U.S. Congress. (1996). *The personal responsibility and work opportunity reconciliation act of 1996.* (Public Law 104-193.) 104th Congress, 2nd session, August 1996.

Van Loon, A.J., Brug, J., Goldbohm, R.A., van den Brandt, P.A., and Brug, J. (1995). Differences in cancer incidence and mortality among socio-economic groups. *Scand J Soc Med,* 23:110–20.

Wilson, W.J. (1996). *When work disappears: the world of the new urban poor.* New York: Knopf.

Wise, P.H, and Meyers, A. (1988) Poverty and child health. *Pediatr Clin North Am,* 35(6):1169–86.

Youngclaus, J. (1998). All politics is legal. *Capital Eye,* 5(2):1,4–5.

Index

Page numbers followed by *f* and *t* indicate figures and tables, respectively.